Atlas of Operative Oral and Maxillofacial Surgery

ATLAS OF OPERATIVE ORAL AND MAXILLOFACIAL SURGERY

Edited by

Christopher J. Haggerty
Private Practice
Lakewood Oral and Maxillofacial Surgery Specialists
Lees Summit, Missouri, USA
Clinical Assistant Professor
Department of Oral and Maxillofacial Surgery
University of Missouri–Kansas City
Kansas City, Missouri, USA

Robert M. Laughlin
Chairman
Department of Oral and Maxillofacial Surgery and Hospital Dentistry
Director of Oral and Maxillofacial Surgery Residency Program
Department of Oral and Maxillofacial Surgery
Director of Microvascular Surgical Training
Naval Medical Center San Diego
San Diego, California, USA

WILEY Blackwell

This edition first published 2015
© 2015 by John Wiley & Sons, Inc.

Editorial offices: 1606 Golden Aspen Drive, Suites 103 and 104, Ames, Iowa 50010, USA
The Atrium, Southern Gate, Chichester, West Sussex, PO19 8SQ, UK
9600 Garsington Road, Oxford, OX4 2DQ, UK

For details of our global editorial offices, for customer services and for information about how to apply for
permission to reuse the copyright material in this book please see our website at www.wiley.com/wiley-blackwell.

Library of Congress Cataloging-in-Publication Data
Atlas of operative oral and maxillofacial surgery / edited by Christopher J. Haggerty, Robert M. Laughlin.
    p. ; cm.
  Includes bibliographical references and index.
  ISBN 978-1-118-44234-0 (pbk.)
  I. Haggerty, Christopher J., editor.   II. Laughlin, Robert M. (Robert Minard), 1969-, editor.
  [DNLM: 1. Oral Surgical Procedures—methods—Atlases.   2. Face—surgery—Atlases.
3. Head—surgery—Atlases.   4. Maxillofacial Injuries—surgery—Atlases.   5. Neck—surgery—
Atlases.   6. Reconstructive Surgical Procedures—methods—Atlases.   7. Stomatognathic Diseases—surgery—
Atlases. WU 600.7]
  RK529
  617.5'22059—dc23

                                                                                2014040039

A catalogue record for this book is available from the British Library.

Wiley also publishes its books in a variety of electronic formats. Some content that appears in print may not
be available in electronic books.

Cover image: iStock / © Eraxion
Cover design by Meaden Creative

Set in 10/12pt Meridien LT Std by Aptara Inc., New Delhi, India

1   2015

CONTENTS

Contents

Contents

LIST OF CONTRIBUTORS

Stephen G. Alfano, DDS, MS
Attending Maxillofacial Prosthodontist
Department of Oral and Maxillofacial Surgery
Naval Medical Center San Diego
San Diego, California, USA

Shahid R. Aziz, DMD, MD, FACS
Professor
Department of Oral and Maxillofacial Surgery
Rutgers University School of Dental Medicine
Newark, New Jersey, USA

R. Bryan Bell, MD, DDS, FACS
Medical Director
Oral, Head and Neck Cancer Program
Providence Cancer Center
Attending Surgeon
Trauma Service/Oral and Maxillofacial Surgery Service
Legacy Emanuel Medical Center
Affiliate Professor
Oregon Health and Science University
Head and Neck Surgical Associates
Portland, Oregon, USA

Remy H. Blanchaert, DDS, MD
Private Practice
Oral and Maxillofacial Surgery Associates
Wichita, Kansas, USA

Hani F. Braidy, DMD, FRCD(C)
Associate Professor
Department of Oral and Maxillofacial Surgery
Rutgers University School of Dental Medicine
Rutgers University
Newark, New Jersey, USA

Matthew T. Brigger, MD, MPH
Chief, Pediatric Otolaryngology
Director of Otolaryngology—Head and Neck Surgery
    Residency Program
Department of Otolaryngology—Head and Neck Surgery
Naval Medical Center San Diego
Assistant Professor of Surgery
Uniformed Services of the Health Sciences University
San Diego, California, USA

Eric R. Carlson, DMD, MD, FACS
Professor and Kelly L. Krahwinkel Chairman
Director of Oral and Maxillofacial Surgery Residency
    Program
Director of Oral/Head and Neck Oncologic Surgery
    Fellowship Program
Department of Oral and Maxillofacial Surgery
University of Tennessee Medical Center
University of Tennessee Cancer Institute
Knoxville, Tennessee, USA

Michael Carson, DDS
Attending Surgeon
Department of Oral and Maxillofacial Surgery
Naval Medical Center Portsmouth
Portsmouth, Virginia, USA

Christopher Choi, DDS, MD
Private Practice
Inland Empire Oral and Maxillofacial Surgeons
Rancho Cucamonga, California, USA
Assistant Professor
Department of Oral and Maxillofacial Surgery
Loma Linda School of Dentistry
Loma Linda, California, USA

Daniel Clifford, DMD, MD
Attending Surgeon
Department of Oral and Maxillofacial Surgery
Naval Medical Center San Diego
San Diego, California, USA

Scott A. Curtice, DMD
Attending Orthodontist
Department of Oral and Maxillofacial Surgery
Naval Medical Center San Diego
San Diego, California, USA

L. Angelo Cuzalina, MD, DDS
Cosmetic Surgery Fellowship Director
American Academy of Cosmetic Surgery
Tulsa, Oklahoma, USA

Thaer Daifallah, DDS
Associate Professor
Department of Oral and Maxillofacial Surgery
University of Missouri–Kansas City
Kansas City, Missouri, USA

Bart C. Farrell, DDS, MD
Private Practice
Carolinas Center for Oral and Facial Surgery
Charlotte, North Carolina, USA
Assistant Clinical Professor
Department of Oral and Maxillofacial Surgery
Louisiana State University Health Sciences Center
New Orleans, Louisiana, USA

Brian B. Farrell, DDS, MD
Private Practice
Carolinas Center for Oral and Facial Surgery
Charlotte, North Carolina, USA
Assistant Clinical Professor
Department of Oral and Maxillofacial Surgery
Louisiana State University Health Sciences Center
New Orleans, Louisiana, USA

Curtis W. Gaball, MD
Vice Chairman
Chief, Facial Plastic Surgery
Department of Otolaryngology—Head and Neck Surgery
Naval Medical Center San Diego
Adjunct Associate Professor of Surgery
Uniformed Services of the Health Sciences University
San Diego, California, USA

Ghali E. Ghali, DDS, MD, FACS
Gamble Professor and Chairman
Oral and Maxillofacial Surgery
Head and Neck Surgery
Louisiana State University School of Medicine
Shreveport, Louisiana, USA

Michael Grau, Jr., DMD
Assistant Program Director, Oral and Maxillofacial
    Surgery Training Program
Department of Oral and Maxillofacial Surgery
Naval Medical Center San Diego
San Diego, California, USA

Christopher J. Haggerty, DDS, MD
Private Practice
Lakewood Oral and Maxillofacial Surgery Specialists
Lees Summit, Missouri, USA
Clinical Assistant Professor
Department of Oral and Maxillofacial Surgery
University of Missouri–Kansas City
Kansas City, Missouri, USA

Christopher M. Harris, DMD, MD
Attending Surgeon
Director of Oral and Maxillofacial Surgery Residency
    Program
Chief, Head and Neck Oncology/Reconstruction
Department of Oral and Maxillofacial Surgery
Naval Medical Center Portsmouth
Portsmouth, Virginia, USA

Matthew W. Hearn, DDS, MD, RM
Private Practice
Valparaiso, Indiana, USA

Dustin M. Heringer, MD
Clinical Assistant Professor
Department of Ophthalmology
University of Arizona
Tucson, Arizona, USA

Markus S. Hill, DMD, MS Ed
Resident OMS
Department of Oral and Maxillofacial Surgery
Naval Medical Center
San Diego, California, USA

Matthew Robert Hlavacek, DDS, MD
Private Practice
Kansas City Surgical Arts
Liberty, Missouri, USA
Clinical Assistant Professor
Department of Surgery and Oral and Maxillofacial
    Surgery
University of Missouri–Kansas City
Kansas City, Missouri, USA

Eric P. Hoffmeister, MD
Chairman
Director of Hand Surgery
Department of Orthopedic Surgery
Attending Surgeon Microvascular
    Surgical Training
Naval Medical Center San Diego
Assistant Professor of Surgery
Uniformed Services University of
    the Health Sciences
San Diego, California, USA

Jon D. Holmes, DMD, MD, FACS
Private Practice
Clark Holmes Oral and Facial Surgery
Associate Clinical Professor
Department of Oral and Maxillofacial Surgery
University of Alabama
Birmingham, Alabama, USA

Reem Hamdy Hossameldin, BDS, MSc
Assistant Lecturer
Department of Oral and Maxillofacial
  Surgery
Faculty of Dental Medicine
Cairo University
Cairo, Egypt
Research Scholar, PhD Scholar
General Surgery Department
Herbert Wertheim College of Medicine
Florida International University
Miami, Florida, USA

Michael J. Isaac, DDS
Chief Resident
Department of Oral and Maxillofacial Surgery
University of Missouri–Kansas City
Kansas City, Missouri, USA

Jason Jamali, DDS, MD
Assistant Professor
Department of Oral and Maxillofacial Surgery
College of Dentistry
University of Illinois Chicago
Chicago, Illinois, USA

Terence E. Johnson, MD
Chairman
Department of Otolaryngology
Naval Medical Center San Diego
San Diego, California, USA

Neil C. Kanning, DMD, MS
Private Practice
Kanning Orthodontics
Liberty, Missouri, USA

Matthew Keller, MD
Physician
Department of Otolaryngology—Head and
  Neck Surgery
Naval Medical Center San Diego
San Diego, California, USA

Brian W. Kelley, DDS, MD
Private Practice
Carolinas Center for Oral and Facial Surgery
Charlotte, North Carolina, USA
Assistant Clinical Professor
Department of Oral and Maxillofacial
  Surgery
Louisiana State University Health Sciences
  Center
New Orleans, Louisiana, USA

John N. Kent, DDS, FACD, FICD
Boyd Professor and Head
Departments of Oral and Maxillofacial Surgery
Louisiana State University Health Science
  Centers
New Orleans 1973-2008 and Shreveport
  1978–2003

Arnett Klugh III, MD
Vice Chairman
Department of Neurosurgery
Chief, Pediatric Neurosurgery
Naval Medical Center San Diego
San Diego, California, USA

Antonia Kolokythas, DDS, MSc
Assistant Professor and Director of Research
  Department of Oral and Maxillofacial Surgery
College of Dentistry
University of Illinois
Chicago, Illinois, USA

Robert M. Laughlin, DMD
Chairman
Department of Oral and Maxillofacial Surgery and
  Hospital Dentistry
Director of Oral and Maxillofacial Surgery Residency
  Program
Department of Oral and Maxillofacial Surgery
Director of Microvascular Surgical Training
Naval Medical Center San Diego
San Diego, California, USA

Andrew Lee, DDS, MD
Fellow
Department of Oral and Maxillofacial Surgery
University of Tennessee Medical Center
University of Tennessee Cancer Institute
Knoxville, Tennessee, USA

Ray Lim, DDS, MD
Department of Oral and Maxillofacial Surgery
Louisiana State University
New Orleans, Louisiana, USA

Patrick J. Louis, DDS, MD
Director
Advanced Educational Program in Oral and Maxillofacial
  Surgery
Professor, School of Dentistry
Professor, School of Medicine
Department of Oral and Maxillofacial
  Surgery
University of Alabama
Birmingham, Alabama, USA

Patrick Lucaci, DDS, MD
Chief Resident
Department of Oral and Maxillofacial
  Surgery
University of Missouri–Kansas City
Kansas City, Missouri, USA

James MacDowell, DDS
Chief Resident
Department of Oral and Maxillofacial
  Surgery
Naval Medical Center
San Diego, California, USA

Lester Machado, DDS, MD, MS, FRCS(Ed)
Co-Chair
Division of Oral and Maxillofacial Surgery
Rady Children's Hospital of San Diego
San Diego, California, USA

Michael R. Markiewicz, DDS, MPH, MD
Resident
Department of Oral and Maxillofacial
  Surgery
Oregon Health and Science University
Portland, Oregon, USA

Joseph P. McCain, DMD
Private Practice of Oral and Maxillofacial Surgery
  Chief of Oral and Maxillofacial Surgery
Baptist Health Systems
Clinical Associate Professor
Oral and Maxillofacial Surgery
Herbert Wertheim College of Medicine
Florida International University
Miami, Florida, USA
Adjunct Professor of Oral and Maxillofacial
  Surgery
Nova Southeastern School of Dental
  Medicine
Fort Lauderdale, Florida, USA

Andrew T. Meram, DDS, MD
Resident
Department of Oral and Maxillofacial Surgery
Louisiana State University Health Sciences
  Center
Shreveport, Louisiana, USA

Michael Miloro, DMD, MD, FACS
Professor and Chairman
Department of Oral and Maxillofacial Surgery
College of Dentistry
University of Illinois
Chicago, Illinois, USA

Dale J. Misek, DMD
Private Practice
Carolinas Center for Oral and Facial Surgery
Charlotte, North Carolina, USA
Clinical Professor
Department of Oral and Maxillofacial Surgery
Louisiana State University Health Sciences Center
New Orleans, Louisiana, USA

Allen O. Mitchell, MD
Chairman
Otolaryngology—Head and Neck Surgery
Naval Medical Center Portsmouth
Portsmouth, Virginia, USA

Anthony B.P. Morlandt, MD, DDS
Assistant Professor
Oral/Head and Neck Oncology and Microvascular
  Reconstructive Surgery
Department of Oral and Maxillofacial Surgery
University of Alabama
Birmingham, Alabama, USA

Patrick B. Morrissey, MD
Department of Orthopedic Surgery
Naval Medical Center
San Diego, California, USA

Robert A. Nadeau, DDS, MD
Attending Surgeon and Associate Professor
Director of Resident Education
Department of Oral and Maxillofacial Surgery
University of Missouri–Kansas City Schools of Medicine
  and Dentistry
Kansas City, Missouri, USA

Brenda L. Nelson, DDS, MS
Chairman, Anatomic Pathology
Department of Pathology
Naval Medical Center San Diego
San Diego, California, USA

Bart Nierzwicki, DMD, MD, PhD, FACS
Private Practice
Millennium Surgical
Chicago, Illinois, USA

Eric Nordstrom, MD, DDS
Physician/Surgeon
Department of Oral and Maxillofacial Surgery
Oregon Health and Science University
Head and Neck Surgical Associates
Portland, Oregon, USA
Department of Oral and Maxillofacial Surgery
Anchorage Oral and Maxillofacial Surgery
Anchorage, Alaska, USA

Celso F. Palmieri, Jr., DDS
Assistant Professor
Department of Oral and Maxillofacial Surgery
Louisiana State University Health Sciences
    Center
Shreveport, Louisiana, USA

Antoine J. Panossian, DMD, MD
Private Practice
Panossian Oral and Maxillofacial Surgery
Massapequa, New York, USA

Earl Peter Park, DMD, MD
Resident
Department of Oral and Maxillofacial Surgery
Louisiana State University Health Sciences
    Center
New Orleans, Louisiana, USA

Min S. Park, MD
Attending Surgeon
Department of Neurosurgery
Naval Medical Center San Diego
San Diego, California, USA

Jeremiah Jason Parker, DMD, MD, FACS
Private Practice
Oral and Maxillofacial Surgery Associates
Montgomery, Alabama, USA

Stavan Patel, DDS, MD
Resident
Department of Oral and Maxillofacial Surgery
Louisiana State University Health Sciences Center
Shreveport, Louisiana, USA

Jon D. Perenack, MD, DDS
Associate Professor
Director of Oral and Maxillofacial Surgery Residency
    Program
Department of Oral and Maxillofacial Surgery
Louisiana State University Health Sciences Center
New Orleans, Louisiana, USA

J. Michael Ray, DDS
Private Practice
DFW Facial and Surgical Arts
Dallas, Texas, USA

Craig Salt, MD
Department of Plastic Surgery
Naval Medical Center
San Diego, California, USA

Anil N. Shah, MD
Resident
Department of Otolaryngology—Head and Neck
    Surgery
Naval Medical Center San Diego
San Diego, California, USA

Vincent Slovan, DMD
Staff Surgeon
Naval Hospital Okinawa
Okinawa, Japan

Nathan Steele, DDS, MD
Private Practice
Cheyenne Oral and Maxillofacial Surgery
Cheyenne, Wyoming, USA

Joshua Stone, DDS, MD
Chief Resident
Department of Oral and Maxillofacial Surgery
University of Missouri-Kansas City
Kansas City, Missouri, USA

**Andrew B.G. Tay, FDS RCS (Edinburgh), FAM
(Singapore)**
Senior Consultant and Director
Department of Oral and Maxillofacial Surgery
National Dental Centre
Singapore

Gabriel C. Tender, MD
Associate Professor
Department of Neurosurgery
Louisiana State University Health Science
    Center
New Orleans, Louisiana, USA

Myron R. Tucker, DDS
Retired
Private Practice
Carolinas Center for Oral and Facial Surgery
Charlotte, North Carolina, USA
Adjunct Clinical Professor
Department of Oral and Maxillofacial Surgery
Louisiana State University Health Sciences
    Center
New Orleans, Louisiana, USA

Billy Turley, DMD
Staff Surgeon
Department of Oral and Maxillofacial
    Surgery
Naval Hospital Camp Lejeune
Jacksonville, North Carolina, USA

Luis Vega, DDS
Associate Professor and Oral and Maxillofacial Surgery
    Residency Program Director
Department of Oral and Maxillofacial Surgery
Vanderbilt University Medical Center
Nashville, Tennessee, USA

Christopher T. Vogel, DDS
Resident
Department of Oral and Maxillofacial Surgery
University of Missouri–Kansas City
Kansas City, Missouri, USA

Brent B. Ward, DDS, MD, FACS
Associate Professor
Oral/Head and Neck Oncologic
Director, Microvascular Reconstructive Surgery Program
Department of Oral and Maxillofacial Surgery
University of Michigan Hospital
Ann Arbor, Michigan, USA

Jennifer Elizabeth Woerner, DMD, MD
Assistant Professor
Department of Oral and Maxillofacial Surgery
Louisiana State University Health Sciences Center
Shreveport, Louisiana, USA

Melvyn S. Yeoh, DMD, MD
Assistant Professor
Department of Oral and Maxillofacial Surgery
Louisiana State University Health Sciences
    Center
Shreveport, Louisiana, USA

Shahrouz Zarrabi, DDS, MD
Resident
Department of Oral and Maxillofacial Surgery
Louisiana State University Health Sciences
    Center
Shreveport, Louisiana, USA

Vincent B. Ziccardi, DDS, MD, FACS
Professor, Chair, and Residency Director
Department of Oral and Maxillofacial Surgery
Rutgers University School of Dental Medicine
Newark, New Jersey, USA

John R. Zuniga, DMD
Professor and Chairman
Department of Oral and Maxillofacial Surgery
University of Texas Southwestern Medical
    Center
Dallas, Texas, USA

FOREWORD

The explosion of new and modified surgical techniques and technological advancements of the maxillofacial region within recent years is the impetus for the generation of *Atlas of Operative Oral and Maxillofacial Surgery*. Christopher J. Haggerty and Robert M. Laughlin have created a contemporary, multidisciplinary reference source for students, residents, recent graduates and yes, experienced surgeons to refresh, update, and gain new knowledge as they contemplate their selection of Oral and Maxillofacial Surgery (OMS) approaches and procedures. This *Atlas* will prove to be an invaluable resource for recent OMS graduates preparing for their board certification examination and for those preparing for their recertification examinations. The readers will enjoy the atlas format, as the high yield clinical vignettes supplemented with over 1,000 color images quickly and concisely deliver pertinent information to the reader.

The editors and contributors comprehensively deliver the indications, contraindications, regional anatomy, procedure selection, post-operative management, complications and key points to the reader in an interesting and contemporary manner. This *Atlas* will become a staple of Oral and Maxillofacial Surgery and as such, will be located in conference rooms, offices, and student/resident backpacks as well as in the library. Like a manual of therapeutic drugs, it can be used as an immediate source of information and teaching. The *Atlas* includes a comprehensive review of oral and maxillofacial surgery procedures and is organized by section to include: dentoalveolar and implant surgery, odontogenic head and neck infections, maxillofacial trauma surgery, orthognathic surgery, temporomandibular joint surgery, facial cosmetic surgery, and pathology and reconstructive surgery. In addition to covering these core oral and maxillofacial surgery procedures, the *Atlas* also includes expanded scope maxillofacial surgery such as head and neck ablative surgery, microvascular surgery, advanced facial cosmetic surgery, reconstructive temporomandibular joint surgery and craniofacial surgery.

The review of key surgical procedures with their associated indications and contraindications will aid in procedure selection and improve surgical outcomes. Key surgical anatomy, techniques and surgical alternatives are knowledgeably described and applicable. Many techniques are in such detail that they read as a well thought out and described operative dictation. Patient follow-up details are discussed in the immediate and long-term post-operative periods. Case reports by expert contributors walk the reader through their favorite operative technique with steps, high resolution color illustrations, and photographs at surgery that depict incision locations, planes of anatomical dissection, and key pre, intra, and postoperative images. The *Atlas* can become a reference source during conversation when the resident and experienced surgeon discuss and compare a case in the *Atlas* with their own recent operative experience. Therein lies the birth of new knowledge, the modifications of surgical techniques, which improve patient outcome and advance scope for the student, instructor, and even the contributors to the *Atlas*. Elective and non-elective surgical techniques, not thought of just a few decades ago, are now commonplace in numbers that are sometimes difficult for a single practitioner to assimilate. In this day of advancing surgical techniques, with more and more subspecialization and cross over care between specialties, delivery of new surgical technique knowledge clearly requires this atlas format.

Four Decade History of Oral and Maxillofacial Surgery Growth and the Birth of Expanded Scope

Oral and maxillofacial surgery (OMS) has had remarkable advancement in the education of residents over the past 4 decades. By 1972, the specialty required a three-year residency, which included medicine and a core year of general surgery and other surgical specialties and anesthesia. At LSU, a 3–4 month rotation on Neurosurgery was begun and remains today a favorite experience by both OMS and Neurosurgery. By 1978, the length of training at LSU was extended to a 4-year program, mostly due to an increase in surgical scope and required numbers of inpatient and outpatient procedures and anesthesia experience. The word "competence" was bandied about by all specialties at that time and most specialties were trying to achieve some degree of competence with an increase in residency training and procedures. OMS was dominant in Orthognathic Surgery and Facial Trauma patient care and research as early as the late 70s and early 80s. In the late 80s, LSU and other institutions initiated the 6-year OMS-MD residency, an experience which had previously been used for many years at only a few institutions such as Harvard, Alabama, and Nebraska. The reason for seeking the integrated advanced standing MD program was to improve residency education and patient care, and delivery of that care that came with expanded scope.

Today, nearly half of U.S. oral and maxillofacial surgery residencies and nearly all of the European training sites offer OMS-MD training. The core year of general surgery, surgical specialists rotations, and anesthesia with at least 30 months of OMS training today is common to both the standard 4-year OMS residency and 6-year OMS-MD residency. This advanced level of surgical training and patient care validates oral and maxillofacial surgery as a major contributor to the surgical and medical management of head and neck patients. Simultaneously, in the late 80s there was an increase of OMS scope in cosmetic surgery, cancer and reconstructive surgery, and the treatment of cleft lip/palate following years of orthognathic surgery. The very surgical technique basis of orthognathic surgery served as a natural springboard into all three areas. In fact, significant contributions by OMS in all three of these areas soon followed. Fellowships in these areas soon followed in not only ENT and Plastic Surgery, but OMS as well.

The educational and surgical scope contribution by OMS on behalf of head and neck patients is unparalleled over the past 40 years, understanding that most surgical specialties that treat head and neck patients have also had significant success. Within the scope of OMS, several areas of advancement are recognized: 1) Even before the treatment of facial injuries during and after major wars, dentists, physicians with dental degrees and oral surgeons were destined to shape the future of today's OMS. Their experiences led to dramatic improvement of both functional and aesthetic aspects in primary and secondary correction of facial injuries. Understanding and recognizing the nature of war time facial fractures led to the development of elective surgical techniques by Obwegeser, Tessier, and other pioneers which are used today in orthognathic and craniofacial surgery. Most patients requiring correction of facial deformities today receive that correction within the private OMS practice or the OMS training centers. OMS offers several cleft and craniofacial surgery fellowships and a significant number of OMS are involved with accredited ACLP teams. 2) After the bloom and dominance by the OMS specialty with orthognathic surgery, facial aesthetic surgery was one of the first areas of expanded scope in the mid 80s. There is no doubt that OMS entrance into facial aesthetic surgery is a logical and orderly consequence following its success in orthognathic surgery and the success of transcutaneous techniques in facial trauma. The very nature of dental reconstruction and OMS education is unequaled in surgical education when assessing oral and facial aesthetic needs of patients. Throughout dental school and OMS training, facial balance and aesthetic needs are a part of daily education. Clearly, that is what orthognathic surgery and orthodontics are all about. Augmenting this education are head and neck anatomy with a cadaver dissection course, cephalometric evaluation courses, and the treatment of hundreds of patients in the dental school and hospital as a part of these dental specialty residencies. Several aesthetic procedures were already a daily part of orthognathic surgery such as facial implants, liposuction, and rhinoplasty. Facial aesthetic fellowship is now common, those approved by AAOMS and other organizations. 3) Thanks to the pioneering work by Drs. Adrian Hubbell and his mentor, John Lundy, an anesthesiologist, and others, intravenous drugs with outpatient sedation and general anesthesia techniques have been used with increasing frequency and safety in OMS offices for decades. This is the basis for much of the OMS surgery done in the U.S. OMS residency training today requires 5 months of general anesthesia as well as periodic BLS, ACLS, and ATLS certification to support the efficacy and safety of delivery of outpatient anesthesia. 4) OMS has long embraced a supportive if not active participating role in care of the oral and head and neck cancer patient. With all the advances in orthognathic surgery techniques as well as in preprosthetic surgery by the late 80s, before the age of dental implants, it was only reasonable to use those surgical experiences to begin performing excision of select cancer lesions and reconstruct with techniques already in use with secondary correction of facial injuries. Oral and Maxillofacial Surgeons have provided significant primary and secondary soft tissue and bony care and sometimes the majority of care of trauma patients during war time conflicts abroad. That experience was the origin of cancer reconstruction. Surgical specialties of the head and neck are indebted to Phillip Boyne (bone grafting research and techniques) and Robert Marx (soft and hard tissue reconstruction and HBO protocols). Today, OMS fellowships are offered in the resection of cancer, reconstruction, or microvascular techniques.

The following list is just a few of services/procedures germane to the specialty of Oral and Maxillofacial Surgery. Those where the specialty is a leader and has made significant contributions include: 1) osteointegration of dental and facial implants, 2) hyperbaric oxygen protocol of the head and neck area, 3) arthroscopy and reconstruction of the temporomandibular joint with total joint prostheses, 4) orthognathic and craniofacial surgery, 5) virtual surgical techniques in orthognathic and reconstruction surgery of the head and neck, 6) distraction of the facial bone, 7) implementation of bone plating techniques in facial trauma and facial deformity patients, 8) improved diagnostic techniques with surgical intervention on sleep apnea patients, 9) maxillofacial cone beam computed tomography, 10) reconstruction in the head and neck areas with soft and hard tissue flaps.

Acknowledgment

The growth of Louisiana Oral and Maxillofacial Surgery over the past 4 decades, as was seen in other states, is a testimony to the specialty growth across the U.S. Expanded scope in orthognathic and craniofacial surgery, pathology and reconstruction of the head/neck areas, and TMJ reconstruction were led by LSU OMS chairs Jack Kent, DDS, G.E. Ghali, DDS, MD, FACS, Dan Lew, DDS, and program directors Mike Zide, DMD, Dale Misiek, DMD, Jon Perenack, DDS, MD, and David Kim, DDS, MD. As a result of their training, 25 former LSU residents and faculty have furthered their education with fellowship training in aesthetic surgery, cleft and craniofacial surgery, and head and neck oncologic/microvascular reconstruction. Many have generously contributed to the *Atlas*.

Continuing education is one of the hallmarks of LSU Oral and Maxillofacial Surgery. Multiple, yearly courses devoted to core and expanded scope topics are helpful to the OMS practitioner just as this *Atlas* should be. For those preparing for Board examinations or those wishing to review and update knowledge, the LSU OMS department has offered a week long full scope Review Course over 40 years and a 3-day Advanced Cosmetic lecture with hands on cadaver course for 20 years. To that extent I wish to thank those that contributed to the education of LSU trainees and so many practitioners. They include G. E. Ghali, DDS, MD, FACS, current chairman of LSUSM Oral and Maxillofacial Surgery at Shreveport and President of the American Board of Oral and Maxillofacial Surgery, Michael Block, DMD, for 30 years of research and dental implant leadership and education at LSU and on behalf of AAOMS Dental Implant Conferences; Michael Zide, DMD, a favorite teacher on daily rounds at Charity Hospital in New Orleans; Dale Misiek, DMD, Brian Farrell, DDS, MD, and Dan Spagnoli, DDS, PhD,

for clinical direction to the LSU residents at New Orleans and Charlotte; and Jon Perenack, DDS, MD, for being a leader and teacher of facial aesthetic surgery in Louisiana. Further contribution to LSU OMS expanded scope came from Michael Kinnebrew, DDS, MD, Randall Wilk, DDS, MD, PhD, and John Neary, DDS, MD, FACS, current chairman of LSUSD Oral and Maxillofacial Surgery at New Orleans.

I wish to thank 4 past presidents of AAOMS, all from Louisiana: Jack Gamble, DDS, Ronald Marks, DDS, Dan Lew, DDS, and the most recent president, Eric Geist, DDS, who was also President of the American Board of Oral and Maxillofacial Surgery, who have contributed enormously to the educational, political, and patient care goals of the Oral and Maxillofacial Surgery specialty. Twenty contributors to the *Atlas* are graduates/faculty of LSU New Orleans or Shreveport Oral and Maxillofacial Surgery Residency Programs. I wish to congratulate, commend, and thank them and all contributors, but especially the two editors, Chris Haggerty, DDS, MD and Rob Laughlin, DMD, two of my former LSU Oral and Maxillofacial Surgery residents, for their creative contribution to the education of all surgeons, and most importantly, to the benefit of patient outcome.

John N. Kent, DDS, FACD, FICD
Boyd Professor and Head
Departments of Oral and Maxillofacial Surgery
LSU Health Sciences Centers
New Orleans 1973–2008 and Shreveport 1978–2003

ACKNOWLEDGMENTS

I would like to sincerely thank the oral and maxillofacial surgery programs of Louisiana State University and the University of Missouri–Kansas City for their commitment and support of this project.

I would like to thank Jack Kent, Michael Block, Jon Perenack, Randy Malloy, and Gabriel Tender for their dedication, patience, and guidance and for teaching me the artistry of surgery and patient management.

I would like to thank Ashley for her perpetual encouragement, exuberance and willingness to endure my long hours with this project, with similar projects, and at the hospitals. I am truly blessed to have you in my life.

I would like to thank my sister Jennifer for her advice and insight, and for being someone who I can always depend on. I would like to thank my brother Nick for always keeping me grounded and for sharing his living room and advice with me on Sundays.

I would like to thank my long-term friend and collaborating editor, Rob Laughlin. Rob, when you have been through as much as you and I have together, we are more family than friends.

Finally, I would like to thank my parents, Ed and Jean Haggerty, for their unconditional and eternal understanding, encouragement, and support. Your unprecedented benevolence, selflessness, and sacrifice have made us who we are today.

Christopher J. Haggerty

This surgical atlas would not have been possible without the hard work and efforts of so many. I would like to thank my family, friends, mentors, residents, and colleagues.

Thank you to the programs at Louisiana State University, New Orleans, and the University of Michigan for the outstanding training and support over the years.

To my mentors, John "Jack" Kent, Michael Block, Randy Malloy, and Joseph Helman, for the numerous hours you have invested in me and the specialty.

To my parents, Ralph and Dianne Laughlin, who made the opportunities possible.

To my Navy family, DC, MG, KF, AC, SA, SC, HC, AB, MB, and GG, thank you.

To the many contributors of oral and maxillofacial surgery, head and neck surgery, and reconstruction, who have demonstrated a commitment to excellence in education, patient care, and the advancement of the specialty.

Lastly, I would like to thank my coeditor and best friend, Chris Haggerty, for his extraordinary efforts.

Robert M. Laughlin

A special thanks to Bill Winn for providing the vast majority of the medical illustrations for this project.

Bill, you are truly the most accomplished and talented oral and maxillofacial, head and neck, and plastic and reconstructive surgery medical illustrator of all time. Thank you very much for all of your efforts with this project and for putting up with all of our changes along the way.

Christopher and Robert

PART ONE

DENTOALVEOLAR AND IMPLANT SURGERY

Anatomical Considerations in Dentoalveolar Surgery

Jason Jamali, Antonia Kolokythas, and Michael Miloro
Department of Oral and Maxillofacial Surgery, College of Dentistry, University of Illinois Chicago, Chicago, Illinois, USA

An understanding of the anatomical relations within the region of intervention is critical to minimize surgical complications. Radiographic imaging assists in the assessment of anatomical variation and allows for risk stratification and predictable treatment outcomes.

Mandible

Lingual Nerve

The lingual nerve provides sensation to the anterior two-thirds of the tongue. The lingual nerve is at risk for injury with the extraction of third molars and with procedures involving the floor of the mouth. Within the third molar region, the lingual nerve is located, on average, 3.0 mm apical to the crest of the alveolar ridge and 2.0 mm medially from the lingual cortical plate. In 17.6% of the population, the lingual nerve is at or above the crest of the alveolar bone. In 22% of the population, the lingual nerve contacts the lingual cortex adjacent to the third molar region. Within the second molar region, the lingual nerve is located, on average, 9.5 mm inferior to the cementoenamel junction (CEJ). Within the first molar and second premolar regions, the average vertical distances from the CEJ lingually are 13.0 mm and 15.0 mm, respectively. The lingual nerve begins to course toward the tongue between the first and second molar regions.

Inferior Alveolar Nerve

As the inferior alveolar nerve (IAN) descends from the base of the skull, it traverses the pterygomandibular space and enters the mandibular foramen approximately 1.5–2.0 cm inferior to the sigmoid notch. Within the corpus of the mandible, the course of the mandibular canal in the buccal–lingual dimension tends to follow one of three general patterns:

- Type 1: in the majority of the population (approximately 70%), the canal follows the lingual plate within the ramus–body region.
- Type 2: in 15% of the population, the canal initially runs within the middle of the ramus when posterior to

the second molar, and then follows the lingual plate as it passes through the region of the second and first molars.
- Type 3: in 15% of the population, the canal is positioned in the middle to lingual third of the mandible along its entire course.

In addition:

- In approximately 80% of the population, the inferior alveolar artery courses above the nerve within the bony canal.
- Older patients have been shown to have less distance between the buccal cortex of the mandible and the lateral aspect of the canal.
- In relation to impacted third molars, the inferior alveolar canal is located:

> Lingual to the third molar in 49% of the population
> Buccal to the third molar in 17% of the population
> Inferior to the third molar in 19% of the population
> Interradicular in 15% of the population.

In general, the risk of exposure of the inferior alveolar canal during third molar removal is greater in patients with lingual, rather than buccal, canal positioning. Among molars in the posterior mandible, the distance from the buccal cortex to the canal tends to be greatest within the region of the second molar.

Mental Nerve

The mental foramen typically lies between the first and second premolars in line corresponding with a vertical reference from the infraorbital foramen. Variability in the vertical distance of the foramen may be problematic in edentulous mandibles with excessive alveolar bone resorption. The mental nerve courses superiorly before exiting the mental foramen. Additionally, the mental nerve commonly loops anteriorly (genu) before its exit from the mental foramen in approximately 48% of the population. The average length of the anterior loop (genu) is 0.89 mm with a range of up to 5.7 mm or more. However, only 5% of individuals have an anterior loop length longer than 3.0 mm and only 2% have an anterior loop length greater than 4.0 mm.

Atlas of Operative Oral and Maxillofacial Surgery, First Edition. Edited by Christopher J. Haggerty and Robert M. Laughlin
© 2015 John Wiley & Sons, Inc. Published 2015 by John Wiley & Sons, Inc.

Maxilla

Nasal Cavity

The palatal process of the maxilla contributes to the anterior three-fourths of the nasal floor. The posterior one-fourth of the nasal floor is comprised from the horizontal process of the palatine bone. Care must be taken during placement of anterior maxillary implants to avoid violating this region.

Maxillary Sinus

The maxillary sinus is the largest of the paranasal sinuses. It is pyramidal in shape with its apex oriented toward the zygoma. It lies within the posterior maxilla bounded by the infratemporal fossa, lateral nasal wall, and floor of the orbit. As a result of pneumatization, extensive variation exists; however, the average volume in adults is roughly 15 mL's. Additionally, the maxillary sinus cavity may occasionally be divided by septae. The maxillary sinus ostium is located along the superior aspect of the medial wall of the sinus and drains into the middle meatus of the nasal cavity.

Key Points

1. Panoramic indicators of inferior alveolar nerve proximity include darkening of the third molar root, interruption of the white line of the mandibular canal (see Figure 1.6 in Case Report 1.2), diversion or displacement of the mandibular canal (see Figure 1.3 in Case Report 1.1), abrupt deflection of the third molar roots, and abrupt narrowing of the tooth root.
2. Cone beam computed tomography (CBCT) scanners have aided greatly in the visualization and avoidance of neurovascular structures during dentoalveolar surgery and implant placement. (See Figures 1.1 and 1.2.)

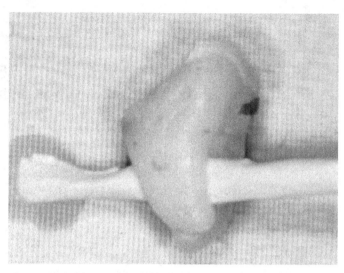

Figure 1.2. Lower wisdom tooth extracted from the patient in Figure 1.1. The yellow paper represents the location of the inferior alveolar nerve through the inferior third of the wisdom tooth.

Case Reports

Case Report 1.1. A 63-year-old patient presents with a chief complaint of pain, foul taste, persistent food impaction, and chronic localized infection to site #32. Based on the patient's age, nerve anatomy, and potential for permanent neurosensory damage, the decision was made to remove the coronal aspect (clinical crown) of the impacted tooth without extracting the root tips (i.e., a **coronectomy**). See Figures 1.3, 1.4, and 1.5.

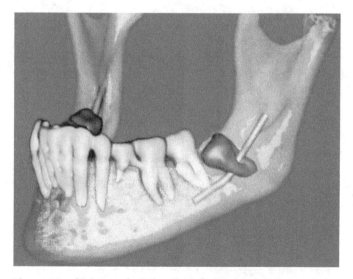

Figure 1.1. 3D image depicting the inferior alveolar nerve coursing directly through an impacted lower wisdom tooth.

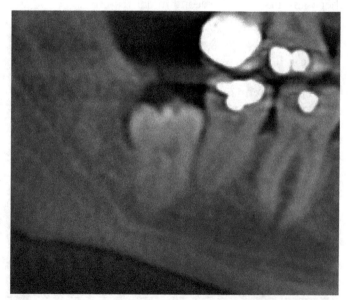

Figure 1.3. 2D film demonstrates impacted tooth #32 with diversion of the mandibular canal at the apex of the tooth.

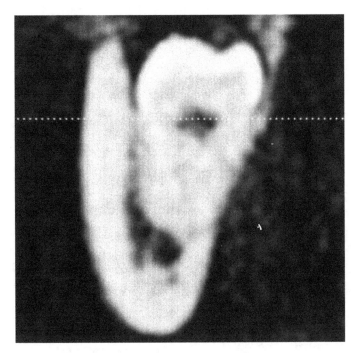

Figure 1.4. Cone beam computed tomography coronal view demonstrating the inferior alveolar nerve coursing through the apical third of tooth #32.

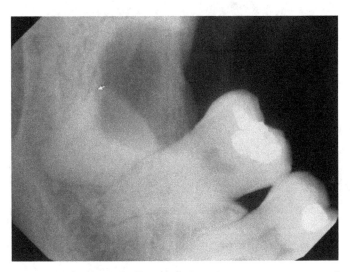

Figure 1.5. Periapical film demonstrating a coronectomy of tooth #32. Note that the entire clinical crown was removed by sectioning the tooth apical to the CEJ to ensure no residual enamel remained and the roots were trimmed 3–4 mm below the bony margin.

Case Report 1.2. A 57-year-old patient presents with a chief complaint of persistent local pain, referred pain, and documented deep probing depths to site #32. See Figures 1.6, 1.7, and 1.8.

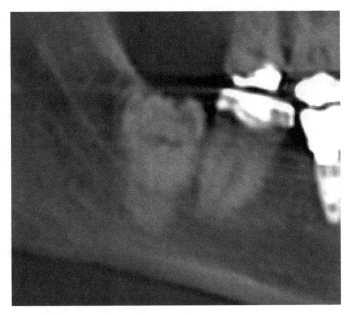

Figure 1.6. 2D film demonstrating interruption of the white lines of the mandibular canal.

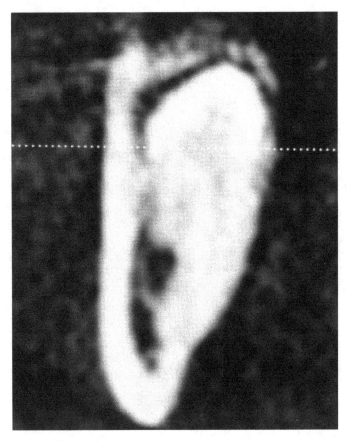

Figure 1.7. Cone beam computed tomography coronal view demonstrating the inferior alveolar nerve coursing through the middle third of the third molar root.

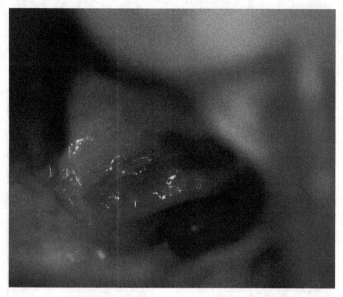

Figure 1.8. Tooth #32 extraction site demonstrating an intact inferior alveolar nerve along the lingual plate.

References

Apostolakis, D., 2012. The anterior loop of the inferior alveolar nerve: prevalence, measurement of its length and a recommendation for interforaminal implant installation based on cone beam CT imaging. *Clinical Oral Implants Research*, 23, pp. 1022–30.

Chan, H-L., 2010. Significance of the lingual nerve during periodontal/implant surgery. *Journal of Periodontology*, 81, pp. 372–7.

Ghaeminia, H., 2009. Position of the impacted third molar in relation to the mandibular canal: diagnostic accuracy of cone beam computed tomography compared with panoramic radiography. *International Journal of Oral and Maxillofacial Surgery*, 38, pp. 964–71.

Janfaza, P., 2011. *Surgical anatomy of the head and neck.* Cambridge, MA: Harvard University Press.

Kim, S.T., 2009. Location of the mandibular canal and topography of its neurovascular structures. *Journal of Craniofacial Surgery*, 20, pp. 936–9.

Levine, M.H., 2007. Location of inferior alveolar nerve position: a clinical and radiographic study. *Journal of Oral and Maxillofacial Surgery*, 65, pp. 470–74.

2

Exposure and Bonding of an Impacted Tooth

Neil C. Kanning,[1] Scott A. Curtice,[2] and Christopher J. Haggerty[3]

[1]*Private Practice, Kanning Orthodontics, Liberty, Missouri, USA*
[2]*Department of Oral and Maxillofacial Surgery, Naval Medical Center San Diego, San Diego, California, USA*
[3]*Private Practice, Lakewood Oral and Maxillofacial Surgery Specialists, Lees Summit; and Department of Oral and Maxillofacial Surgery, University of Missouri–Kansas City, Kansas City, Missouri, USA*

A method of facilitating the eruption of severely impacted and/or malpositioned teeth with orthodontic guidance.

Indications

1. Appropriate arch length to accommodate the impacted tooth within the alveolar arch
2. Appropriate interdental space for the incorporation of the impacted tooth within the alveolus
3. Erupted or impacted tooth on the contralateral side of the arch to provide appropriate symmetry
4. Appropriately developed impacted tooth with no associated malformations or pathology

Contraindications

1. When repositioning impacted teeth will create a structural weakness in the roots of adjacent teeth
2. When other structures (i.e., adjacent roots, supernumerary teeth, and odontomas) are in the path of the anticipated distraction vector
3. Impacted teeth that appear malformed or associated with pathology

Technique

1. Local anesthesia is administered in the form of blocks and infiltration. Subperiosteal injection into the area of the anticipated mucoperiosteal flap will hydro-dissect the tissue and aid in hemostatic flap reflection.
2. Primary teeth in the path of distraction and/or functioning as a space maintainer are extracted.
3. A crestal incision is created within the area of the edentulous space or extraction site of the retained deciduous tooth. Incisions are designed to bisect the attached tissue overlying the alveolar ridge. This will allow the impacted tooth to be distracted through keratinized tissue and will lead to optimal periodontium supporting the tooth.
4. A full-thickness mucoperiosteal flap is raised, with or without distal releasing incisions depending on the access needed to locate the impacted tooth (see Figure 2.6 in Case Report 2.1 and Figure 2.16 in Case Report 2.2).
5. The impacted tooth is frequently identified as an area with a bulge and/or by the identification of the dental follicle. Thin superficial bone overlying the impacted tooth can be removed with a periosteal elevator (see Figure 2.16 in Case Report 2.2). If significant bone removal is required to expose the clinical crown of the impacted tooth, a small round bur with copious irrigation is utilized.
6. Once the clinical crown of the impacted tooth is exposed, the dental follicle is removed with cautery (see Figure 2.7 in Case Report 2.1 and Figure 2.17 in Case Report 2.2). Cautery allows for quick and easy removal of the follicle and greatly adds to hemostasis.
7. If needed, local anesthesia containing a vasoconstrictor can be injected into the surrounding tissue and around the clinical crown of the tooth to aid in hemostasis.
8. A suction tip is placed at the tooth–bone interface to further enhance hemostasis and to aid in the creation of a dry field. A dry field is paramount to ensuring that the composite adheres and has a strong bond.
9. Once a dry field is established and maintained, the bracket is placed toward the incisal or occlusal tip of the impacted tooth in the position of the ideal vector for the distraction of the tooth into the space created by the orthodontist or within the space created by the extraction of the primary tooth.
10. Once the bracket is secured in the appropriate position, the chain attached to the bracket is tested with cotton pliers or pickups to ensure a strong bond between the composite and the impacted tooth. Excessive composite flange is removed with a round bur with copious irrigation.
11. The chain is secured to the orthodontic archwire with 4-0 silk sutures. Excessive chain links are removed in order to minimize slack within the chain (see Figure 2.11 in Case Report 2.1 and Figure 2.18 in Case Report 2.2) as excessive chain slack can lead to bracket detachment.

Atlas of Operative Oral and Maxillofacial Surgery, First Edition. Edited by Christopher J. Haggerty and Robert M. Laughlin

12. The area is closed primarily with interrupted 4-0 chromic sutures (see Figure 2.13 in Case Report 2.1).

Postoperative Management

1. Analgesics are prescribed based on the invasiveness of the procedure.
2. Antibiotics are not routinely prescribed.
3. Patients return to their normal activities the next day.
4. Orthodontic traction should begin as soon as possible after exposure, typically between 5 and 21 days post exposure. Immediate traction is initiated for teeth that have been luxated to address ankylosis.

Complications

Early Complications

1. **Bleeding**: Often from not identifying bleeding tissue on closure. Alternatively, since most expose and bond patients are very young, this may represent an underlying, undiagnosed coagulation disorder.
2. **Bracket detachment**: From inadequate moisture control during the use of composite. It is important to reattach the bracket within 72 hours before extensive healing of the mucoperiosteal flap occurs.
3. **Infection**: Rare. Treated with antibiotics and oral rinses such as Peridex. If an abscess is identified on examination or with radiographs, an incision and drainage procedure is indicated.

Late Complications

1. **Bracket detachment**: Frequently due to an ankylosed tooth or excessive force by the orthodontist.
2. **Failure of tooth movement (ankylosed tooth)**: Treatment options include re-exposure of the impacted tooth with more aggressive bone removal, attempted luxation of the tooth with a dental elevator, and the creation of a bony tunnel through the alveolus to facilitate movement. Care should be taken during surgical exposure to avoid trauma to the cementoenamel junction (CEJ) and the periodontal ligament. Damage to these structures may result in potential periodontal defects and subsequent ankylosis. If the above fails, consider tooth removal and closure of the space via orthodontic means or with a dental implant.
3. **Periodontal defects**: Less likely with conservative flap elevation, the use of orthodontic brackets, conservative bone removal around only the clinical crown, and distracting the impacted tooth through attached keratinized gingiva. Utilizing a bonded bracket to engage the impacted tooth instead of ligating a steel wire around the CEJ will discourage periodontal defects and promote a more optimal periodontal result.

Key Points

1. Radiographs allow the operator to know the exact position of the impacted tooth, its labial or lingual-palatal position, any interferences caused by other structures (i.e., adjacent teeth roots, supernumerary teeth, or odontomas), and whether the tooth is malformed or associated with a pathologic condition. Radiographs should include any combination of orthopantomograms, periapical films, occlusal films, and/or cone beam computed tomography (CBCT) imaging. When utilizing periapical and occlusal films, it is important to understand Clark's rule (i.e., the SLOB rule, for "same lingual; opposite buccal").
2. Communication with the orthodontist is important prior to the ligation of the bracket. Having a clear concept of the overall orthodontic treatment plan and the eruption vectors will lead to more precise bracket placement and ideal treatment outcomes.
3. Some orthodontists prefer to have the expose and bond procedure completed several weeks prior to the placement of full orthodontics. In these instances, the impacted tooth is exposed and bonded, and the silk suture is tied around the teeth adjacent to the site where the tooth will be distracted. For example, for an impacted maxillary canine, the silk suture is tied below the CEJ of the adjacent lateral incisor.
4. The more vertically upright the impacted tooth is positioned, the higher the success rate for distraction into the alveolus and the less chance of ankylosis.
5. Incisions are always crestal. All incisions are designed to bisect the attached tissue overlying the alveolar ridge. This will allow the impacted tooth to be distracted through keratinized tissue and will lead to optimal periodontal support of the tooth. Incisions placed within alveolar mucosa may lead to the eruption of the impacted tooth through unattached tissue and compromise the periodontal support of the tooth once it is aligned within the alveolus.
6. Adequate clinical crown exposure and a dry field are keys to the success of the bonding of the composite to the impacted tooth. It is also paramount to select a composite specifically designed for orthodontic bonding.
7. The bracket should be placed so that when the chain is activated by the orthodontist, the vector of the chain pull coincides with the anticipated path of eruption of the impacted tooth. The bracket should also be placed close to the incisal or occlusal tip of the impacted tooth in order to give the orthodontist optimal control over the movement of the tooth.
8. Orthodontic traction should begin as soon as possible after exposure, but no later than 3 weeks post exposure. Immediate traction should be initiated for teeth that have been luxated to address ankylosis.

9. The technique described above is often referred to as the closed eruption technique because the technique involves full flap closure after exposure and bonding of the bracket to the impacted tooth. Alternatively, an open eruption technique can be employed. The open eruption technique is primarily utilized for palatally impacted maxillary canines when there is concern of adjacent root resorption from the vector of distraction from a closed technique. The open eruption technique involves creating an incision that bisects the attached mucosa and removing sufficient bone to expose the clinical crown of an impacted tooth just as in the closed eruption technique. Next, the flap is repositioned over the impacted tooth, and a perforation is created within the tissue overlying the impacted tooth's clinical crown. The tissue perforation is packed with a surgical packing (typically, a periodontal pack; Coe-Pak, GC American Inc., Alsip, IL, US) or an appliance (a cleat, bracket, or chrome steel crown), and the tooth is allowed to erupt autonomously to the level of the occlusal plane.

Case Reports

Case Report 2.1. Palatally positioned impacted teeth. A 14-year-old female presents with impacted teeth #6 and 11 and retained primary teeth c and h. The patient has been in full orthodontics for 9 months in order to align teeth and alleviate anterior crowding. (See Figures 2.1 through 2.13.)

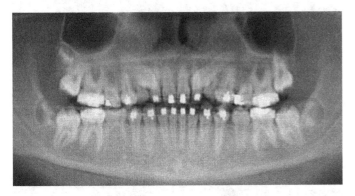

Figure 2.1. Orthopantomogram demonstrating retained primary teeth c and h and impacted teeth #6 and #11.

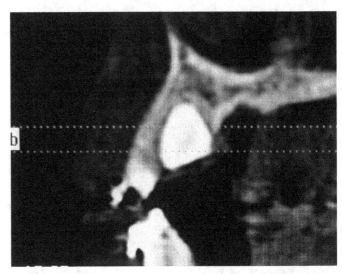

Figure 2.2. Cone beam computed tomography sagittal view demonstrating the palatal position of tooth #6.

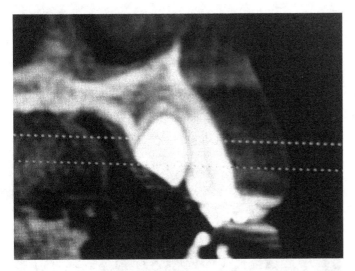

Figure 2.3. Cone beam computed tomography sagittal view demonstrating the palatal position of tooth #11.

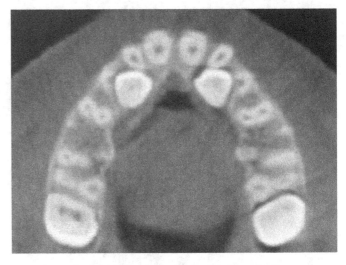

Figure 2.4. Occlusal view of impacted teeth #6 and #11.

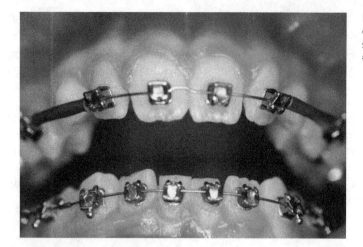

Figure 2.5. 14-year-old patient in full orthodontics with c and h acting as space maintainers for impacted teeth #6 and #11.

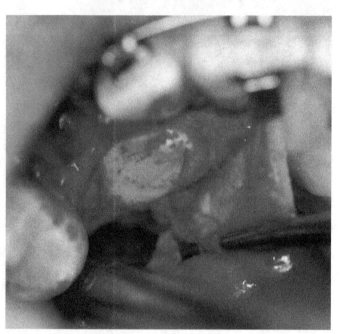
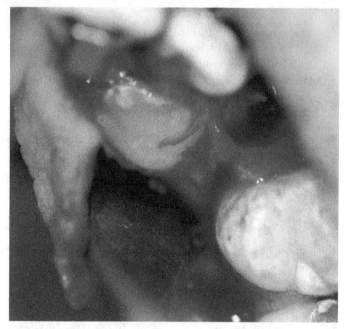

Figure 2.6. Extraction of primary teeth c and h. Crestal incision and reflection of full-thickness mucoperiosteal flaps to expose teeth #6 and #11. The flaps are not connected within the midline in order to preserve the integrity of the incisive canal and of its contents.

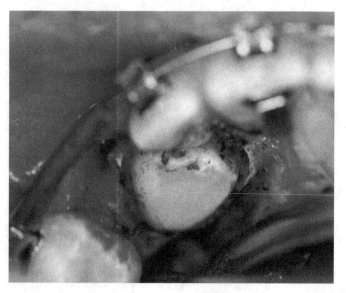
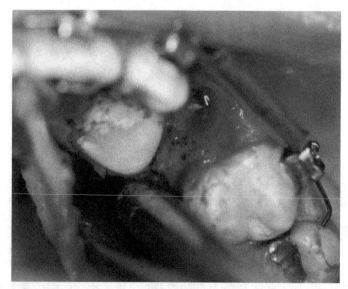

Figure 2.7. Removal of the dental follicles and surrounding bone to expose the clinical crowns of teeth #6 and #11.

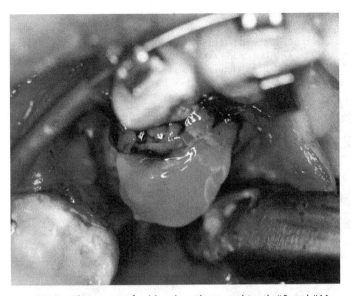

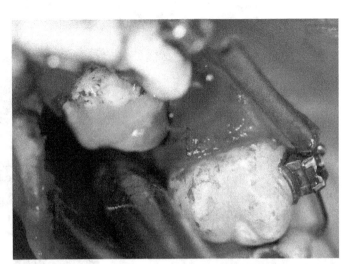

Figure 2.8.   Placement of acid etch on impacted teeth #6 and #11.

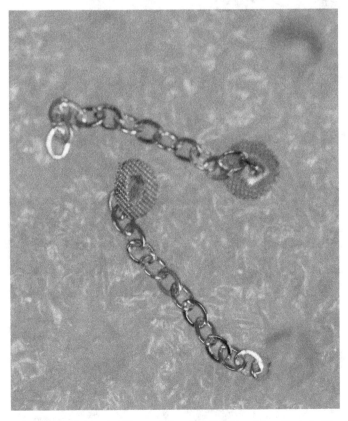

Figure 2.9.   A low-profile mesh bracket is utilized to attach to the impacted teeth (Cusp-Lok Chain and Mesh, Xemax Surgical Products, Inc., Napa, CA, USA). The mesh allows for greater adherence of the composite to the bracket, and the low-profile design helps to prevent external forces from displacing the bracket.

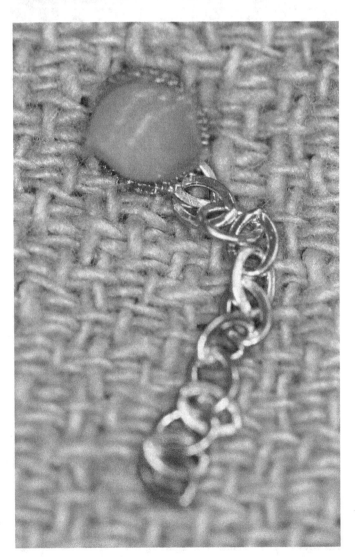

Figure 2.10.   A very small amount of composite is utilized, as excessive composite does not aid in adherence and creates a plaque trap.

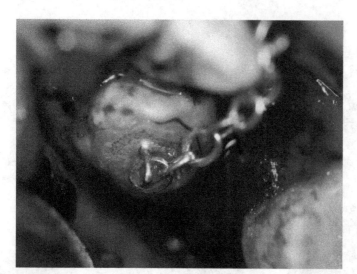

Figure 2.11. The bracket is bonded to impacted tooth #11, excessive composite has been removed with a round bur, additional gold chain links have been removed to eliminate potential slack, and the chain has been secured to the orthodontic wire with 4-0 silk sutures.

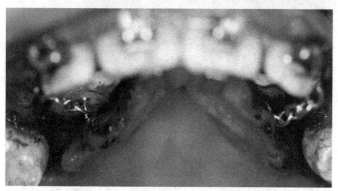

Figure 2.12. Gold chains secured to the orthodontic archwire using 4-0 silk sutures.

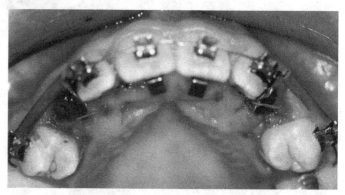

Figure 2.13. Bilateral palatal flaps are closed with interrupted 4-0 chromic sutures placed over the primary canine extraction sites and within the interproximal embrasures.

Case Report 2.2. Labially positioned impacted tooth. A 15-year-old female presents with failure of spontaneous eruption of tooth #11. The patient has been in full orthodontics for 6 months and has already lost all of her primary dentition. The orthodontist has created sufficient space for the orthodontic redirection of tooth #11. (See Figures 2.14, 2.15, 2.16, 2.17, and 2.18.)

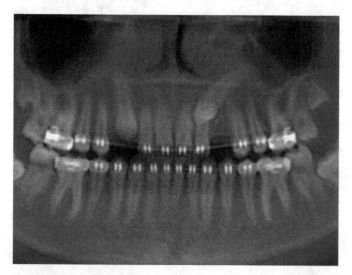

Figure 2.14. Orthopantomogram demonstrating vertically erupting tooth #6 and impacted tooth #11.

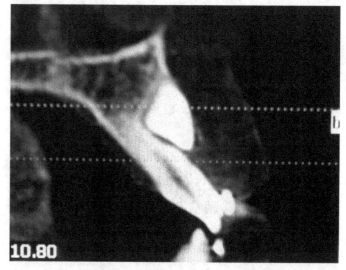

Figure 2.15. Cone beam computed tomography sagittal view demonstrating the labial position of tooth #11.

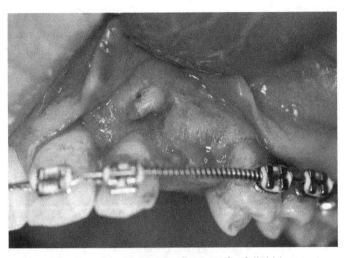

Figure 2.16.   Crestal incision and reflection of a full-thickness muco-periosteal flap to expose tooth #11. A periosteal elevator has been used to locate the tooth by removing a small piece of thin overlying bone.

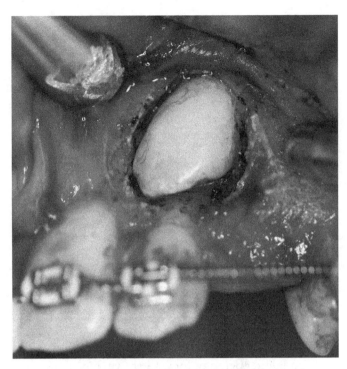

Figure 2.17.   Removal of the dental follicle and surrounding bone to expose the clinical crown of tooth #11.

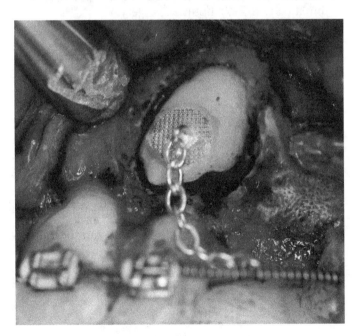

Figure 2.18.   Placement of bracket, removal of excessive composite flash, removal of excess chain links, and securing the chain to the orthodontic archwire with 4-0 silk sutures.

References

Caminiti, M.F., Sandor, G.K., Giambattistini, C. and Tompson, B., 1998. Outcomes of the surgical exposure, bonding and eruption of 82 maxillary canines. *Journal of the Canadian Dental Association*, 64, pp. 576–59.

Chaushu, S., Becker, A., Zeltser, R., Branski, S., Vasker, N. and Chaushu, G., 2005. Patient's perception of recovery after exposure of impacted teeth: a comparison of closed versus open eruption techniques. *Journal of Oral and Maxillofacial Surgery*, 63, pp. 323–9.

Kurol, J., Erikson, S. and Andreasen, J.O., 1997. The impacted maxillary canine. In: J.O. Andreasen, J.K. Petersen and D. Laskin, eds. 1997. *Textbook and color atlas of tooth impactions*. Copenhagen: Munksgaard.

Kokick, V.G., 2010. Preorthodontic uncovering and autonomous eruption of palatally impacted maxillary canines. *Seminars in Orthodontia*, 16, 205–11.

3

Pre-Prosthetic Surgery

Daniel Clifford

Department of Oral and Maxillofacial Surgery, Naval Medical Center San Diego, San Diego, California, USA

Procedure: Fibrous Tuberosity Reduction

A procedure performed to reduce excessive soft tissue from the maxillary tuberosities.

Indications

1. Excessive soft tissue tuberosity
2. Interference with prosthetic rehabilitation
3. Infection, ulceration, and/or pain
4. Masticatory dysfunction or trauma

Contraindications

1. Adequate topography for a retentive and stable prosthesis
2. Adequate space for prosthetic fabrication

Surgical Technique: Wedge Reduction

1. The tissue to be excised is marked with a sterile marking pen based on the prosthodontic treatment plan (see Figure 3.1 in Case Report 3.1).
2. Local anesthesia containing a vasoconstrictor is administered via posterior superior alveolar and greater palatine nerve blocks. Additional local anesthesia containing a vasoconstrictor is injected directly within the fibrous tuberosity to aid in hemostasis.
3. A full-thickness elliptical incision is initiated over the posterior alveolar ridge in the area of desired tissue reduction. The intervening wedge of tissue is removed (Figure 3.2, Case Report 3.1). If additional tissue reduction is necessary after the initial wedge resection, additional tissue may be removed from the buccal and/or lingual flaps until the desired reduction is accomplished (Figure 3.3, Case Report 3.1).
4. The area is checked for adequacy of reduction and for hemostasis. Tension-free primary closure is performed utilizing 3-0 resorbable sutures (Figure 3.4, Case Report 3.1).

Postoperative Management

1. Analgesics are prescribed based on the amount of tissue removed.
2. A clear liquid diet is recommended for 24 hours, with the patient advancing to a regular diet as tolerated.
3. Saltwater rinses are begun three times a day beginning the day of surgery.
4. For patients receiving an immediate prosthesis, denture adjustments or relines to the prosthesis are initiated within 72 hours of surgery.

Complications

1. **Hemorrhage**: Arterial bleeding from the greater or lesser palatine arteries is controlled with constant, direct pressure.
2. **Infection**: Occurs from poor oral hygiene, food impaction, and necrotic tissue resulting from an ill-fitting prosthesis. Treated with improved oral hygiene, chlorhexidine gluconate 0.12% oral rinses, and oral antibiotics.
3. **Tissue necrosis**: Typically occurs from a poor-fitting maxillary prosthesis. Treatment involves the relining or removal of the offending prosthesis and the debulking of necrotic tissue.

Atlas of Operative Oral and Maxillofacial Surgery, First Edition. Edited by Christopher J. Haggerty and Robert M. Laughlin
© 2015 John Wiley & Sons, Inc. Published 2015 by John Wiley & Sons, Inc.

Case Report 3.1. A 54-year-old patient presents after a prosthodontic consultation with a referral for the removal of excessive soft tissue from the left maxillary tuberosity in preparation for a removable partial denture. (See Figures 3.1, 3.2, 3.3, and 3.4.)

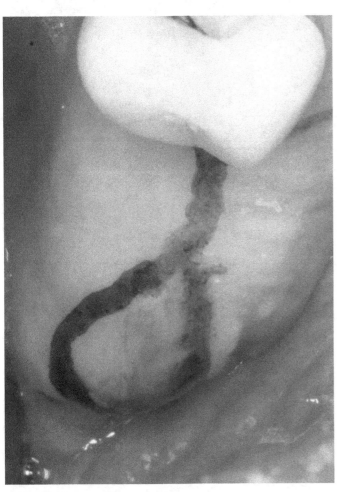

Figure 3.1.   The area of tissue to be excised is determined, and the incision outline is marked.

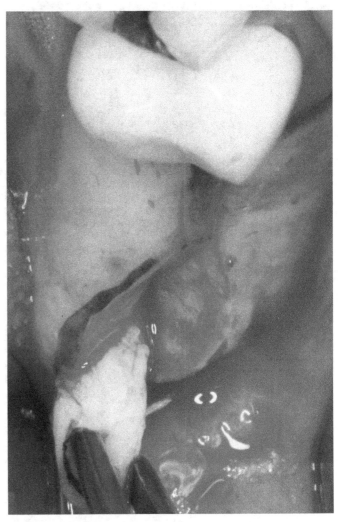

Figure 3.2.   A full-thickness elliptical incision is created, and the intervening wedge of tissue is removed.

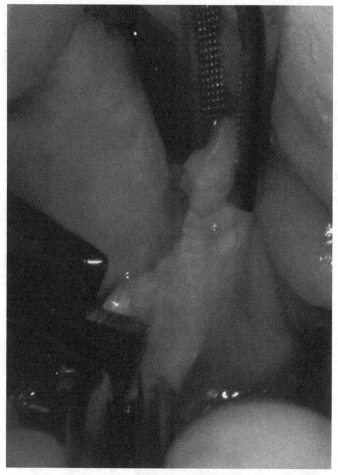

Figure 3.3.   Additional tissue may be removed by undermining the buccal and/or lingual tissue flaps.

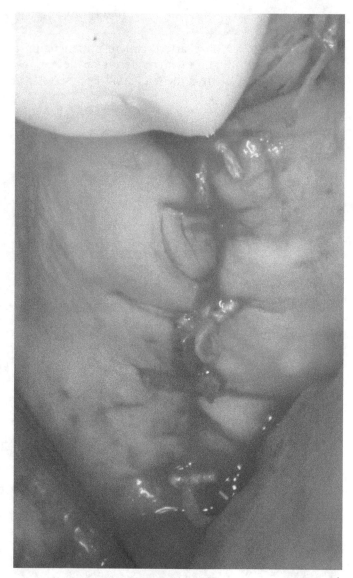

Figure 3.4.   The site is closed primarily in a tension-free manner with resorbable sutures.

Procedure: Torus Mandibularis Reduction

A procedure performed to reduce or recontour a bony protuberance, or torus, of the mandible.

Indications

1. Interference with prosthetic rehabilitation
2. Infection or ulceration of overlying tissues due to trauma
3. Pain or impingement of the lingual frenum
4. Masticatory dysfunction
5. Negative impact on speech

Contraindications

1. Asymptomatic torus mandibularis
2. Adequate skeletal relationship and soft and hard tissue architecture for stable and satisfactory prosthetic device fabrication
3. Systemic factors that influence bone and tissue healing (intravenous bisphosphonates, head and neck radiation, etc.)

Anatomy

Torus mandibularis are present in 7.75% to 15% of the population and are found bilaterally in up to 80% of cases. Mandibular tori occur above the mylohyoid ridge and are typically located within the canine and premolar regions.

Surgical Technique

1. Torus mandibularis or mandibular tori reductions may be performed with local anesthesia alone or combined with moderate sedation or general anesthesia. Local anesthesia is performed with inferior alveolar and lingual nerve blocks. Additional local anesthesia containing a vasoconstrictor is injected directly into the mucosa overlying the tori in order to hydro-dissect the thin tissue from the tori.
2. Depending on the presence of dentition, a full-thickness lingual circumdental (sulcular) or crestal incision is created within the area of the tori. The incision may be extending anteriorly and posteriorly to allow for complete and tension-free exposure of the tori.
3. A full-thickness mucoperiosteal flap is elevated, and a subperiosteal retractor is placed. The retractor is positioned along the inferior aspect of the torus and reflects the tongue, the contents of the floor of the mouth, and the full-thickness tissue flap medially.
4. Large mandibular tori are typically reduced by scoring the entire superior length of the torus with a fissured bur to a depth of one-half to three-fourths of the vertical dimension of the tori. While maintaining a retractor beneath the tori and providing jaw support, an osteotome is used to cleave the tori from the lingual aspect of the mandible in a controlled fashion.

Any remaining irregularities after tori reduction are smoothed with an acrylic bur, a bone file, or a rasp. Smaller tori are reduced with an acrylic bur alone.
5. The surgical site is irrigated, inspected for hemostasis, and closed primarily with resorbable sutures. Flap tears are managed with interrupted resorbable sutures.
6. Immediate placement of a postoperative stent or tissue-conditioned prosthesis is beneficial for large tori reduction.

Key Points

1. Appropriate placement of a lingual subperiosteal retractor will aid in visualization of the mandibular tori, minimize iatrogenic tissue damage to the mucoperiosteal tissue flap, and protect the tongue and floor-of-the-mouth contents during the procedure.
2. Care should be taken to remove all sharp edges of bone, particularly at the inferior aspect of the mylohyoid ridge, in order to prevent secondary revisions and a painful prosthesis.

Procedure: Torus Palatinus Reduction

A procedure performed to reduce or recontour bony protuberances of the midline palate.

Indications

1. Traumatized mucosa overlying the torus
2. Interference with speech or deglutition
3. Torus with deep undercuts resulting in food impaction and halitosis
4. Masticatory dysfunction
5. Interference with prosthetic rehabilitation
6. Torus that extends beyond the dam area, preventing prosthetic seal
7. Pain
8. Removal prior to the initiation of intravenous bisphosphonates and/or head and neck radiation

Contraindications

1. Asymptomatic torus
2. Presence of torus with minimal or no impact on the planned prosthesis
3. No masticatory impact
4. No interference with speech or deglutition
5. Systemic factors that influence bone and tissue healing (intravenous bisphosphonates, head and neck radiation, etc.)

Anatomy

Maxillary palatal tori occur in approximately 20% of the population and are characteristically located within the midline of the hard palate.

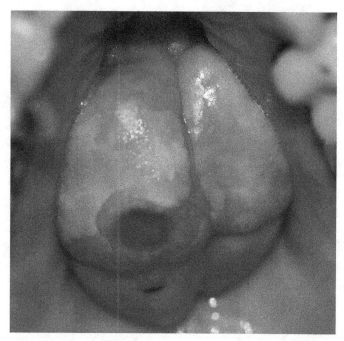

Figure 3.5. Patients with large palatal tori typically develop food impaction, halitosis, pain, and chronic ulcerations to the thin overlying mucosa.

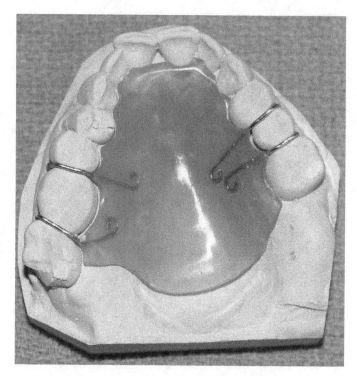

Figure 3.6. A palatal prosthesis fabricated for the patient in Figure 3.5. The prefabricated temporary prosthesis is inserted at the time of tori reduction to aid in tissue hemostasis, increase patient comfort and encourage optimal soft tissue healing.

Surgical Technique

1. Maxillary tori reduction may be performed with local anesthesia alone or combined with moderate sedation or general anesthesia. Local anesthesia is performed with incisive and bilateral greater palatine nerve blocks. Additional local anesthesia containing a vasoconstrictor is injected directly into the mucosa overlying the tori in order to hydro-dissect the thin tissue from the tori.
2. A double-"Y" incision is outlined along the midline of the torus with anterior and posterior releasing incisions (see Figure 3.7 in Case Report 3.2).
3. A subperiosteal dissection is performed to expose the entire torus and adjacent bone (Figure 3.8, Case Report 3.2). Bilateral subperiosteal retractors are placed in order to minimize iatrogenic damage to the tissue flaps.
4. Large tori may be reduced utilizing a 701 bur to divide the tori into smaller subunits using a grid pattern. A mallet and curved osteotome are used to remove the smaller subunits. Smaller tori are reduced with an acrylic bur alone.
5. Any remaining irregularities after tori reduction are smoothed with an acrylic bur, a bone file, or a rasp (Figure 3.9, Case Report 3.2).
6. The surgical site is irrigated, inspected for hemostasis, and primarily closed with resorbable sutures (Figure 3.10, Case Report 3.2). Flap tears are managed with interrupted resorbable sutures.
7. Immediate placement of a postoperative stent or tissue-conditioned prosthesis is beneficial for large tori reduction (Figures 3.5 and 3.6).

Complications of Mandibular and Maxillary Tori Reductions

1. **Wound dehiscence**: The mucoperiosteum overlying the tori is frequently thin and friable. Postoperative tissue breakdowns are managed with excellent oral hygiene and saline rinses throughout the day and following meals. If a prosthesis is suspected to have contributed to wound dehiscence, the prosthesis is relieved, and a tissue conditioner is placed or the prosthesis is discontinued until healing is completed.
2. **Hematoma formation**: Managed within the immediate postoperative period with direct pressure and prosthesis placement. Managed after 24 hours with needle aspiration or exploration with incision and drainage, based on the size of the presenting hematoma.

Key Points

1. Prefabricated prostheses in the form of a complete denture or a palatal prosthesis (Figure 3.6) are beneficial with large tori reductions to minimize postoperative patient discomfort and food impaction, to apply pressure to the surgical site, and to encourage optimal soft tissue healing.

Case Report 3.2. A 46-year-old patient presents for the removal of her palatal tori prior to the fabrication of a maxillary complete removable denture. (See Figures 3.7, 3.8, 3.9, and 3.10.)

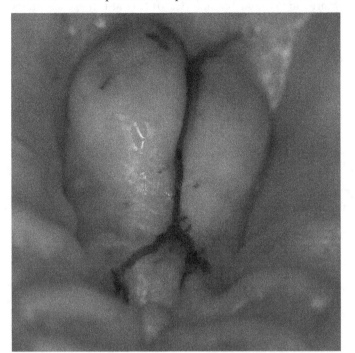

Figure 3.7.   A double-"Y" incision is outlined over the midline palatal tori.

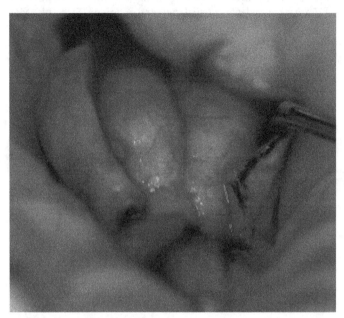

Figure 3.8.   Elevation of a full-thickness mucoperiosteal tissue flap and complete exposure of the palatal tori and adjacent bone.

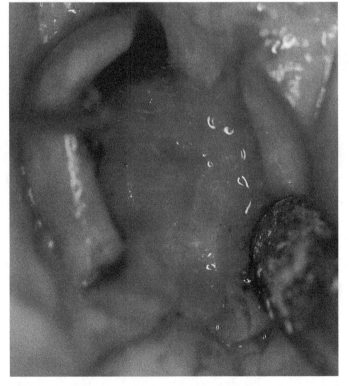

Figure 3.9.   Adequate reduction of the palatal tori and removal of all bone irregularities.

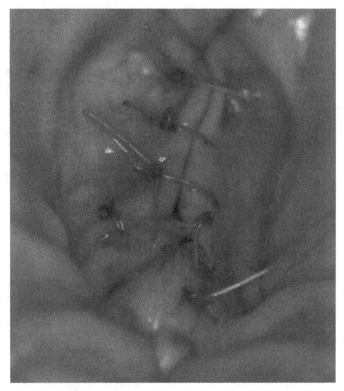

Figure 3.10.   Primary closure is obtained with interrupted resorbable sutures.

References

Gahleitner, A., Hofschneider, U., Tepper, G., Pretterklieber, M., Schick, S., Zauza, K. and Watzek, G., 2001. Lingual vascular canals of the mandible: evaluation with dental CT. *Radiology*, 220, 180–89.

Guernsey, L.H., 1984. Preprosthetic surgery. In: G.O. Kruger, ed. *Textbook of oral and maxillofacial surgery*. 6th ed. St. Louis, MO: Mosby. pp. 106–66.

Haug, R.H. 2012. Microorganisms of the nose and paranasal sinuses. *Oral and Maxillofacial Surgery Clinics of North America*, 24(2), 191–6.

Kolas, S., Halperin, V., Jefferis, K.R., Huddleston, S. and Robinson, H.B., 1953. The occurrence of torus palatinus and torus mandibularis in 2,478 dental patients. *Oral Surgery*, 6, 1134–43.

Morrison, M. and Tamimi, F., 2012. Oral tori are associated with local mechanical and systemic factors: a case-control study. *Journal of Oral and Maxillofacial Surgery*, 71(1), 14–22.

Scott, R.F. and Olson, R.A.J., 1995. Minor preprosthetic procedures. In: R.J.Fonseca and W.H.Davis, eds. *Reconstructive preprosthetic oral and maxillofacial surgery*. 2nd ed. Philadelphia: W.B. Saunders. pp. 733–42.

CHAPTER

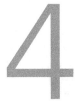

Extraction Site (Socket) Preservation

Christopher Choi,[1] Ray Lim,[2] and Dale J. Misek[2]

[1]Private Practice, Inland Empire Oral and Maxillofacial Surgeons, Rancho Cucamonga, California, USA
[2]Private Practice, Carolinas Center for Oral and Facial Surgery, Charlotte, North Carolina, USA; and
Department of Oral and Maxillofacial Surgery, Louisiana State University Health Science Center, New Orleans,
Louisiana, USA

A method of preserving and augmenting bone height and width immediately after tooth extraction for future dental implant placement.

Indications

1. Prevention of alveolar ridge atrophy after tooth extraction
2. Restoration of bony defects caused by infection, trauma, and/or traumatic extractions

Contraindications

1. Sites where future implant placement is unachievable
2. Medical conditions that preclude implant placement

Technique

1. Preoperative antibiotics and chlorhexidine rinses are administered immediately prior to extraction.
2. Atraumatic exodontia is performed to maintain the buccal cortical plate and septal bone (see Figure 4.3 in Case Report 4.1).
3. All periapical and granulation tissue is curetted from the extraction site.
4. The extraction site is copiously irrigated, and doxycycline paste is applied to the extraction socket walls for 5 minutes.
5. A particulate grafting medium is placed and compacted within the defect.
6. A collagen membrane is placed (see Figure 4.4 in Case Report 4.1) to stabilize the graft and to guide tissue regeneration. A resorbable figure-of-eight suture is used to secure the collagen membrane and to close tissue elevations.

Postoperative Management

1. Postoperative discomfort is managed with analgesics or nonsteroidal anti-inflammatory drugs.
2. Patients are instructed to minimize pressure to the grafted area. Patients are asked to refrain from using straws, avoid masticating on the area of the graft and to maintain a soft diet for one week postoperatively.
3. Gentle saltwater rinses are begun after 48 hours and are continued until mucosalization of the graft site occurs.
4. Smoking cessation is encouraged during the recovery period.

Complications

1. Graft loss
2. Inadequate graft consolidation
3. Infection

Key Points

1. Not all extraction sockets require grafting, particularly those without wall defects and with thick buccal walls.
2. Recombinant human bone morphogenic protein 2 has received US Food and Drug Administration approval for alveolar ridge augmentation for defects associated with extraction sockets.
3. After tooth extraction, predictable alveolar ridge atrophy occurs. Tan et al. (2012) reported 29–63% horizontal bone loss and 11–22% vertical bone loss 6 months following tooth extractions without socket preservation grafting.

Atlas of Operative Oral and Maxillofacial Surgery, First Edition. Edited by Christopher J. Haggerty and Robert M. Laughlin

Case Report 4.1. A 39-year-old male presents for the extraction of tooth #30 and socket preservation grafting to optimize the opportunity for future dental implant placement. Clinical and radiographic examination demonstrate a hopeless tooth #30 with buccal root exposure, buccal and lingual plate defects, significant gingival recession, and abscess formation. (See Figures 4.1, 4.2, 4.3, 4.4, and 4.5.)

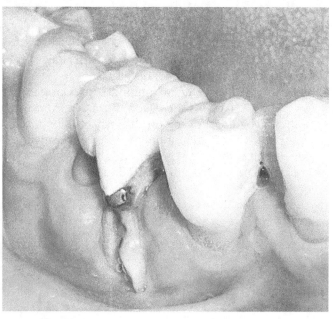

Figure 4.1. Buccal cortical defect and gingival recession associated with tooth #30.

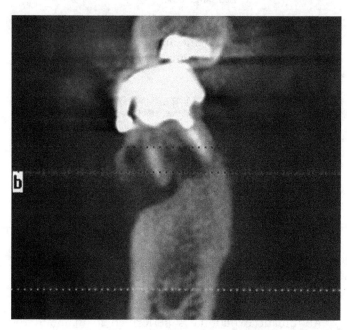

Figure 4.2. Cone beam computed tomography view demonstrating buccal and lingual plate defects and abscess formation.

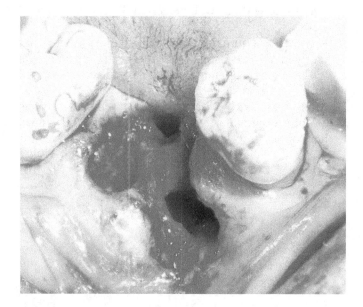

Figure 4.3. Tooth #30 is extracted atraumatically, and the site is curetted to remove all granulation and infected tissue.

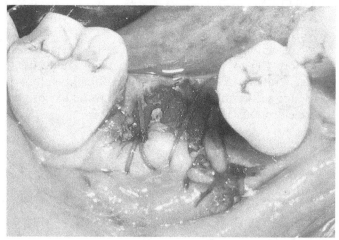

Figure 4.4. The particulate graft is compacted within the extraction site, and a collagen membrane is placed and secured with 4-0 chromic sutures.

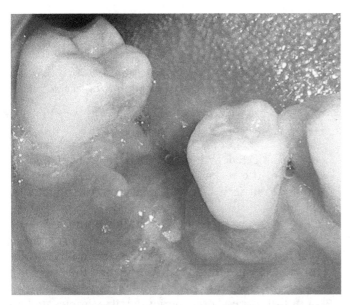

Figure 4.5. Site #30 shown 4 weeks post extraction and socket preservation grafting.

References

Barone, A., Aldini, N.N., Fini, M., Giardino, R., Calvo Guirado, J.L. and Covani, U., 2008. Xenograft versus extraction alone for ridge preservation after tooth removal: a clinical and histomophometric study. *Journal of Periodontology*, 79, 1370–77.

Block, M.S., 2004. Treatment of the single tooth extraction site. *Oral and Maxillofacial Surgery Clinics of North America*, 16, 41–63.

Cardaropoli, G., Araujo, M. and Lindhe, J., 2003. Dynamics of bone tissue formation in tooth extraction sites: an experimental study in dogs. *Journal of Clinical Periodontology*, 30, 809–18.

Cawood, J.I. and Howell, R.A., 1988. A classification of the edentulous jaws. *International Journal of Oral and Maxillofacial Surgery*, 17, 232–6.

Fiorellini, J.P., Howell, T.H., Cochran, D., Malmquist, J., Lilly, L.C., Spagnoli, D., Toljanic, J., Jones, A. and Nevins, M., 2005. Randomized study evaluating recombinant human bone morphogenetic protein-2 for extraction socket augmentation. *Journal of Periodontology*, 76, 605.

Froum, S., Cho, S.C., Rosenberg, E., Rohrer, M. and Tarnow, D., 2002. Histological comparison of healing extraction sockets implanted with bioactive glass or demineralized freeze-dried bone allograft: a pilot study. *Journal of Periodontology*, 73, 94–102.

Tan, W.L., Wong, T.L., Wong, M.C. and Lang, N.P., 2012. A systematic review of post-extractional alveolar hard and soft tissue dimensional changes in humans. *Clinical Oral Implants Research*, 23(Suppl. 5), 1–21.

Trombelli L., Farina, R., Marzola, A., Bozzi, L., Liljenberg, B. and Lindhe, J., 2008. Modeling and remodeling of human extraction sockets. *Journal of Clinical Periodontology*, 35, 630–39.

CHAPTER

5 Onlay Bone Grafting

Michael Grau, Jr.[1] and Christopher J. Haggerty[2]

[1]Department of Oral and Maxillofacial Surgery, Naval Medical Center San Diego, San Diego, California, USA
[2]Private Practice, Lakewood Oral and Maxillofacial Surgery Specialists, Lees Summit; and Department of Oral and Maxillofacial Surgery, University of Missouri–Kansas City, Kansas City, Missouri, USA

Procedure: Onlay Bone Grafting

A method of augmenting the hard tissue of the mandible and/or maxilla to facilitate the placement of endosseous implants.

Indications

1. Inadequate available bone width and/or height for the placement of dental implants in an ideal restorative position
2. Adequate space in relation to vital structures allowing for the placement of fixation screws

Contraindications

1. Inadequate restorative space for the fabrication of the final prosthesis
2. Intravenous bisphosphonate therapy
3. Immunosuppressed patients
4. Previous radiation therapy to the site of grafting and implant placement
5. Relative contraindications include uncontrolled diabetes mellitus, cigarette smoking, alcoholism, active periodontal disease, and chronic corticosteroid therapy

Intraoral Alveolar Ridge Augmentation Technique

1. Preoperative models and radiographs are used to estimate the amount of bone augmentation required.
2. The risks, benefits, and alternatives of the procedure and the type of graft material utilized are discussed with the patient. The graft material (autogenous or allogenous) is selected based on defect size, defect location, patient desires, and the surgeon's preference.
3. The procedure may be performed under local anesthesia, intravenous sedation, or general endotracheal sedation depending on the amount of bone augmentation required, the donor site, the patient's anxiety level, and the patient's medical history.
4. Antibiotic prophylaxis is administered 30 minutes preoperatively. The oral cavity is prepped with chlorohexidine and/or betadine solution.
5. Local anesthesia is administered within the augmentation site, utilizing nerve blocks for the mandible and local infiltration for the maxilla. Local anesthesia is also injected within the attached and unattached tissue of the recipient site to aid in hemostasis and to hydro-dissect the periosteum from the underlying bone.
6. A #15 blade is utilized to bisect the keratinized tissue overlying the atrophic alveolar ridge. Vertical releasing incisions are frequently necessary to obtain adequate exposure of the surgical site and to allow for a tension-free closure over the augmented area.
7. A full-thickness mucoperiosteal flap is elevated to expose the atrophic alveolar site (see Figures 5.1 and 5.8 in the Case Reports) and the osseous defect is measured. The defect size determines the amount of allograft required or the amount of autogenous bone to be extracted from the harvest site.
8. For block grafting, the recipient site is contoured (Figure 5.2, Case Report 5.1) with a round bur to allow for passive and even contact of the graft to the underlying alveolus.
9. A 701 bur may be utilized to create perforations within the buccal cortex to stimulate blood flow to the area. The periosteum is released with a #15 blade (Figure 5.8, Case Report 5.2) in order to allow for added mobility of the mucoperiosteal flap and a tension-free closure.
10. The graft (block or particulate) is placed with the recipient site. For block grafts, the graft should be flush with the underlying bone, should have a passive fit, should completely fill the area to be grafted, and should have no sharp protruding edges or corners. Block grafts are fixated to the recipient site with a minimum of two positional screws (see Figures 5.4 and 5.23 in the Case Reports). Particulate grafting may be utilized to fill any residual defects between the graft and the recipient bed (Figure 5.23, Case Report 5.3).
11. The full-thickness mucoperiosteal flap is advanced and checked for passivity. Membranes are placed (Figure 5.11, Case Report 5.2) based on the surgeon's preference, the ability to achieve a tension-free primary closure of the augmented surgical site, and the presence of tears within the overlying mucoperiosteal flap.
12. The surgical site is closed in a tension-free manner (Figure 5.12, Case Report 5.2) with 3-0 or 4-0 sutures.

Atlas of Operative Oral and Maxillofacial Surgery, First Edition. Edited by Christopher J. Haggerty and Robert M. Laughlin.
© 2015 John Wiley & Sons, Inc. Published 2015 by John Wiley & Sons, Inc.

Transcutaneous Mandibular Augmentation Technique

1. Preoperative models and films are used to estimate the amount of bone augmentation required.
2. Preoperative intravenous antibiotics, antisialagogues, and steroids are given. The patient is orally intubated. Both the donor and the graft site are prepped with betadine scrub and paint and outlined with sterile towels. The patient is draped, and anatomical markings are drawn with a sterile pen.
3. Local anesthesia containing a vasoconstrictor is deposited within the site of the proposed skin incisions. For augmentation posterior to the corner of the mouth, the local anesthesia should be injected superficial to the platysma muscle, long-acting paralytics should be avoided, and a nerve stimulator should be employed.
4. The inferior border of the mandible is exposed in a subperiosteal plane (Figure 5.20, Case Report 5.3). Care is taken to avoid unnecessary periosteal elevation along the lingual and superior aspects of the mandible.
5. A block of bone wax can be shaped to mimic the amount of desired augmentation (Figure 5.21, Case Report 5.3). The bone wax can be used as a guide (Figure 5.22, Case Report 5.3) to determine the amount of bone harvested from the autogenous donor site and to shape the autogenous graft prior to placement.
6. The block graft and the recipient site are contoured to allow for a flush fit with even contacts and no sharp edges. The block graft is positioned with positional screws placed in sites where future dental implants will not be placed (Figure 5.23, Case Report 5.3). Care is taken to ensure that the positional screws engage the inferior border of the atrophic mandible but do not penetrate the oral mucosa.
7. Particulate grafting may be performed around the periphery of the block graft to minimize voids (Figure 5.23, Case Report 5.3). The site is closed in a layered fashion, and a pressure dressing is placed.

Postoperative Management

1. Analgesics and antibiotics are prescribed.
2. A liquid diet is recommended for the first 48 hours. The diet is then advanced to a soft mechanical diet for the first week. Patients are to avoid masticating at the site of the graft.
3. Oral hygiene is maintained with gentle brushing of any teeth adjacent to the surgical site and the utilization of saltwater rinses three times daily until all intra oral incision sites are healed.
4. Patients are to avoid the wearing of any prosthesis that will place pressure on the graft site for a minimum of 14 days. Preexisting or temporary dentures may be relined to alleviate pressure on the augmented ridges.
5. Patients are to avoid strenuous activity until evaluated at 7 days postoperatively.

Complications

1. **Wound dehiscence**: Incision line dehiscences result from failure to obtain a tension-free closure, failure to remove sharp edges from block grafts, and placing too much grafting material within the recipient site. Dehiscences result in contamination of the graft, delayed healing, and partial or complete loss of the graft. Dehiscences are treated with meticulous oral hygiene, chlorhexedine rinses, and the addition of systemic antibiotics as indicated. Exposed, loose particulate grafting material should be removed with a curette, and areas of exposed block grafts should be removed with a handpiece with copious irrigation. The above techniques may allow for the partial retention of the underlying, unexposed graft.
2. **Infection**: Infections typically occur from intraoperative wound contamination and/or postoperative wound dehiscence. Infections are treated with prompt incision and drainage, removal of the source of the infection (infected hardware and mobile graft), chlorohexidine rinses, and systemic antibiotics.
3. **Loss of graft**: Partial or complete loss of bone graft may occur secondary to infection or wound dehiscence. Significant graft loss may require additional augmentation.
4. **Nerve damage**: The inferior alveolar nerve may be damaged during the harvest of lateral ramus grafts, during the exposure of the parasymphysis region of the mandible, and during the placement of position screws to secure block grafts. Nerve damage can be minimized with a thorough evaluation of preoperative radiographs and attention to detail. Close monitoring, testing, and documentation are performed until resolution of symptoms. Patients who fail to improve should be referred for evaluation from a microvascular nerve specialist.
5. **Graft mobilization**: Graft mobilization may occur secondary to fixation failure or localized infection. Failure to achieve adequate fixation may lead to partial or total graft loss, infection, or fibrous union.

Key Points

1. A thorough evaluation and calibration of preoperative radiographs will aid the surgeon in determining the amount of bone augmentation required, the type of graft needed, and will minimize the potential for nerve injury.
2. Block grafts require contouring prior to placement to maximize bone contact, allow an even and passive fit, and to remove all sharp edges and corners.
3. Immobility of the graft is key to successful incorporation. Two-point fixation is necessary with block grafting to minimize rotation and movement during the healing process. Positional screws are preferred to lag screws in order to minimize iatrogenic fracture of the block graft.

Case Report 5.1. A 48-year-old male presents 12 months post extraction of tooth #7 desiring a dental implant. On review of the cone beam computed tomography images, there was insufficient alveolar ridge height and width for

the placement of a dental implant. The decision was made to augment the horizontal and vertical dimensions of site #7 with a lateral ramus onlay graft. (See Figures 5.1, 5.2, 5.3, and 5.4.)

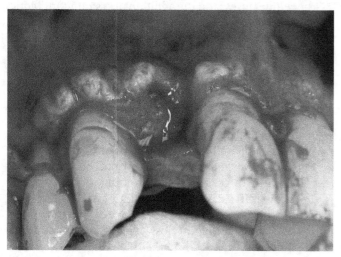

Figure 5.1. Mucoperiosteal flap reflection revealed alveolar ridge bony exostosis and a combined vertical and horizontal bone deficiency.

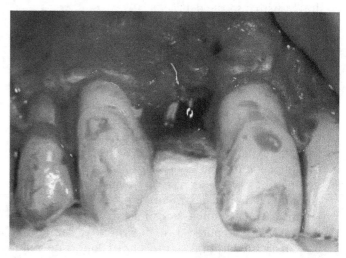

Figure 5.2. The recipient site is recontoured to remove areas of bony exostosis and to allow for even contact of the onlay graft.

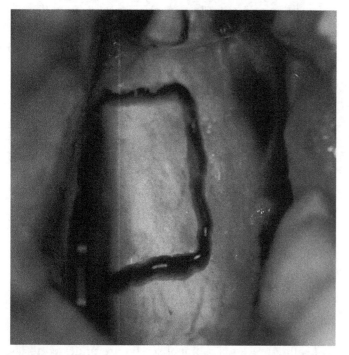

Figure 5.3. The lateral ramus is osteotomized posterior to the dentition.

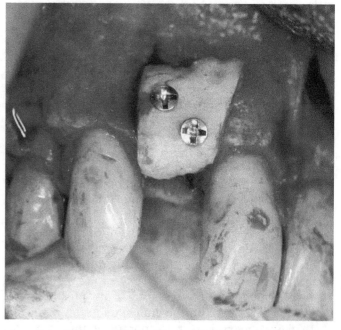

Figure 5.4. The ramus block onlay graft is secured to the donor site with positional screws. All sharp edges of the graft will be removed, and particulate bone will be packed around the periphery of the graft prior to closing the site.

Case Report 5.2. A 64-year-old female presents with a chief complaint of a failing 20-year-old four-unit fixed bridge from abutment teeth #7 and #10. Tooth #7 with gross marginal decay, and tooth #10 with a perapical abscess and a vertical root fracture. Teeth #7 and #10 were extracted, and socket preservation grafting was performed. Due to the inability to place large-diameter implants (lack of ridge width to sites #7 and #10) for an implant-supported fixed bridge and the span of the edentulous area, the restoring doctor requested the placement of three or more dental implants within the edentulous area. Due to the amount of anterior maxillary alveolus atrophy, the decision was made to augment the anterior maxillary alveolus with a particulate onlay graft. (See Figures 5.5 through 5.18.)

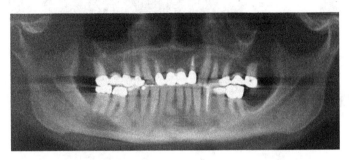

Figure 5.5.   Orthopantomogram depicting failing teeth #7 and #10 with associated four-unit bridge.

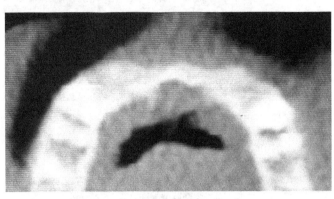

Figure 5.6.   Axial cone beam computed tomography image depicting anterior maxillary alveolar resorption.

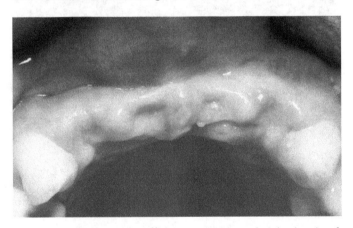

Figure 5.7.   Patient with sufficient vertical bone height, but insufficient bone width for the placement of dental implants.

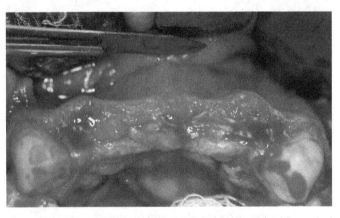

Figure 5.8.   A mucoperiosteal tissue flap is elevated with vertical releases posterior to the canines. The periosteum is released with a #15 blade to allow for a tension-free closure.

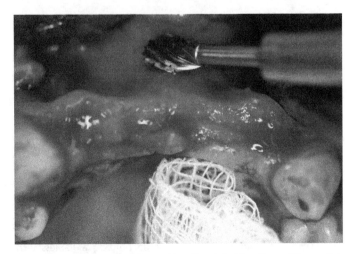

Figure 5.9.   A round bur is used to stimulate bleeding of the recipient site prior to graft placement.

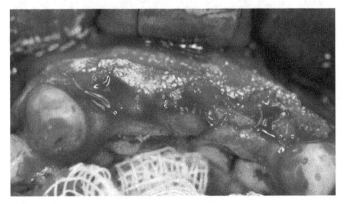

Figure 5.10.   A particulate graft consisting of bovine bone and fibrin sealant is placed. The fibrin sealant aids in particulate graft retention and minimizes graft displacement.

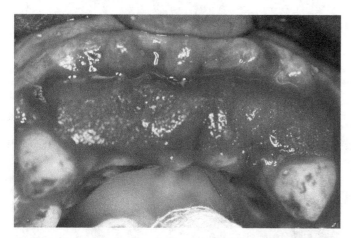

Figure 5.11.   A resorbable membrane is placed over the particulate graft.

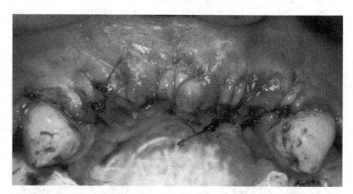

Figure 5.12.   The recipient site is closed in a tension-free manner with resorbable sutures.

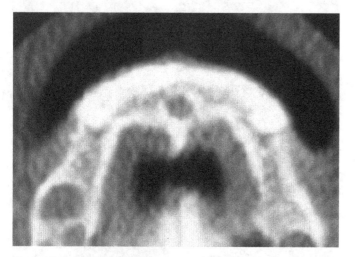

Figure 5.13.   Axial cone beam computed tomography image six months after bone grafting demonstrating sufficient horizontal bone augmentation for the placement of dental implants.

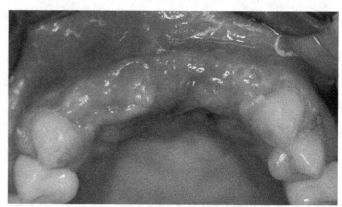

Figure 5.14.   Tissue condition and ridge width after six months of healing.

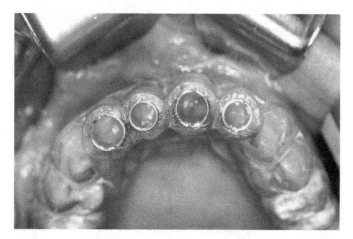

Figure 5.15.   Cone beam computed tomography–generated guide is fabricated to allow for the placement on dental implants within the grafted anterior maxilla.

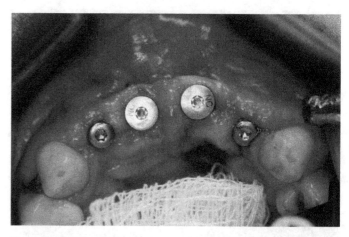

Figure 5.16.   Dental implants are placed utilizing a flapless technique to minimize periosteal striping and postoperative patient discomfort.

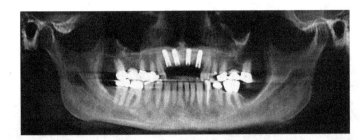

Figure 5.17. Postoperative orthopantomogram depicting the placement of dental implants into grafted anterior maxilla.

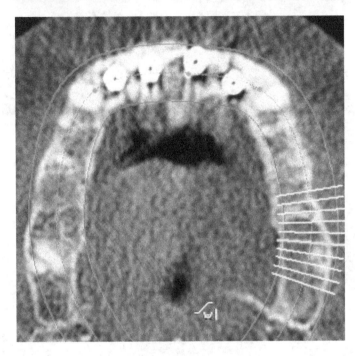

Figure 5.18. Postoperative axial cone beam computed tomography image demonstrating bone augmentation and implant placement.

Case Report 5.3. A 68-year-old female presents with an ill-fitting mandibular denture, a mobile transosseus mandibular implant, and severe mandibular atrophy. Due to the patient's anterior mandibular atrophy, the decision was made to remove her transosseus implant and reconstruct the vertical height of the anterior mandible with an anterior iliac crest onlay graft to allow for future anterior mandibular endosseus implant placement. The intraoral prongs were removed 8 weeks prior to the removal of the transosseus implant in order to allow for complete mucosal healing to minimize the contamination of the graft site with oral microbes. (See Figures 5.19 through 5.25.)

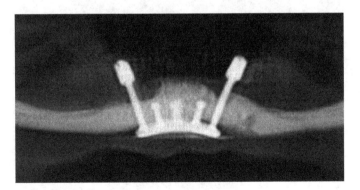

Figure 5.19. Orthopantomogram demonstrating atrophic mandible with failing transosseus implant.

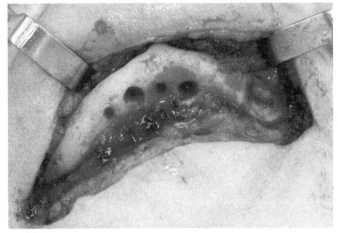

Figure 5.20. Transcutaneous exposure of the anterior mandible and removal of the transosseus implant. Care is taken to minimize periosteal reflection from the lingual and alveolar surfaces of the atrophic mandible.

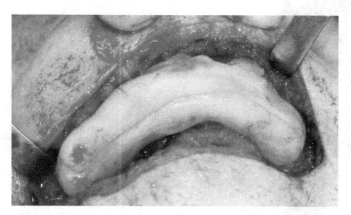

Figure 5.21. A block of bone wax is shaped to mimic the amount of onlay graft required.

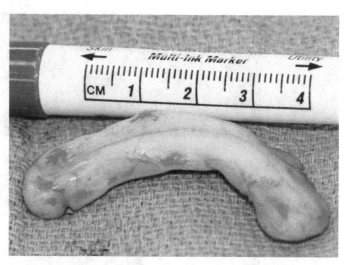

Figure 5.22. The bone wax template is used to determine the size of the bone block removed from the donor site.

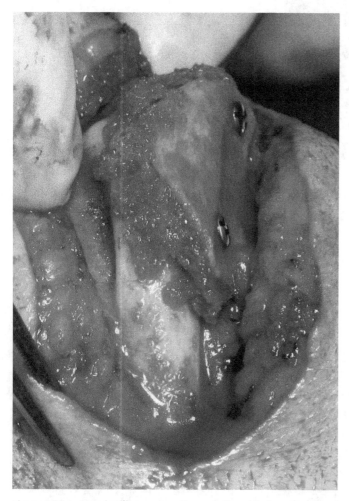

Figure 5.23. Anterior iliac crest corticocancellous block graft secured to the inferior border of the mandible with positional screws in locations where future endosseus implants will not be placed. All bony edges of the block onlay graft are smoothed, and marrow is packed around the periphery of the block graft.

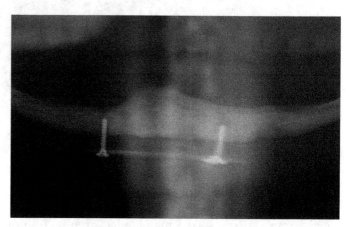

Figure 5.24. Postoperative orthopantomogram illustrating significant vertical augmentation of the anterior mandible.

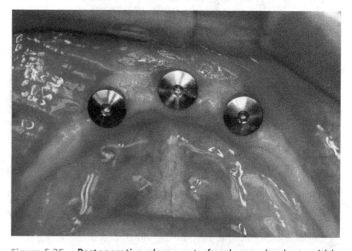

Figure 5.25. Postoperative placement of endosseus implants within the reconstructed anterior mandible five months after inferior border onlay grafting.

References

Cha, J-K., Kim, C.S., Choi, S.H., Cho, K.S., Chai, J.K. and Jung, U.W., 2012. The influence of perforating the autogenous block bone and the recipient bed in dogs. Part II: histologic analysis. *Clinical Oral Implants Research*, 23, 987–92.

Levin, L., Herzberg, R., Dolev, E. and Schwartz-Arad, D., 2004. Smoking and complications of onlay bone grafts and sinus lift operations. *International Journal of Maxillofacial Implants*, 19, 369–73.

Li, J. and Wang, H-L., 2008. Common implant-related advanced bone grafting complications: classification, etiology, and management. *Implant Dentistry*, 17, 389–97.

Lindeboom, J., Tuk, J.G., Kroon, F.H. and van den Akker, H.P., 2005. A randomized prospective controlled trial of antibiotic prophylaxis in intraoral bone grafting procedures: single dose clindamycin versus 24-hour clindamycin prophylaxis. *Mund-, Kiefer- und Gesichtschirurgie*, 9, 384–88.

Louis, P.J., 2011. Bone grafting in the mandible. *Oral and Maxillofacial Surgery Clinics of North America*, 23, 209–27.

Misch, C.M., 2011. Maxillary autogenous bone grafting. *Oral and Maxillofacial Surgery Clinics of North America*, 23, 229–38.

Oh, K-C., Cha, J.K., Kim, C.S., Choi, S.H., Chai, J.K. and Jung, U.W., 2011. The Influence of perforating the autongenous block bone and the recipient bed in dogs. Part I: a radiographic analysis. *Clinical Oral Implants Research*, 22, 1298–302.

Schwartz-Arad, D., Levin, L. and Sigal, L., 2005. Surgical success of intraoral autogenous block onlay bone grafting for alveolar ridge augmentation. *Implant Dentistry*, 14, 131–6.

Spin-Neto, R., Stavropoulos, A., Coletti, F.L., Faeda, R.S., Pereira, L.A. and Marcantonio, E., Jr., 2014. Graft incorporation and implant osseointegration following the use of autologous and fresh-frozen allogenic block bone grafts for lateral ridge augmentation. *Clinical Oral Implants Research*, 25(2), 226–33.

6

Sinus Lift Grafting

Christopher Choi[1] and Dale J. Misek[2]

[1]Private Practice, Inland Empire Oral and Maxillofacial Surgeons, Rancho Cucamonga, California, USA
[2]Private Practice, Carolinas Center for Oral and Facial Surgery, Charlotte, North Carolina, USA; and Department of Oral and Maxillofacial Surgery, Louisiana State University Health Science Center, New Orleans, Louisiana, USA

A procedure designed to augment the vertical height of the maxillary sinus to facilitate implant placement in patients with pneumatized sinuses.

Indications

1. Pneumatized maxillary sinus with a lack of vertical osseous support (<10 mm) for dental implant(s) placement within the posterior maxilla

Contraindications

1. Chronic and acute maxillary sinusitis
2. Odontogenic infection
3. Maxillary sinus pathology (cysts, tumors, or polyps)
4. Medical comorbidities:

   A. Coagulopathy or patients on anticoagulants
   B. Uncontrolled systemic disease
   C. Heavy smoking

Anatomy

Pneumatization of the maxillary sinus refers to the enlargement of the sinus cavity that occurs with advancing age and tooth loss. The maxillary alveolus resorbs, and the sinus walls thin with loss of masticatory forces and function. The Schneiderian membrane lines the sinus cavity and contains ciliated epithelium, which propel sinus contents against gravity through an ostium located along the medial wall of the maxillary sinus, which drains into the middle meatus of the nose. Membrane thickness varies from 0.13 to 0.5 mm. Bony septae are variable in size and can be found emanating from the sinus floor, dividing the sinus cavity into multiple compartments. The blood supply to the maxillary sinus originates from three arteries—the infraorbital artery, the posterior superior alveolar artery, and the posterior lateral nasal artery—all of which are branches of the maxillary artery. Intraosseous, and sometimes extraosseous, anastomoses between the infraorbital and posterior superior alveolar arteries give off networks of fine branches toward the alveolus.

Technique: Lateral Wall Technique

1. Antibiotic prophylaxis is recommended prior to any invasive sinus procedure. Intravenous sedation is typically utilized for prolonged cases, sinuses requiring extensive grafting, or anxious patients. For smaller grafting procedures and for procedures lasting less than 45 minutes, local anesthesia alone is frequently sufficient.
2. Local anesthetic is infiltrated within the maxillary vestibule and the alveolar mucosa. Infraorbital and posterior superior alveolar blocks are recommended. Injection into the greater palatine canal provides profound anesthesia to the sinus cavity.
3. The patient's face is prepped with betadine, and sterile towels are placed to isolate the oral cavity. The teeth and gingiva are brushed with betadine or chlorhexidine to disinfect the oral cavity.
4. Adjacent to the edentulous region, a full-thickness semilunar incision is made at the mucogingival junction with extension into the vestibule. A subperiosteal dissection is performed to expose the maxillary antral wall at the proposed site of entry into the maxillary sinus (see Figure 6.2 in Case Report 6.1).
5. A round diamond bur with copious irrigation is used to create an oval window (Figure 6.3, Case Report 6.1) within the area of the proposed bone graft. Care is taken to not perforate the Schneiderian membrane during removal of the antral bone window. An island of bone (Figure 6.4, Case Report 6.1) may be left in the center of the sinus window, which will be elevated with the Schneiderian membrane. Piezosurgical manipulation can be used as well, but with a thick lateral sinus wall, bone removal can be tedious.
6. Various instruments are used to carefully lift the Schneiderian membrane from the walls of the maxillary sinus (Figure 6.5, Case Report 6.1). Once initially freed, the membrane is elevated from the floor and medial wall of the maxillary sinus. The anterior boundary of the sinus cavity should be determined with instrument palpation. The membrane should be freed in all directions to allow

---

Atlas of Operative Oral and Maxillofacial Surgery, First Edition. Edited by Christopher J. Haggerty and Robert M. Laughlin
© 2015 John Wiley & Sons, Inc. Published 2015 by John Wiley & Sons, Inc.

for the placement of sufficient grafting material. The sinus window can be enlarged with the use of a Kerrison rongeur (Figure 6.6, Case Report 6.1), if needed.

7. The bone graft of choice is placed and compacted within the sinus cavity without perforating the Schneiderian membrane (Figure 6.7, Case Report 6.1). To minimize voids, the graft should be packed anteriorly and medially first (Figure 6.8, Case Report 6.1). With simultaneous implant placement (Figure 6.9, Case Report 6.1), the implants are placed after initial medial and anterior packing, and then additional grafting material is packed lateral (Figure 6.10, Case Report 6.1) to the implants.

8. A membrane may be placed lateral to the graft, but it is not mandatory. The mucosal incision is primarily closed with 4-0 chromic gut sutures.

Postoperative Management

1. Analgesics are prescribed based on the invasiveness of the procedure.
2. Oral antibiotics are prescribed for coverage of sinus microorganisms. A clindamycin–saline mouth rinse (clindamycin 900 mg mixed into 1 liter of saline) is prepared for the patient with instructions to swish and spit 10 mL's orally twice daily for 7–10 days.
3. Sinus precautions are recommended and include restricting smoking, spitting, nose blowing, heavy lifting, and valsalva maneuvers. Sneezing is allowed with an open mouth only to minimize sinus pressure and graft displacement.
4. Expected postoperative sequelae include moderate facial edema, light epistaxis, ecchymosis, and discomfort. The extent of the postoperative sequelae varies depending on the invasiveness of the procedure, the graft material employed, and the patient's medical history and age.

Complications

Intraoperative and Early Complications

1. **Sinus perforation**: Risk factors include irregularities of the sinus floor (septae), tooth root formations, scar tissue from prior sinus surgeries, lower residual alveolar ridge height, acute angles between the medial and lateral walls, and an inexperienced operator. Minor perforations are managed with the use of resorbable membranes. Major perforations may require abandonment of the procedure and reattempting the procedure after 6 months of healing. However, the use of rhBMP-2 will typically succeed even with large perforations.
2. **Hemorrhage**: The intraosseous artery is commonly located 16–19 mm from the alveolar ridge and is closer in more resorbed ridges. The posterior lateral nasal artery may be encountered with vigorous curettage of the posterior lateral wall of the sinus.

Late Complications

1. Infection
2. Bone graft failure
3. Non-integration of the implant(s)

Key Points

1. Multiple episodes of sinusitis warrant an evaluation of the patency of the maxillary ostium with a computed tomography (CT) scan (traditional or cone beam CT [CBCT]) and/or via nasal endoscopy.
2. Prior sinus surgery, such as closure of an oral antral fistula after tooth extraction or Caldwell Luc procedure, may result in scarring and confluence of the sinus and oral mucosa.
3. Anticoagulants should be held prior to surgery to minimize the risk of hemorrhage, as there are no effective local hemostatic measures to control anticoagulant bleeding with the sinus cavity. Anticoagulant suspension should be performed only after discussion with the primary care physician or prescribing physician.
4. Smokers should refrain from smoking 2 weeks prior to surgery and 6 weeks after surgery to avoid its deleterious effects on wound healing.
5. The restorative treatment plan (the type of prosthesis, and the number and location of implants) will dictate the volume of sinus graft augmentation.
6. CBCT is recommended prior to sinus augmentation to determine sinus anatomy, to identify anatomic variations such as septae, to identify the presence of pathology, and to quantify the amount of vertical augmentation required.
7. Sinus augmentation techniques are selected based on the amount of augmentation needed. General guidelines are as follows:

   A. Internal osteotome technique (sinus bump): 1–2 mm of vertical augmentation
   B. Lateral wall technique: >3 mm of vertical augmentation
   C. Le Fort 1 osteotomy with interpositional graft: severely atrophic, edentulous maxilla.

8. Simultaneous implant placement requires initial primary stability of the implant. Implant techniques may be modified, such as under preparation of the osteotomy, to ensure stability.
9. Perforations usually occur during instrumentation and are best avoided by initial circumferential membrane elevation of at least 5 mm to prevent tension during floor and medial-wall membrane elevation.
10. Bone grafts should be allowed to heal for 4–6 months prior to placement and/or uncovering of implants. Unless extreme sinus atrophy is present, most situations allow for simultaneous grafting and implant placement.

Case Report 6.1. A 54-year-old female presents for implant reconstruction of her right posterior maxilla. The patient denies any history of sinus disease or prior surgeries to the area. Her medical history is noncontributory. The restorative plan involves placing implants in the areas of the upper right first molar and second premolar, and replacing the first premolar with a fixed prosthesis. The surgical plan involves the atraumatic extraction of tooth #5; right maxillary sinus augmentation with a particulate graft containing tetracycline, rhBMP-2 (XS kit), and freeze-dried, mineralized, corticocancellous bone (FDMCB) using the lateral wall approach; and the simultaneously placement of implants into sites #3, #4, and #5. Figures 6.1 through 6.12 illustrate this process.

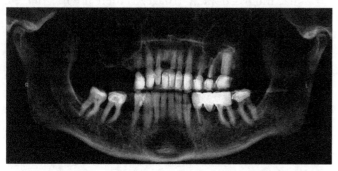

Figure 6.1. Preoperative cone beam computed tomography (CBCT) showing a pneumatized right maxillary sinus. There is approximately 1 mm of vertical bone height in the area of the first molar. No sinus pathology or anatomic abnormalities are noted on CBCT evaluation.

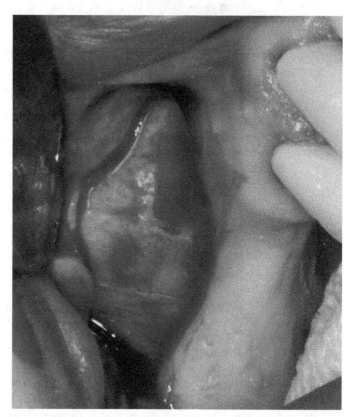

Figure 6.2. A semilunar incision is made at the mucogingival junction, followed by subperiosteal elevation to expose the lateral antral wall.

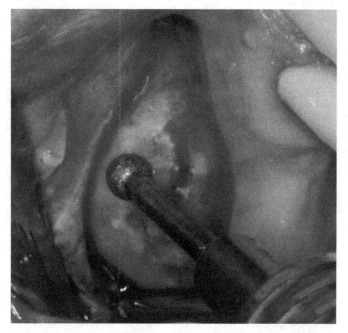

Figure 6.3. Creation of an oval window using a large diamond bur.

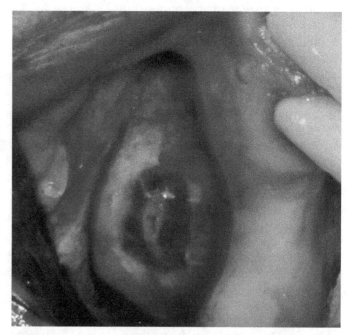

Figure 6.4. The Schneiderian membrane is exposed, and a sinus window with a central bony island is created along the lateral wall of the sinus.

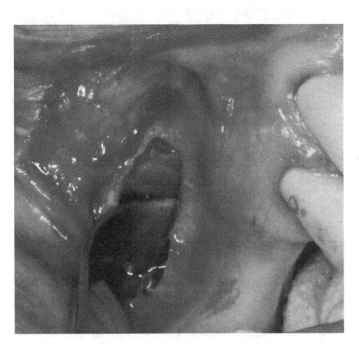

Figure 6.5.   The sinus membrane is elevated from the floor and walls of the sinus using blunt instruments (i.e., a J freer elevator, a Woodson periosteal elevator, and/or any combination of curved or angled sinus elevators).

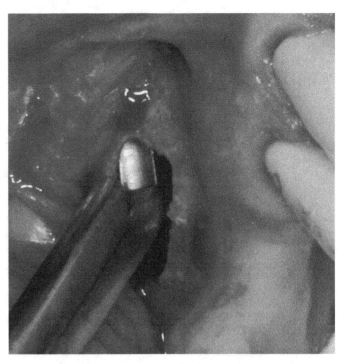

Figure 6.6.   The initial sinus window is enlarged by removing bone with a Kerrison rongeur.

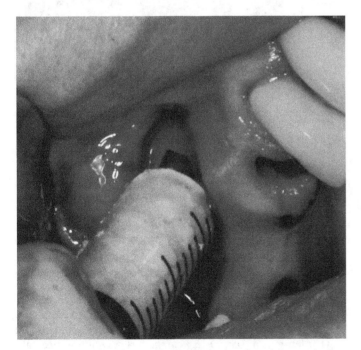

Figure 6.7.   Tooth #5 is atraumatically extracted, and the particulate graft is placed within a syringe delivery system and deposited within the sinus.

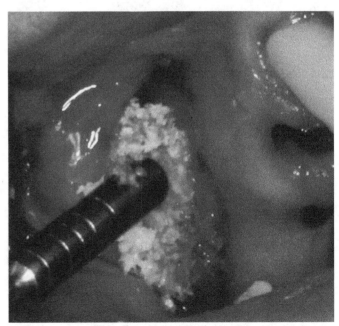

Figure 6.8.   The graft is compacted against the medial and anterior walls of the sinus.

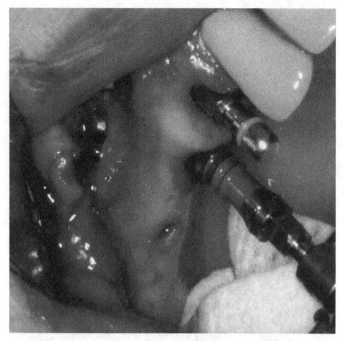

Figure 6.9. Implant osteotomies are carried to completion through the gingiva utilizing a flapless technique. In the areas of thin residual alveolus (<3 mm), the osteotomies are underprepared to ensure initial implant stability, and the implants are placed.

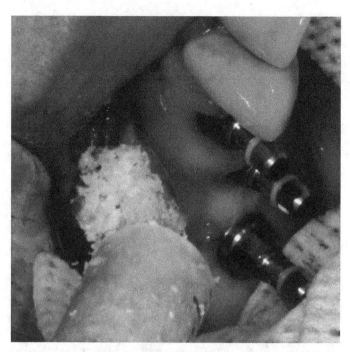

Figure 6.10. Additional particulate graft is placed and compacted lateral to the implants.

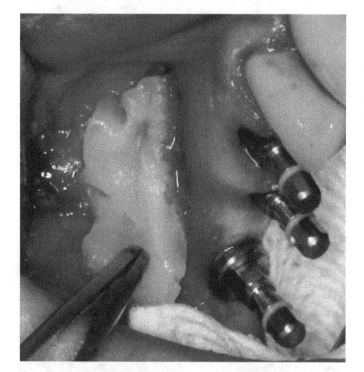

Figure 6.11. A rhBMP–collagen sponge is placed along the lateral wall of the sinus, and the mucosal incision is closed.

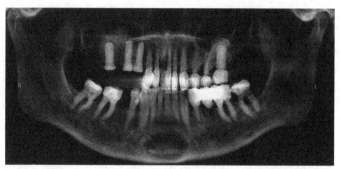

Figure 6.12. Postoperative cone beam computed tomography illustrating sufficient right maxillary sinus augmentation with simultaneous implant placement.

Tatum, H., Jr., 1986. Maxillary and sinus implant reconstructions. *Dental Clinics of North America*, 30, 207.

Triplett, R.G., Nevins, M., Marx, R.E., Spagnoli, D.B., Oates, T.W., Moy, P.K. and Boyne, P.J., 2009. Pivotal, randomized, parallel evaluation of recombinant human bone morphogenetic protein-2/absorbable collagen sponge and autogenous bone graft for maxillary sinus floor augmentation. *Journal of Oral and Maxillofacial Surgery*, 67(9), 1947–60.

Watzek, G.W., Ulm, C.W. and Haas, R., 1998. Anatomic and physiologic fundamentals of sinus floor augmentation. In: O.T. Jensen, ed. *The sinus bone graft*. Berlin: Quintessence Publishing Company, Inc. Pp. 31–45.

Zijderveld, S.A., Van Den Berg, J.P.A., Schulten, E.A.J.M. and Bruggenkate, C.M.T., 2008. Anatomical and surgical findings and complications in 100 consecutive maxillary sinus floor elevation procedures. *Journal of Oral and Maxillofacial Surgery*, 66, 1426–38.

References

Boyne, P.J. and James, R.J., 1980. Grafting of the maxillary sinus floor with autogenous marrow and bone. *Journal of Oral Surgery*, 38, 613.

7 Immediate Implant-Supported Restoration of the Edentulous Arch

Stephen G. Alfano and Robert M. Laughlin

Department of Oral and Maxillofacial Surgery, Naval Medical Center San Diego, San Diego, California, USA

A method of transitioning a patient with complete edentulism or a nonrestorable dentition to an implant-supported fixed restoration without the use of an interim removable prosthesis.

Indications

1. Adequate bone volume for the placement of dental implants
2. Adequate interarch distance for a fixed prosthesis
3. Properly motivated patient to maintain a fixed prosthesis

Contraindications

1. Uncontrolled systemic disease
2. Retrognathic jaw relationship

Technique (Surgical)

1. The procedure may be undertaken using local, intravenous, or general anesthesia.
2. Extraction of the remaining dentition is carefully completed, making sure to preserve alveolar bone.
3. The alveolar bone is curetted to debride granulation tissue, periapical pathology, and fistulous tracts.
4. The residual edentulous maxillary arch is leveled and reduced to ensure the interface between the abutment, and the final restoration is superior to the lip line during animation (see Figure 7.2 [all figures are in Case Report 7.1]).
5. The residual edentulous mandibular arch is leveled to achieve a uniform flat surface topography to provide the proper width for the placement of dental implants and sufficient vertical space to allow for restorative materials (Figures 7.5 and 7.6).
6. Posterior implants are placed to ensure proper distal angulation to avoid violating vital structures (mental nerve, and maxillary sinuses) (Figures 7.3 and 7.5). Anterior implants are placed along the long axis of the anterior alveolus (Figure 7.6).
7. Alveolar bone interfering with the seating of the abutments is removed.
8. Abutments are seated and torqued to manufacturer recommendations.
9. Healing caps are placed on the abutments, and the incisions are closed in a tension-free manner with resorbable sutures (Figures 7.4 and 7.7).
10. Postsurgical films are taken to ensure appropriate implant position and complete seating of abutments.

Note: These procedures are typically performed in conjunction with the restoring prosthodontist, and the interim prosthesis is placed and adjusted immediately after implant placement.

Technique (Restorative)

1. If intravenous or general anesthesia is utilized, the patient is allowed to recover prior to the restorative phase of the procedure.
2. The restorative phase is initiated with the removal of the healing caps and the placement of the impression copings (Figure 7.8).
3. Floss is threaded around the impression copings to provide a scaffold for the impression.
4. A low-flow bis-acryl bite registration material is used to connect the impression copings.
5. A medium-viscosity impression material is flowed under the bis-acryl registration material and onto the tissue (Figure 7.9).
6. A rigid-bite registration material is placed over the bis-acryl and medium-viscosity impression material to complete the impression (Figure 7.10). Care is made to avoid covering the screws with impression material.
7. The impression is removed and poured.
8. The impression is completed for the opposing arch and poured.
9. The interim dentures are relieved to allow complete, passive seating over the abutments.
10. Impression material is placed on the intaglio surface of the denture, and the denture is placed in the mouth to identify the exact location of the abutments (Figure 7.11).
11. Access holes are placed at two locations within each denture, allowing the full seating of the denture. Temporary cylinders and copings are placed on two of the abutments (Figure 7.12).
12. A rubber dam is placed over the sutures and extraction sites to prevent the extravagation of the

---

Atlas of Operative Oral and Maxillofacial Surgery, First Edition. Edited by Christopher J. Haggerty and Robert M. Laughlin.
© 2015 John Wiley & Sons, Inc. Published 2015 by John Wiley & Sons, Inc.

impression material into the surrounding tissues or extraction sites (Figure 7.12).

13. Self-cure acrylic resin is used to connect the temporary cylinders to the denture (Figure 7.13).
14. The process is repeated for the opposing arch, if applicable.
15. The remaining temporary cylinders are connected to the abutments, which creates a fixed restoration.
16. The dentures are placed (Figures 7.15 and 7.16), and retaining screws are torqued to 15 NCm.
17. The access holes are filled with a silicone material.
18. Final occlusal adjustments are made with the dentures seated.
19. A final film is obtained (Figure 7.19).

Postoperative Management

1. Analgesics and antibiotics are prescribed based on the invasiveness of the procedure.
2. Continued follow-up with both the surgeon and the restoring prosthodontist is key to patient comfort and prosthesis success.

Complications

1. **Lack of primary stability of the implants**: Care is taken in the site preparation to prepare the site according to the bone density. Softer bone requires minimal site preparation and/or the use of dental implants with a more aggressive thread pitch.
2. **Inability to fully seat the abutment**: The use of a bone mill or bone profile is required to ensure the bone does not interfere with seating the abutment. Full seating must be visually confirmed during surgery.
3. **Sinus location prevents adequate anterior-posterior spread of implants**: Preoperative evaluation is critical in case selection. The use of zygomatic implants can be used to extend the anterior-posterior spread of the maxilla.
4. **Inadequate inter-arch distance to properly fabricate restorations**: Adequate bone removal is necessary prior to implant placement to ensure the appropriate amount of inter-arch distance.
5. **Transition of prosthesis to tissue is evident during animation**: Evaluation of the smile line is a key component in the preoperative evaluation. The bone level must be superior to the smile line for this type of restoration. If this is not possible, alternative restorations should be considered.
6. **Fracture of the provisional prosthesis**: Adequate thickness of the provisional restoration and/or additional substructure support may be necessary.

Key Points

1. The smile line must be evaluated and bone level determined prior to surgery.

2. The required inter-arch distance and amount of reduction required must be determined prior to surgery.
3. An adequate anterior-posterior spread is required.
4. An implant insertion torque of 35 NCm must be obtained.
5. Verification that the abutments are fully seated must be visually and radiographically confirmed prior to beginning the restorative phase.
6. Restoration must be cleansable.
7. A substructure support may be necessary if a large span is present.
8. A sufficient number of implants should be placed to avoid a pontic span greater than 15 mm.

Case Report

Case Report 7.1. A 62-year-old male presents with a chief complaint of failing dentition and the inability to tolerated removable partial dentures. The decision was made to extract the remaining dentition, place immediate dental implants and fabricate immediate maxillary and mandibular implant-supported restorations.

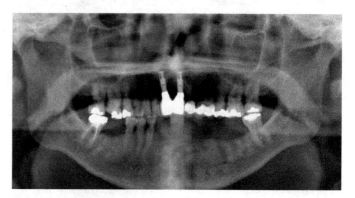

Figure 7.1.   Pretreatment panoramic radiograph; note existing anterior maxillary dental implants.

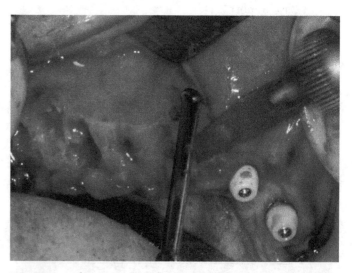

Figure 7.2.   After extraction, the maxillary alveolus is leveled with a reciprocating saw.

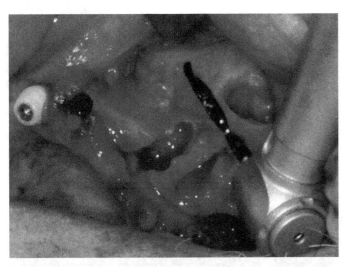

Figure 7.3. The sinus is located. The drill demonstrates the proposed angle of the distal implant to engage the medial sinus wall.

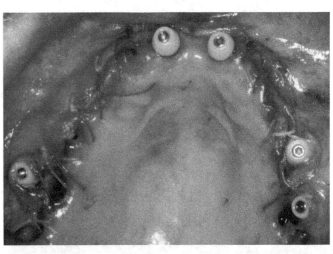

Figure 7.4. Maxilla immediately post-surgery and prior to the restorative process.

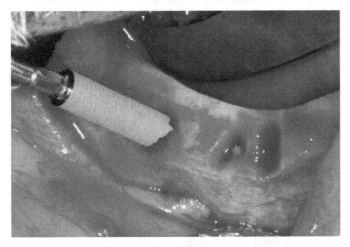

Figure 7.5. Mandibular arch after extraction of teeth and the creation of a flat broad table for implant placement. The mental nerve is identified, and the posterior implant is angled distally to avoid contact with the mental nerve and to maximize the anterior-posterior (A-P) spread of implants.

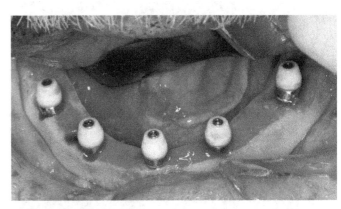

Figure 7.6. Mandibular arch post implant placement demonstrating the abutment locations and the anterior-posterior (A-P) spread. Both distal implants are angulated to increase the A-P spread.

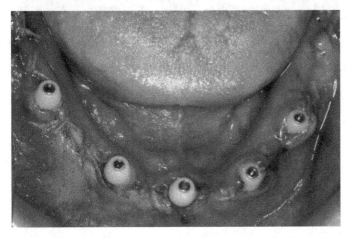

Figure 7.7. Mandible immediately post-surgery and prior to the restorative procedure.

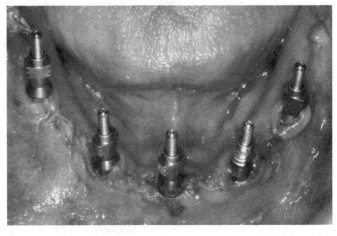

Figure 7.8. Impression copings placed within the mandibular arch.

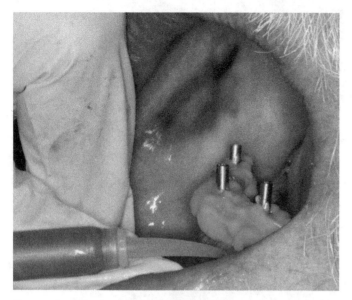

Figure 7.9. Injection of a medium-body impression material under the bis-acryl resin to impress the tissue surface.

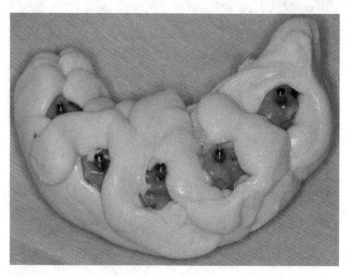

Figure 7.10. A rigid-bite registration material completes the impression.

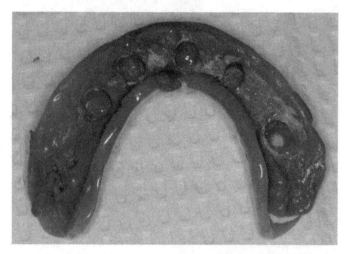

Figure 7.11. A heavy-body impression material is used to locate the abutments, and the denture is relieved to allow for complete seating.

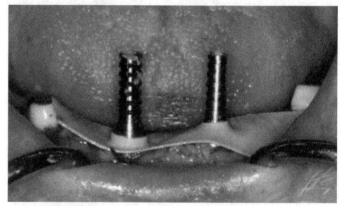

Figure 7.12. Temporary cylinders are in place, and a rubber damn is placed over the tissue to protect suture ties and extraction sockets from the acrylic resin.

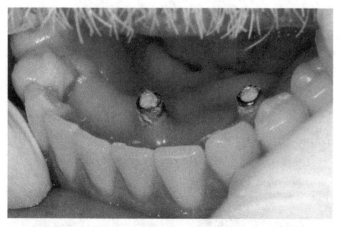

Figure 7.13. The mandibular denture is completely seated and held in place as the resin cures and connects the temporary cylinders to the denture.

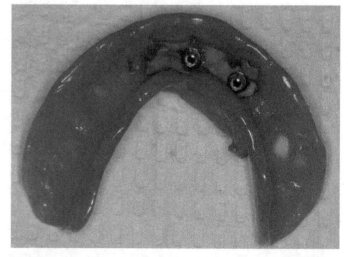

Figure 7.14. Intaglio surface of the mandibular denture after the pickup of the temporary cylinders.

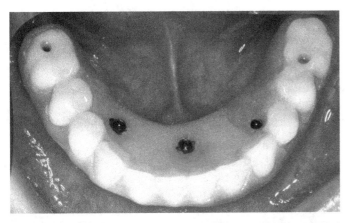

Figure 7.15   Occlusal view of the completed mandibular provisional restoration.

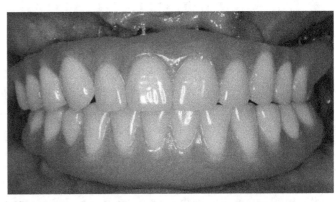

Figure 7.16.   Retracted frontal view of completed restorations.

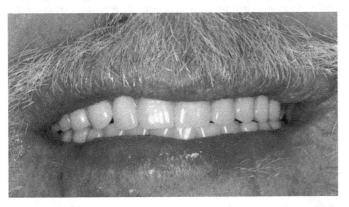

Figure 7.17.   Completed restorations upon animation.

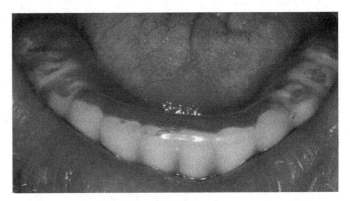

Figure 7.18.   A 3 mm soft mouth guard provides cushioning during occlusal force while the patient sleeps.

Figure 7.19.   Postoperative panoramic radiograph demonstrates ideal implant placement. The interim fixed restorations are in place, and a titanium mesh substructure is used to support areas of excessive pontic span.

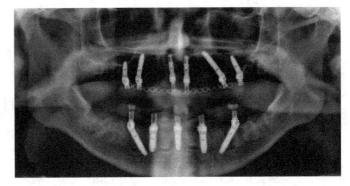

References

Balshi, T.J. and Wolfinger, G.J., 1997. Immediate loading of Brånemark implants in edentulous mandibles. A preliminary report. *Implant Dentistry*, 6, 83–8.

Maló, P., Rangert, B. and Nobre, M., 2003. "All-on-4" immediate-function concept with Brånemark system implants for completely edentulous mandibles: a retrospective clinical study. *Clinical Implant Dentistry and Related Research*, 5(Suppl. 1), 2–9.

Parel, S. and Phillips, W., 2011. A risk assessment treatment planning protocol for the four implant immediate loaded maxilla: preliminary findings. *Journal of Prosthetic Dentistry*, 106, 359–66.

Schnitman, P.A., Wöhrle, P.S., Rubenstein, J.E., DaSilva, J.D. and Wang, N.H. 1997. Ten-year results for Brånemark implants immediately loaded with fixed prostheses at implant placement. *International Journal of Oral and Maxillofacial Implants*, 2, 495–503.

CHAPTER

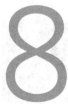

Zygomatic Implants

Luis Vega[1] and Patrick J. Louis[2]
[1]Department of Oral and Maxillofacial Surgery, Vanderbilt University Medical Center, Nashville, Tennessee, USA
[2]Department of Surgery, University of Alabama, Birmingham, Alabama, USA

Procedure: Zygomatic Implants

A zygomatic implant is a long implant (30–62.5 mm) that obtains its main anchorage from the zygoma bone in the presence or absence of maxillary alveolar bone. Zygomatic implants were designed by Per-Ingvar Brånemark to allow for implant-supported prosthesis placement where maxillary bony support for prosthetic rehabilitation is inadequate.

Indications

1. Severe atrophy of the posterior maxilla with sufficient bone support for dental implants within the anterior maxilla
2. Generalized severely atrophic maxilla
3. Acquired maxillary bony defects (benign or malignant pathological ablation, infectious debridement, and avulsive trauma)
4. Congenital maxillary bony defects (cleft lip and palate)
5. Previous failed dental implant and/or bony reconstructions

Contraindications

1. Medically compromised patient
2. Acute sinusitis
3. Adequate maxillary alveolar bone for conventional dental implants
4. Severe trismus (relative contraindication)
5. Previous history of head and neck radiation treatment (relative contraindication)

Anatomy

The zygoma bone has a mean anterior-posterior length that ranges from 14.1 to 25.4 mm and a mean mediolateral thickness that ranges from 7.6 to 9.5 mm. When the zygoma bone is measured along the potential implant axis, the bone-to-implant contact ranges from 14 to 16.5 mm, and approximately 36% of the implant is in contact with the zygoma bone. Although poor trabecular bone density has been described, the zygoma bone has a strong cortex, which provides the primary stability of the zygomatic implant. The placement of zygomatic implants was originally described using an intrasinus approach. The main disadvantage of this approach is the palatal emergence of the implant platforms. The palatal emergence occurs because during the process of maxillary resorption, the residual maxillary basal bone is in a more posterior position than the alveolar bone, whereas the position of the zygoma bone remains unchanged. The palatal emergence of the zygomatic implant requires the fabrication of a bulkier prosthesis that is difficult to restore and requires greater buccal cantilevers. Several modifications have been described within the literature that allow for more favorable implant placement, and these are described in this chapter.

Implant Anatomy

Numerous companies have designed and market zygomatic implants worldwide. The implant most commonly used in the United States is available in eight different lengths (30, 35, 40, 42.5, 45, 47.5, 50, and 52.5). All implants have a diameter of 5 mm in the coronal third and 4 mm in the apical two-thirds. The difference of diameters within the coronal and apical portions compensates for the potential widening of the maxillary implant bed that occurs during the determination of the proper trajectory of the drill to engage the zygoma bone. Finally, a 45° platform allows the inclined insertion of the zygomatic implant and its restoration.

Original Surgical Technique

1. This procedure is typically performed with either general anesthesia or intravenous deep sedation. Local anesthesia is given intraorally within the maxillary vestibule and the posterior hard palate to block the superior alveolar, infraorbital, and greater palatine nerves and to control bleeding during dissection. When the procedure is performed under deep sedation, additional extraoral anesthesia is infiltrated around the zygoma prominence.

Atlas of Operative Oral and Maxillofacial Surgery, First Edition. Edited by Christopher J. Haggerty and Robert M. Laughlin
© 2015 John Wiley & Sons, Inc. Published 2015 by John Wiley & Sons, Inc.

2. A crestal incision is initiated from tuberosity to tuberosity bisecting the keratinized gingiva. Vertical releases are placed posteriorly along the maxillary buttress and anteriorly within the midline region.

3. Mucoperiosteal flap elevation is used to expose the alveolar crest, the lateral maxilla, the maxillary antral wall, the infraorbital nerve, the zygomaticomaxillary complex, and the lateral surface of the zygomatic bone cephalically to the incisura (the point between the lateral and medial surfaces of the frontal process of the zygomatic bone and the zygomatic arch; see Figures 8.2 and 8.9 in the Case Reports). Exposure of the infraorbital nerve is important as it serves as the anterior limit for implant placement in cases in which two ipsilateral zygomatic implants are placed. Exposure of the infraorbital rim is not necessary. The palatal mucosa is elevated due to the palatal emergence of the zygomatic implants.

4. A zygoma retractor is placed at the incisura. The zygoma retractor is used to retract the soft tissues and to assist with implant angulation during implant placement. Care must be taken to properly insert the zygoma retractor at the incisura as it can be easily malpositioned along the infraorbital rim.

5. A sinus window is created within the supero-lateral portion of the maxillary sinus. The window should allow for the elevation of the sinus mucosa, providing direct vision to the roof of the sinus and the base of the zygoma bone. No special effort is made to keep the sinus membrane intact. A larger, trapezoid-shaped window is used when two ipsilateral zygomatic implants are indicated (Figure 8.2, Case Report 8.1).

6. Determination of the implant trajectory is performed with the aid of a properly placed zygoma retractor and direct visualization of the base of the zygoma bone and sinus roof. For better orientation of the implant trajectory, the measuring device or the drill bit can be placed over the lateral maxillary wall prior to initiating the drilling protocol. The zygomatic implant platforms generally emerge within the areas of the second bicuspid or first molar (Figure 8.12, Case Report 8.2) and within the canine region if a second ipsilateral zygomatic implant is placed (Figure 8.4, Case Report 8.1). The implant osteotomies are planned as far posteriorly as possible and with the crestal emergence located as close to the alveolar crest as possible.

7. A 105° zygomatic implant hand piece with a round bur is used to enter the residual maxillary bone, penetrating through the atrophic maxillary alveolus and maxillary sinus and marking the area of the sinus roof and the base of the zygoma bone that the implant will engage. A 2.9 mm twist drill is used to penetrate both cortices of the zygoma bone. The zygoma bone osteotomy is enlarged using a 3.5 mm

final drill. This final drill provides the implant site with the final width of the zygomatic implant.

8. The osteotomy depth is measured using a specially designed depth gauge. The device utilizes a small hook to engage the superior cortex, and depth measurements are made with the aid of 5 mm markings along the depth gauge.

9. Implant placement can be performed manually or by using a hand piece. During implant placement, soft tissue frequently wraps around the body of the implant. Care must be taken to avoid embedding these tissues within the osteotomy site as this may impede osseointegration of the zygomatic implant. The tip of the implant is placed 2 mm beyond the superior cortex of the zygoma bone, and the platform is placed as close as possible to the maxillary bone. Care should be taken to position the 45° platform parallel to the occlusal plane.

10. The implant mount is retrieved, and cover screws are placed.

11. Additional traditional dental implants are placed within the anterior maxilla. Anterior traditional implants are desirable but not necessary with the placement of two ipsilateral zygomatic implants.

12. Wounds are evaluated for hemostasis, copious irrigation is applied, and primary closure is performed with 3-0 Vicryl sutures.

Two-Zygomatic-Implant Placement

Special considerations when placing two ipsilateral zygomatic implants include:

1. A larger sinus window is required to better identify the area in which both of the implants will be placed (Figure 8.2, Case Report 8.1).

2. Implants are not placed parallel to each other. Instead, they are convergent in the apices. This allows for a better anterior-posterior spread to minimize cantilever forces. The most posterior implant should be placed as close as possible to the posterior lateral wall of the maxillary sinus, and the anterior implant should be placed as anterior as the infraorbital nerves permit.

Modifications of the Original Protocol

Several modifications of the original protocol have been described in the literature, including:

1. **Sinus slot technique**: Simplifies the technique by eliminating the need for a sinus window, and improves the orientation of the zygomatic implant.

2. **Change implant design to a 55° platform**: Uses a specially designed device to improve the orientation of the implant. The new implant platform decreases buccal cantilevers up to 20%.

3. **Immediate loading**: Allows immediate function.

4. **Quad-zygomas**: Placement of four zygomatic implants without traditional dental implants and immediate loading with a fixed prosthesis.
5. **Extrasinus implant placement**: The remaining maxillary alveolar ridge is not engaged and the zygomatic implant completely bypasses the maxillary sinus, minimizing sinus complications and improving buccal cantilevers.
6. **Maxillary wall and sinus membrane preservation**: The maxillary wall is preserved to protect the sinus membrane. Advantages of this technique include extra bone formation around the implant.
7. **Zygoma anatomy-guided approach (ZAGA)**: An anatomical- and prosthetically driven approach in which the preparation of the zygomatic implant osteotomy site is guided by the anatomy of the zygoma bone and the ideal site of the implant platform (Figure 8.9).

Postoperative management

Postoperative management is similar to that for patients who have undergone maxillary implant placement with a simultaneous sinus lift:

1. Analgesics
2. Antibiotics and chrohexidine mouth rinses
3. Sinus precautions
4. A soft diet

Complications

Intrasurgical Complications

1. **Invasion into orbit**: Avoided by the proper placement of the zygoma retractor into the incisura.
2. **Invasion into the temporal fossa**: Occurs when the trajectory of the implant is located too posterior at the base of the zygoma or when inadequate zygoma bone is present, especially if two implants are planned. This is corrected with repositioning of the implant bed into a more anterior location.

Postoperative Complications

1. **Sinusitis**: Three different etiopathogenic mechanisms have been proposed: (i) a zygoma implant represents invasive surgery for the sinus, (ii) a zygoma implant is an intrasinusal foreign body, and (iii) a zygoma implant could create a oroantral communication. Sinusitis is typically treated via medical therapy with antibiotics and nasal decongestants. Failed medical management or recurrent events are better treated surgically via functional endoscopic sinus surgery (FESS).
2. Oroantral communication.
3. Peri-implantitis.
4. Loss of implant.

Key Points

1. Zygomatic implant reconstruction of the severely atrophic maxilla for acquired or congenital maxillary defects is a safe, predictable, and cost-effective treatment modality. Advantages of zygomatic implant reconstruction versus traditional implant reconstruction include shorter treatment time frames, avoidance of the need for bone grafting and its associated morbidity, fewer total implants required for a fixed prosthesis, and the fact that zygomatic implants allow the potential for immediate functioning. Disadvantages of zygomatic implants include the need for general or deep sedation, plus the facts that implant failures are more difficult to treat and the procedure is very technique sensitive.
2. The single most important factor for treatment success is a team approach between the surgeon and the restorative dentist. As with any pre-prosthetic surgery, the treatment plan should be prosthetically driven. When possible, the placement of one or two extra traditional dental implants will improve the distribution of forces and increase the support of the final prosthesis.
3. In cases with limited mouth opening, a contra-angle hand piece allows for improved access for osteotomy preparation and implant placement.

Case Reports

Case Report 8.1. A 74-year-old male with a severely atrophic maxilla desires a fixed dental restoration without having to undergo multiple reconstructive surgeries and the associated treatment time. Due to extreme combined anterior and posterior maxillary atrophy and the lack of sufficient vertical anterior maxillary bone for the placement of traditional implants, the decision was made to place four zygomatic implants via the intrasinus approach. (See Figures 8.1, 8.2, 8.3, 8.4, and 8.5.)

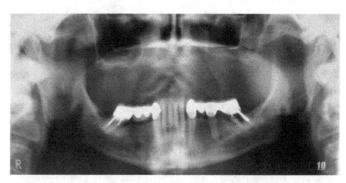

Figure 8.1. Preoperative orthopantomogram demonstrating pneumatized maxillary sinuses and inadequate maxillary bone for the placement of traditional dental implants.

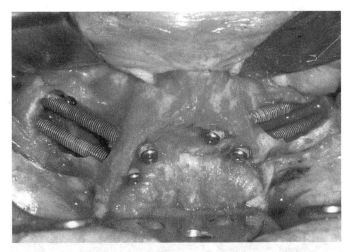

Figure 8.2. Quad-zygomas placed using the original technique via the intrasinus approach.

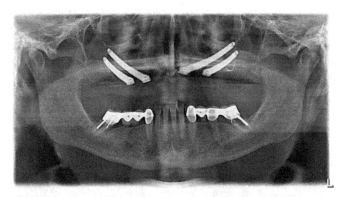

Figure 8.3. Postoperative orthopantomogram demonstrating ideal implant position.

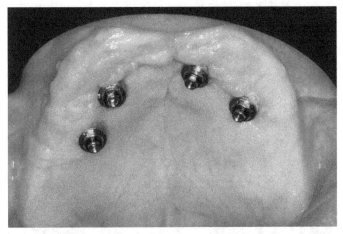

Figure 8.4. Implants are uncovered and healing abutments are placed after 4 months of integration. Notice the palatal location of the implants.

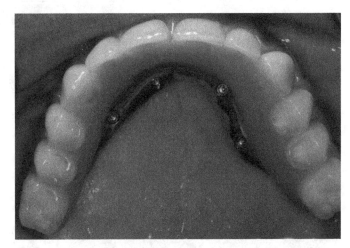

Figure 8.5. Final prosthesis in place (courtesy of Dr William Gielincki, prosthodontist).

Case Report 8.2. A 48-year-old edentulous female presents to clinic desiring maxillary and mandibular implants for fixed dental restorations. Preoperative computed tomography scans demonstrated sufficient bone for the placement of six maxillary implants with sinus augmentation. The patient rejected traditional reconstructive approaches, as she wanted to be restored as soon as possible. (See Figures 8.6 through 8.13.)

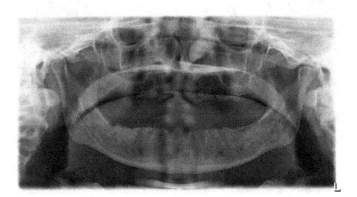

Figure 8.6. Preoperative orthopantomogram demonstrating adequate maxillary bone for the placement of six maxillary implants with sinus augmentation.

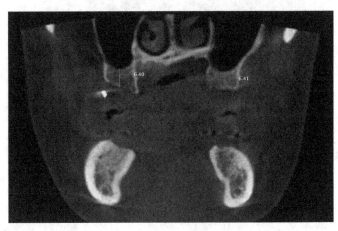

Figure 8.7. Computed tomography (CT) scan demonstrating a lack of bone height in the areas of the second premolar and first molar.

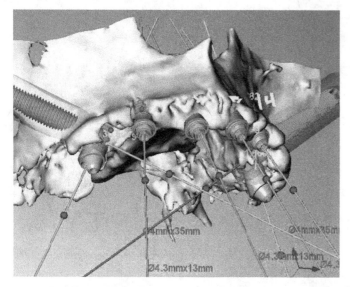

Figure 8.8. Computer-assisted virtual treatment planning showing the potential location of the zygomatic implants.

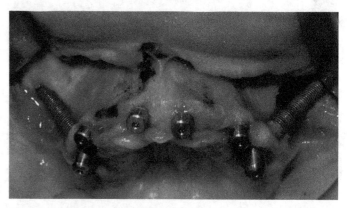

Figure 8.9. Placement of four anterior traditional dental implants and two zygomatic implants. No sinus window was used on the right zygoma implant as it was placed using the zygoma anatomy-guided approach (ZAGA) principal.

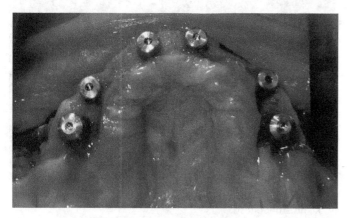

Figure 8.10. Occlusal view of implant placement. Note the crestal location of the implants.

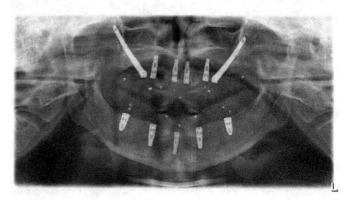

Figure 8.11. Postoperative orthopantomogram demonstrating the ideal placement of implants.

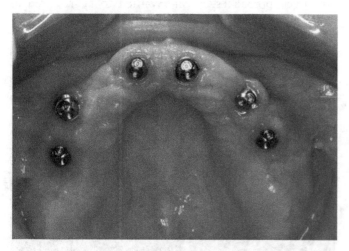

Figure 8.12. Implants are uncovered and healing abutments are placed after 4 months of integration. Note the difference of the implant emergence compared to the original technique (Figure 8.4).

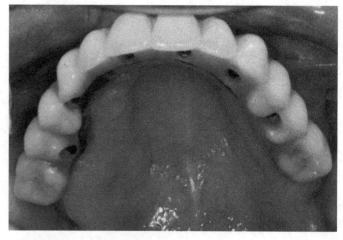

Figure 8.13. Final fixed-hybrid prosthesis in place (courtesy of Dr William Gielincki, prosthodontist).

References

Aparicio, C., 2011. A proposed classification for zygomatic implant patient based on the zygoma anatomy guided approach (ZAGA): a cross-sectional survey. *European Journal of Oral Implantology*, 4(3), 269–75.

Balshi, T.J., Wolfinger, G.J., Shuscavage, N.J. and Balshi, S.F., 2012. Zygomatic bone-to-implant contact in 77 patients with partially or completely edentulous maxillas. *Journal of Oral and Maxillofacial Surgery*, 70, 2065–9.

Brånemark, P-I., Gröndahl, K., Ohrnell, L-O., Nilsson, P., Petruson, B., Svensson, B., Engstrand, P. and Nannmark, U., 2004. Zygoma fixture in the management of advanced atrophy of the maxilla: technique and long-term results. *Scandinavian Journal of Plastic and Reconstructive Surgery and Hand Surgery*, 38, 70–85.

Davó, R., Malevez, C., López-Orellana, C., Pastor-Beviá, F. and Rojas, J., 2008. Sinus reactions to immediately loaded zygoma implants: a clinical and radiological study. *European Journal of Oral Implantology*, 1(1), 53–60.

Vega, L., Gielincki, W. and Fernandes, R., 2013. Zygoma implant reconstruction of acquired and maxillary bony defects. *Oral and Maxillofacial Surgery Clinics of North America*, 25, 223–39.

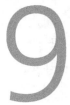

CHAPTER

9

Cone Beam CT-Guided Dental Implant Surgery

Christopher J. Haggerty

Private Practice, Lakewood Oral and Maxillofacial Surgery Specialists, Lees Summit; and Department of Oral and Maxillofacial Surgery, University of Missouri–Kansas City, Kansas City, Missouri, USA

The placement of dental implants with the use of custom guides generated from specific computed tomography (CT) scanning protocols and software.

Indications

1. Placement of dental implants where bone height, width, or shape is limited
2. Placement of dental implants near anatomical structures (inferior alveolar nerve, mental foramen, etc.)
3. Flapless implant surgery
4. Placement of dental implants in areas of bone atrophy resistant to grafting
5. Placement of multiple dental implants
6. Placement of dental implants in areas of significant adjacent root dilacerations
7. When ideal prosthetics are required for the aesthetic zone

Contraindications

1. Insufficient bone height, width, or shape for the placement of dental implants
2. Poor bone quality
3. Systemic issues (previous radiation therapy, intravenous bisphosphonates, and chronic immunosuppression)
4. Bone pathology, infection, and gross periodontal disease
5. Skeletal immaturity
6. Psychological disorders

Technique

1. Patients are consulted regarding implant and grafting materials, potential complications, the implant-to-crown timeline, the workup and surgical procedure, the healing period, and realistic final results.
2. A cone beam CT (CBCT) scan, dental models, and a bite registration are taken. Any intraoral scanner that exports stereolithography (STL) files can be used. Additionally, scans of the stone models can be utilized if intraoral scanners are not available.

3. The CBCT and STL files are merged using surface-mapping technology (see Figures 9.3 and 9.23 [all figures are in Case Reports 8.1 and 8.2]). The patient's bony anatomy, soft tissue anatomy, and teeth are evaluated in a layered 3D environment. Anatomical structures are highlighted (mandibular canal, mental foramen, and sinuses).
4. Implant treatment planning is performed virtually using restoration-guided implant planning (a crown-down approach) (Figures 9.2 and 9.22). Most software programs contain the majority of commercial-grade implants preloaded within their software package. The implant (or implants) is selected and is placed within the edentulous region. Manipulation of the implant position is performed with the aid of axial, sagittal, and coronal views; serial slices; and custom cross-sections. The surgeon must be cognizant of the location of vital structures, the opposing dentition, and the anticipated location of the final crown. The decision is made as to whether the crown would be best restored with a screw-retained or cement-retained prosthesis. For screw-retained prostheses, implants are planned palatal so that the screw can be positioned along the cingulum of the crown. For cement-retained prostheses, implants are centered parallel to the long axis of the crown. If multiple implants are to be placed, the implants should be placed as parallel as possible, and spacing should be optimized. Most programs have paralleling tools for this type of application.
5. The final 3D treatment plan is approved, and a surgical guide is fabricated (Figures 9.4 and 9.24).
6. The guide is placed prior to the administration of local anesthesia to ensure a proper fit (Figures 9.5 and 9.26). The guide should interdigitate with the occlusal third of the clinical crowns, should be rigid, and should not rock or bend. Any potential for movement of the surgical guide will be translated into drilling errors and unplanned implant placement.
7. Local anesthesia is administered in the form of infiltration only. Sedations and nerve blocks are typically

Atlas of Operative Oral and Maxillofacial Surgery, First Edition. Edited by Christopher J. Haggerty and Robert M. Laughlin.
© 2015 John Wiley & Sons, Inc. Published 2015 by John Wiley & Sons, Inc.

not utilized for mandibular implant surgery as the vibration of the drill as it nears the inferior alveolar nerves adds an additional layer of safety during mandibular osteotomy preparation. Depending on the clinical situation and the operator's experience, the decision is made for creating a mucoperiosteal tissue flap or performing flapless surgery.

8. In flapless surgery, the guide is placed, and the appropriate drill sleeve is placed for the pilot drill (Figure 9.6). The pilot drill is taken to the predetermined depth using drill stops and/or external measurements. The surgical guide is removed, and a parallel pin (or pins) is placed to confirm the depth and angulation of the osteotomy (Figure 9.7). The patient is asked to partially bite down in order to assess the placement of the parallel pin (or pins) against the opposing dentition. If the parallel pin (or pins) position does not correlate with the presurgical work-up, a periapical radiograph or CBCT may be taken to confirm parallel pin position prior to enlarging the osteotomy.

9. The parallel pin (or pins) are removed and the surgical guide is placed. The osteotomy is enlarged to the preplanned size using sequential drill sleeves and drills with copious irrigation.

10. Once the preplanned implant osteotomy depth and diameter are reached, a bone probe is placed into the osteotomy site in order to confirm 360° of bone contact around the circumference of the osteotomy site.

11. Based on the surgeon's preference and the guide design, the implant may be placed with the guide in place or removed.

12. Based on the bone quality, either a cover screw, a healing abutment (Figure 9.9), or a provisional prosthesis (Figure 9.11) is placed. For anterior cases, immediate or early loading with prefabricated temporary crowns is recommended to shape tissue architecture.

Postoperative Management

1. Patients are prescribed analgesics based on the invasiveness of the procedure. With the flapless approach, patient pain is minimal.
2. Patients are instructed to begin twice-daily saltwater rinses beginning the day after surgery.
3. Follow-up appointments are typically at 2, 8, and 14 weeks.

Complications

1. Complications are associated with non-ideal implant placement, implant failure, and damage to adjacent structures.

Key Points

1. Complications do occur with the placement of guided dental implants. Errors can occur in the planning stage; these include errors in the dental or digital impression, scanning and software errors, and planning errors. Late errors include guide fabrication errors, ill-fitting guides, insufficient irrigation due to the thickness of the guide, implants placed too superficially, implants placed without complete bone coverage, and implants that violate adjacent anatomical structures.
2. A surgical guide that is not rigid and/or does not fit ideally will cause inaccuracies with implant placement during guided surgery.
3. The patient's maximum vertical opening (MVO) will determine if the placement of posterior implants is possible using a guide. In patients with a limited MVO, it is difficult to place the surgical guide, drill sleeves, and hand piece and orient them appropriately.

Case Reports

Case Report 9.1. An 18-year-old patient presents status post orthodontic treatment with a congenitally missing left lateral incisor and a peg lateral for the right maxillary lateral incisor. On review of the cone beam computed tomography (CBCT), there is minimal space for the placement of a dental implant due to severe bone atrophy and the dilaceration of the root of the central incisor. A treatment plan was developed with the patient's restoring dentist for the placement of a CBCT-guided implant, custom abutment, and final prosthesis that matched the contralateral peg lateral. (See Figures 9.1 though 9.20.)

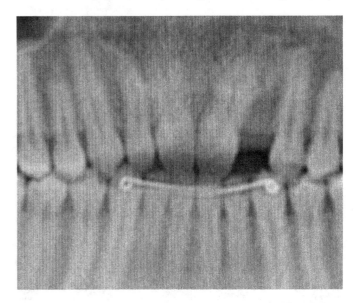

Figure 9.1. Limited mesial-distal space to site #10 due to severe dilaceration of the central incisor. Note contralateral peg lateral #7.

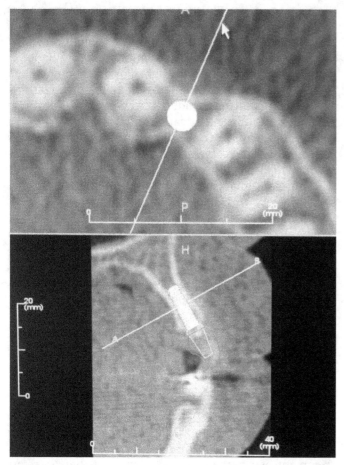

Figure 9.2. Alveolar bone atrophy associated with congenitally missing lateral incisor. Restoration-guided treatment planning is performed using implant-specific software (Anatomage, Los Angeles, California, USA).

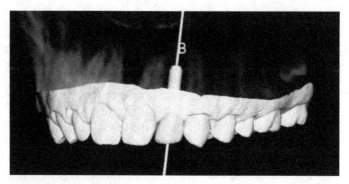

Figure 9.3. The white area represents the surface topography of the dentition and adjacent soft tissue collected with the i-Tero intra oral digital scanner (Align Technology, Inc, San Jose, CA, USA). A virtual crown is placed to ensure ideal final prosthetics.

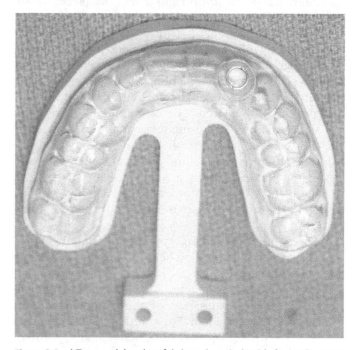

Figure 9.4. i-Tero model and prefabricated surgical guide for implant #10.

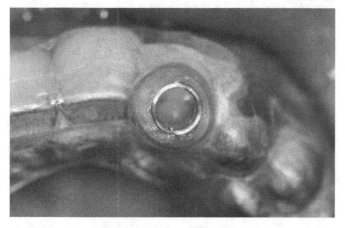

Figure 9.5. Tooth-supported surgical guide in place.

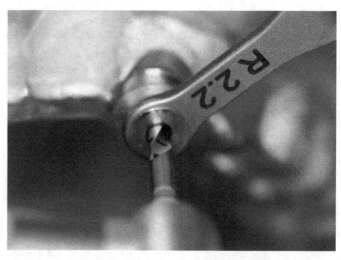

Figure 9.6. Drill sleeve in place and pilot drill placed to the predetermined depth.

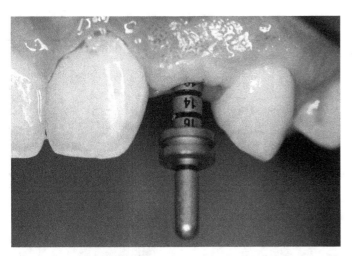

Figure 9.7.   Parallel pin in place to a depth of 13 mm. The site is planned for a 10 mm implant. Three millimeters of soft tissue is measured intraoperatively.

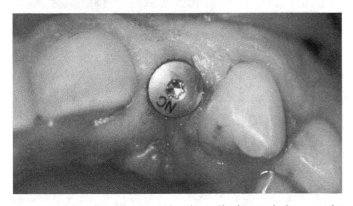

Figure 9.9.   Healing abutment in place. Flapless technique results in minimal postoperative discomfort and maintenance of soft tissue architecture.

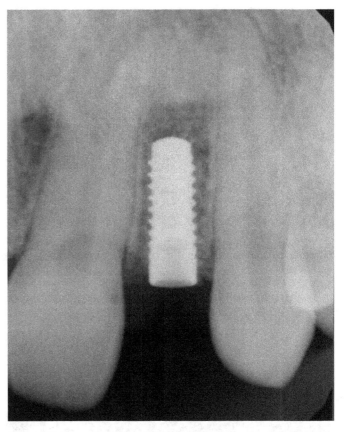

Figure 9.8.   A periapical radiograph is taken to ensure appropriate bone level of the implant.

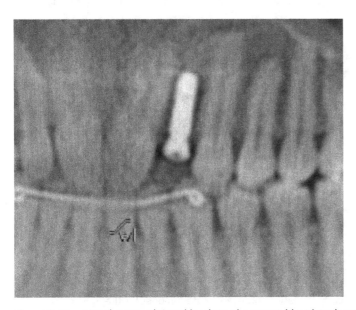

Figure 9.10.   Actual versus planned implant placement (the virtual crown was software generated).

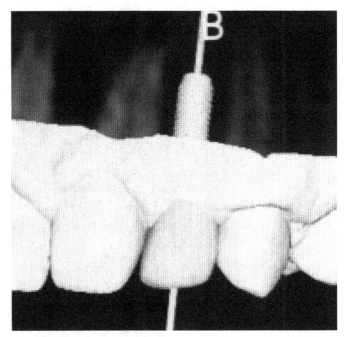

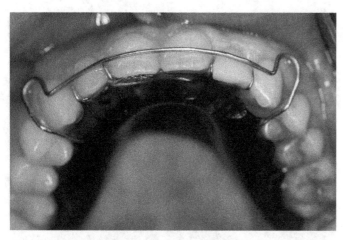

Figure 9.11.   The patient's preexisting orthodontic retainer is modified to avoid vertical (shearing) forces on the implant and healing abutment.

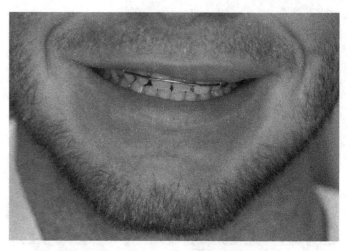

Figure 9.12.   The patient's modified orthodontic retainer acts as a provisional prosthesis.

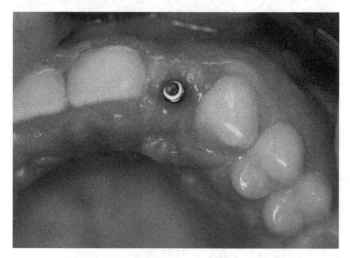

Figure 9.13.   The patient presents 4 months after implant placement for the placement of a scan body and a new i-Tero scan. Note 3.5 mm of soft tissue depth.

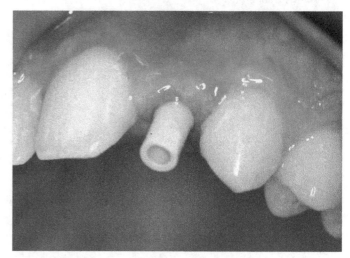

Figure 9.14.   The scan body is secured to the implant and will serve as a reference for the implant position during the i-Tero scan.

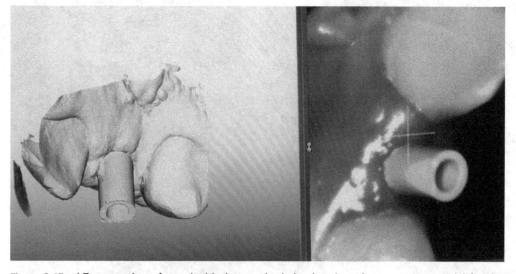

Figure 9.15.   i-Tero scan is performed with the scan body in place in order to create a model for the fabrication of the final custom abutment and crown.

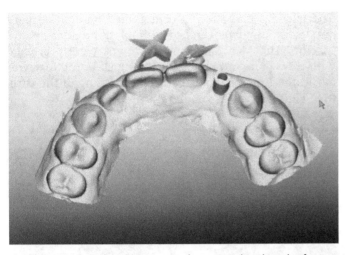

Figure 9.16. Completed i-Tero scan demonstrating dental reference points (dentition and adjacent soft tissue) and the scan body.

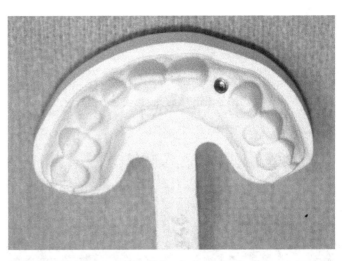

Figure 9.17. i-Tero model with implant analog in place.

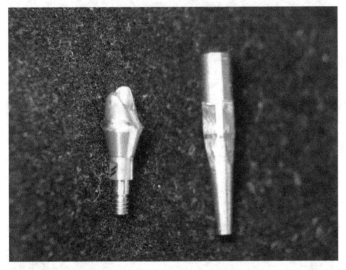

Figure 9.18. A custom abutment is made from the data collected from the i-Tero digital scan. Shown above: the custom abutment and implant analog.

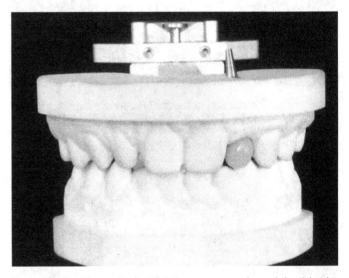

Figure 9.19. The articulated i-Tero generated model with the implant analog, custom abutment, and final peg lateral crown.

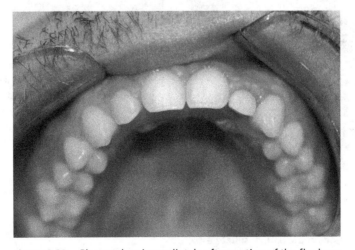

Figure 9.20. Photo taken immediately after seating of the final peg lateral crown to site #10.

Case Report 9.2. A 42-year-old patient presents after a fall resulting in a comminuted anterior maxillary alveolar ridge fracture with avulsion and fracture of teeth #7, #8, #9, and #10. Within 24 hours of the incident, the fractured teeth were removed and the alveolar process was grafted for future implant placement. The decision was made to perform guided implant surgery due to the importance of ideal implant angulation and spacing. The ideal anatomical crowns were recreated with a wax-up and a barium sulfate essix retainer was fabricated to aid in the treatment planning of the case. (See Figures 9.21 through 9.35.)

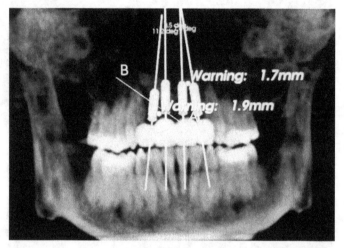

Figure 9.21.   Cone beam computed tomography image with the barium sulfate essix in place. The implants are virtually placed, and warnings are set to demonstrate the proximity of anatomical structures and adjacent implants or teeth.

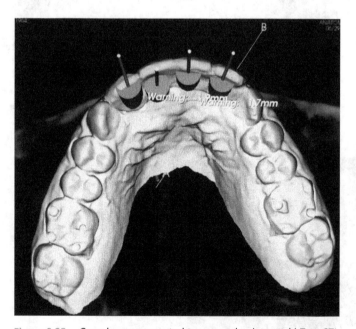

Figure 9.23.   Cone beam computed tomography data and i-Tero STL files are uploaded into implant-specific planning software (Anatomage). The white area represents the dentition and tissue topography collected with the i-Tero digital scanner, the brown represents the ideal position of the final crowns based on the barium sulfate essix, and the green represents the projection of the planned implants in relation to the anticipated crown locations.

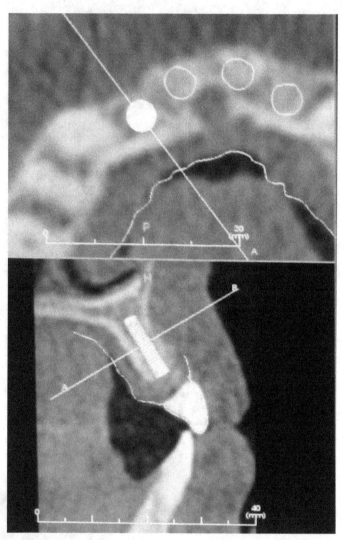

Figure 9.22.   Barium sulfate essix retainer in place to aid in the ideal placement of the implants. Implants are spaced ideally, positioned within available bone, designed for individual screw-retained prostheses, and placed away from vital structures.

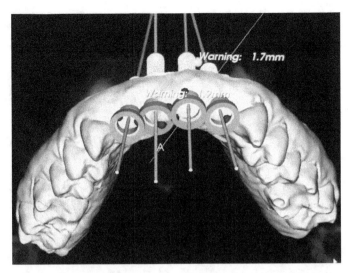

Figure 9.24. Image depicting the exact location of the drill sleeves prior to the fabrication of the surgical guide.

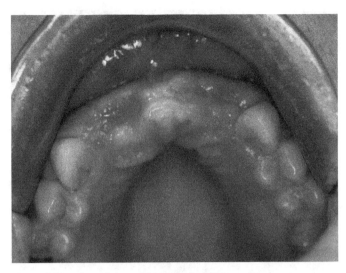

Figure 9.25. Anterior maxilla 4 months after grafting.

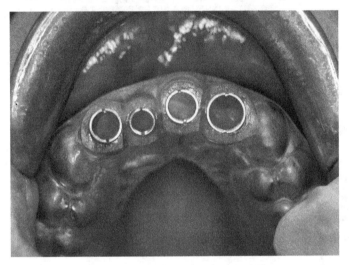

Figure 9.26. Placement of prefabricated surgical guide.

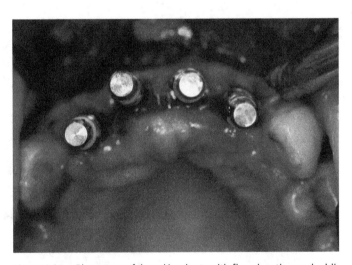

Figure 9.27. Placement of dental implants with flap elevation and additional bone grafting preplanned from the implant-specific software.

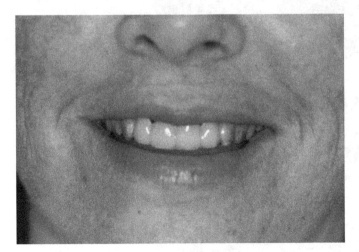

Figure 9.28. The patient is immediately provisionalized using a prefabricated essix retainer.

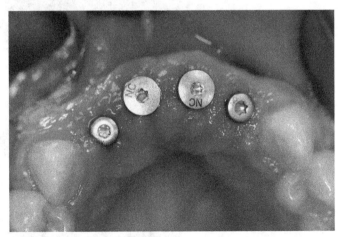

Figure 9.29. After 14 weeks, the implants are uncovered, and diameter-appropriate healing abutments are placed.

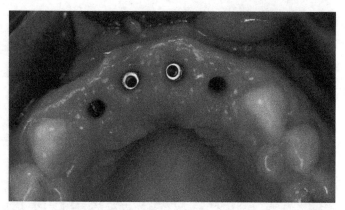

Figure 9.30. Patient with 3–4 mm of keratinized tissue and integrated implants.

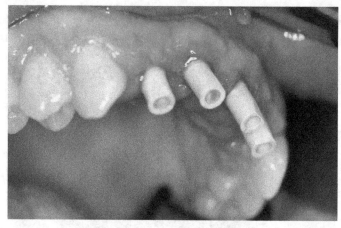

Figure 9.31. Scan bodies are placed 18 weeks after insertion of implants.

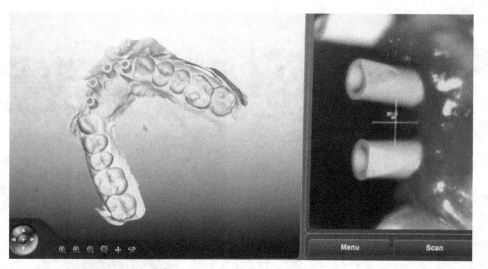

Figure 9.32. An i-Tero is taken with scan bodies in place in order to fabricate a model for the fabrication of a temporary restoration.

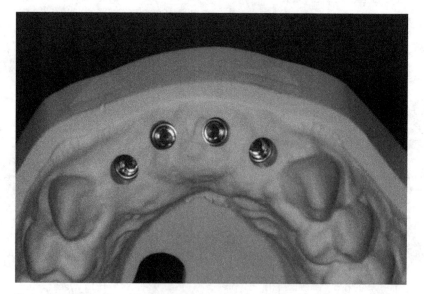

Figure 9.33. i-Tero model with implant analogs in place.

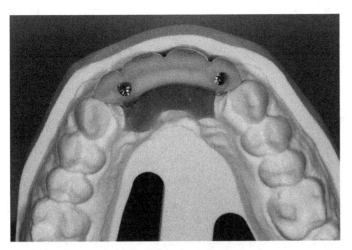

Figure 9.34.   Soft tissue replica material is added to the i-Tero model, and a screw-retained temporary prosthesis is created to allow for shaping of the soft tissue prior to the fabrication of the final crowns.

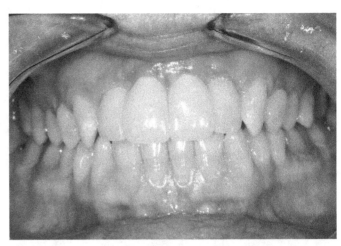

Figure 9.35.   After the recreation of papillae, a second i-Tero is taken. Final crowns fabricated from an i-Tero model (courtesy of Dr Susan Widick, DDS).

References

Bedard, J.F., 2009. Enhanced cast-based guided dental implant placement for ultimate esthetics: concept and technical procedures. *Journal of Oral and Maxillofacial Surgery*, 67, 108.

Block, M.S. and Chandler C., 2009. Computed tomography-guided surgery: complications associated with scanning, processing, surgery, and prosthetics. *Journal of Oral and Maxillofacial Surgery*, 67, 13.

PART TWO

ODONTOGENIC HEAD AND NECK INFECTIONS

Review of Spaces

Matthew W. Hearn,[1] Christopher T. Vogel,[2] Robert M. Laughlin,[3] and Christopher J. Haggerty[4]

[1]*Private Practice, Valparaiso, Indiana, USA*
[2]*Department of Oral and Maxillofacial Surgery, University of Missouri–Kansas City, Kansas City, Missouri, USA*
[3]*Department of Oral and Maxillofacial Surgery, Naval Medical Base San Diego, San Diego, California, USA*
[4]*Private Practice, Lakewood Oral and Maxillofacial Surgery Specialists, Lees Summit; and Department of Oral and Maxillofacial Surgery, University of Missouri-Kansas City, Kansas City, Missouri, USA*

> *Never let the sun rise or set on pus.*
> —Matt Hearn

General Principles of Surgical Infection Management

1. Incisions should be placed within non-involved skin and mucosa when possible. Incisions placed within necrotic or inflamed tissues result in delayed healing and unaesthetic scars.
2. Incisions should be placed within aesthetic areas when possible. Incisions should parallel resting skin tension lines and should be placed within natural skin creases.
3. Incisions should be placed to allow for gravity-dependent drainage when possible.
4. Sharp dissection is recommended within the superficial layers only (skin, subcutaneous tissues, and mucosa). Blunt dissection is continued through the deeper layers to minimize damage to vital structures. Dissection patterns should parallel vessels and nerves to minimize iatrogenic damage to these structures.
5. Each space should be explored completely to ensure complete disruption and evacuation of purulence and to avoid compartmentalization of the space.
6. All explored spaces require drain placement. The exception is the peritonsillar space.
7. Drains should be removed when they become non-productive. Drains are removed based on the patient's physical examination and drainage output. Drains are typically left in place for 72–120 hours. Nonproductive drains left in place for extended periods of time may lead to recontamination of the space.
8. Wound margins are cleaned daily to remove blood clots, debris, and discharge.

Vestibular Space

Boundaries

Superior: Buccinator muscle
Inferior: Buccinator muscle
Anterior: Intrinsic lip musculature
Posterior: Buccinator muscle
Lateral: Vestibular mucosa
Medial: Mandible or maxilla with overlying periosteum
Contents: Areolar connective tissue, parotid duct, long buccal, and mental nerves
Connections: Canine (infraorbital) space and buccal space
Signs and symptoms: Vestibular fluctuance
Approach: Drainage is achieved via an incision parallel to and in the depth of the vestibule, ideally at the height of fluctuance. Blunt dissection is utilized to explore the vestibular space. Vertical incisions are utilized in the region of the mental foramen to avoid injury to the mental nerve (Figure 10.1).

Key Points

The vestibular space is a potential space between the vestibular mucosa and the underlying muscles of facial expression.

Atlas of Operative Oral and Maxillofacial Surgery, First Edition. Edited by Christopher J. Haggerty and Robert M. Laughlin
© 2015 John Wiley & Sons, Inc. Published 2015 by John Wiley & Sons, Inc.

Intraoral Incisions

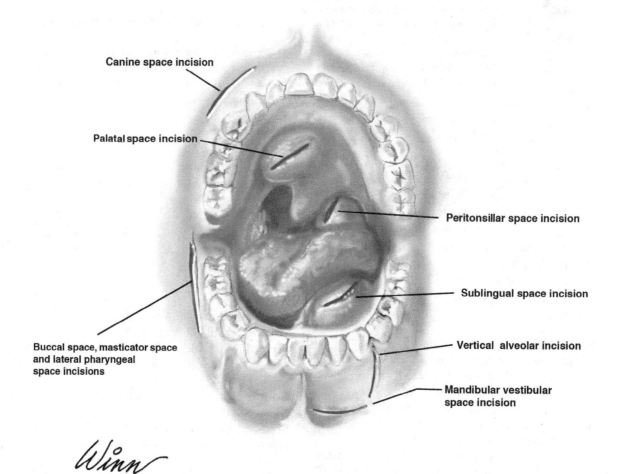

Canine space incision

Palatal space incision

Peritonsillar space incision

Sublingual space incision

Buccal space, masticator space
and lateral pharyngeal
space incisions

Vertical alveolar incision

Mandibular vestibular
space incision

Winn

Figure 10.1.   Intraoral drainage incision sites.

Buccal Space (Buccinator Space)

Boundaries

Superior: Zygomatic arch
Inferior: Lower border of the mandible
Anterior: Labial musculature (zygomatic and depressor muscles at the angle of the mouth)
Posterior: Pterygomandibular raphe
Lateral: Skin of the cheek
Medial: Buccinator muscle and the overlying buccopharyngeal fascia
Contents: Buccal fat pad, Stensen's duct, transverse facial artery and vein, and the anterior facial artery and vein

Connections: Canine space, submandibular space, masticator space, and infratemporal space
Signs and symptoms: Cheek edema (Figure 10.2)
Approach: The buccal space may be drained intraorally or extraorally. Intraoral drainage is best accomplished via a mandibular or maxillary vestibular incision with dissection through the buccinator muscle (Figure 10.1). Extraoral drainage is achieved via a submandibular incision (Figure 10.3). Blunt dissection is directed superiorly and superficial to the buccinator muscle to enter the buccal space (Figure 10.4).

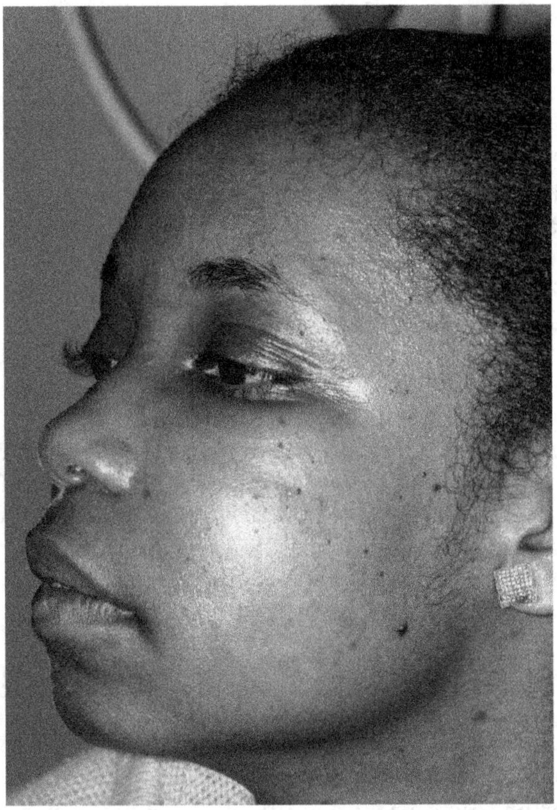

Buccal and Palatal Spaces

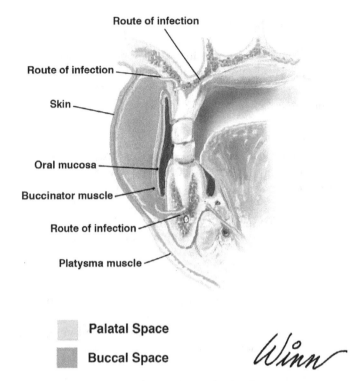

Figure 10.2. Typical presentation of a buccal space abscess with marked cheek edema anterior to the masseter.

Figure 10.4. Anatomy of the buccal and palatal spaces.

Standard Extraoral Incisions

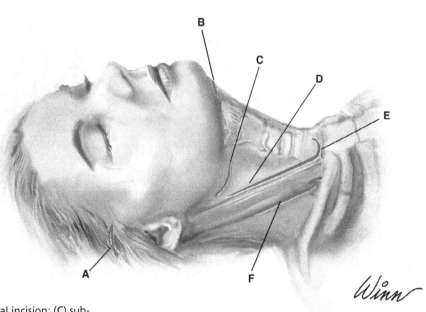

Figure 10.3. (A) Gillies incision; (B) submental incision; (C) submandibular incision; (D) anterior sternocleidomastoid muscle (SCM) incision; (E) transcervical mediastinum incision; and (F) posterior SCM incision.

Key Points

1. Isolated buccal space abscesses do not cause trismus. Trismus, in the presence of a buccal space abscess, is an important and ominous finding that should alert the clinician to the posterior spread of infection.
2. In the pediatric population (age 3 months–3 years), it is important to differentiate between a true buccal space abscess of odontogenic origin and from *Haemophilus influenzae* cellulitis.

Palatal Space

Boundaries

Superior: Palate
Inferior: Periosteum
Anterior: Alveolar process of the maxilla
Posterior: Periosteal attachment to the palate and the maxilla
Lateral: Maxillary alveolus
Medial: Midline space (however, abscesses are typically contained laterally due to firm periosteal attachment)
Contents: Greater palatine nerve, artery, and vein, and nasopalatine nerve
Connections: None
Signs and symptoms: Localized palatal swelling
Approach: Drainage is achieved via an incision through palatal mucosa into the abscess cavity that parallels the regional vasculature, in particular the greater palatine neurovascular bundle (Figure 10.1).

Key Points

Palatal space infections typically arise from the palatal roots of maxillary molars and premolars (Figure 10.4).

Canine Space (Infraorbital Space)

Boundaries

Superior: Infraorbital rim
Inferior: Oral mucosa
Anterior: Quadratus labii superioris muscles (levator labii superioris alaeque nasi, levator labii superioris, zygomaticus minor, and zygomaticus major)
Posterior: Levator anguli oris (caninus) muscle
Lateral: Buccal space
Medial: Nasal cartilages and subcutaneous tissue
Contents: Angular artery and vein and the infraorbital nerve
Connections: Vestibular space and buccal space
Signs and symptoms: Obliteration of the nasolabial fold and periorbital edema
Approach: Intraoral drainage is accomplished via an incision located within the depth of the vestibule, immediately adjacent to the abscessed tooth (Figure 10.1). Blunt dissection is carried superiorly through the levator anguli oris (caninus) muscle and into the canine space.

Key Points

1. Canine space infections typically arise when an anterior maxillary periapical abscess (typically from a canine) erodes through the buccal plate superior to the attachment of the caninus muscle.
2. Care must be taken to avoid damage to the infraorbital nerve during exploration of the canine space.
3. The facial veins are generally valveless (allowing bidirectional flow). Infections of the canine space can result in septic thrombophlebitis or emboli of the angular vein. Cavernous venous sinus thrombosis can result from ascension from the angular vein, to the inferior ophthalmic vein, and into the cavernous sinus. Prompt and aggressive treatment of canine space infections are necessary to avoid this exceeding rare, but potentially devastating sequela.

Submental Space

Boundaries

Superior: Mylohyoid muscle
Inferior: Superficial (investing) layer of the deep cervical fascia
Anterior: Inferior border of the mandible
Posterior: Hyoid bone
Lateral: Anterior bellies of the digastric muscles
Medial: No true medial border as it is a midline space
Contents: Anterior jugular veins and lymph nodes
Connections: Submandibular space
Signs and symptoms: Submental edema and erythema (Figure 10.5)

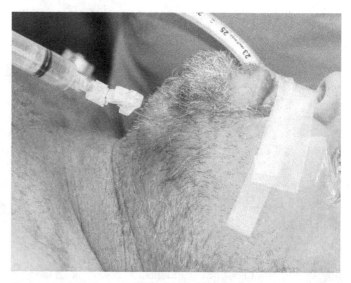

Figure 10.5. Typical submental abscess presentation with obvious edema and erythema of the submental region. Prior to surgical drainage, a sterile aspirate is obtained for culture and sensitivity.

Submental Space

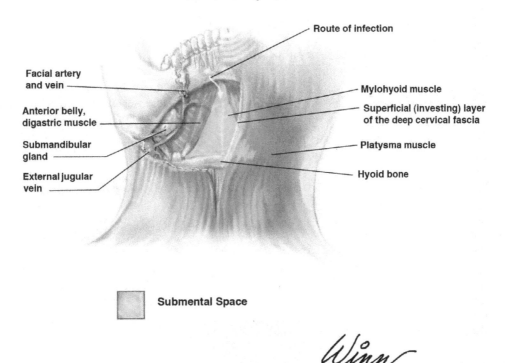

Figure 10.6.   Anatomy of the submental space.

Approach: Drainage is accomplished via a horizontal midline incision just anterior to the hyoid bone within the submental skin crease (Figure 10.3). Incisions placed near the hyoid bone provide gravity dependent drainage as the hyoid bone is the most inferior boundary of the submental space (Figure 10.6). Blunt dissection is directed superiorly through skin, subcutaneous tissue, and the platysma muscle to enter the submental space. Care must be taken to avoid the anterior jugular veins. The submental space may also be drained intraorally via a vestibular incision continued through the mentalis muscle. The intraoral approach fails to provide dependent drainage.

Key Points

1. The submental space is commonly involved via medial extension of submandibular space infections. Other potential sources of infection include direct spread from the mandibular incisors and symphyseal fractures.
2. The spread of infection from the submental space posterolateral to the anterior digastric muscles allows for direct bilateral extension of infections to the submandibular and sublingual spaces. Bilateral brawny cellulitis of the submental, sublingual, and submandibular spaces is termed Ludwig's angina.

Submandibular Space (Submaxillary Space, Submylohyoid Space)

Boundaries

Superior: Inferior and lingual surfaces of the mandible and the mylohyoid muscle
Inferior: Investing fascia with the digastric tendon at the apex
Anterior: Anterior belly of the digastric muscle
Posterior: Posterior belly of the digastric muscle and the stylohyoid muscle
Lateral: Platysma muscle and investing fascia
Medial: Hyoglossus and mylohyoid muscles
Contents: Facial artery and vein, marginal mandibular nerve, mylohyoid nerve, submandibular gland, and lymph nodes
Connections: Lateral pharyngeal space, submental space, sublingual space, and buccal space
Signs and symptoms: Swelling at the inferior border of the mandible that extends medially to the anterior digastric muscle and posteriorly to the hyoid bone
Approach: Drainage is accomplished via an extraoral submandibular approach (Figure 10.3). A 2–4 cm incision is placed 2–3 cm caudal to the inferior border of the mandible, parallel to the resting skin tension lines at the level of the hyoid bone and at the point that will allow for maximum gravity-dependent drainage (see Figure 10.10 in Case Report 10.1). A hemostat is

introduced through the skin incision and is directed toward the inferior border of the mandible. The hemostat is then directed lingual to the mandible to enter the submandibular space. Blunt dissection continues superiorly along the lingual aspect of the body of the mandible and is continued superiorly to the mylohyoid muscle.

Key Points

The submandibular approach provides extraoral access to the sublingual, submandibular, buccal, masticator (pterygomandibular and masseteric), and lateral pharyngeal spaces.

Sublingual Space

Boundaries

Superior: Oral mucosa of the floor of the mouth
Inferior: Mylohyoid muscle
Anterior: Mandible
Posterior: Open
Lateral: Lingual cortex of the mandible
Medial: Muscles of the tongue
Contents: Sublingual gland, lingual nerve, Wharton's duct, hypoglossal nerve, and the sublingual artery and vein
Connections: Submandibular space and the lateral pharyngeal space
Signs and symptoms: Floor of the mouth and tongue elevation, dysphasia, and sialorrhea

Approach: Drainage is best accomplished via an extraoral submandibular approach (Figure 10.3). Once the submandibular space is explored, blunt dissection continues superiorly along the lingual aspect of the body of the mandible and is continued through the mylohyoid muscle to enter the sublingual space. Nondependent drainage can be achieved via an intraoral incision placed at the anterior and lateral portion of the floor of the mouth, parallel and lateral to the submandibular duct (Figure 10.1). Blunt dissection proceeds through the oral mucosa and directly into the sublingual space.

Key Points

1. Infections of the sublingual space are typically odontogenic in origin. Whether an odontogenic infection occurs within the sublingual space or the submandibular space is a result of the spread of the infection in relation to the attachment of the mylohyoid muscle (Figure 10.7). Infections originating superior to the attachment of the mylohyoid muscle (teeth anterior to the second molar) will occur within the sublingual space. Infections originating inferior to the attachment of the mylohyoid muscle (second and third molars) will present within the submandibular space.
2. Posteriorly, the sublingual space is contiguous with the submandibular space, allowing for rapid spread of infection.

Sublingual and Submandibular Spaces

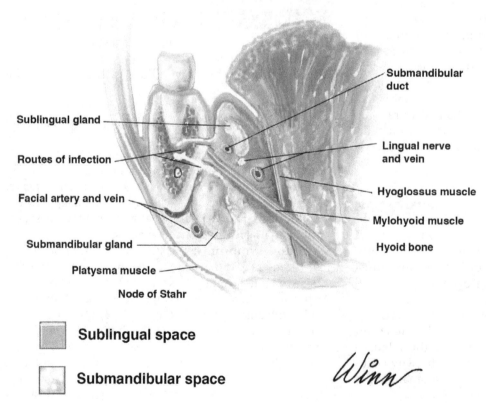

Figure 10.7.   Anatomy of the sublingual and submandibular spaces.

Sublingual gland

Routes of infection

Facial artery and vein

Submandibular gland

Platysma muscle

Node of Stahr

Submandibular duct

Lingual nerve and vein

Hyoglossus muscle

Mylohyoid muscle

Hyoid bone

Sublingual space

Submandibular space

Winn

Case Report 10.1. A 27-year-old male presents with a chief complaint of right-sided facial edema, floor-of-mouth elevation and tenderness, right posterior mandibular pain, and a history of dental abscesses. (See Figures 10.8 through 10.13.)

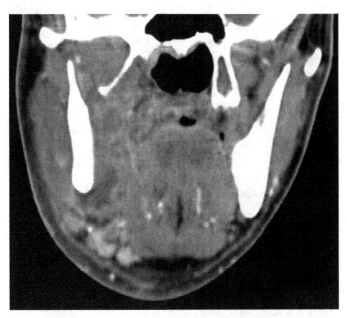

Figure 10.8. Coronal contrast-enhanced computed tomography scan demonstrating a combined submandibular-sublingual space abscess.

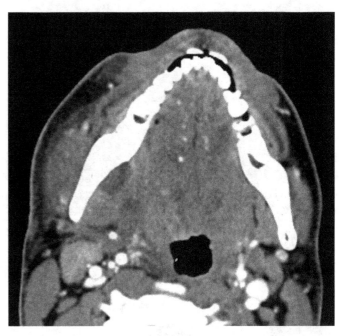

Figure 10.9. Axial contrast-enhanced computed tomography scan demonstrating a combined submandibular-sublingual space abscess.

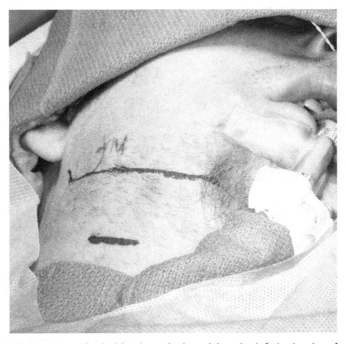

Figure 10.10. The incision is marked caudal to the inferior border of the mandible, parallel to the resting skin tension lines, at the level of the hyoid bone, and in an area that will allow for maximum dependent drainage.

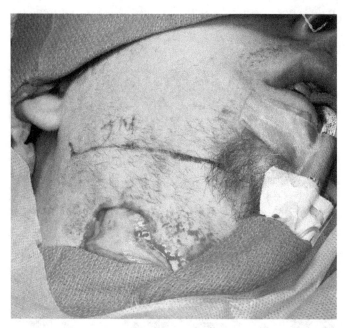

Figure 10.11.   Purulence is expressed once the submandibular space is entered.

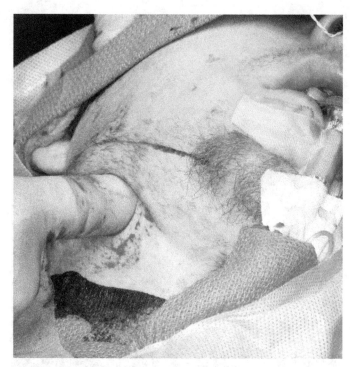

Figure 10.12.   Blunt finger dissection is utilized to ensure that the entire submandibular and sublingual spaces have been explored.

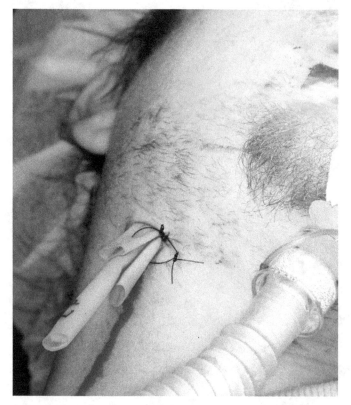

Figure 10.13.   Drain placement within the right submandibular, sublingual, and lateral pharyngeal spaces.

Masticator Space (Masticatory Space, Masseter–Mandibulopterygoid Space)

The masticator space consists of four subspaces:

Masseteric (submasseteric) space
Pterygomandibular space
Superficial temporal space
Deep temporal space

Boundaries

Superior: Temporal crest

Inferior: Pterygomasseteric sling and the inferior border of the mandible

Anterior: Orbital rim and the anterior border of the ramus

Posterior: Posterior border of the mandible

Lateral: Parotideomasseteric fascia (superficial layer of the deep cervical fascia)

Medial: The greater wing of the sphenoid bone, the squamous portion of the temporal bone, and the superficial layer of the deep cervical fascia deep to the medial pterygoid

Contents: Muscles of mastication (temporalis, masseter, medial, and lateral pterygoids), internal maxillary artery, mandibular division of the trigeminal nerve, and the buccal fat pad

Connections: All subspaces are interconnected (Figure 10.14). Connections also exist between the buccal, lateral pharyngeal, and infratemporal spaces.

Signs and symptoms: Trismus and edema

1. The masticator space contains the masseteric (submasseteric), pterygomandibular, deep, and superficial temporal spaces (Figure 10.14).
2. Individual subspaces will be discussed in detail in the following four subsections.

Masseteric (Submasseteric) Space

Boundaries

Superior: Zygomatic arch
Inferior: Inferior border of the mandible
Anterior: Anterior border of the ramus
Posterior: Posterior border of the ramus

Lateral: Parotideomasseteric fascia (superficial layer of the deep cervical fascia)
Medial: Vertical ramus of the mandible
Contents: Masseter muscle, masseteric artery, and vein
Connections: Superficial temporal space and pterygomandibular space
Signs and symptoms: Trismus and posterior mandibular angle edema
Approach: Drainage is best accomplished via an extraoral submandibular approach to allow for gravity dependent drainage (Figure 10.3). After entering the submandibular space, blunt dissection is continued posteriorly through the pterygomasseteric sling to enter the masseteric space located between the body of the masseter

Masticator Spaces

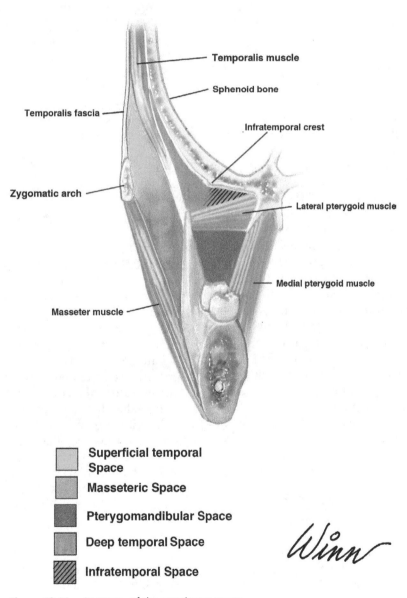

- Superficial temporal Space
- Masseteric Space
- Pterygomandibular Space
- Deep temporal Space
- Infratemporal Space

Figure 10.14.   Anatomy of the masticator space.

and the lateral ramus of the mandible. Alternatively, the masseteric space may be accessed intraorally (Figure 10.1) via a vertical incision lateral and parallel to the pterygomandibular raphe. Sharp dissection is carried through the buccinator muscle, and blunt dissection is continued to enter the masseteric space.

Key Points

1. Common sources of infection include pericoronitis, third molar abscesses, and mandibular angle fractures.
2. The intraoral approach is often impractical due to the presence of trismus and the inability to establish dependent drainage.

Pterygomandibular Space

Boundaries

Superior: Lateral pterygoid muscle
Inferior: Pterygomasseteric sling
Anterior: Anterior border of the ramus
Posterior: Posterior border of the ramus
Lateral: Ascending ramus
Medial: Superficial layer of the deep cervical fascia
Contents: Inferior alveolar artery, vein, and nerve; lingual and mylohyoid nerves
Connections: Masseteric space, infratemporal space, and lateral pharyngeal space
Signs and symptoms: Trismus
Approach: Extraoral drainage is accomplished via a submandibular approach (Figure 10.3). Once the inferior border of the mandible is reached, blunt dissection proceeds posteriorly through the pterygomasseteric sling to enter the pterygomandibular space located between the body of the medial pterygoid muscle and the medial ramus of the mandible. Intraorally, the space may be accessed through an incision placed lateral and parallel to the pterygomandibular raphe through the buccinator muscle (Figure 10.1). Blunt dissection is carried into the pterygomandibular space on the medial side of the mandible. In addition, the intraoral approach may be carried inferiorly through the pterygomandibular space, passing through the pterygomasseteric sling into the submandibular space. This may then be connected to a submandibular approach, and a through-and-through intraoral-extraoral drain can be passed with resulting gravity-dependent drainage.

Key Points

1. Common sources of infection include pericoronitis, third molar abscesses, mandibular angle fractures, and needle track infections caused by inferior alveolar nerve blocks.

2. Symptoms of needle track infections include pain, trismus, and localized abscess formation visible on computed tomography (CT) scan.

Superficial Temporal Space (Superficial Temporal Pouch)

Boundaries

Superior: Temporal crest
Inferior: Zygomatic arch
Anterior: Lateral orbital rim
Posterior: Fusion of the temporalis fascia with the pericranium at the temporal crest
Lateral: Temporalis fascia
Medial: Temporalis muscle
Contents: Middle temporal artery and vein
Connections: Masseteric space and deep temporal space
Signs and symptoms: Trismus and temporal swelling
Approach: Refer to deep temporal space.

Key Points

1. The temporal space is divided into superficial and deep spaces by the temporalis muscle.
2. The temporal spaces are commonly involved by the secondary spread of infection from neighboring contiguous spaces.

Deep Temporal Space (Deep Temporal Pouch)

Boundaries

Superior: Attachment of the temporalis muscle to the temporal crest
Inferior: Superior surface of the lateral pterygoid muscle
Anterior: Infratemporal surface of the maxilla and the posterior surface of the orbit
Posterior: Attachment of the temporalis muscle to the cranium
Lateral: Temporalis muscle
Medial: Greater wing of the sphenoid bone and squamous portion of the temporal bone (terminating at the infratemporal crest)
Contents: Deep temporal artery and vein
Connections: Pterygomandibular space, and superficial temporal and infratemporal spaces
Signs and symptoms: Trismus and temporal swelling
Approach: Drainage of both the superficial and deep temporal spaces is achieved via a Gillies approach (Figure 10.3). A 2–4 cm horizontal temporal incision is made posterior to the hairline and 3 cm inferior to the anterior temporal crest. The incision is carried through the scalp, temporoparietal fascia and deep to the temporalis fascia to expose the temporalis muscle and enter the superficial temporal space. Dissection can be carried bluntly through the temporalis muscle to enter the deep temporal space if necessary. Blunt dissection is carried inferiorly along the superficial or deep surface of the temporalis muscle to explore

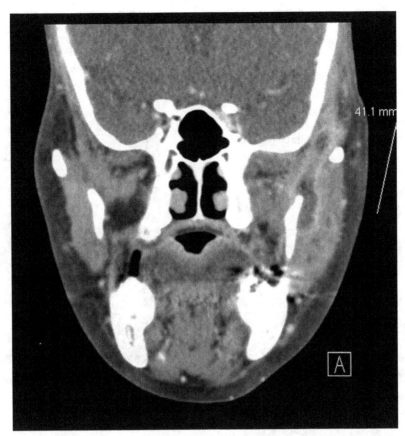

Figure 10.15. Coronal contrast enhanced computed tomography scan demonstrating a left temporal space abscess.

the spaces. When draining the superficial temporal space, it is best to combine the Gillies approach with a mandibular posterior vestibular incision with dissection superficial to the temporalis tendon. A through-and-through drain can be passed from the scalp incision to the intraoral incision to allow for dependent drainage.

Key Points

Infections within the temporal spaces are able to communicate freely around the temporalis muscle (Figure 10.15).

Infratemporal Space (Postzygomatic Space)

Boundaries

Superior: Infratemporal surface of the greater wing of the sphenoid and temporal bones, extending laterally to the infratemporal crest
Inferior: Open to pterygomandibular space
Anterior: Posterior surface of the maxillary tuberosity
Posterior: Temporomandibular joint and the deep lobe of the parotid gland
Lateral: Deep surface of the temporalis muscle and the coronoid process of the mandible
Medial: Lateral pterygoid plate and the lateral pterygoid muscle

Contents: Middle (muscular) division of the internal maxillary artery, mandibular division of the trigeminal nerve, posterior portion of the buccal fat pad, and pterygoid plexus of veins
Connections: Deep temporal space, pterygomandibular space, buccal space, and orbital space (via inferior orbital fissure)
Signs and symptoms: Trismus
Approach: The infratemporal space can be drained utilizing an intraoral or extraoral incision. When only the infratemporal portion of the masticator space is involved, a posterior maxillary vestibular incision is made through the buccinator muscle and carried posteriorly around the maxillary tuberosity to enter the infratemporal space. Blunt dissection is important within the infratemporal space to avoid hemorrhage from the maxillary arteries and their associated branches. When the pterygomandibular space is involved, both spaces may be drained via a submandibular incision, with dissection medial to the mandible through the pterygomasseteric sling. The infratemporal space may also be accessed via a Gillies approach extending through the deep temporal space, with a through-and-through drain passing deep to the temporalis muscle and entering the oral cavity through the posterior maxillary vestibular incision.

1. The infratemporal space is the medial extension of the deep temporal space.
2. In addition, the infratemporal space provides a potential source for the posterior spread of infection to the cavernous sinus.
3. Infections of the infratemporal space most often result from secondary spread; however, maxillary dental and sinus infections are known etiologies.

Case Report

Case Report 10.2. A 12-year-old male presents with moderate left-side facial edema, left-side facial pain, trismus, fever, and marked leukocytosis. (See Figures 10.16 through 10.25.)

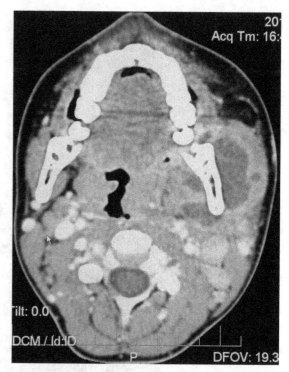

Figure 10.17.   Axial contrast-enhanced computed tomography scan demonstrating involvement of the left masticator space. Airway deviation is noted.

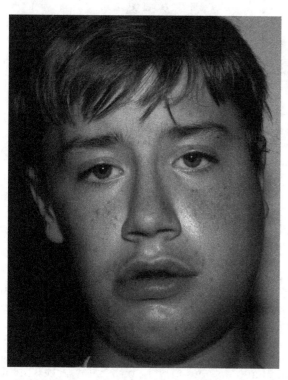

Figure 10.16.   12-year-old patient with obvious left masticator space edema, discomfort, and trismus.

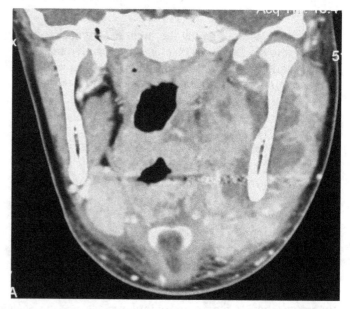

Figure 10.18.   Coronal contrast-enhanced computed tomography scan demonstrating involvement of the left masseteric, pterygomandibular, and lateral pharyngeal spaces.

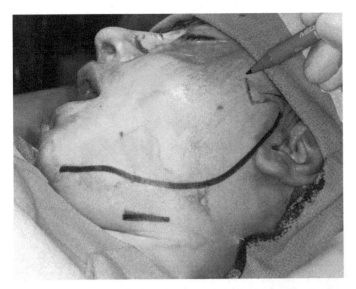

Figure 10.19. Anatomical markings to include the inferior border of the mandible, the condyle–coronoid complex, and the site of proposed drainage located 3 cm caudal to the inferior border of the mandible to allow for dependent drainage.

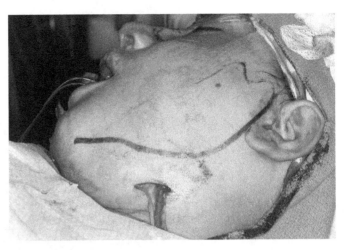

Figure 10.20. Purulence was identified once the masticator space was entered.

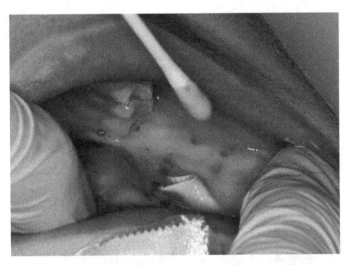

Figure 10.21. A through-and-through drain (buccal vestibule–submandibular incision) was placed. Purulence was evacuated, involved teeth were extracted, and cultures were taken.

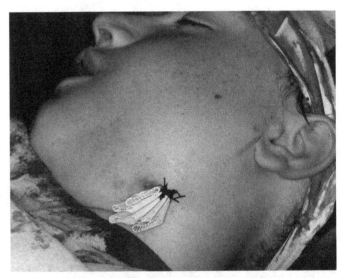

Figure 10.22. Drains were placed within the left masseteric space, pterygomandibular space, lateral pharyngeal space, along the posterior aspect of the ascending ramus to the level of the skull base, and a single intraoral through-and-through drain was placed.

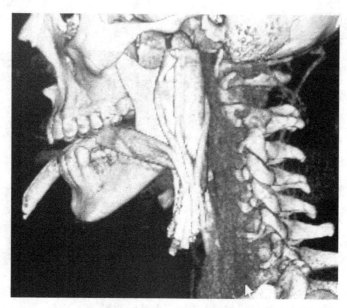

Figure 10.23. 3D image depicting drain placement. Drains are located along the medial, lateral, and posterior aspect of the mandible. A drain was placed within the lateral pharyngeal space, and a through-and-through drain was placed as well.

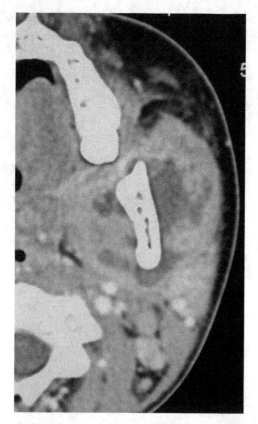 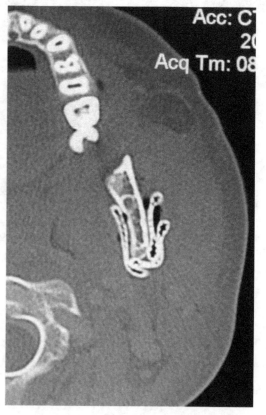

Figures 10.24. and 10.25. Axial computed tomography scans comparing preoperative (Figure 10.24) and postoperative images (Figure 10.25). Figure 10.25 demonstrates the placement of drains along the medial and lateral border of the ascending ramus within the masseteric and pterygomandibular compartments of the masticator space.

Peritonsillar Space (Paratonsillar Space)

Boundaries

Superior: Hard palate
Inferior: Piriform fossa
Anterior: Anterior tonsillar pillar (palatoglossus muscle)
Posterior: Posterior tonsillar pillar (palatopharyngeus muscle)
Lateral: Superior pharyngeal constrictor
Medial: Oropharyngeal mucosa
Contents: Loose connective tissue
Connections: Lateral pharyngeal space via perforation of the superior constrictor and buccopharyngeal fascia
Signs and symptoms: "Hot potato" voice, odynophagia, drooling, uvular deviation, palatal asymmetries, and medial displacement of the tonsil
Approach: Treatment of peritonsillar abscess includes aspiration and incision and drainage (Figure 10.26). When a peritonsillar abscess is suspected, aspiration confirms the diagnosis and evacuates purulence. An 18-gauge needle is inserted into the pointing area, the pharyngeal mucosa is penetrated, and aspiration is performed. If purulence is detected on aspiration, an incision-and-drainage procedure is performed. A #15 blade is utilized to create a

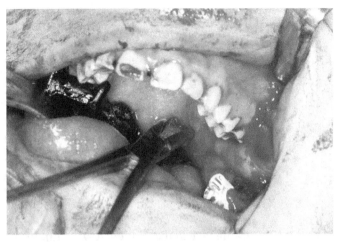

Figure 10.27. Exploration of the peritonsillar space with a blunt-ended hemostat.

curvilinear incision along the perimeter of the tonsillar capsule (Figure 10.1) and through the point from which purulence was evacuated. A blunt hemostat is inserted into the incision and opened widely (Figure 10.27). The entire peritonsillar space is explored with blunt dissection with the hemostat. The peritonsillar space is then copiously irrigated with saline.

Key Points

1. When performing aspiration, the needle is advanced less than 1 cm in order to prevent injury to the glossopharyngeal nerve and the internal carotid artery, which may be aberrantly located within the parapharyngeal space.
2. A drain is typically not placed within the peritonsillar space.
3. Irrigating the peritonsillar space with half-strength hydrogen peroxide may aid in hemostasis.

Pharyngeal Spaces (Lateral and Retropharyngeal Spaces)

Lateral Pharyngeal Space (Parapharyngeal Space, Pharyngomaxillary Space, Pterygopharyngeal Space, Pharyngopterygoid Space, Peripharyngeal Space)

Boundaries

Superior: Skull base on the sphenoid bone
Inferior: Hyoid bone
Anterior: Pterygomandibular raphe
Posterior: Prevertebral division of the deep cervical fascia and the carotid sheath at the posterolateral corner
Lateral: Superficial layer of the deep cervical fascia overlying the mandible, the medial pterygoid, and the parotid gland

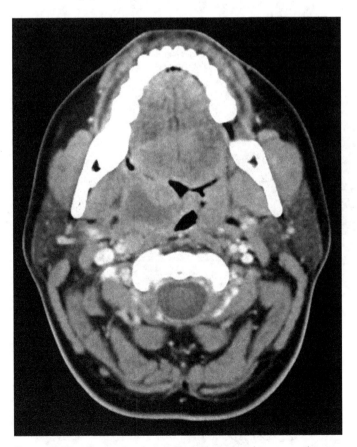

Figure 10.26. Contrast-enhanced axial computed tomography scan demonstrating a right peritonsillar abscess.

Medial: Visceral division of the middle layer of the deep cervical fascia (buccopharyngeal fascia) encasing the pharyngeal constrictors

Contents: *Prestyloid*: Fat, loose connective tissue; lymph nodes

Poststyloid: CN IX, CN XI, CN XII, carotid sheath, sympathetic chain, and lymph nodes

Connections: Masticator space, retropharyngeal space, carotid sheath, and submandibular and sublingual spaces (see Figures 10.28 and 10.29)

Signs and symptoms: Trismus, dysphonia, dysphagia, odynophagia, posturing, dyspnea, inability to control oral secretions, medial displacement of the lateral pharyngeal wall, uveal deviation, and edema

Approach: Drainage can be achieved via numerous approaches. Drainage via the submandibular approach (Figure 10.3) involves dissection through the submandibular space (see "Approach" in the "Submandibular Space" section) with blunt dissection continued posteriorly and cephalically until the styloid process is palpated. Blunt finger dissection is directed medially

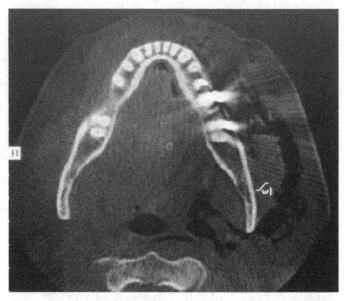

Figure 10.28. Axial computed tomography scan demonstrating a combined masticator space, lateral pharyngeal space, and retropharyngeal space infection.

Pharyngeal Spaces

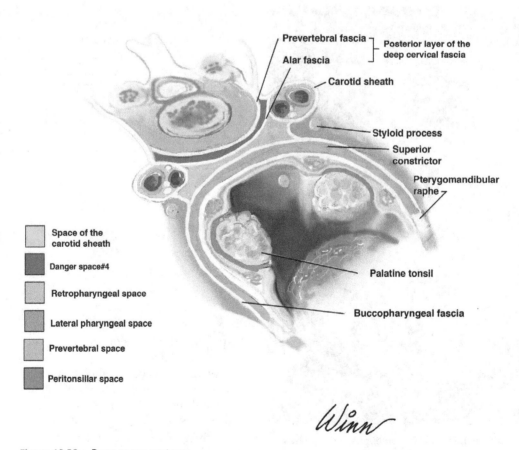

Figure 10.29.   Deep space anatomy.

toward the posterior tonsillar pillar. The space is fully explored by continued posteromedial dissection and palpation of the ipsilateral transverse process, posterior carotid sheath, and skull base. Drainage via an intraoral approach (Figure 10.1) involves an incision placed within the posterior mandibular vestibule. Blunt dissection continues through the buccinator muscle and lateral and parallel to the pterygomandibular raphe. Dissection proceeds medially and superiorly, deep to the medial pterygoid muscle to enter the lateral pharyngeal space. Care must be taken during dissection to avoid the ascending pharyngeal artery located on the superficial surface of the superior constrictor muscle.

Key Points

1. The lateral pharyngeal space is shaped like an inverted cone with its base at the skull and apex at the hyoid bone (see Figure 10.31 in Case Report 10.3).
2. The aponeurosis of Zuckerkandl and Testut divides the lateral pharyngeal space into anterior (prestyloid) and posterior (poststyloid) compartments and provides a barrier to the spread of infection.
3. Due to its location, nearly all life-threatening odontogenic infections will pass through this space before entering the deeper, more inferior spaces of the neck.
4. An arteriogram is indicated if coagulated blood or old blood clots are encountered within the lateral pharyngeal space, as these are signs of carotid sheath involvement.

Retropharyngeal Space (Retroesophageal Space, Retrovisceral Space, Posterior Visceral Space, Retropharyngeal Part of Visceral Compartment): Posterior Aspect of Grodinsky and Holyoke's Space 3

Boundaries

Superior: Base of the skull
Inferior: To the fusion of the visceral (buccopharyngeal) and alar fascia at a variable level between C-6 and T-4, typically at the level of tracheal bifurcation
Anterior: Visceral (buccopharyngeal) fascia
Posterior: Alar fascia
Lateral: Continuous with the lateral pharyngeal space from the base of the skull to the hyoid bone. Inferior to the hyoid, the carotid sheath forms the lateral boundary.
Medial: Midline structure
Contents: Areolar connective tissue and lymphatic drainage from Waldeyer's ring
Connections: Lateral pharyngeal space, pretracheal space, danger space 4, the space of the carotid sheath, and the mediastinum

Signs and symptoms: Dysphagia, dyspnea, sepsis, neck pain, kyphotic curve posturing, widening of retrotracheal tissues, and symptoms of carotid sheath involvement
Approach: Drainage can be achieved via numerous approaches. The most common approach to the retropharyngeal space involves an incision placed either anterior or posterior to the sternocleidomastoid muscle (SCM) (Figure 10.3). These approaches can also be used to access the pretracheal, visceral, danger space 4, and prevertebral spaces. The anterior SCM approach involves a linear incision made at the anterior border of the sternocleidomastoid muscle from the hyoid bone to a point just superior to the sternum. Sharp dissection proceeds to the superficial layer of the deep cervical fascia. The sternocleidomastoid muscle, hyoid bone, cricoid cartilage, and carotid sheath are identified. The sternocleidomastoid muscle and carotid sheath are retracted posterolaterally, while the thyroid gland, superior thyroid vessels, and superior laryngeal nerve are retracted medially. If necessary, the inferior thyroid artery, middle thyroid vein, and omohyoid muscle may be sectioned for access. Blunt dissection proceeds between the medial side of the carotid sheath and the pharyngeal constrictor muscles to enter the retropharyngeal space. The retropharyngeal space is explored by finger dissection, and soft drains are placed.

The posterior SCM approach involves a linear incision placed along the posterior border of the SCM muscle from the level of the hyoid bone to the omohyoid muscle. Sharp dissection proceeds to the superficial layer of the deep cervical fascia. The SCM muscle and carotid sheath are retracted anteriorly, taking care to identify and protect the cervical sympathetic chain attached to the posterior surface of the carotid sheath. The alar fascia is divided to enter the retropharyngeal space. The brachial plexus is protected by keeping the dissection above the omohyoid muscle. The retropharyngeal space is explored, and soft drains are placed

Key Points

1. The retropharyngeal space is regarded as the main pathway for the spread of odontogenic infections to the mediastinum. As such, infections involving the retropharyngeal space should be managed aggressively, often with the establishment of a surgical airway. Retropharyngeal abscesses extending below the superior mediastinum are an indication for prompt thoracotomy.
2. The posterior approach to the retropharyngeal space avoids the branches of the carotid artery and internal jugular vein.
3. An intraoral surgical approach is acceptable for localized retropharyngeal infections in the pediatric population.

Case Report 10.3. A 26-year-old male presents with trismus, dysphonia, dysphagia, posturing, difficulty controlling secretions, uvula deviation, facial edema, and marked leukocytosis. (See Figures 10.30, 10.31, 10.32, and 10.33.)

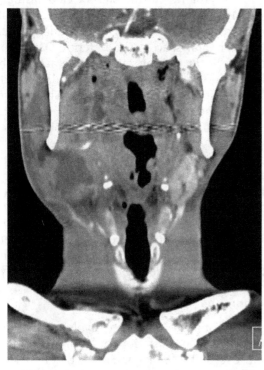

Figure 10.30. Coronal contrast-enhanced computed tomography scan demonstrating abscess formation within the right masticator space and lateral pharyngeal space.

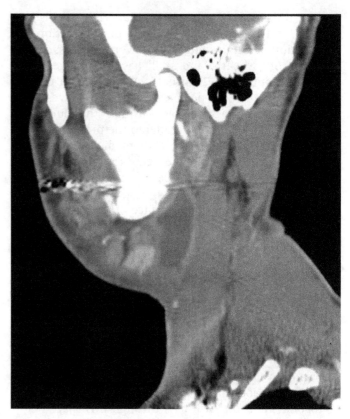

Figure 10.31. Sagittal contrast-enhanced computed tomography scan demonstrating a pyramid-shaped abscess extending from the hyoid bone superiorly toward the skull base.

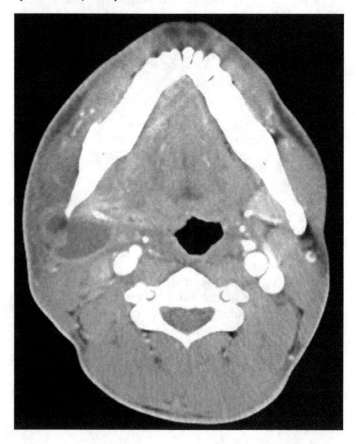

Figure 10.32. Axial contrast-enhanced CT scan demonstrating a right lateral pharyngeal space abscess.

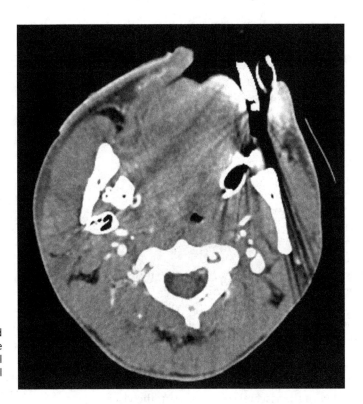

Figure 10.33. Axial contrast-enhanced CT scan demonstrating appropriate drain placement within the right lateral pharyngeal space at the base of the skull and just lateral to the carotid sheath.

Pretracheal Space (Perivisceral Space, Paravisceral Space, Paratracheal Space, Anterior Visceral Space, Prevertebral Part of Visceral Compartment): Anterior Aspect of Grodinsky and Holyoke's Space 3

Boundaries

Superior: Fusion of the middle and pretracheal (visceral) fascia at the level of the hyoid and thyroid cartilage

Inferior: Anterior portion of the superior mediastinum

Anterior: The middle (sternothyroid–thyrohyoid) division of the middle layer of the deep cervical fascia

Posterior: The visceral fascia (deep division of the middle layer of the deep cervical fascia) that encloses the thyroid, trachea, and esophagus. Inferior to the level of the inferior thyroid artery, the pretracheal space is separated from the retropharyngeal space by a dense connective-tissue band extending from the lateral esophagus to the wall of the carotid sheath.

Lateral: Carotid sheath

Medial: Midline structure

Contents: Thyroid gland, trachea, esophagus, and recurrent laryngeal nerves

Connections: Mediastinum and the retropharyngeal space

Signs and symptoms: Dysphagia, dyspnea, dysphonia, odynophagia, airway obstruction, anterior neck swelling, and overlying tissue erythema

Approach: Drainage is achieved via an incision placed anterior to the SCM muscle (Figure 10.3) carried through skin, subcutaneous tissue, platysma muscle, and the superficial and the muscular division of the middle layer of the deep cervical fascia. The carotid sheath is identified and retracted posterolaterally with the overlying SCM muscle. The larynx, trachea, and esophagus are identified and explored to expose the abscess for drainage. If necessary, the visceral fascia can be divided to enter the visceral space.

Key Points

1. The pretracheal space communicates posterolaterally with the retropharyngeal space via a bridge extending around the sides of the thyroid gland, trachea, and esophagus.
2. The bridge's superior boundary is the oblique line of the thyroid cartilage, and the inferior boundary is the inferior thyroid artery.

Visceral Space

Boundaries

Superior: The anterior aspect of the visceral space begins superiorly at the thyroid cartilage, while the posterior aspect originates at the base of the skull.
Inferior: Mediastinum
Anterior: Visceral fascia
Posterior: Visceral fascia
Lateral: Visceral fascia
Medial: Midline structure
Contents: Pharynx, larynx, trachea, esophagus, and thyroid glands
Connections: Retropharyngeal space, pretracheal space, and mediastinum
Signs and symptoms: Dysphagia, dyspnea, dysphonia, odynophagia, and airway obstruction
Approach: The surgical approach to the visceral space is an extension of the approach to the pretracheal space previously described.

Key Points

Often confused with the visceral compartment, the visceral space is located deep to the surrounding visceral fascia.

Space of the Carotid Sheath (Visceral Vascular Space, Grodinsky and Holyoke's Space 3A, "Lincoln's Highway of the Neck")

Boundaries

Superior: Base of the skull
Inferior: Root of the neck
Anterior: Carotid sheath
Posterior: Carotid sheath
Lateral: Carotid sheath
Medial: Carotid sheath
Contents: Carotid artery, internal jugular vein, and vagus nerve
Connections: Lateral pharyngeal space, retropharyngeal space, pretracheal space, and the mediastinum
Signs and symptoms: Ipsilateral Horner's syndrome, acute deficits of CN-IX through CN-XII, "herald bleeds," septic shock, hematoma of surrounding tissues, and variations in heart rate or speech function
Approach: Drainage is achieved via a transcervical approach along the anterior aspect of the SCM (Figure 10.3). Once identified, the carotid sheath is opened with an incision placed along the anterior surface between the internal jugular vein laterally and the internal carotid artery medially. After visualization of the contents of the carotid sheath, the carotid sheath can be thoroughly explored for suppuration.

Key Points

1. The space of the carotid sheath is formed from the confluens of the three layers of the deep cervical fascia.
2. Superior to the hyoid, the space of the carotid sheath communicates with the posterolateral compartment of the lateral pharyngeal space.
3. Arteriography, venography, or contrast-enhanced CT are utilized to determine which vessels are at risk, fluid collections, and whether collateral flow to or from the brain is present.
4. "Herald bleeds" are defined as recurrent unexplained hemorrhaging from the mouth, nose, and/or ear.

Danger Space #4 (Grodinsky and Holyoke's Space 4)

Boundaries

Superior: Base of the skull
Inferior: Posterior mediastinum to the level of the diaphragm
Anterior: Alar division of the deep layer of the deep cervical fascia
Posterior: Prevertebral division of the deep layer of the deep cervical fascia
Lateral: Fusion of the alar and prevertebral fascia at the transverse process of the vertebrae
Medial: Midline structure
Contents: Loose connective tissue
Connections: Retropharyngeal space, prevertebral space, and the mediastinum
Signs and symptoms: Mediastinitis, empyema, and sepsis
Approach: Drainage is achieved either via a transcervical approach anterior or posterior to the SCM (Figure 10.3) or via open thoracotomy (Figure 10.34). With the transcervical approaches, once the retropharyngeal space has been entered, blunt finger dissection is carried posteriorly through the alar fascia to enter the danger space. After exploration and drainage, a large soft drain is inserted into the space.

Key Points

1. The danger space contains only loose connective tissue, and its two fascial layers (alar and prevertebral) are easily separated, allowing for rapid spread of infection to the posterior mediastinum.
2. As this is a closed space, oropharyngeal infections occurring within the danger space originate from the retropharyngeal space.

Prevertebral (Grodinsky and Holyoke's Space 5)

Boundaries

Superior: Base of the skull
Inferior: Coccyx

Approaches to the Mediastinum

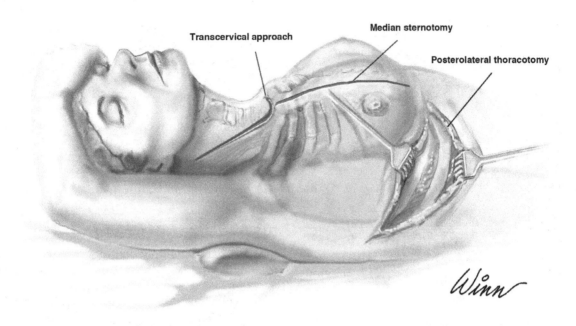

Figure 10.34.   Approaches to the mediastinum.

Anterior: Prevertebral division of the deep layer of the deep cervical fascia

Posterior: Vertebral bodies

Lateral: Fusion of the prevertebral fascia with the transverse processes of the vertebral bodies

Medial: Midline structure

Contents: Potential space

Connections: Danger space

Signs and symptoms: Neck and back pain and symptoms of deep neck infections

Approach: See "Approach" in the "Retropharyngeal Space" section.

Key Points

1. Rarely involved with head and neck infections.
2. Infections of this space most commonly arise from adjacent vertebral bodies, not from oropharyngeal sources (Figure 10.35).

Mediastinum

Boundaries

Superior: First rib
Inferior: Diaphragm
Anterior: Sternum
Posterior: Vertebral column
Lateral: Pleura
Medial: Midline structure

Contents: Carotids, subclavians, aortic arch, thoracic duct, vagus nerves, trachea, esophagus, phrenic nerves, thoracic aorta, superior and inferior venae cavae, azygos vein, splanchnic nerves, the heart, and the lungs

Connections: Retropharyngeal space, pretracheal space, space of the carotid sheath, and danger space #4

Signs and symptoms: Pleural and pericardial effusions (tamponade), aspiration pneumonia, bronchial erosion, pyopneumothorax, purulent pericarditis, and esophageal necrosis and rupture

Approach: Drainage of the mediastinum can be achieved via numerous approaches depending on which compartments are involved. Access to the mediastinum includes the transcervical, the median sternotomy, and the posterolateral thoracotomy approaches (Figure 10.34). The transcervical approach involves an incision anterior and parallel to the anterior border of the SCM muscle and is extended across the midline anteriorly, over the suprasternal notch. If necessary, tracheotomy tube placement can be incorporated within this incision. The superior portion of the incision is used to drain involved spaces to include the lateral pharyngeal space, the retropharyngeal space, the pretracheal space, and the space of the carotid sheath. At the inferior extent of the incision (overlying the suprasternal notch), the pretracheal space is entered, and blunt finger dissection proceeds substernally into the superior mediastinum to the level of the tracheal bifurcation. A posterior finger sweep is performed around the paraesophageal

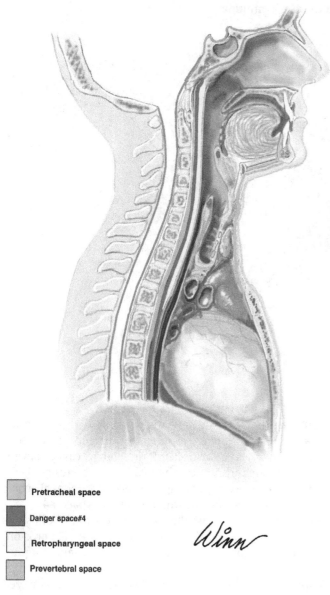

Pretracheal space

Danger space#4

Winn

Retropharyngeal space

Prevertebral space

Figure 10.35.   Sagittal view of the deep spaces of the neck.

structures. Finger dissection continues posterior to the esophagus, the alar fascia is penetrated, and danger space 4 is entered. The superior division of the mediastinum can be effectively explored to the level of T-4. After drainage, debridement, and irrigation, soft silicone rubber suction drains are placed to avoid erosion of vital structures. Drains are placed to closed suction. Thoracotomy tubes may be inserted to rule out empyema. The median sternotomy approach (Figure 10.34) involves a vertical incision from the sternal notch to the xiphoid process. The sternum is divided and spread to allow access to both the right and left thorax. The pleura is opened in its anteromedial aspect. This approach is used for infections involving the anterior mediastinum. The posterolateral thoracotomy approach

(Figure 10.34) involves placing the patient in a lateral decubitus position. An incision is made obliquely between the spinous processes and the medial border of the scapula inferiorly to approximately one finger breadth below and in front of the tip of the scapula. The latissimus dorsi muscle may be divided; however, many surgeons prefer to spare this muscle and mobilize its lateral and inferior edge to facilitate additional exposure. The serratus anterior muscle is typically not divided, but is simply mobilized along its lateral border. The chest is entered through the fifth intercostal space. The posterior portion of the sixth rib is often divided to facilitate exposure and to minimize the risk of breaking the rib. This approach is used for infections involving the posterior mediastinum.

Key Points

1. The overwhelming majority of cases of oropharyngeal mediastinitis originate from retropharyngeal and peritonsillar abscesses, are polymicrobial in nature, and involve both aerobic and anaerobic bacteria.
2. In patients with descending mediastinitis from odontogenic origin, the spread of the infection begins at a level superior to the hyoid bone. Drains are placed into all involved spaces and extend from the skull base to the mediastinum. Skin edges are loosely closed to allow for additional drainage.
3. Treatment of descending mediastinitis involves early and aggressive surgical drainage, definitive airway management, and intravenous broad-spectrum antibiotic therapy directed at both aerobic and anaerobic bacteria.
4. The transcervical approach allows access to the superior division of the mediastinum only. Once the infection has extended beyond the retropharyngeal space, involves the posterior mediastinum, or spreads inferior to the level of T-4 or tracheal bifurcation, the transcervical approach should be combined with transthoracic drainage. In general, there should be a low threshold for combining transcervical and transthoracic exploration.
5. Patients who have undergone previous transcervical mediastinum drainage and who develop sepsis or fail to improve should undergo prompt transthoracic drainage.
6. The median sternotomy allows for drainage of infections that have spread inferior to the carina or the T-4 level and involve the anterior mediastinum. The posterolateral thoracotomy allows for drainage of infections that involve the posterior mediastinum.
7. Postoperative spiral CT scans of the head and chest with contrast should be used to evaluate drain placement. Additional drainage procedures are required in patients with undrained purulence, in patients whose purulent collections reaccumulate

Periorbital Spaces

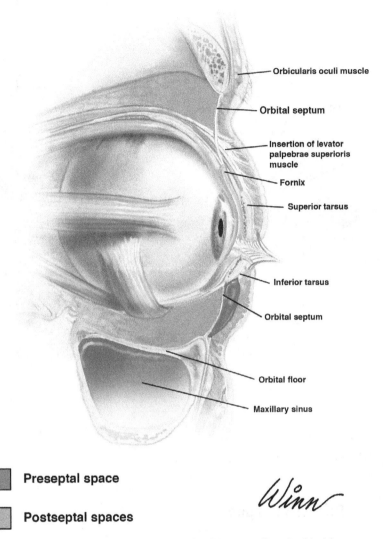

— Orbicularis oculi muscle

— Orbital septum

— Insertion of levator palpebrae superioris muscle

— Fornix

— Superior tarsus

— Inferior tarsus

— Orbital septum

— Orbital floor

— Maxillary sinus

◼ **Preseptal space**

◻ **Postseptal spaces**

Winn

Figure 10.36.   Sagittal view of the periorbital (preseptal) and orbital (postseptal) spaces.

and in patients whose clinical symptoms fail to improve.

Periorbital Space (Preseptal Space)

Boundaries

Superior: The periosteal attachment of the orbicularis oculi muscle

Inferior: The periosteal attachment of the orbicularis oculi muscle

Anterior: Orbicularis oculi muscle

Posterior: Orbital septum

Lateral: The periosteal attachment of the orbicularis oculi muscle

Medial: The periosteal attachment of the orbicularis oculi muscle

Contents: Fat and areolar connective tissue

Connections: Canine space and orbital space

Signs and symptoms: Periorbital edema and ecchymosis

Approach: Drainage of the lower lid is achieved via an intraoral approach. An incision is placed within the maxillary buccal vestibule. Blunt dissection proceeds cephalically through the canine space (Figure 10.1) to the orbital rim. The periorbital space is entered with a hemostat and explored. A dependent drain is placed and exits through the transoral incision. The preseptal space may also be approached via the orbital space. (See the "Orbital Space" section.)

Orbital Space

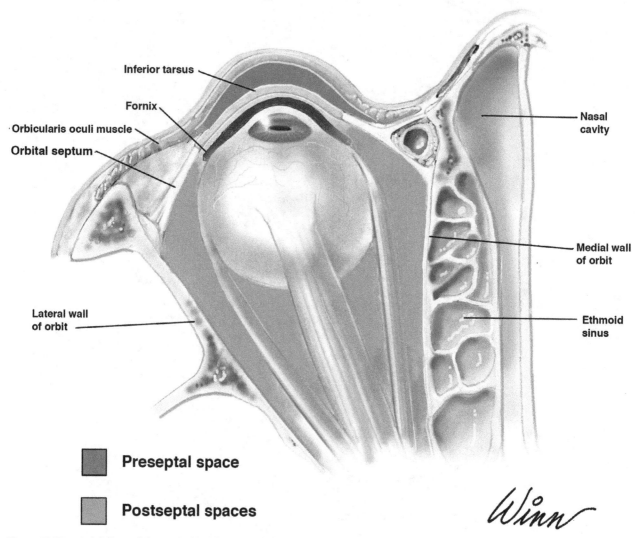

Inferior tarsus

Fornix

Orbicularis oculi muscle

Orbital septum

Nasal cavity

Medial wall of orbit

Lateral wall of orbit

Ethmoid sinus

■ **Preseptal space**

■ **Postseptal spaces**

Winn

Figure 10.37. Axial view of the periorbital (preseptal) and orbital (postseptal) spaces.

Key Points

1. Infections of the periorbital space are most commonly from contiguous spread from the canine space.
2. Periorbital space infections require urgent drainage to avoid spread to the cavernous sinus.

Orbital Space (Postseptal Space)

Boundaries

Superior: Bony orbit
Inferior: Bony orbit
Anterior: Orbital septum
Posterior: Bony orbit
Lateral: Bony orbit

Medial: Bony orbit
Contents: Orbital contents (Figures 10.36 and 10.37)
Connections: Paranasal sinuses, cavernous sinus, periorbital space, and the infratemporal space
Signs and symptoms: Proptosis, superior orbital fissure syndrome (CN III, IV, V1, and VI, and ophthalmic veins), and orbital apex syndrome (CN II, III, IV, V1, and VI)
Approach: Drainage is achieved via a lateral canthotomy with posterior dissection along the orbital floor and orbital walls.

Key Points

Infections of the orbital space frequently originate from paranasal sinusitis.

References

Bullock, J.D. and Fleishman, J.A., 1985. The spread of odontogenic infections to the orbit: diagnosis and management. *Journal of Oral and Maxillofacial Surgery*, 43, 749–55.

Caccamese, J.F. and Coletti, D.P., 2008. Deep neck infections: clinical considerations in aggressive disease. *Oral and Maxillofacial Surgery Clinics of North America*, 20, 367–80.

Carrau, R.L., Cintron, F.R. and Astor, F., 1990. Transcervical approaches to the prevertebral space. *Archives of Otolaryngology—Head and Neck Surgery*, 116, 1070–73.

Dzyak W.R. and Zide, M.F., 1984. Diagnosis and treatment of lateral pharyngeal space infections. *Journal of Oral and Maxillofacial Surgery*, 42, 243–9.

Flynn, T.R., 1994. Anatomy and surgery of deep fascial space infections of the head and neck. In: J.P.W.Kelly, ed. *Oral and maxillofacial surgery knowledge update*. Vol. 1. Rosemont, IL: American Association of Oral and Maxillofacial Surgeons.

Flynn, T.R., 2000. Surgical management of orofacial infections. *Atlas of Oral and Maxillofacial Surgery Clinics of North America*, 8, 77–100.

Gaughran, G.R.L., 1957. Fascia of the masticator space. *Anatomical Record*, 129, 383–400.

Granite, E.L., 1976. Anatomic considerations in infections of the face and neck: review of the literature. *Journal of Oral Surgery*, 34, 31–4.

Grodinsky, M., 1939. Retropharyngeal and lateral pharyngeal abscesses: an anatomic and clinical study. *Annals of Surgery*, 110, 177–99.

Grodinsky, M. and Holyoke, E., 1938. The fasciae and fascial spaces of the head, neck, and adjacent regions. *American Journal of Anatomy*, 63, 367–408.

Haug, R.H., Wible, R.T. and Lieberman, J., 1991. Measurement standards for the prevertebral region in the lateral soft-tissue radiograph on the neck. *Journal of Oral and Maxillofacial Surgery*, 49, 1149–51.

Hollinshead, W.H., 1982. *Anatomy for surgeons, 1: the head and neck*. 3rd ed. Philadelphia: Harper & Row.

Jayasekera, B.A.P., Dale, O.T. and Corbridge, R.C., 2012. Descending necrotizing mediastinitis: a case report illustrating a trend in conservative management. *Case Reports in Otolaryngology*, 2012, 1–4.

Jones, J.L. and Candelaria, L.M., 2000. Head and neck infections. In: R.J. Fonseca, T.P. Williams, and J.C.B. Stewart, eds. *Oral and maxillofacial surgery: surgical pathology*. Philadelphia: W.B. Saunders.

Kinzer, S., Pfeiffer, J., Becker, S. and Ridder, G.J., 2009. Severe deep neck space infections and mediastinitis of odontogenic origin: clinical relevance and implications for diagnosis and treatment. *Acta Oto-Laryngologica*, 129, 62–70.

Landa, L.E., Tartan, B.F., Acartuk, A., Skouteris, C.A., Gordon, C. and Sotereanos, G.C., 2003. The transcervical incision for use in oral and maxillofacial surgical procedures. *Journal of Oral and Maxillofacial Surgery*, 61, 343–46.

Laskin, D.M., 1964. Anatomic considerations in diagnosis and treatment of odontogenic infections. *Journal of the American Dental Association*, 69, 308–16.

Lazlow, S.K., 2000. Necrotizing fasciitis and mediastinitis. *Atlas of Oral and Maxillofacial Surgery Clinics of North America*, 8, 101–19.

Levine, T.M., Wurster, C.F. and Krespi, Y.P., 1986. Mediastinitis occurring as a complication of odontogenic infections. *Laryngoscope*, 96, 747–50.

Levitt, G.W., 1970. Cervical fascia and deep neck infections. *Laryngoscope*, 80, 409–35.

Levitt, G.W., 1970. The surgical treatment of deep neck infections. *Laryngoscope*, 81, 403–11.

Limongelli, W.A., Clark, M.S. and Williams, A.C., 1977. Panfacial cellulitis with contralateral orbital cellulitis and blindness after tooth extraction. *Journal of Oral Surgery*, 35, 38–43.

Lypka, M. and Hammoudeh, J., 2011. Dentoalveolar infections. *Oral and Maxillofacial Surgery Clinics of North America*, 23, 415–24.

McGurk, M., 2003. Diagnosis and treatment of necrotizing fasciitis in the head and neck region. *Oral and Maxillofacial Surgery Clinics of North America*, 15, 59–67.

Mihos, P, Potaris, K., Gakidis, I., Papadakis, D. and Rallis, G., 2004. Management of descending necrotizing mediastinitis. *Journal of Oral and Maxillofacial Surgery*, 62, 966–72.

Mitz, V. and Peyronie, M., 1976. The superficial musculoaponeurotic system (SMAS) in the parotid and cheek area. *Plastic and Reconstructive Surgery*, 58, 80–88.

Moncada, R., Warpeha, R., Pickleman, J., Spak, M., Cardoso, M., Berkow, A. and White, H., 1978. Mediastinitis from odontogenic and deep cervical infection: atomic pathways of propagation. *Chest*, 73, 497–500.

Mosher, H., 1929. The submaxillary fossa approach to deep pus in the neck. *Transactions of the Annual Meeting of the American Academy of Ophthalmology and Otolaryngology*, 34, 19–36.

O'Ryan, F., Diloreto, A., Barber, D. and Bruckner, R., 1988. Orbital infections: clinical and radiographic diagnosis and surgical treatment. *Journal of Oral and Maxillofacial Surgery*, 46, 991–97.

Osborn, T.M., Assael, L.A. and Bell, R.B., 2008. Deep space neck infection: principles of surgical management. *Oral and Maxillofacial Surgery Clinics of North America*, 20, 353–65.

Peterson, L.J., 1993. Contemporary management of deep infections of the neck. *Journal of Oral and Maxillofacial Surgery*, 51, 226–31.

Potter, J.K., Herford, A.S. and Ellis, E., 2002. Tracheotomy versus endotracheal intubation for airway management in deep neck space infections. *Journal of Oral and Maxillofacial Surgery*, 60, 349–54.

Reynolds, S.C. and Chow, A.W., 2007. Life-threatening infections of the peripharyngeal and deep fascial spaces of the head and neck. *Infectious Disease Clinics of North America*, 21, 567–76.

Roccia, F., Pecorari, G.C., Oliorio, A., Passet, E., Rossi, P., Nadalin, J., Garzino-Demo, P. and Berrone, S., 2007. Ten years of descending necrotizing mediastinitis: management of 23 cases. *Journal of Oral and Maxillofacial Surgery*, 65, 1716–24.

Sarna, T., Sengupta, T., Miloro, M. and Kolokythas, A., 2012. Cervical necrotizing fasciitis with descending mediastinitis: literature review and case report. *Journal of Oral and Maxillofacial Surgery*, 70, 1342–50.

Sicher, H. and DuBrul, E.L., 1975. *Oral Anatomy*. 6th ed. St. Louis, MO: Mosby.

Som, P.M. and Curtin, H.D., 2011. Fascia and spaces of the head and neck. In: P.M. Som and H.D. Curtin, eds. *Head and neck imaging*. 5th ed. St. Louis, MO: Mosby.

Som, P.M. and Curtin, H.D., 2011. Parapharyngeal and masticator space lesions. In: P.M. Som and H.D. Curtin, eds. *Head and neck imaging*. 5th ed. St. Louis, MO: Mosby.

Spilka, C.J., 1966. Pathways of dental infections. *Journal of Oral Surgery*, 24, 111–24.

Stuzin, J.M., Wagstrom, L., Kawamoto, H.K. and Wolfe, S.A., 1989. Anatomy of the frontal branch of the facial nerve: the significance of the temporal fat pad. *Plastic and Reconstructive Surgery*, 83, 266–71.

Tagliareni, J.M. and Clarkson, E.I., 2012. Tonsillitis, peritonsillar and lateral pharyngeal abscesses. *Oral and Maxillofacial Surgery Clinics of North America*, 24, 197–204.

Topazian, R.G., Goldberg, M.H. and Hupp, J.R., 2002. *Oral and maxillofacial infections*. 4th ed. Philadelphia: W.B. Saunders.

Vieira, F., Allen, S.M., Stocks, R.M.S. and Thompson, J.W., 2008. Deep neck infection. *Otolaryngology Clinics of North America*, 41, 459–83.

Wheatley, M.J., Stirling, M.C., Kirsh, M.M., Gago, O. and Orringer, M.B. 1990. Descending necrotizing mediastinitis: transcervical drainage is not enough. *Annals of Thoracic Surgery*, 49, 780–84.

11 Osteomyelitis

Matthew W. Hearn,[1] Christopher T. Vogel,[2] Robert M. Laughlin,[3] and Christopher J. Haggerty[4]

[1]Private Practice, Valparaiso, Indiana, USA
[2]Department of Oral and Maxillofacial Surgery, University of Missouri–Kansas City, Kansas City, Missouri, USA
[3]Department of Oral and Maxillofacial Surgery, Naval Medical Center San Diego, San Diego, California, USA
[4]Private Practice, Lakewood Oral and Maxillofacial Surgery Specialists, Lees Summit; and Department of Oral and Maxillofacial Surgery, University of Missouri-Kansas City, Kansas City, Missouri, USA

Osteomyelitis: Inflammation of the osseous medulla.

General Principles of Management of Osteomyelitis (Acute and Chronic)

1. A definitive diagnosis of osteomyelitis can only be made via bone biopsy with histopathological examination and staining, and microbiologic culture (including *actinomyces* and *nocardia*) and sensitivities.
2. All forms of osteomyelitis are managed with a combination of removal of the source of the infection, bone removal or resection to healthy, bleeding bone margins, reestablishment of blood flow to the involved area, and antibiotic therapy.
3. All potential sources of infection are eradicated. Decayed and mobile teeth within the involved area should be extracted, all fixation plates and screws should be removed, and intraoral and cutaneous fistulae are resected.
4. All necrotic and involved bone must be completely removed to expose healthy bleeding bone. Bone that does not freely bleed from its marrow cavity is avascular bone, will interfere with antibiotic penetration of the involved area, will serve as a nidus for future infections, and will prevent adequate blood flow to the involved area. The removal of involved bone will frequently lead to continuity defects.
5. Initial antibiotic coverage includes broad-spectrum antibiotics with both aerobic and anaerobic coverage.
6. Bone biopsy culture and sensitivities will ultimately guide antibiotic selection.
7. Cases that do not respond to initial surgical debridement and antibiotic therapy require more aggressive surgical intervention, the extraction of adjacent teeth, infectious disease consultation, and peripherally inserted central catheter (PICC) line placement for long-term intravenous antibiotic management.
8. Due to the inflammatory nature of osteomyelitis, anti-inflammatory medications such as nonsteroidal anti-inflammatory drugs and corticosteroids are beneficial in the management of symptoms both before and after surgical intervention.

Acute osteomyelitis: Clinical symptoms present for less than 4 weeks. Radiographic findings are typically absent.

Chronic osteomyelitis: Clinical symptoms present for 4 weeks or longer. Commonly has radiographic findings. Subclassifications include suppurative and non-suppurative forms.

Clinical symptoms of osteomyelitis: Pain, edema, mobile teeth, suppuration, induration, paresthesia or anesthesia, tissue erythema, and exposed bone (Figure 11.1). Acute osteomyelitis frequently presents as a facial abscess with symptoms specific to the space involved (i.e., trismus).

Radiographic findings of osteomyelitis: Altered areas of bone density, including areas of osteosclerosis, osteolysis, periosteal reaction (periostitis ossificans), sequestrum, and cortical and trabecular defects (see Figures 11.2, 11.3, 11.4, and 11.5).

Surgical Treatment Options for Osteomyelitis

Saucerization

Saucerization involves the removal of involved bone to expose the medullary cavity and the smoothing of surrounding bone.

Saucerization Technique

1. This procedure may be performed under local or general anesthesia.
2. Mobile teeth and loose segments of bone are removed.
3. The exposed or involved bone is removed with a combination of a ronguer and a round bur. The depth of the saucerization terminates within bleeding bone marrow. All margins should involve healthy, bleeding bone. All removed segments of bone and tissue are sent for histopathologic examination.

Atlas of Operative Oral and Maxillofacial Surgery, First Edition. Edited by Christopher J. Haggerty and Robert M. Laughlin
© 2015 John Wiley & Sons, Inc. Published 2015 by John Wiley & Sons, Inc.

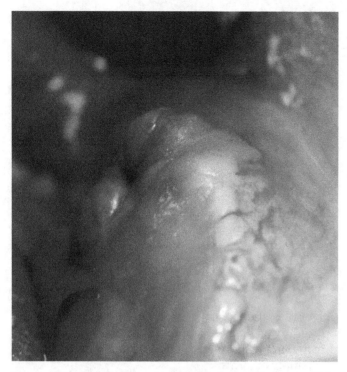

Figure 11.1.   Suppurative osteomyelitis of the anterior mandible. Note fistula formation, edema, and overlying tissue erythema.

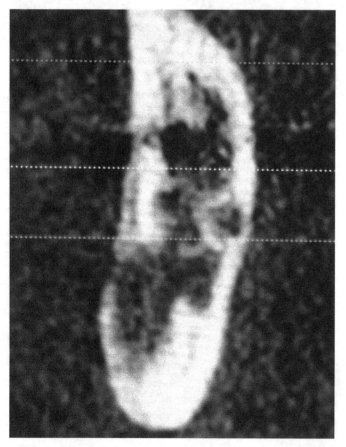

Figure 11.3.   Coronal cone beam computed tomography scan demonstrating alternating areas of osteosclerosis and osteolysis of the posterior mandible.

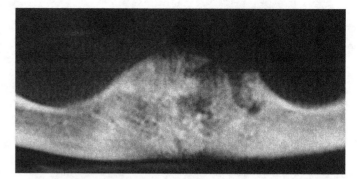

Figure 11.2.   Cone beam computed tomography scan of the patient in Figure 11.1. Radiograph demonstrates areas of osteolysis and trabecular defects within the anterior mandible.

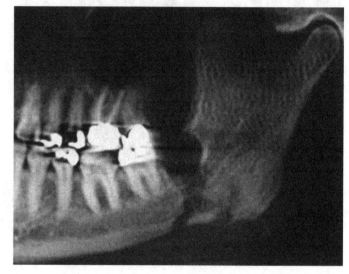

Figure 11.4.   Orthopantomogram of the left posterior mandible demonstrating areas of cortical defects and osteolysis extending to the inferior border.

4. All bony edges are smoothed, and the surgical site is copiously irrigated.
5. The surgical site is packed with ribbon gauze. The gauze is changed every 2–3 days in order to stimulate the formation of a healthy tissue bed with eventual epithelization of the surgical site.

Key Points

1. Saucerization is the most conservative form of surgical treatment for osteomyelitis and, as such, has the highest recurrence rate.
2. Saucerization is only indicated for relatively superficial forms of osteomyelitis.

Decortication

Decortication involves the removal of the involved cortical bone to expose the underlying inflamed marrow.

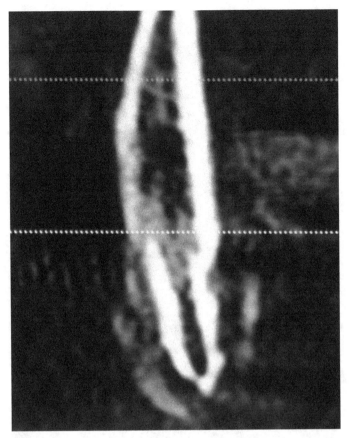

Figure 11.5. Coronal cone beam computed tomography scan of the patient in Figure 11.4 demonstrating a periosteal reaction associated with osteomyelitis of the posterior mandible.

Decortication Technique

1. The procedure is typically performed under general anesthesia.
2. An intraoral incision with a buccal release is placed over the area of involved bone. A full-thickness mucoperiosteal tissue flap is elevated to gain wide surgical access to the affected area. If the lingual plate is uninvolved, the lingual periosteal attachment is preserved to allow blood supply to the lingual cortex.
3. Loose segments of bone and adjacent, involved, and mobile teeth are removed.
4. Curettes are used to remove nonviable, inflammatory, and necrotic soft tissue.
5. A ronguer is used to remove the involved cortices of the mandible. Curettes are used to remove involved marrow.
6. A round bur with copious irrigation is used to remove any sharp or irregular pieces of bone and to remove all necrotic bone. Bone removal is complete when all margins are within healthy bleeding bone. All removed bone and tissue are sent for histopathological evaluation and culture and sensitivities.
7. The surgical site is copiously irrigated.
8. The tissue is closed around the defect in a tension-free manner to allow for complete coverage of the surgical site.

1. Decortication may be achieved through either an intraoral or extraoral approach. Intraoral approaches are preferred for areas involving the alveolar crest or lateral cortex of the mandible and for patients with intraoral fistulae. Extraoral approaches are preferred for areas involving the inferior cortex of the mandible and for percutaneous fistulae. Fistulectomies are performed at the time of decortication.
2. All margins should be within bleeding bone in order to ensure complete removal of necrotic bone and to stimulate blood flow to the surgical site.
3. The tension-free closure of the surgical site will allow coverage of the surgical site with vascularized tissue (muscle and mucosa), which will transform into periosteum and aid in the blood supply to the area.
4. Depending on the extent of bone removal, a period of maxillomandibular fixation (MMF) may be required to prevent pathologic fracture. It is not advised to place internal fixation to the surgical site.
5. During decortication procedures involving the inferior third of the mandible, it is important to be cognizant of the inferior alveolar nerve.

Resection involves the removal of significant hard tissue (cortical bone and marrow) resulting in sizable hard tissue defects.

Resection Technique

1. This procedure is performed under general anesthesia.
2. Wide surgical access of the involved bone is obtained via either an intraoral approach or a combined intraoral-extraoral approach. Fistulae are incorporated into the incision design and excised.
3. Involved bone is resected to areas of healthy, bleeding bone.
4. Involved teeth are removed en bloc within the surgical specimen.
5. Complete tissue coverage is obtained over the resected site.
6. For marginal resections placing the mandible at risk for pathologic fracture, a period of MMF is employed. For continuity defects, the segments are stabilized prior to definitive reconstruction with either MMF or external skeletal fixation.

1. Hard tissue defects are reconstructed after a 4–6-month symptom-free period.
2. Immediate reconstruction is not recommended due to the decreased vascular supply of the recipient tissue bed and the potential for recurrence of the infection.

Case Report

Case Report 11.1. A 13-year-old patient presents with a chief complaint of recurrent swelling to his left posterior mandible 5 weeks after the extraction of teeth #29–31 due to tooth mobility, infection, and pain. The patient with a medical history significant for multiple autoimmune disorders. The patient's medication list consisted of infliximab, methotrexate, and prednisone for severe bouts of Crohn's disease requiring frequent hospitalizations. The patient was initially treated with the extraction of mobile and symptomatic teeth, an incision and drainage procedure, a bone and tissue biopsy, cultures and sensitivities, infectious disease consultation, and weight-appropriate intravenous Unasyn (ampicillin-sulbactam) (Phizer Inc, New York, USA). Based on cultures and sensitivity results, the patient was continued on inpatient intravenous Unasyn and outpatient oral Augmentin (amoxicillin-clavulanic acid) (GlaxoSmith Kline, Brentford, London, UK). The patient underwent an uneventful postoperative course and was followed closely for several asymptomatic postoperative appointments until he developed a recurrent swelling some 5 weeks postoperatively. An orthopantomogram (Figure 11.6) was taken that demonstrated an inconsistent appearance of the bone of the left posterior mandible. A computed tomography scan was obtained that depicted distinct areas of altered bone density to include areas of osteosclerosis and osteolysis (Figures 11.7 and 11.8) of the left posterior mandible, including the parasymphysis, body, angle, ascending ramus, condyle, and coronoid process. The glenoid fossa and the skull base were free from radiographic abnormalities. The patient was taken to the operating room for a deep bone biopsy. At the time of deep bone biopsy, drains were placed for irrigation of the posterior mandible. Bone biopsy results confirmed the diagnosis of osteomyelitis, and cultures and sensitivities suggested that Unasyn was an appropriate antibiotic for the causative bacteria. The patient was taken to the operating room for lateral nerve repositioning (Figure 11.10; see also Figures 11.9 and 11.11) and for the removal of all necrotic and involved bone. A PICC line was placed for the administration of long-term antibiotics, and a drain was left in place for 1 week postoperatively for continued irrigation of the site (Figure 11.12). Definitive reconstruction of the mandibular defect will be undertaken after complete resolution of the infection.

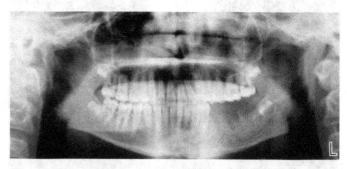

Figure 11.6. Orthopantomogram taken 5 weeks post extraction of mobile teeth #29–31 and incision and drainage procedure. The orthopantomogram depicts areas of altered bone density.

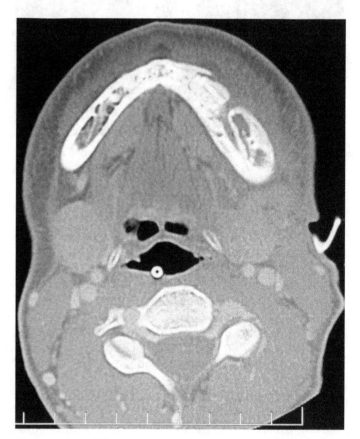

Figure 11.7. Axial computed tomography scan demonstrating the involved left posterior mandible with areas of alternating osteosclerosis and osteolysis.

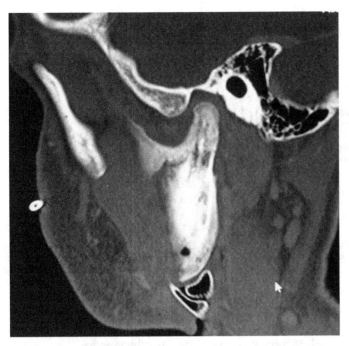

Figure 11.8. Sagittal computed tomography scan demonstrating the involved left posterior ascending ramus, condyle, and coronoid process. Irrigation drains are in place at the inferior border of the angle of the mandible.

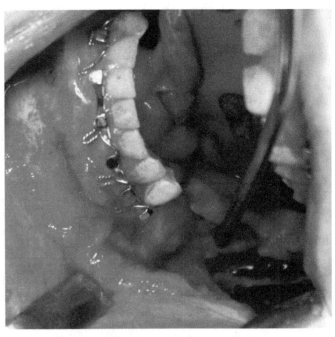

Figure 11.9. The left posterior mandible is exposed via an intraoral incision. All involved sclerotic and avascular bone is removed until normal, bleeding bone is encountered.

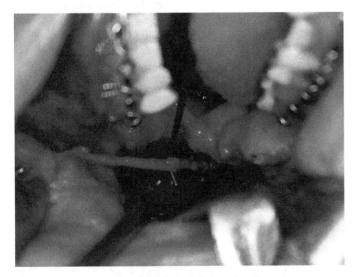

Figure 11.10. Lateralization of the inferior alveolar nerve.

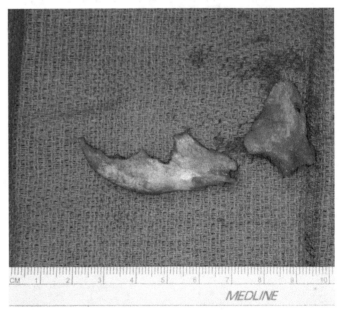

Figure 11.11. Involved sclerotic and avascular bone from the inferior border of the left mandible and the coronoid process.

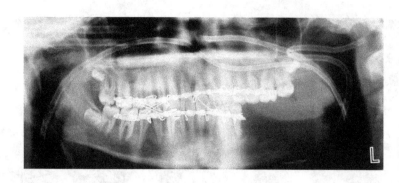

Figure 11.12. Postoperative ortho-pantomogram showing a left hemi-mandiblectomy with irrigation drains in place.

An antibiotic chart can be found in Appendix 1 for reference.

References

An, C.H., An, S.Y., Choi, B.R., Huh, K.H., Heo, M.S., Yi, W.J., Lee, S.S. and Choi, S.C., 2012. Hard and soft tissue changes of osteomyelitis of the jaws on CT images. *Oral Surgery, Oral Medicine, Oral Pathology, Oral Radiology, and Endodontology*, 114, 118–26.

Baltensperger, M.M. and Eyrich, G.K., 2009. Osteomyelitis therapy – general considerations and surgical therapy. In: M.M. Baltensperger and G.K. Eyrich, eds. *Osteomyelitis of the Jaws*. Leipzig: Springer.

Bevin, C.R., Inwards, C.Y. and Keller, E.E., 2008. Surgical management of primary chronic osteomyelitis: a long-term retrospective analysis. *Journal of Oral and Maxillofacial Surgery*, 66, 2073–85.

Goldberg, M.H., 2003. Diagnosis and treatment of cervicofacial actinomycosis. *Oral and Maxillofacial Surgery Clinics of North America*, 15, 51–58.

Koorbusch, G.F. and Deatherage, J.R., 2011. How can we diagnose and treat osteomyelitis of the jaws as early as possible? *Oral and Maxillofacial Surgery Clinics of North America*, 23, 557–67.

Krakowiak, P.A., 2011. Alveolar osteitis and osteomyelitis of the jaws. *Oral and Maxillofacial Surgery Clinics of North America*, 23, 401–13.

Kushner, G.M. and Alpert, B., 2004. Osteomyelitis and osteoradionecrosis. In: M. Miloro, G.E. Ghali, P. Larsen and P. Waite, eds. *Peterson's Principles of Oral and Maxillofacial Surgery*. 2nd ed. Shelton: Peoples Medical Publishing House.

Marx, R.E., 1991. Chronic osteomyelitis of the jaws. *Oral and Maxillofacial Surgery Clinics of North America*, 3, 367–81.

Montonen, M. and Lindqvist, C., 2003. Diagnosis and treatment of diffuse sclerosing osteomyelitis of the jaws. *Oral and Maxillofacial Surgery Clinics of North America*, 15, 69–78.

Sharkawy, A.A., 2007. Cervicofacial actinomycosis and mandibular osteomyelitis. *Infectious Disease Clinics of North America*, 21, 543–56.

Topazian, R.G., Goldberg M.H. and Hupp J.R., 2002. *Oral and Maxillofacial Infections*. 4th ed. Philadelphia: W.B. Saunders.

Wallace-Hudsom, J., 2000. Osteomyelitis and osteoradionecrosis. In: R.J. Fonseca, T.P. Williams and J.C.B. Stewart, eds. *Oral and Maxillofacial Surgery: Surgical Pathology*. Philadelphia: W.B. Saunders.

PART THREE

MAXILLOFACIAL TRAUMA SURGERY

12 Surgical Management of the Airway

Christopher J. Haggerty

Private Practice, Lakewood Oral and Maxillofacial Surgery Specialists, Lees Summit; and Department of Oral and Maxillofacial Surgery, University of Missouri–Kansas City Kansas City, Missouri, USA

Surgical Cricothyrotomy

An emergent airway when other methods of securing an airway have failed or are not possible.

Indications

When an acute emergent airway is indicated and oral and nasal intubation devices are not available or are not possible due to a mechanical airway obstruction such as an expanding hematoma, hypopharyngeal obstruction, angioedema, retropharyngeal abscess, or laryngeal edema.

Contraindications

1. Pediatric patients under the age of 10. In pediatric patients, surgical cricothyrotomy can damage the cricoid cartilage and lead to subglottic stenosis
2. Relative contraindications include complete or partial transection of the airway, laryngeal fracture and injury to the cricoid cartilage

Anatomy

Cricothyroid space: The cricothyroid space is located between the inferior border of the thyroid cartilage and the superior border of the cricoid cartilage. The cricothyroid space spans 20–30 mm in its horizontal dimension and 8–10 mm in its vertical dimension. Within this space lies the cricothyroid membrane (Figure 12.1). There are no large vessels, glandular structures, or complex fascial or muscular layers overlying the cricothyroid membrane.

Cricothyrotomy Landmarks

1. The greater prominence of the thyroid cartilage
2. The lesser prominence of the cricoid cartilage
3. Between these two landmarks is the cricothyroid space.

Cricothyrotomy Layers

1. Skin
2. Subcutaneous tissue
3. Cervical fascia
4. Cricothyroid membrane

Surgical Cricothyrotomy Technique

1. The patient is positioned with hyperextension of the neck (if no cervical spine injuries) for better visualization of the thyroid and cricoid cartilages.
2. The skin is prepped, and local anesthetic containing a vasoconstrictor is injected to aid in pain control and hemostasis. Avoid excessive local anesthetic as this will obscure landmarks.
3. If time permits, transtracheal injections are performed to decrease cough reflex (for an awake patient).
4. With the nondominant hand, stabilize the thyroid cartilage between the thumb and middle finger, and palpate the cricothyroid space with the index finger. With the dominant hand, make a 3–4 cm vertical midline incision over the inferior portion of the thyroid cartilage extending inferiorly to the inferior border of the cricoid cartilage (see Figure 12.2 in Case Report 12.1). A vertical incision is utilized in an emergent situation to decrease the risk of vascular injury and to decrease the operating time from the skin to the cricothyroid membrane. The incision extends through the skin, subcutaneous tissue, and cervical fascia to the thyroid and cricoid cartilage, exposing the cricothyroid membrane. The thumb and middle finger are used to apply a slight downward pressure to separate the skin edges after the incision. The incision should be made in a single, continuous swipe. If arterial bleeding is encountered, suspect the cricothyroid branches of the superior thyroid artery, which enter the cricothyroid membrane superiorly.
5. Incise through the cricothyroid membrane in a horizontal manner, and place a scalpel handle or scissors/hemostat to enlarge the cricothyrotomy opening (Figure 12.3, Case Report 12.1).
6. Place a pediatric uncuffed tracheotomy tube or lubricated tracheotomy tube (Shiley number 4) into the trachea through the cricothyroid space (Figure 12.4, Case Report 12.1).

Atlas of Operative Oral and Maxillofacial Surgery, First Edition. Edited by Christopher J. Haggerty and Robert M. Laughlin

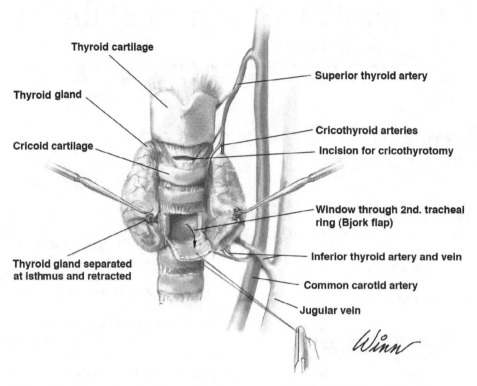

Thyroid cartilage

Thyroid gland

Cricoid cartilage

Superior thyroid artery

Cricothyroid arteries

Incision for cricothyrotomy

Window through 2nd. tracheal ring (Bjork flap)

Thyroid gland separated at isthmus and retracted

Inferior thyroid artery and vein

Common carotid artery

Jugular vein

Winn

Figure 12.1.   Illustration depicting trachea anatomy and the ideal locations of cricothyrotomy and tracheotomy placement.

7. Attach the anesthesia circuit, check for end-tidal CO_2, and perform bilateral chest auscultation.
8. Secure the tube to the skin with sutures and a cloth tie around the neck, or convert the cricothyrotomy to an open tracheotomy. Do not close the skin incision as this can lead to subcutaneous emphysema.

Complications

Cricothyrotomy complications coincide with tracheotomy complications.

Key Points

1. With any emergent surgical airway procedure, a midline vertical incision allows for faster access to the trachea and minimizes the risk of arterial and venous bleeding.
2. There is no definitive evidence to support the conversion of a cricothyrotomy to a tracheotomy. Because most cricothyrotomies are performed in acute obstructive situations (anaphylactic edema, expanding hematoma, and abscess formation), the need for prolonged mechanical ventilation is often unnecessary.
3. A true surgical cricothyrotomy is contraindicated in children under the age of 10 years or in patients who weigh less than 40 kg. In pediatric emergent

airway situations, a needle cricothyrotomy should be utilized. There are numerous commercial needle cricothyrotomy kits available. Some utilize 12–14-gauge needles that can be inserted directly into the cricothyroid space and attached to a jet ventilation apparatus. Other kits allow for the placement of a needle into the cricothyroid space and allow for the changing of a specific catheter over a guide wire. All needle cricothyrotomies need to be converted to a definitive airway immediately as they are highly unstable due to dislodgement of the needle and loss of the airway.

References

DiGiacomo, C.J., Neshat, K., Angus, L.D.G., Simpkins, C.O., Sadoff, R.S. and Shaftan, G.W., 2003. Emergency cricothyrotomy. *Military Medicine*, 168, 541–4.

Hart, K.L. and Thompson, S.H., 2010. Emergency cricothyrotomy. *Oral and Maxillofacial Surgery Clinics of North America*, 18, 29–38.

Macdonald, J.C. and Tien, H.C.N., 2008. Emergency battlefield cricothyrotomy. *Canadian Medical Association Journal*, 178, 1133–5.

OMFS Knowledge Update. Available from http://www.aaoms.org/members/meetings-and-continuing-education/oms-knowledge-update/

Case Report 12.1. Patient presents with impending airway obstruction due to expanding floor-of-mouth hematoma after a gunshot wound to the anterior mandible.

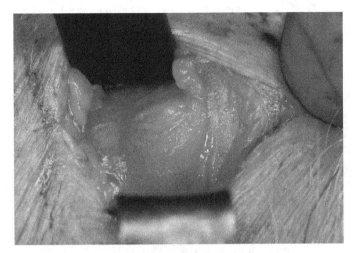

Figure 12.2.   A 3–4 cm vertical midline incision is initiated over the inferior portion of the thyroid cartilage and extended caudally to the cricoid cartilage.

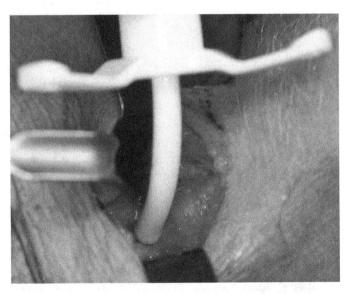

Figure 12.4.   An airway device is inserted into the cricothyroid space.

Tracheotomy

A definitive surgical airway for utilization in both emergent and non-emergent (elective) situations.

Indications

1. Upper airway obstruction (edema, expanding hematomas, infections, and facial trauma resulting in mechanical airway obstruction)
2. Significant facial injuries requiring maxillomandibular fixation (MMF) when nasal intubation is

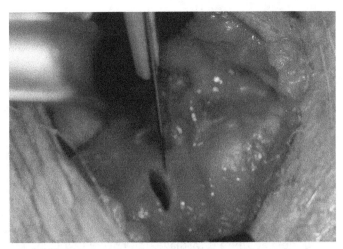

Figure 12.3.   The cricothyroid membrane is identified between the thyroid and cricoid cartilages. A #15 blade is used to penetrate the cricothyroid membrane, and an osteum is created.

contraindicated (ie. combined mandibular and NOE type fractures)
3. Head and neck tumor patients
4. Inability to intubate
5. Prolonged intubation or positive ventilation requirements
6. Failure to wean from mechanical ventilation
7. Loss of normal laryngeal function as a result of trauma or oncologic surgery
8. Pulmonary insufficiency from either acute or chronic respiratory failure
9. Severe obstructive sleep apnea

Contraindications

1. There are no absolute contraindications for tracheostomy
2. Relative contraindications include tracheal infection and significant burn injuries

Anatomy

Tracheotomy Landmarks

1. The greater prominence of the thyroid cartilage
2. The lesser prominence of the cricoid cartilage
3. Sternal notch

Tracheotomy Layers

1. Skin
2. Subcutaneous tissue
3. Platysma muscle
4. The superficial (investing) layer of the deep cervical fascia, which splits to invest the SCM and trapezius muscles
5. The midline infrahyoid linea alba which is formed from the fusion of the superficial (investing) and the middle (pretracheal) cervical fasciae

6. The thyroid isthmus may be identified at the level of the second tracheal ring
7. The pretracheal (middle) layer of the deep cervical fascia which invests the infrahyoid (strap) muscles, thyroid gland, trachea and esophagus
8. Tracheal rings

Tracheotomy Procedure

1. The patient's head is placed in the midline of the table with cervical hyperextension (unless c-spine injury is suspected).
2. The patient is prepped and draped from the inferior mandible to a point several centimeters below the sternal notch.
3. A sterile marking pen is used to mark the inferior border of the thyroid cartilage, the cricoid cartilage, and the sternal notch.
4. A 3–4 cm horizontal line is drawn with a sterile marking pen 2 cm inferior to the cricoid cartilage or midway between the cricoid cartilage and the sternal notch (Figure 12.6). This line will represent the skin incision and corresponds to the level of the second and third tracheal rings.
5. Local anesthetic is injected under the horizontal line of the marker superficial to the platysma muscle. In an emergent situation with an awake patient, a transtracheal injection is used to decrease the cough reflex.
6. A 3–4 cm horizontal skin incision is placed over the horizontal line (Figure 12.7). The incision initially transverses skin, subcutaneous tissue and the platysma muscle (if present). Electrocautery is used for hemostasis of subcutaneous bleeding. In elective tracheotomy, a horizontal skin incision has the advantage of improved cosmesis following secondary revision. Excessive lateral extension of the incision can lead to severance of the anterior jugular veins. In an emergent tracheotomy, a midline vertical incision allow for faster access to the trachea and minimizes the chance of arterial and venous bleeding.
7. After transecting the platysma muscle, a vertical incision is performed through the superficial (investing) layer of the deep cervical fascia.
8. Loose connective tissue is retracted laterally, and the linea alba and strap muscles are identified.
9. Blunt dissection is carried through the midline avascular linea alba separating the strap muscles of the anterior neck until the thyroid isthmus and the pretracheal fascia are identified (Figure 12.8). If the thyroid isthmus is noted to cross over the second and third tracheal rings, it is divided with electrocautery. Failure to cauterize the transected thyroid isthmus can lead to postoperative bleeding. Failure to stay within the midline (within the avascular linea alba) during the initial dissection can result in muscle bleeding and lateral dissection of the trachea. The lateral sulcus between the trachea and esophagus contains the recurrent laryngeal nerves. Damage to this nerve results in impaired vocal cord function.
10. Kittner pledgets are used to remove the pretracheal fascia and to expose the cricoid cartilage and tracheal rings.
11. The tracheotomy cuff is lubricated and tested (inflated) prior to tracheal ring incision to ensure that the cuff works appropriately. Occasionally, the tracheotomy tube may be torn upon insertion into the trachea or may be too large for passive insertion into the surgical stoma. A second, smaller tracheotomy tube is always available as a backup.
12. A cricoid hook is used to engage and elevate the cricoid cartilage upward and superiorly to gain better visibility of the tracheal rings.
13. Prior to entering the trachea, it is paramount that the incision site is hemostatic in order to improve visualization and to minimize postoperative bleeding.
14. The anesthetic gases are stopped, and the FiO_2 is decreased to less than 30% to minimize the opportunity for airway fire.
15. The ideal placement of the tracheal incision is through tracheal rings 2 and 3. Numerous types of tracheal incisions can be utilized. A simple "T" or cross incision can be made through tracheal rings 2 and 3 with an #11 blade, and a tracheal dilator can be used to enlarge the size of the surgical stoma. Alternatively, a Bjork flap (inverted U-flap) can be placed through tracheal rings 2 and 3 (Figure 12.9). The width of the base of the Bjork flap should be one-third of the tracheal diameter. 2-0 stay sutures are placed within the nonhinged border of the cartilage window. Appropriately positioned stay sutures will aid in the retraction of the Bjork flap during tube insertion. The stay sutures may be tied to the skin incision to reflect the flap open, or they can be taped to the patient's anterior chest wall with steri-strips at the completion of the procedure. The Bjork flap has the advantage of creating a stable tract for tube reinsertion should accidental decannulation occur in a noncontrolled setting. For patients requiring prolonged or permanent mechanical ventilation, a permanent surgical stoma can be created by removing a wedge of cartilage the size of the Bjork flap from the anterior tracheal wall at the level of tracheal rings 2–3.
16. After creation of a surgical stoma through tracheal rings 2 and 3, the anesthesia team is asked to slowly pull back the endotracheal tube (Figure 12.9). Once the endotracheal tube has moved superior to the surgical stoma, an unfenestrated tracheotomy tube with its obturator is placed into the tracheal stoma with gentle inferior pressure and following the natural curvature of the trachea (Figure 12.10). The obturator

is removed, and the inner cannula is inserted. The tracheotomy tube cuff is inflated, and the anesthesia circuit is attached (Figure 12.11).

17. The anesthesia team is asked to check for end-tidal CO_2 and bilateral breath sounds.

18. The tracheotomy flange is secured with a cloth tie around the neck and to the skin with 2-0 sutures (Figure 12.11). The previously placed stay sutures are secured to the skin of the anterior chest wall with steri-strips if they were not secured to the skin incision. A split gauze dressing is placed between the tube collar and the skin to protect the wound and to absorb venous bleeding.

19. The skin, subcutaneous tissue, and muscle layers are not closed in order to minimize the risk of subcutaneous emphysema, which can result from positive pressure ventilation and a tightly closed tracheotomy incision.

20. An immediate chest film is obtained in order to confirm tracheal tube placement and to assess the lung fields to rule out pneumothorax. The ideal position of a tracheotomy tube should be a minimum of 2 cm above the carina so that inadvertent main stem cannulation does not occur.

Postoperative Management

1. Tracheotomy dressings (split sheet) are changed as they become saturated, or at least once per day.

2. The surgical site or stoma is cleaned daily to remove secretions and coagulated blood, and to clean the surrounding skin edges.

3. Prior to tracheotomy tube removal, an air leak test is performed to evaluate breathing around the tracheotomy tube. If indicated, a computed tomography scan can also be obtained to evaluate airway space. Prior to extubation, make sure to have all appropriate equipment and personnel ready to place a new tracheotomy tube if the patient begins to desaturate bedside. After extubation, the patient is closely observed in a monitored setting for several hours. One hour after extubation, an arterial blood gas (ABG) is obtained to assess for adequate ventilation.

Complications

Immediate or Early Tracheotomy Complications

1. **Bleeding**: Sources of early bleeding include the anterior jugular veins, thyroid ima artery, inferior thyroid arteries and veins, highly vascular thyroid parenchyma, innominate artery, external jugular veins, and thyroid isthmus. Arterial bleeding should be explored in a controlled setting (operating room). Venous bleeding is common and can be controlled by local measures bedside.

2. **Subcutaneous emphysema**: Occurs from tight closure of the skin incision, from a small skin incision, or from false passage of the tracheotomy tube into the pretracheal tissue. Subcutaneous emphysema can also occur when the posterior wall of the trachea is inadvertently perforated (more common with percutaneous tracheotomy). Symptoms occur after positive pressure ventilation is attached to the tracheotomy tube and air dissects within the pretracheal subcutaneous tissue. Air emphysema can further dissect within the subcutaneous tissues of the head, neck, face, and thorax (mediastinal emphysema and pneumomediastinum). Subcutaneous emphysema will resolve once its source is identified and corrected.

3. **Inappropriate tracheotomy tube placement**: The tracheotomy tube can be inadvertently placed (false passage) into the subcutaneous tissue plane between the trachea and the sternum. This will result in loss of airway and subcutaneous emphysema. The tracheotomy tube can also be incorrectly positioned within the trachea itself. If inappropriately positioned within the trachea, the tracheotomy tube can place unwanted pressure on the tracheal walls resulting in dysphagia, ulceration, and fistulae formation.

4. **Loss of airway**: Results from a false passage of the tracheotomy tube or from inadequately securing of the tracheotomy tube in the operating room.

5. **Damage to adjacent structures**: Structures damaged may include the cricoid cartilage, thyroid cartilage, posterior tracheal wall, esophagus, vocal cords, and recurrent laryngeal nerves. Inadvertent lateral tracheal dissection can occur when the midline is lost or obscured during the surgical dissection. Dissection along the lateral sulcus of the trachea can damage the recurrent laryngeal nerve and result in vocal cord paralysis and dysphonia.

6. **Perforation of the posterior trachea**: Occurs more commonly with percutaneous tracheostomy than with open tracheostomy. This is frequently caused during percutaneous dilation tracheotomy when the guide wire is poorly stabilized and perforates the posterior tracheal wall. Symptoms include subcutaneous emphysema, decreased arterial saturation, and decreased breath sounds, often proceeding toward tension pneumothorax.

7. **Pneumothorax or hemothorax**: Inadvertent perforation or laceration of the posterior wall of the trachea may also penetrate into the pleural spaces, leading to pneumothorax or hemothorax. Note that the pleural cavity is not limited to the lateral aspects of the trachea, but extends around the lateral walls of the trachea to the posterior wall of the trachea, and that there is a short distance between the dorsal tracheal wall and the pleural cavity.

8. **Tracheal tube obstruction**: Initial tracheotomy tube obstruction is commonly with mucous or blood. These obstructions are frequently due to the placement of a small-diameter tracheotomy tube and/or poor daily tracheotomy tube care.

9. **Accidental decannulation**: Accidental decannulation can occur from increased pulmonary secretions, the patient changing position in bed, lack of clinically indicated limb restraints, and an improperly secured tracheotomy tube. Accidental decannulation is more common in the pediatric population.

10. **Aspiration pneumonia**: Symptoms include tachycardia, tachypnea, cough, chest pain, sputum production, rales, cyanosis, wheezing, fever, and leukocytosis, or may be completely asymptomatic. Chest films demonstrate pulmonary infiltrates specific to the segments of the lobes involved.

11. **Airway fire**: This extremely rare but catastrophic complication can be minimized by avoiding the use of electrocautery to enter the trachea and by minimizing the use of volatile anesthetic gases and decreasing the FiO_2 to less than 30% prior to incising the trachea.

Late Tracheotomy Complications

1. **Erosion of the tube into adjacent structures**: Erosion into the tracheal or laryngeal cartilages will cause chondromalacia and ultimately stenosis. Erosion through the posterior wall will cause a tracheo-esophageal fistula. Erosion into vessels will cause bleeding and tracheo-arterial fistulae development.

2. **Fistula formation**: Fistulae may form between the trachea and either the esophagus (tracheo-esophageal fistula) or the innominate artery (tracheo-arterial fistula). Tracheo-esophageal fistulae are a rare complication that can occur at the time of tracheostomy or from improper positioning of the tracheostomy tube. Treatment involves tracheal resection and anastomosis plus esophageal closure, with or without a muscle interposition. Tracheo-arterial fistulae are the most lethal late complication of tracheotomy (they occur in 0.6–0.7% of patients). Tracheo-arterial fistulae can occur between 30 hours and several years after tracheotomy. However, 70% occur within the first 3 weeks postoperatively. Symptoms include sentinel bleeding and a pulsating tracheotomy tube. The innominate artery is the most common site, but left innominate vein, aortic arch, and right common artery fistulae can also occur. Tracheo-arterial fistulae occur owing to erosion of the anterior tracheal wall from the tracheostomy cuff or tip. Treatment involves early identification, occlusive pressure, and urgent surgical exploration.

3. **Stomal infection**: Stomal infections result from contamination of the surgical site at surgery or contamination of the wound in the postoperative period.

4. **Formation of granulation tissue**: Granulation tissue typically grows in the areas of tube irritation. These growths can cause airway obstruction, interfere with vocal cord function, interfere with decannulation, and ultimately lead to tracheal or laryngeal stenosis. Treatment is with steroid injections and/or excision.

5. **Tracheal and/or subglottic stenosis**: Symptoms (stridor, cough, dyspnea, shortness of breath, and malaise) typically do not occur until the luminal diameter is reduced by 50%. Stenosis often occurs above or at the stoma and below the vocal cords. Stenosis can be prevented by limiting the size of the stomal opening, avoiding cartilage fracture, preventing mechanical irritation of the tube on the trachea, preventing infections, and maintaining cuff pressures of 20 mm Hg or less. Treatment of stenosis is with surgery, most commonly with tracheal resection with end-to-end anastomosis, tracheal dilation, and trancheobronchial airway stenting.

6. **Tracheomalacia**: Tracheomalacia is rare and presents as necrosis and destruction of the supporting cartilage. Treatment involves using a longer tracheotomy tube to bypass the area of necrosis, bronchoscopic stenting, surgical resection, and tracheoplasty.

7. **Persistent tracheal stoma (>3 months after tube removal)**: Persistent tracheal stomas occur from prolonged cannulation, which allows the tracheostomy tract to epithelialize. Treatment includes tract excision and a layered closure, with or without a muscle flap.

Key Points

1. **Tracheotomy tube selection**: The size of the tracheotomy tube coincides with the internal diameter of the tube. Men require an internal diameter of 7.0 to 8.5. Women require an internal diameter of 6.0 to 7.5. In children, the size of the tube should be the size of the child's little finger. In toddlers and infants, an uncuffed tube is recommended because the trachea is so small that the tracheotomy tube will create an adequate seal without a cuff.

2. In the acute trauma situation, unfenestrated tubes should be utilized. After initial placement of an unfenestrated tube, secondary placement of a fenestrated tube for phonation and weaning is appropriate.

3. Bleeding is the most common complication in tracheotomy. Bleeding can be minimized with a 2–4 cm incision. Longer, more lateral incisions risk inadvertent damage to the great vessels (anterior, external, and internal jugular veins and carotid arteries). Bleeding can also be minimized by maintaining a midline dissection and by dividing the strap muscles rather than transecting them. Finally, postoperative bleeding can be minimized by using electrocautery to divide the thyroid isthmus instead of transecting with a blade. Alternatively, the thyroid isthmus can be left intact and retracted superiorly to provide access to the tracheal rings.

4. After division of the strap muscles, army-navy retractors are placed on either side of the trachea in order to keep the trachea within the midline. Dissection lateral to the trachea can lead to damage of the recurrent laryngeal nerve and paralysis of the vocal cords, resulting in hoarseness.

5. The ideal placement of the surgical stoma is between tracheal rings 2 and 3. The cricoid cartilage and the first tracheal ring should never be cut or injured. The surgical stoma should never extend below the fourth tracheal ring. The surgical stoma should not extend more than one-half of the circumference of the tracheal lumen (less than one-third is preferred).

6. The advantage of the Bjork flap is that if unintentional decannulation occurs, the inverted U-flap provides an ideal pathway for recannulation, especially if stay sutures are utilized.

7. Patients with thick necks or obese patients may require an extended tracheotomy tube. This decision should be made by assessing lateral neck films before tracheotomy. Alternatively, adjustable tracheotomy tubes are utilized in this patient population.

8. With obese patients, it is easy to become anatomically disoriented and dissect too far inferiorly (around the sternal notch or beneath the sternum). Be cognizant of low dissections as this increases the risk of encountering the innominate artery and thus increases the risk of development of a tracheo-innominate artery fistulae.

9. Tracheotomy in the pediatric population differs from the adult population in that the procedure is technically more demanding and is associated with a higher morbidity and mortality. Most pediatric tracheotomy tubes are cuffless and nonfenestrated (Figure 12.12).

References

Antonelli, M., Michetti, V., Di Palma, A., Conti, G., Pennisi, M.A., Arcangeli, A., Montini, L., Bocci, M.G., Bello, G., Almadori, G., Paludetti, G. and Proietti, R., 2005. Percutaneous translaryngeal versus surgical tracheostomy: a randomized trial with 1-yr double-blind follow-up. *Critical Care Medicine*, 33, 1015–20.

Bernard, A.C. and Kenady, D.E., 1999. Conventional surgical tracheostomy as the preferred method of airway management. *Journal of Oral and Maxillofacial Surgery*, 57, 310–15.

Deutsch, E.S., 2010. Tracheostomy: pediatric considerations. *Respiratory Care*, 55, 1082–90.

Engels, P.T., Bagshaw, S.M., Meier, M. and Brindley, P.G., 2009. Tracheostomy: from insertion to decannulation. *Canadian Journal of Surgery*, 52, 427–33.

Fattahi, T., Vega, L., Fernandes, R., Goldman, N., Steinberg, B. and Schare, H., 2012. Our experience with 171 open tracheostomies. *Journal of Oral and Maxillofacial Surgery*, 70, 1699–702.

Fikkers, B.G., van Veen, J.A., Kooloos, J.G., Pickkers, P., van den Hoogen, F.J., Hillen, B. and van der Hoeven, J.G., 2004. Emphysema and pneumothorax after percutaneous tracheostomy: case reports and an anatomic study. *Chest*, 125, 1805–14.

Gelman, J.J., Aro, M. and Weiss, S.M., 1994. Tracheoinnominate artery fistula. *Journal of the American College of Surgeons*, 179, 626–34.

Gilyoma, J.M., Balumuka, D.D. and Chalya, P.L., 2011. Ten-year experiences with tracheostomy at a university teaching hospital in northwest Tanzania: a retrospective review of 214 cases. *World Journal of Surgery*, 6, 1–7.

Haspel, A.C., Coviello, V.F. and Stevens, M., 2012. Retrospective study of tracheostomy indications and perioperative complications on oral and maxillofacial surgery service. *Journal of Oral and Maxillofacial Surgery*, 70, 890–95.

Melloni, G., Muttini, S., Gallioli, G., Carretta, A., Cozzi, S., Gemma, M. and Zannini, P., 2002. Surgical tracheostomy versus percutaneous dilational tracheostomy: a prospective-randomized study with long-term follow-up. *Journal of Cardiovascular Surgery (Torino)*, 43, 113–21.

O'Connor, H.H. and White, A.C., 2010. Tracheostomy decannulation. *Respiratory Care*, 55, 1076–81.

OMFS Knowledge Update. Available from http://www.aaoms.org/members/meetings-and-continuing-education/oms-knowledge-update/

Ridley, R.W. and Zwischenberger, J.B., 2006. Tracheoinnominate fistula: surgical management of an iatrogenic disaster. *Journal of Laryngology and Otology*, 120, 676–80.

Rowshan, H.H. and Baur, D.A., 2010. Surgical tracheotomy. *Oral and Maxillofacial Surgery Clinics of North America*, 18, 39–50.

Shen, K.R. and Mathisen, D.J., 2003. Management of persistent tracheal stoma. *Chest Surgery Clinics of North America*, 13, 369–73.

Sue, R.D. and Susanto, I., 2003. Long-term complications of artificial airways. *Clinics in Chest Medicine*, 24, 457–71.

Sviri, S., Samie, R., Roberts, B.L. and van Heerden, P.V., 2003. Long-term outcomes following percutaneous tracheostomy using Griggs technique. *Anaesthesia and Intensive Care*, 31, 401–7.

Trotter, S.J., Hazard, P.B., Sakabu, S.A., Levine, J.H., Troop, B.R., Thompson, J.A. and McNary, R., 1999. Posterior tracheal wall perforation during percutaneous dilation tracheostomy. *Chest*, 115, 1383–9.

Case Report

Case Report 12.2. A 23-year-old male presents after a motor vehicle accident. The patient sustained multiple injuries to include a Le Fort III fracture, a right zygomaticomaxillary complex fracture, nasal bone fractures, maxillary palatal fractures, bilateral condylar neck fractures, a left parasymphysis fracture, multiple orthopedic fractures, rib fractures, and pulmonary contusions. Due to the extensive midface fractures, the need for maxillomandibular fixation, and the need for prolonged intubation, the decision was made to perform an open tracheotomy at the time of the repair of the patient's facial fractures. (See Figures 12.5 through 12.11.)

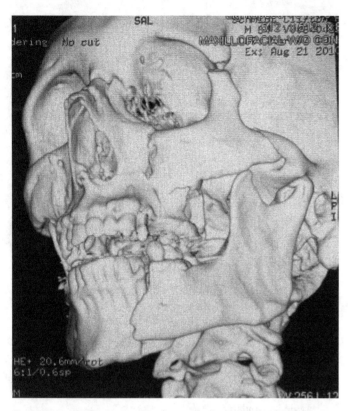

Figure 12.5. 3D reconstruction demonstrating extensive facial fractures.

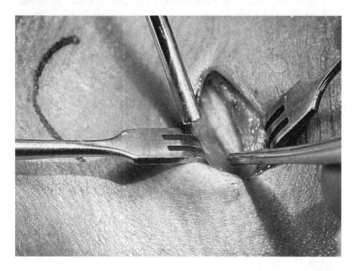

Figure 12.7. Horizontal incision through skin, subcutaneous tissue and platysma muscle to reveal the superficial layer of the deep cervical fascia.

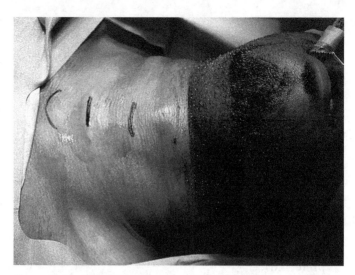

Figure 12.6. A sterile marking pen is used to draw a 3-4 cm horizontal line 2 cm inferior to the cricoid cartilage or midway between the cricoid cartilage and the sternal notch.

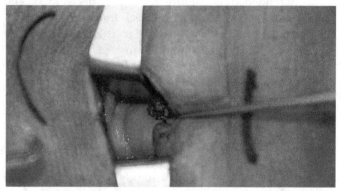

Figure 12.8. The pretracheal fascia overlying the trachea is exposed. Army-navy retractors are placed to retract the subcutaneous tissues and strap muscles, and to keep the trachea midline.

Figure 12.9. A #11 blade is used to create an inferiorly based Bjork flap through tracheal rings 2 and 3, and stay sutures are placed. The endotracheal tube is deflated and is slowly pulled cephalically until it is just above the Bjork flap.

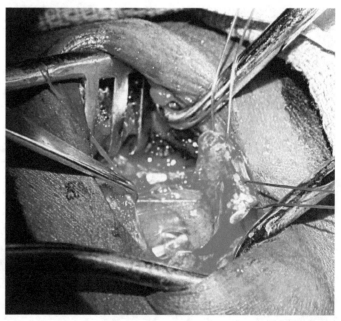

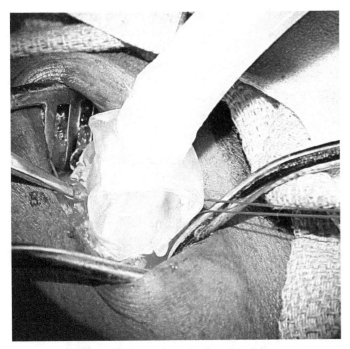

Figure 12.10.   Once the endotracheal tube is cephalic to the Bjork flap, the tracheotomy tube is inserted into the tracheal stoma with gentle inferior pressure and following the natural curvature of the trachea.

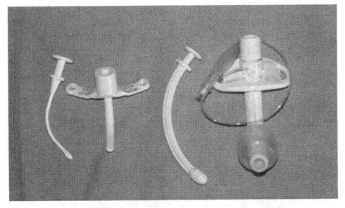

Figure 12.12.   (Left) A 4.0 Shiley pediatric tracheotomy tube uncuffed and unfenestrated with obturator. (Right) An 8.0 Shiley adult tracheotomy tube cuffed and unfenestrated with obturator.

Submental Intubation

An alternative to tracheotomy when short-term ventilation is required.

Indications for Submental Intubation

1. Maxillofacial trauma patients who require maxillomandibular fixation and dental occlusal references when nasal intubation is contraindicated (i.e., mandibular fractures with associated midface fractures and/or skull-based fractures) and postoperative mechanical ventilation is not necessary or will be of short duration

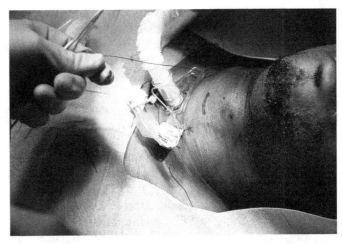

Figure 12.11.   The anesthesia circuit is connected, the tracheotomy tube cuff is inflated, and tube placement is confirmed with end-tidal CO_2 readings and bilateral chest auscultation. The tracheotomy tube flange is secured to the skin with 2-0 silk sutures and a cloth neck tie.

2. Patients requiring a short-term definitive airway for elective craniomaxillofacial reconstructive surgery where a reference to the dental occlusion is required with a desire to avoid the complications of tracheotomy (i.e., orthognathic surgery where nasal intubation is not possible, cleft lip–palate patients, and maxillomandibular advancement with concurrent nasal surgery for sleep apnea)
3. In situations where nasal intubation cannot be achieved (lack of operator experience, lack of fiber optic equipment, and intranasal pathology)

Anatomy

Submental Intubation Landmarks

1. Submental crease
2. Midline floor of mouth

Submental Intubation Layers

1. Skin
2. Subcutaneous tissue
3. Platysma muscle
4. Deep cervical fascia
5. Mylohyoid muscle
6. Geniohyoid muscle
7. Genioglossus muscle
8. Oral mucosa

Submental Intubation Procedure

1. The patient is orally intubated with a semirigid oral tube and a bite block is placed.
2. The skin is prepped to include the anterior neck, chin, and floor of mouth.
3. The patient is drapped from midface to sternal notch.
4. The submental crease is identified and injected with local anesthetic containing a vasoconstrictor (Figure 12.15).

5. A 2–3 cm incision is created 2 mm posterior to the submental crease. The incision transects skin, subcutaneous tissue, and platysma only. Superficial bleeds are controlled with electrocautery.

6. A Kelley clamp is used to bluntly dissect from the skin incision through the deep cervical fascia and muscles of the floor of the mouth into the midline of the oral cavity under the ventral aspect of the tongue (Figure 12.13).

7. The pilot tube cuff is inserted into the beaks of the Kelley clamp. The Kelley clamp is used to pull the pilot cuff from the oral cavity through the submental incision (Figure 12.16).

8. The endotracheal tube connector is removed. The Kelley clamp is reinserted from the submental incision into the oral cavity, and the semirigid oral endotracheal tube is grasped and pulled through the submental incision (Figure 12.17). The connector is reattached, and the anesthesia circuit is reconnected (Figure 12.19).

9. The endotracheal tube is secured to the skin of the submental region with 2-0 silk sutures (Figure 12.18). A 24-gauge wire can be used to secure the rigid endotracheal tube to the lingual aspect of the first molar below the occlusal plane so that it does not interfere with the ability to check dental occlusal references during the procedure.

10. At the completion of the procedure, the patient can be left submentally intubated, or the submental intubation can be converted to a traditional oral intubation (Figure 12.20).

Submental Intubation Complications

Immediate Submental Intubation Complications

1. Floor-of-mouth edema
2. Floor-of-mouth hematoma
3. Injury to the sublingual duct, submandibular duct, or lingual nerve or vessels
4. Detachment of or damage to the pilot balloon

Late Submental Intubation Complications

1. Infection of submental incision from oral contamination
2. Accidental extubation
3. Oral cutaneous fistula formation
4. Abscess formation in the floor of the mouth
5. Salivary fistula formation
6. Mucocele or ranula formation
7. Hypertrophic scarring

Key Points

1. Submental intubation is *not* a replacement for open tracheostomy. Submental intubation is indicated in select cases of facial trauma and reconstructive surgery where postoperative mechanical ventilation is not required or will be of a short duration.

2. As with all airways procedures, the airway must be secured in a stable manner. With submental intubation,

this is with skin sutures and/or with a 24-gauge wire secured circumferentially to a molar tooth.

3. Although submental intubation is a secure airway, it is not indicated for prolonged periods of intubation. Submental intubations are typically converted to oral intubations immediately after surgery. Alternatively, when short periods of intubation are required and the need for long-term ventilatory support is not required, submental intubation is an appropriate alternative to open tracheostomy.

4. Prior to initiating the surgical procedure (i.e., Naso-Orbito-Ethmoid [NOE] fracture reduction), end-tidal CO_2 readings, bilateral chest auscultation, and chest movement are assessed to ensure that displacement of the endotracheal tube did not occur during the submental intubation procedure.

5. Although paramedian skin incisions have been described in the literature, these incisions increase the risk of damage to the sublingual glands and facial nerve and result in a more difficult tube passage. The midline approach for submental intubation is preferred as there are few anatomic structures to damage and the scar is well hidden within the submental crease.

6. Submental intubation is a quick, simple, and safe procedure that is associated with fewer complications and postoperative management issues when compared to open tracheotomy.

7. Metal-reinforced endotracheal tubes are used to reduce the risk of tube kinking during manipulation through the submental tract.

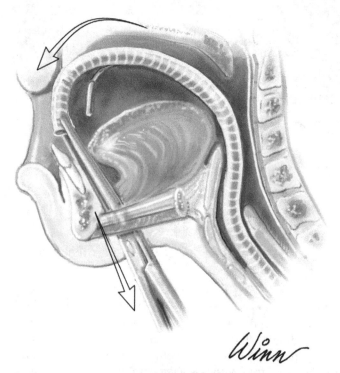

Figure 12.13. A Kelley clamp is inserted through the submental incision into the oral cavity to grasp the semirigid oral endotracheal tube. The oral endotracheal tube is pulled through the submental incision.

Case Report

Case Report 12.3. An 11-year-old male presents after a motor vehicle accident with extensive comminuted facial fractures to include basilar skull fractures, cribriform plate fractures, Le Fort II fractures, cerebrospinal fluid (CSF) rhinorrhea, bilateral orbits floor fractures, hard-palate fractures, and displaced mandibular fractures. The patient received a right decompressive craniectomy due to a large intracranial bleed. Maxillomandibular fixation (MMF) was necessary to reestablish the anterior-posterior dimension of the facial skeleton, to establish appropriate occlusion, and to reduce and fixate the comminuted facial fractures. The presence of the comminuted NOE fracture, basilar skull fracture, cribriform plate fracture, and CSF rhinorrhea prohibited nasal endotracheal intubation. Because the patient demonstrated no airway edema and no pulmonary trauma, and thus did not require long-term ventilation, the decision was made for a submental intubation in order to avoid the potential complications associated with an open tracheotomy. (See Figures 12.14 through 12.20.)

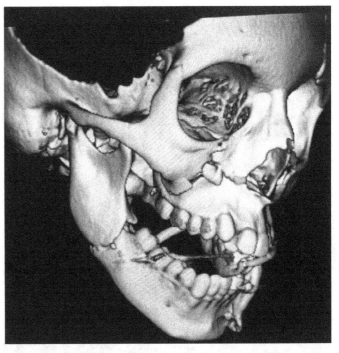

Figure 12.14. 3D reconstruction demonstrating mandibular and panfacial fractures, left-sided basilar skull fractures, and a right craniectomy.

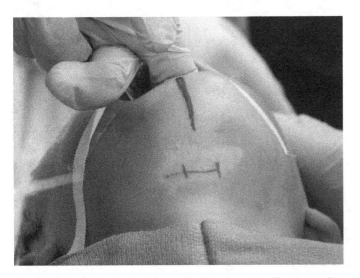

Figure 12.15. The patient is orally intubated in the operating room, and the midline submental crease is identified. A finger is used to palpate the floor of the mouth for the anticipated exit of the tube.

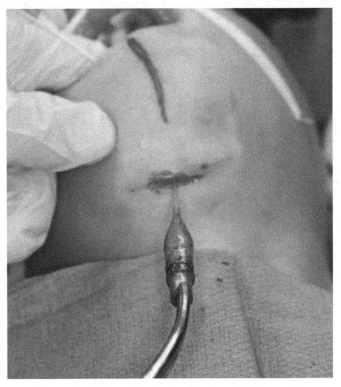

Figure 12.16. A Kelley clamp is used to pull the pilot cuff from the oral cavity through the submental incision.

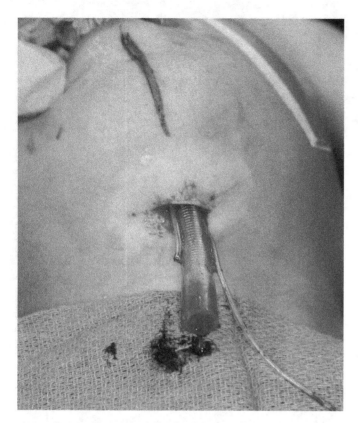

Figure 12.17.   The endotracheal tube connector is removed. The semirigid oral endotracheal tube is grasped and pulled through the submental incision with a Kelley clamp.

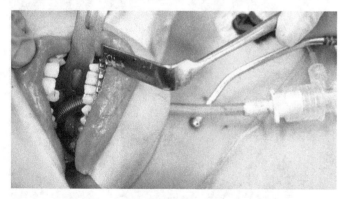

Figure 12.19.   The endotracheal tube connector is reattached, and the anesthesia circuit is reconnected.

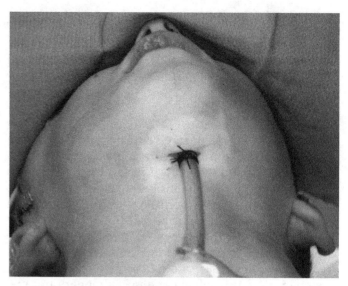

Figure 12.18.   The endotracheal tube is secured to the skin of the submental region with 2-0 silk sutures.

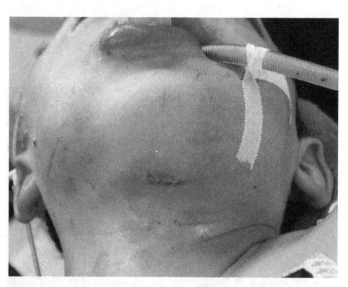

Figure 12.20.   At the completion of the procedure, the submental intubation is converted into a traditional oral intubation, and the incision site is closed. The patient will be placed into MMF with elastic once he is extubated.

References

Agrawal, M. and Kang, L.S., 2010. Midline submental orotracheal intubation in maxillofacial injuries: a substitute to tracheostomy where postoperative mechanical ventilation is not required. *Journal of Anaesthesiology Clinical Pharmacology*, 26, 498–502.

Franco, J., Coppage, J., Fallucco, M. and Ferguson, J.S., 2009. Submental intubation: an alternative to tracheostomy when nasoendotracheal intubation is unsuccessful—a case report. *Canadian Journal of Plastic Surgery*, 17, e37–8.

Kar, C. and Mukherjee, S., 2010. Submental intubation: an alternative and cost-effective technique for complex maxillofacial surgeries. *Journal of Oral and Maxillofacial Surgery*, 9, 266–9.

Lima, S.M., Jr., Asprino, L., Moreira, R.W. and de Moraes, M., 2011. A retrospective analysis of submental intubation in maxillofacial trauma patients. *Journal of Oral and Maxillofacial Surgery*, 69, 2001–5.

Mahmood, S. and Lello, G.E., 2002. Oral endotracheal intubation: median submental (retrogenial) approach. *Journal of Oral and Maxillofacial Surgery*, 60, 473–4.

OMFS Knowledge Update. Available from http://www.aaoms.org/members/meetings-and-continuing-education/oms-knowledge-update/

Schutz, P. and Hamed, H.H. 2008. Submental intubation versus tracheostomy in maxillofacial trauma patients. *Journal of Oral and Maxillofacial Surgery*, 66, 1404–9.

13 Mandibular Fractures

Christopher J. Haggerty

Private Practice, Lakewood Oral and Maxillofacial Surgery Specialists, Lees Summit; and Department of Oral and Maxillofacial Surgery, University of Missouri–Kansas City, Kansas City, Missouri, USA

Surgical Management of Anterior Mandibular Fractures (Symphysis and Parasymphysis)

Indications for Open Reduction of Anterior Mandibular Fractures

1. When closed reduction will not adequately reduce fractures
2. When the fixation of anterior mandibular fractures will allow for alignment of other fractures (condyle or angle fracture)
3. In order to allow for early mobilization of condylar fractures
4. Patients who cannot tolerate maxillomandibular fixation (MMF)

See Figure 13.13 for a comparison of regions of dentate mandible fractures.

Contraindications for Open Reduction of Anterior Mandibular Fractures

1. Fractures that can be reduced with MMF alone

Intraoral Surgical Approach and Open Reduction of the Anterior Mandible

1. The patient is nasally intubated to allow for the placement of MMF. The endotracheal tube is secured, a throat packing is placed, and the patient is prepped and draped in a sterile fashion.
2. Maxillary and mandibular Erich arch bars are adapted and secured in place with either 24- or 26-gauge stainless steel circumdental wires placed below the cingulums of the dentition from first molar to first molar or SMARTLock Hybrid MMF (Stryker, Kalamazoo, Michigan, USA) may be utilized. If Erich arch bars are placed, the incisors may be linked together or abstained if sufficient occlusion results without their incorporation into the arch bars.
3. Local anesthesia containing a vasoconstrictor is injected within the anterior mandibular vestibule to include the mentalis muscle.
4. A mucosal incision is created with sharp scissors, cautery, or a blade (see Figure 13.3 in Case Report 13.1). The mucosal incision is created parallel to the attached gingiva and approximately 15 mm lateral to the attached gingiva.
5. The mentalis muscle and periosteum are transversed between the canines with sharp scissors, cautery, or a blade.
6. The mental foramen and nerves are identified with blunt dissection with a fine hemostat within the pre-molar region. Care is taken to spread the hemostat tines parallel to the anticipated course of the mental nerve. Alternatively, a periosteal elevator can be used to dissect in a subperiosteal plane posterior to the original dissection to locate the mental foramen. Once the mental nerves have been identified, they are dissected free from their surrounding tissue and retracted from the operating site with gentle superior traction.
7. The fracture is aligned with a periosteal elevator, and the patient is placed into MMF with 24- or 26-gauge stainless steel wires and/or heavy elastics. If necessary, the fracture can be temporarily reduced with bone-reducing forceps (Figure 13.5, Case Report 13.1), a 24-gauge intraosseous wire, or a small bone plate.
8. The well-reduced fracture is internally fixated with lag screws (Figures 13.8 and 13.9, Case Report 13.1; see also Figure 13.1), tension plates (Figures 13.11 and 13.12, Case Report 13.1), or a combination of the two. Care is taken to ensure that the fixation plates and screws are placed a safe distance from the apices of the teeth, the inferior alveolar nerve, and the mental foramen.
9. Once internal fixation is applied, the bone-reducing forceps (if utilized) are removed, MMF wires and elastics are removed, and the occlusion is verified.
10. Any changes in the patient's occlusion should be addressed by removing the fixation, identifying areas of interference, and refixating the mandible.
11. Once the ideal pre-trauma occlusion has been verified, the incision site is irrigated and closed in a layered fashion.

Postoperative Management

1. A supportive dressing may be applied to the chin and submental area to provide superior support of the mentalis muscle and to act as a pressure dressing.
2. Arch bar removal and functioning are based upon the surgeon's preferences, the degree of fixation, patient compliance, and the management or fixation of more proximal fractures of the mandible.

Atlas of Operative Oral and Maxillofacial Surgery, First Edition. Edited by Christopher J. Haggerty and Robert M. Laughlin

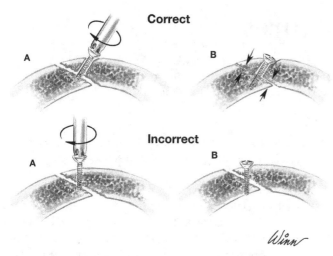

Figure 13.1. Illustration depicting the appropriate and inappropriate placement of lag screws. Note that the gliding osteotomy is larger than the traction osteotomy.

Complications

1. **Ptotic chin (witch's chin)**: From inadequate closure of the mentalis muscle.
2. **Lip perforation**: From inadvertent perforation of the anterior lip during dissection to the inferior border of the anterior mandible. Minimized by placing the non-dominant hand on the outer surface of the lip to detect the level of dissection.

Key Points

1. By placing the mucosal incision 15 mm of more lateral from the attached gingiva, it will permit a sufficient mucosal edge for easy closure, especially in the area of the arch bar.
2. Initial dissection should not extend beyond the canines until the location of the mental foramen and mental nerves have been verified.
3. Appropriate closure of the mentalis muscle can prevent the formation of a ptotic chin (witch's chin), asymmetrical muscle contraction, or dimple formation from placing the deep sutures too superficially.
4. If other mandibular fractures are present (body, angle, and/or condyle), the anterior mandible fractures are typically fixated first.
5. The final step prior to closing any mandible fracture is the verification of the patient's occlusion.

Procedure: Lag Screw Fixation

A form of compression osteosynthesis commonly utilized in the symphysis and parasympysis region

Indications

1. Linear mandibular fractures
2. Fractures within the symphyis and parasympysis region (although lag screws can be placed in other locations)

Contraindications

1. Oblique fractures
2. Comminuted fractures
3. Atrophic, edentulous mandibular fractures
4. Patients with diminished or poor bone quality

Technique

1. Maxillary and mandibular arch bars are placed, and the anterior mandible is exposed from an intraoral approach (Figure 13.3 [all figures in this list appear in Case Report 13.1]).
2. The anterior mandibular fracture is aligned and reduced with a periosteal elevator and MMF is applied with 24 or 26-gauge wires and/or heavy elastics.
3. Bone reduction forceps may be placed within an area that will not interfere with the placement of the lag screws (Figure 13.5).
4. A gliding osteotomy is created. A 2.4 mm drill bit is oriented so that a 30–45 mm screw may be placed perpendicular to the linear fracture. The 2.4 mm drill bit is then drilled to the fracture site (Figure 13.6).
5. A traction osteotomy is created. A drill sleeve is inserted that enters the previous drill site (gliding osteotomy). A 1.8 mm drill bit is utilized to drill distal to the fracture until it exits the cortical bone perpendicular to the linear fracture (Figure 13.7).
6. The gliding osteotomy is countersunk, and the depth of the osteotomy is measured.
7. An appropriate-length screw is placed through the gliding osteotomy, and the traction osteotomy is engaged.
8. As the traction osteotomy is engaged with the lag screw, the fracture site will further compress and reduce (Figure 13.8). If the lag screw does not engage the traction osteotomy ideally, the fracture will become displaced as the lag screw is tightened.
9. An adjacent lag screw is placed in a similar fashion. The second lag screw may course either in the same direction or in the opposite direction (Figure 13.9) of the first lag screw.
10. MMF is removed, and the occlusion is verified prior to closing of the incision in a layered fashion.

Key Points

1. Lag screw fixation has a lower incidence of infection and wound dehiscence when compared to plate fixation.
2. When drilling the traction osteotomy, make sure to keep the 1.8 mm drill bit as perpendicular as possible to avoid flexing and fracture of the drill bit and to allow for compression perpendicular to the fracture.
3. After the placement of lag screw fixation, it is important to exam the lingual aspect of the anterior mandible to ensure that the lingual plate is not splayed. This can be performed by a combination of a conservative dissection of the lingual plate from the inferior border

of the mandible and/or by running a finger along the lingual plate after MMF has been removed.

4. Fracture selection is paramount in lag screw placement. Ideal fractures include noncomminuted, linear fractures in dentate patients.

References

Ellis, E., 1998. Lag screw fixation of mandibular fractures. *Journal of Cranio-Maxillofacial Trauma*, 3, 27.

Ellis, E., 2012. Is lag screw fixation superior to plate fixation to treat fractures of the mandibular symphysis? *Journal of Oral and Maxillofacial Surgery*, 70, 875.

Ellis, E. and Ghali, G.E., 1991. Lag screw fixation of anterior mandibular fractures. *Journal of Oral and Maxillofacial Surgery*, 49, 13.

Tiwana, P.S., Kushner, G.M. and Alpert, B., 2007. Lag screw fixation of anterior mandibular fractures: a retrospective analysis if intraoperative and postoperative complications. *Journal of Oral and Maxillofacial Surgery*, 65, 1180.

Case Reports

Case Report 13.1. Anterior mandibular fracture treated with lag screws. A 16-year-old male presents status post altercation with a linear anterior mandibular fracture. (See Figures 13.2 through 13.9.)

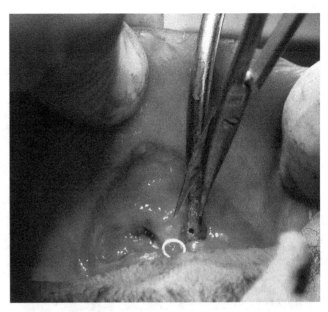

Figure 13.3. Dissection through the mucosa and mentalis muscle with sharp scissors. A finger is placed on the outer lip for support and to detect flap thickness to prevent accidental skin perforation.

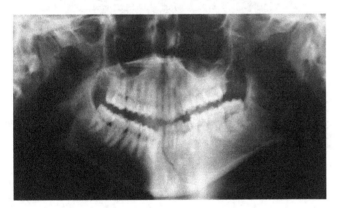

Figure 13.2. Orthopantomogram demonstrating a linear fracture through the mandibular symphysis.

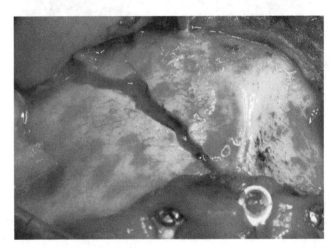

Figure 13.4. Subperiosteal exposure of the anterior mandibular fracture.

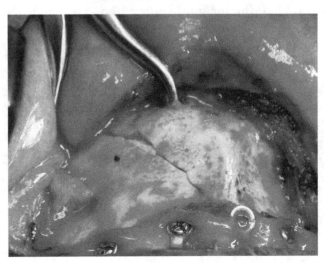

Figure 13.5. Bone reduction forceps are placed at the inferior border of the mandible to reduce the fracture prior to internal fixation.

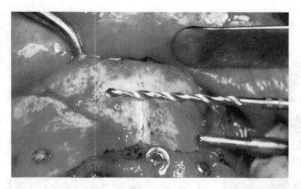

Figure 13.6.   The 2.4 mm drill bit is used prior to drilling to estimate the angle and depth of the gliding osteotomy. The cautery was used to create a burn mark to aim for during the preparation of the gliding and traction osteotomy.

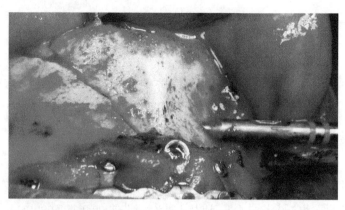

Figure 13.7.   The specialized drill sleeve for the 1.8 mm drill bit is inserted internally into the gliding osteotomy to allow for controlled drilling through the distal cortex (traction osteotomy).

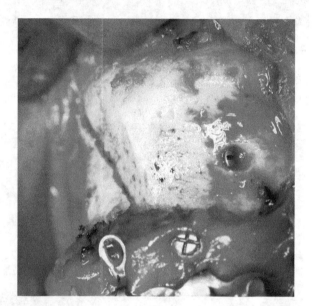

Figure 13.8.   As the lag screw engages the contralateral aspect of the fracture, the fracture compresses and reduces. The gliding osteotomy is countersunk slightly.

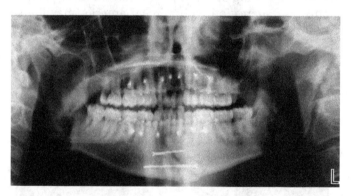

Figure 13.9.   Postoperative orthopantomogram demonstrating Stryker SMARTLock Hybrid MMF and the ideal reduction of the linear symphysis fracture with lag screw internal fixation.

Case Report 13.2. Anterior mandibular fracture treated with bone reduction plate placement. A 17-year-old female presents status post motor vehicle accident resulting in a displaced left parasymphysis fracture and a nondisplaced (greenstick) right angle fracture. (See Figures 13.10, 13.11, and 13.12.)

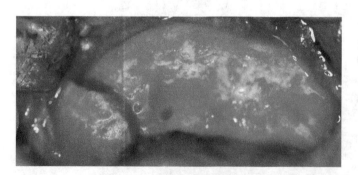

Figure 13.10.   Displaced left parasymphysis fracture of the mandible.

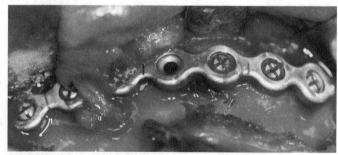

Figure 13.11.   Appropriate adaptation and placement of a 2.8 mm reconstruction plate to the inferior border of the anterior mandible inferior to the mental foramen. The empty plate hole represents the site of the reduced left parasymphysis fracture.

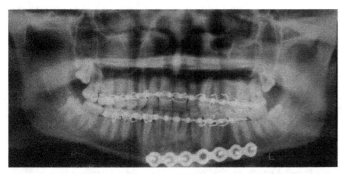

Figure 13.12. Postoperative orthopantomogram showing a well reduced left parasymphysis fracture with appropriate inferior border plate adaptation.

Surgical Management of Posterior Mandibular Fractures (Body and Angle)

Indication for Open Reduction of Posterior Mandibular Fractures

1. Unfavorable fractures
2. Displaced fractures that cannot be adequately reduced with closed reduction alone
3. Flail jaw
4. Contralateral condyle fractures that require early mobilization
5. Patients who cannot tolerate closed reduction
6. Infected fractures
7. Open fractures
8. Patients with other facial fractures that will require using the mandible as a base or starting point for establishing the vertical and anterior-posterior dimensions of the midface

Contraindications for Open Reduction of Posterior Mandibular Fractures

1. Favorable fractures well reduced with MMF alone
2. When damage to the neurovascular bundle is imminent
3. Grossly comminuted fractures with bone segments too small to fixate
4. Patients with significant comorbidities (e.g., elderly, previous head and neck radiation, or bisphosphonate-induced osteonecrosis of the jaw)

Submandibular Approach Layers

1. Skin
2. Subcutaneous tissue
3. Platysma muscle
4. Superficial layer of the deep cervical fascia (SDCF)
5. Pterygomasseteric sling
6. Periosteum
7. Mandible

Anatomy

Platysma muscle: Paired muscle that originates from the superficial fascia of the pectoral and deltoid muscles and runs obliquely to insert at the corner of the mouth and inferior portion of the cheek.

Superficial layer of the deep cervical fascia (SDCF): Located just deep to the platysma muscle. This fascial layer encircles the sternocleidomastoid muscle (SCM) and the trapezius muscle. The SDCF forms the capsule overlying the submandibular gland. The SDCF contains the facial artery, the facial vein, the node of Stahr, and the marginal mandibular and cervical branches of the facial nerve.

Submandibular gland: Located between the anterior and the posterior bellies of the digastric muscle.

Node of Stahr (submandibular lymph node): Typically encountered in the area of the premasseteric notch. Serves as a warning for the location of the facial artery and vein, which lie just anterior to the node of Stahr.

Marginal mandibular nerve: Located above the inferior border of the mandible (80%) or within 2 cm below the inferior border (20%). Lies deep of the platysma muscle along its entire course but becomes more superficial 2 cm lateral to the corner of the mouth. Damage to the marginal mandibular nerve results in paralysis of the depressors of the corner of the mouth (depressor labii inferioris, depressor anguli oris, inferior fibers of the orbicularis oris, and the mentalis).

Cervical nerve: Located inferior to the marginal mandibular nerve and deep to the platysma muscle. Damage to the cervical nerve results in paralysis of the depressor anguli oris and of the platysma muscle.

Intraoral Surgical Approach and Open Reduction of the Posterior Mandible

1. The patient is nasally intubated, the endotracheal tube is secured, a throat pack is placed, and the patient is prepped and draped.
2. Maxillary and mandibular arch bars are placed.
3. Local anesthesia containing a vasoconstrictor is injected within the area of the proposed intraoral incision.
4. A bite block is placed on the contralateral side of the posterior mandibular fracture.
5. A #15 blade or needle-tip cautery is used to create an incision through mucosa parallel to the mucogingival line. The incision is placed at least 15 mm lateral to the mucogingival line in order to allow for uncomplicated closure of the intraoral incision.
6. After mucosal incision, the #15 blade or cautery tip is directed toward the underlying mandible. The submucosa, muscle, and periosteum are sharply transected.

7. A periosteal elevator is used to dissect within a sub-periosteal plane posterior to the sigmoid notch and anteriorly as far as needed. Attention to the location of the mental foramen and mental nerve is key as the dissection proceeds anteriorly.

8. The proximal and distal segments of the fracture are aligned with a periosteal elevator, and the patient is placed into MMF with either 24- or 26-gauge stainless steel wires and/or heavy elastics. If a posterior tooth is located within the line of fracture and if it will not serve as an occlusal reference, it is removed at this time (see Figure 13.15; all figures cited appear in Case Reports 13.3, 13.4, and 13.5).

9. If a trocar is indicated, a local anesthesia needle is inserted through the cheek at the desired location of the intraoral trocar site (Figure 13.16). A #15 blade is used to make a skin incision approximately 4–6 mm in length and parallel to the anticipated direction of the facial nerve. The trocar is bluntly inserted from the extraoral incision into the oral cavity (Figure 13.17).

10. After fixation of the fracture (Figures 13.18 and 13.21), a curved periosteal elevator is run along the inferior border of the mandible to assess for proper alignment. For angle fractures, a periosteal elevator is also used to evaluate the superior aspect of the lingual plate of the mandible to ensure ideal fracture reduction.

11. The patient is removed from MMF, and the occlusion is verified.

12. After occlusal verification, the intraoral incision is closed with interrupted or continuous 4-0 chromic or Vicryl sutures. If a trocar incision was created, it is closed with 5-0 interrupted plain gut sutures.

Submandibular Approach and Open Reduction of the Posterior Mandible

1. The patient is nasally intubated, the endotracheal tube is secured, and maxillary and mandibular arch bars are placed. Short-acting paralytics are used in order to allow for testing of the facial nerve.

2. The patient is prepped and draped. A sterile marking pen is used to mark the site of the proposed skin incision (Figure 13.26).

3. Local anesthesia containing a vasoconstrictor is injected within the subcutaneous tissue superficial to the platysma muscle. If local anesthetic is deposited below the platysma muscle, it may paralyze the cervical and marginal mandibular branches of the facial nerve. Alternatively, injection deep to the platysma may be performed with a vasoconstrictor without local anesthetic. Seven to ten minutes are allowed prior to incision for the ideal hemostatic properties of the vasoconstrictor.

4. The incision is placed at least 2 cm below the inferior border of the mandible within a neck crease or parallel to a neck crease (Figure 13.26). The incision should allow for direct visualization of the fracture(s) and may extend posteriorly to the mastoid region and anteriorly as far as is needed. The initial incision is carried through skin, subcutaneous tissue, and platysma muscle only.

5. The subcutaneous layer is undermined in all directions with a hemostat in order to facilitate a tension-free closure at the end of the procedure.

6. Deep to the platysma muscle is the SDCF. The SDCF can be exposed by utilizing a 4 × 4 gauze and digital pressure once the platysma muscle is transected. The marginal mandibular and cervical branches of the facial nerve are located within or just deep to the SDCF.

7. A nerve stimulator is set on 2 milliamperes (mA) and tested. Blunt dissection through the SDCF is performed with a pair of fine hemostats and a nerve stimulator (Figure 13.27).

8. The submandibular gland is identified. The SDCF forms the investing fascia of the submandibular gland (Figure 13.28). The submandibular gland is retracted inferiorly. The node of Stahr may be encountered within the area of the premasseteric notch and retracted superiorly. The node of Stahr acts as a warning for the proximity of the facial artery.

9. Dissection continues cephalically after developing a plane of dissection deep to the SDCF. The pterygomasseteric sling is encountered and is divided at its avascular plane at the inferior border of the angle of the mandible where the masseter and medical pterygoid muscle intersect.

10. The periosteum is incised,, and the lateral aspect of the mandible is exposed in a subperiosteal plane (Figure 13.29).

11. After fixation of the posterior mandibular fracture (Figure 13.31) and verifying occlusion, closure is performed in the following fashion: the pterygomasseteric sling is tightly approximated with interrupted 3-0 Vicryl sutures, the platysma muscle is closed with 3-0 interrupted or continuous Vicryl sutures, the subcutaneous tissue is closed with interrupted or continuous 4-0 monofilamentous sutures, and the skin is approximated with either steri-strips or 5-0 plain gut sutures (Figure 13.32).

Postoperative Management

1. Patients are placed into MMF using either stainless steel wires or heavy elastics. The duration of MMF is dependent on the degree of fixation, patient compliance, medical issues (e.g., malnourishment, seizures, or mental handicap), patient age, and other associated

fractures (e.g., condyle fractures require earlier mobilization).

2. Elastics may be used to place the patient into heavy MMF or to act as guiding elastics to allow for the early limited functioning and muscle reprogramming. Light or guiding elastics are typically reserved for patients with rigid fixation, younger patients, patients with medical issues contraindicating prolonged MMF, and patients with associated condyle fractures.

3. Pressure dressings are applied based on the surgeon's preference.

4. Appropriate analgesic and antibiotic coverage is warranted for the first 7 days after surgery. Scopolamine transdermal anti-nausea patches are prescribed for patients in MMF. Nutrition consultation is recommended for all patients discharged with MMF for periods greater than 2 weeks.

5. Ice is applied to the fracture site for the first 24 hours.

6. Patients with any form of MMF are discharged with either wire cutters or scissors.

7. Patients are followed at 1 week, 3 weeks, and 6 weeks after surgery.

8. Arch bars are typically removed after 4–6 weeks based on patient exam (occlusion and maximum vertical opening), fixation technique, and compliance.

Complications

1. **Malocclusion**: Caused by failure to appropriately reduce fractures, displaced condyle fractures, inappropriate fixation, or fixation failure. Minor occlusal discrepancies can be corrected with guiding elastic (early) or orthodontics (late). Severe occlusal discrepancies are best treated with reoperation (early) or mandibular osteotomy (late).

2. **Damage to tooth roots**: Caused by placing fixation screws near adjacent teeth roots. Can be minimized by positioning bone reduction plates along the inferior border of the mandible, using monocortical screws, using drills with 4–6 mm stops, and placing screws a minimum of 12 mm inferior to the cementoenamel junction of posterior teeth.

3. **Hypoesthesia**: Can be caused from damage to the mental nerve during fracture exposure or from damage to the inferior alveolar nerve during screw placement. Bicortical screws should only be placed caudal to the mandibular canal. Monocortical screws should be placed along the lateral border of the mandible cephalic to the mandibular canal.

4. **Facial paralysis**: Typically occurs from stretching or transection of the marginal mandibular or cervical nerves during external approaches to the posterior mandible.

5. **Infection**: Infections typically present in the form of wound dehiscence or abscess formation. Infections occur from a variety of reasons. Infections involving hardware should be treated with hardware removal, gross debridement of all nonvital bone and granulation tissue, a period of MMF, and antibiotics. Continuity defects are best treated with grafting procedures after the infection has resolved. Infections can also occur in the areas of teeth left within the line of fracture or from the extraction of teeth within the line fracture (typically third molars). Infections originating from teeth within the line of fracture are treated with tooth extraction and surgical debridement of nonvital bone and granulation tissue and the use of antibiotics. Infections originating from extraction sites are also treated with the removal of nonvital bone and granulation tissue and the use of antibiotics. A short period of MMF is suggested with moderate to severe infections or with fracture mobility.

6. **Wound dehiscence**: Frequently caused by infection, hardware exposure, or smoking abuse. Hardware exposure is initially treated with oral antibiotics and debridement of the site. Areas of hardware exposure that fail to heal after conservative managment or areas with fractured or loose hardware require hardware removal.

7. **Pseudoarthrosis (non-union) or fibrous union**: Typically occur from infection or mobility of the fractured segments. Sources include hardware failure, nonrigid fixation, noncompliance with soft diet or MMF, and underlying medical conditions (diabetes, substance abuse, cigarette abuse, reduced immune system, etc.).

8. **Malunion**: Occurs from inadequate fracture reduction, patient noncompliance, and torsional forces when treating multiple fractures.

9. **Hardware failure**: Hardware fracture can be caused by repeated bending of the plate by the novice surgeon prior to rigid fixation. Loosening of screws is typically caused by improper drilling techniques. Such techniques involve insufficient irrigation, not placing fixation screws perpendicular to the bone reduction plate, and insufficient bone contact when using shorter 4 mm screws. Hardware fracture can also occur from patient noncompliance and additional trauma. All failed hardware should be removed, the site debrided and additional hardware is placed unless sufficient bone union has occurred.

Key Points

1. Wisdom teeth in the line of fracture should be removed to minimize postoperative infection.

2. Patients with multiple mandibular fractures are plated from anterior to posterior and from rigid to nonrigid fixation. For example, if a patient has sustained a symphysis and an angle fracture, the symphysis is typically plated first with rigid internal fixation,

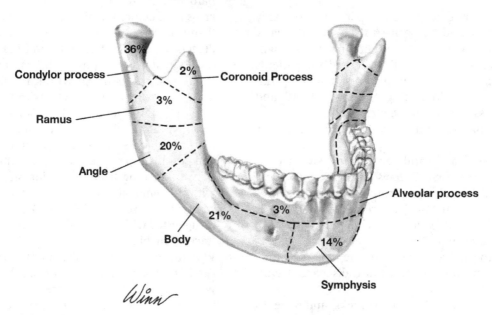

Dentate Fracture Regions(%)

Condylor process — 36%

Coronoid Process — 2%

Ramus — 3%

Angle — 20%

Alveolar process

Body — 21%   3%

14%

Symphysis

Winn

Figure 13.13.   Percentage of dentate mandible fractures by region. Modified from Ochs, MW (2008).

and then the angle is plated with rigid or nonrigid (Champy plate) fixation. If a patient presents with an angle fracture and a condylar fracture, the angle fracture is typically plated first with rigid fixation, and the condylar fracture can be treated closed or with nonrigid or rigid fixation. In the situations discussed here, the more assessable fracture (simpler fracture) is rigidly fixated in order to provide less torsional forces to the more distal (more difficult) fracture. After the application of rigid fixation to the simpler fracture, the more difficult fracture can be treated as if it were an isolated fracture.

3. If fracture reduction is non-ideal, it may be necessary to remove MMF, adjust the proximal and distal segments of the fracture site, and then reapply MMF. Sometimes, MMF can lock out the fracture if MMF is applied early on in the procedure.

References

Ellis, E., 2009. Management of fractures through the angle of the mandible. *Oral and Maxillofacial Surgery Clinics of North America*, 21, 163.

Ellis, E., 2010. A prospective study of 3 treatment methods for isolated fractures of the mandibular angle. *Journal of Oral and Maxillofacial Surgery*, 68, 2743.

Ellis E., 2013. Open reduction and internal fixation of combined angle and body/symphysis fractures of the mandible: how much fixation is enough? *Journal of Oral and Maxillofacial Surgery*, 71, 726.

Fattahi, T., 2006. Surgical anatomy of the mandibular region for reconstructive purposes. *Atlas of Oral and Maxillofacial Surgery Clinics of North America*, 14, 137.

Goyal, M., Marya, K. and Chawla, S., 2011. Mandibular osteosynthesis: a comparative evaluation of two different fixation systems using 2.0 mm titanium miniplates and 3-D locking plates. *Journal of Oral and Maxillofacial Surgery*, 10, 32.

Luyk, N.H., 1992. Principles of management of fractures of the mandible. In: L.J. Peterson, A.T. Indresano, R.D. Marciani and S.M.Roser, eds. *Principles of oral and maxillofacial surgery*. Philadelphia: Lippincott-Raven. Pp. 381–434.

Ochs, M.W., 2008. Fractures of the mandible. In: E. Myers, ed. *Operative otolaryngology*. 2nd ed. Amsterdam: Elsevier. Ch. 92, Fig. 92-1.

Van der Bergh, B., Heymans, M.W., Duvekot, F. and Forouzanfar, T., 2012. Treatment and complications of mandibular fractures: a 10-year analysis. *Journal of Cranio-Maxillofacial Surgery*, 40, e108.

Case Reports

Case Report 13.3. An intraoral approach to a posterior mandibular fracture. A 16-year-old male involved in an altercation presents with a right body fracture and a left angle fracture. (See Figures 13.14 through 13.20.)

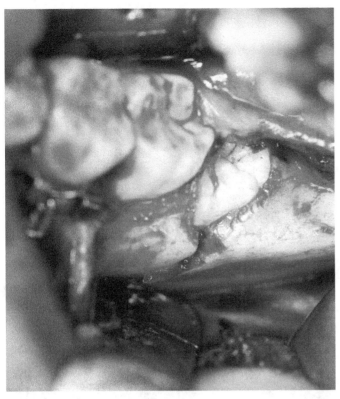

Figure 13.14. Intraoral exposure of the left mandibular angle fracture. The incision was created to incorporate the exposure and extraction of tooth #17 within the line of fracture.

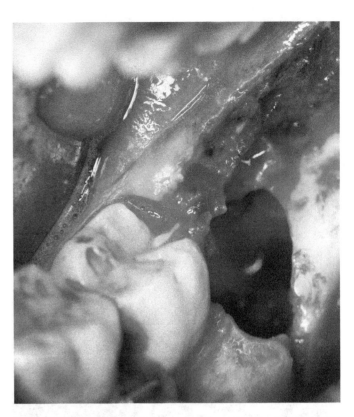

Figure 13.15. Left angle fracture after the extraction of tooth #17. Care was taken to not damage or displace the cortical bone during the extraction.

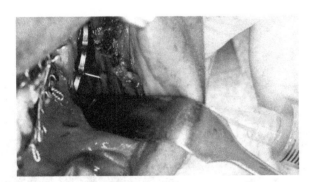

Figure 13.16. Insertion of a local anesthesia needle through the cheek to the oral cavity. By using the local anesthesia needle as a reference, it will allow for the ideal placement of the skin incision and trocar placement.

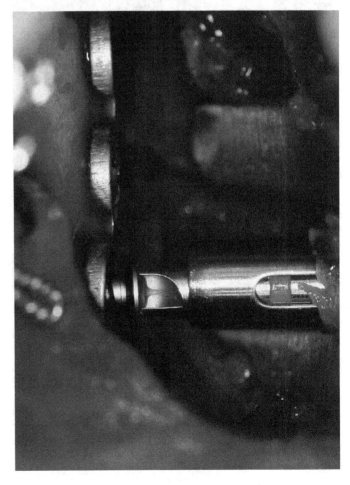

Figure 13.17. Placement of monocortical 2.0 screws through the trocar.

115

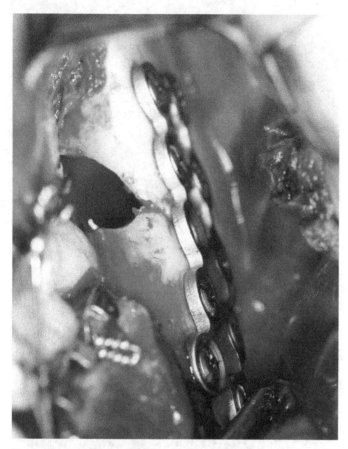

Figure 13.18. Plate secured to the lateral aspect of the posterior mandible with a strut plate and monocortical screws.

Case Report 13.4. An intraoral approach to a posterior mandibular fracture. A 17-year-old male presents after an altercation with a left posterior mandibular angle fracture. The patient was treated with the removal of impacted tooth #17 and the placement of a six-hole 2.0 mm plate at the superior border of the mandible with monocortical screws. The patient was placed into MMF with elastics for 3 weeks and then advanced to a soft diet. (See Figures 13.21 and 13.22.)

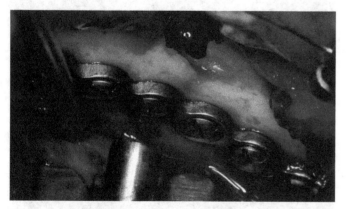

Figure 13.21. Six-hole plate placed at the superior border of the mandibular angle with monocortical screws. Impacted tooth #17 was extracted, and the plate was placed utilizing a percutaneous trocar.

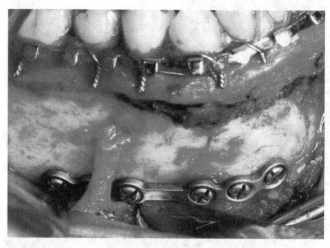

Figure 13.19. Contralateral fracture reduced with six-hole 2.0 plate at the inferior border with bicortical screws.

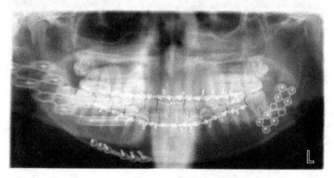

Figure 13.20. Postoperative orthopantomogram demonstrating fracture reductions.

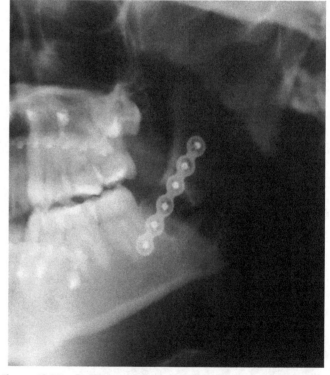

Figure 13.22. Postoperative orthopantomogram showing fracture reduction.

Case Report 13.5. An extraoral approach to a posterior mandibular fracture. A 27-year-old male presents status post altercation resulting in bilateral mandibular angle fractures. The patient was initially treated with the extraction of bilateral lower wisdom teeth and the placement of a strut plate with monocortical screws on the right side and a 2.8 mm reconstruction plate with bicortical screws on the left side. After 2 weeks of MMF, the patient presented with right-sided failed hardware and a subperiosteal facial abscess. The left side showed no signs of hardware failure or infection. (See Figures 13.23 through 13.33.) The patient was treated with the removal of the failed right mandibular angle strut plate through a submandibular incision, the debridement of the surgical site and the placement of a 2.8 mm reconstruction plate with bicortical screws.

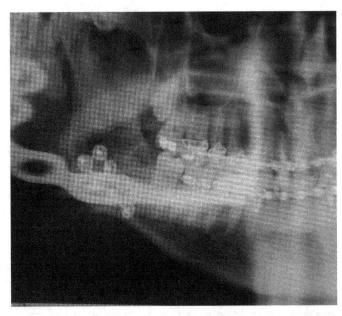

Figure 13.24.   Patient initially treated with the removal of impacted tooth #32 and the placement of a struct plate with monocortical screws.

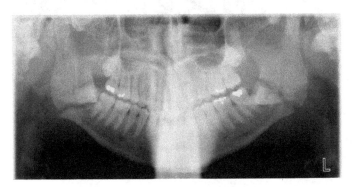

Figure 13.23.   Initial presentation of the patient with bilateral mandibular angle fractures with teeth in the line of the fractures.

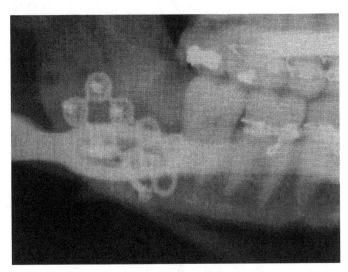

Figure 13.25.   Orthopantomogram 2 weeks postoperative demonstrating hardware failure.

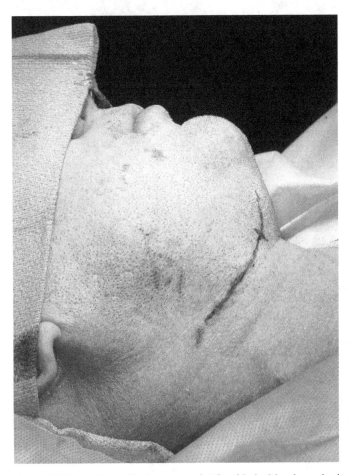

Figure 13.26.   Submandibular approach. The skin incision is marked and positioned within an upper cervical crease greater than 2 cm below the inferior border of the mandible.

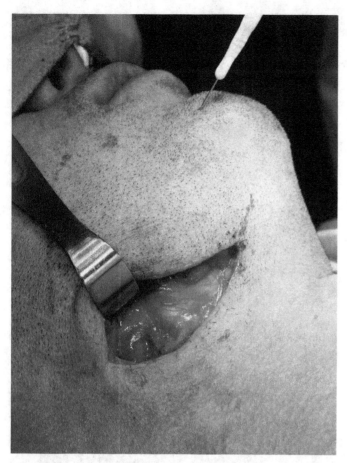

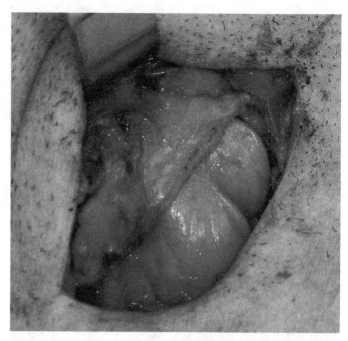

Figure 13.28. Division of the superficial layer of the deep cervical fascia (SDCF) as it courses over the submandibular gland. The marginal mandibular nerve is typically located within the SDCF overlying the submandibular gland.

Figure 13.27. Exposure of the superficial layer of the deep cervical fascia (SDCF) and the placement of a nerve stimulator within the soft tissue of the chin. The SDCF contains the marginal mandibular and the cervical nerves.

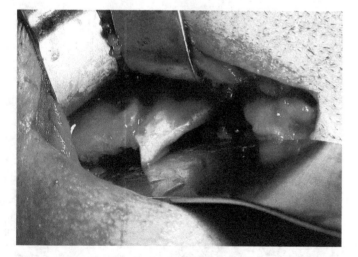

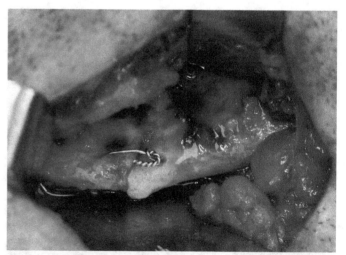

Figure 13.29. The inferior border of the mandible is exposed, the failed hardware is removed and the site is debrided.

Figure 13.30. Placement of a 24-gauge stainless steel intraosseous wire to align the proximal and distal segments of the fracture prior to the placement of rigid internal fixation.

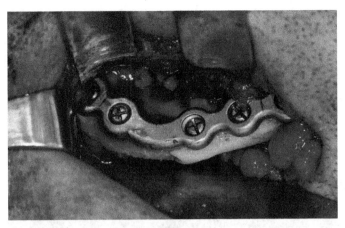

Figure 13.31. Placement of a seven-hole 2.8 mm reconstruction plate at the inferior border of the mandible caudal to the anticipated course of the inferior alveolar nerve.

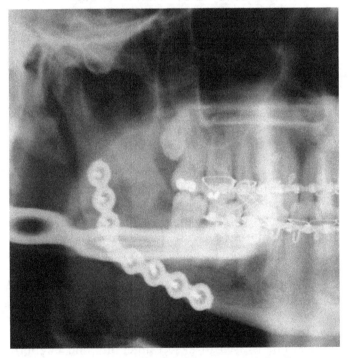

Figure 13.33. Postoperative orthopantomogram showing reconstruction plate placement at the inferior border of the mandible with fracture reduction.

Surgical Management of Mandibular Condyle Fractures (Extracapsular and Intracapsular Fractures)

Indications for Open Reduction of Mandibular Condyle Fractures

1. Inability to achieve pre-traumatic occlusion with manipulation and closed reduction
2. Open fracture with potential for fibrosis
3. Severe hypomobility of the affected joint after one week
4. Lateral extracapsular deviation
5. Foreign body within the joint space

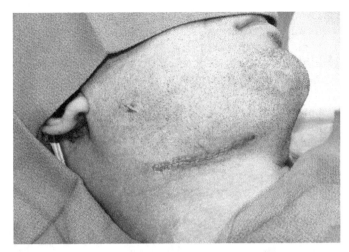

Figure 13.32.   Closure of the submandibular and trocar incisions.

6. Fracture into the middle cranial fossa
7. When stability of the occlusion is limited (e.g., less than three teeth per quadrant, gross periodontal disease, or skeletal abnormality)
8. Conditions that preclude closed reduction (severe chronic obstructive pulmonary disorder [COPD] or emphysema, seizure disorder, alcoholism, substance abuse, status asthmaticus, mental retardation, and psychosis)
9. To reestablish the vertical height of the lower third of the face with bilateral displaced condylar fractures
10. To reestablish anterior-posterior and vertical dimensions of the mandible in order to reconstruct midface crush-type injuries

Contraindications for Open Reduction of Mandibular Condyle Fractures

1. Condylar fractures with little or no dislocation
2. Condylar fractures with little or no fracture displacement
3. Fractures with minor malocclusion
4. Fractures occurring in childhood (below the age of 12 years; author preference)
5. Comminuted fractures or fractured segments too small to fixate
6. Medical conditions that preclude general anesthesia

Retromandibular Approach for Open Reduction of Extracapsular Condylar Fractures

1. The patient is nasally intubated. Short-acting paralytics are used in order to allow for testing of the facial nerve.
2. The patient is prepped from the hairline to the clavicles, and MMF is applied.
3. The head is turned to the side to allow for direct exposure of the ascending ramus. A sterile pen is used to

draw a 1.5–3.0 cm vertical line just posterior to the posterior border of the ascending ramus and originating 5 mm inferior to the ear lobe. The incision area is infiltrated with local anesthetic containing a vasoconstrictor within the subcutaneous tissue only.

4. A #15 blade is used to transect the skin and subcutaneous tissue. Needle-tipped electrocautery is used to control skin bleeders. The subcutaneous tissue is undermined in all directions to facilitate a tension-free closure at the end of the procedure.

5. A fine hemostat is used to dissect through the scant platysma muscle, SDCF (see Figure 13.36 in Case Report 13.6), and superficial musculoaponeurotic system (SMAS) to the parotid capsule. Blunt dissection proceeds anteromedially through the parotid gland to the posterior border of the ascending ramus. Care is taken to spread the tines of the hemostat in a direction parallel to the anticipated course of the facial nerve and to use a nerve stimulator once the parotid gland is reached. When branches of the facial nerve are identified, they are gently freed from surrounding tissue and reflected from the surgical site.

6. Army-navy retractors are used to provide direct visualization of the posterior ascending ramus. A #15 blade is used to transect the periosteum overlying the posterior aspect of the ascending ramus.

7. A periosteal elevator is used to dissect in a subperiosteal plane to expose and reduce the proximal and distal aspect of the subcondylar fracture (Figure 13.37, Case Report 13.6). A towel clip may be used to grasp the inferior aspect of the ramus in order to provide an inferior vector to aid in the reduction of the subcondylar fracture.

8. The fracture is plated (Figure 13.38, Case Report 13.6), the occlusion is verified, and the incision is closed in a tension-free, layered fashion. The parotid capsule is closed with interrupted 5-0 Vicryl sutures, the subcutaneous layer is closed with 4-0 Monocryl, and the skin edges are reapproximated with a running 5-0 plain gut suture.

Key Points for Extracapsular Open Reduction

1. Closed reduction of extracapsular or intracapsular condylar fractures are frequently treated with 10–14 days of MMF followed by aggressive physical therapy. Occlusion should be maintained with guiding elastics, and other mandibular fractures should be rigidly fixated to allow for this early mobilization.

2. Open reduction of indicated condyle fractures results in anatomical repositioning with rigid fixation of displaced segments, increased long-term occlusal stability, restoration of the vertical dimension of the ramus, and rapid return to function.

3. The condyle can be approached through a variety of approaches to include preauricular, submandibular, retromandibular, intraoral, and endoscopic approaches. The retromandibular approach allows for a more direct approach to the condylar neck, more visible exposure, and faster operating times.

4. When plating condylar fractures, the use of two plates provides superior strength and anti-rotational properties compared to the use of a single plate. The overall stability of two parallel plates versus two angulated plates is a highly polarized topic in the literature.

Pre-auricular Approach for Open Reduction of Intracapsular Condylar Fractures

1. The patient is nasally intubated. Short-acting paralytics are used in order to allow for testing of the facial nerve.

2. An ear wick is placed within the external auditory canal. The patient is prepped from the hairline to the clavicles, and MMF is applied. The head is turned to the side to allow for direct exposure of the ear, zygomatic arch, and temporomandibular joint.

3. A sterile pen is used to outline the incision. The incision should be hidden within a natural skinfold anterior to the ear. The incision originates within the hairline and courses caudally to the inferior aspect of the external auditory canal. Further superior and inferior extension is possible if additional exposure is required.

4. Local anesthetic containing a vasoconstrictor is used to infiltrate the subcutaneous tissue. The incision is created with a #15 blade and is carried through skin only. At the superior extent of the incision (above the zygomatic arch), needle-tipped electrocautery is used to cauterize skin bleeders and to transect the subcutaneous tissues and the temporoparietal fascia down to the temporalis fascia. The blunt end of a periosteal elevator is used to dissect anteriorly and inferiorly along the superficial layer of the temporalis fascia.

5. At the root of the zygoma, electrocautery is used to transect the superficial layer of the temporalis fascia, the temporal fat pad, and the periosteum overlying the zygomatic arch.

6. A periosteal elevator is used to dissect anteriorly along the zygomatic arch within a subperiosteal plane until the articular eminence is reached (Figure 13.42, Case Report 13.6). A periosteal elevator is used in a gentle sweeping motion to expose the lateral capsule of the tempomandibular joint.

7. Inferior mandibular traction is placed in order to separate the head of the condyle from the glenoid fossa. An incision is initiated with a #15 blade at the posterior slope of the eminence and proceeds posteriorly to the posterior aspect of the joint space. The #15 blade

is angled at 45° while inferior traction is applied to the mandible in order to avoid damaging the articular disc. A 2–3 mm cuff of tissue is left attached to the root of the zygoma–eminence in order to allow for closure of the lateral capsule.

8. The blunt end of a periosteal elevator is used to enter the superior joint space. The periosteal elevator is used in a sweeping motion to dissect into the anterior and posterior recesses of the superior joint space and medially to the medial pole of the condylar head.

9. The inferior joint space is entered by making an incision with a #15 blade at the inferior aspect of the lateral recess, where the lateral aspect of the articular disc attaches to the capsule.

10. Two periosteal elevators are used to locate and reduce the fractured segments. A towel clip can be used to grasp the inferior border of the angle of the mandible, and inferior traction can be applied to enlarge the joint space.

11. The fractured intracapsular segments are fixated with either a four-hole plate (Figure 13.43, Case Report 13.6) or two to three position screws, depending on the line of the fracture.

12. Once the fracture is fixated, the articular disc is repositioned into its most anatomical position with 5-0 Vicryl sutures.

13. MMF is removed, and the occlusion is assessed. The capsule is closed with 5-0 Vicryl sutures. The subcutaneous tissues are closed with 4-0 Monocryl sutures, and the skin edges are reapproximated with either steri-strips or 5-0 plain gut sutures (Figure 13.44, Case Report 13.6).

Key Points for Intracapsular Open Reduction

1. The tempomandibular joint space can be expanded for additional exposure or fracture reduction by one of three methods. A towel clip can be placed transcutaneously at the inferior angle of the mandible, and inferior traction is applied. Once the joint space is reached through the pre-auricular approach, a gauze packer (wire director) can be placed within the sigmoid notch and a downward vector of traction is applied. Finally, when the retromandibular approach is utilized, a skin hook can be placed within the sigmoid notch and a downward vector of traction is applied.

2. Care is taken to not strip the lateral pterygoid muscle from the condylar head. Care is also taken to not damage the articular cartilage and to not place plates or screws in close proximity to the articular surface.

3. Positional screws should only be used in intracapsular fractures if the screws can be inserted 90° to the fracture. For this reason, most intracapsular fractures are treated with bone reduction plates.

4. With the recent advancements in surgical techniques, instrumentation, and rigid fixation, there has been a recent movement away from traditional closed treatment of extracapsular and intracapsular fractures. Current therapy is based upon the anatomical repositioning of fractured segments with semirigid or rigid fixation, early and aggressive physical therapy, and a rapid return to function. Advantages of open reduction of extracapsular and intracapsular fractures include exact restoration of pretraumatic anatomy, maintenance of the vertical dimension of the ramus, articular disc repositioning and repair, increased occlusal stability, and early return to function without the need for prolonged MMF.

Postoperative Management

1. Appropriate analgesic and antibiotic coverage is warranted for the first 7 days after surgery.

2. Patients are allowed to function immediately after surgery. Patients are instructed to wear guiding elastics during the day for the first 2 weeks. Guiding elastics allow for a full range of motion and help to facilitate an appropriate occlusion. Heavier elastics are placed at night. After 2 weeks, no elastics are utilized unless malocclusion occurs. Mouth-opening exercises are begun on postoperative day 7. Physical therapy is initiated for patients who have hypomobility after 4 weeks.

3. Patients are maintained on a soft, nonchew diet for the first 2 weeks. They are gradually advanced to a full diet in weeks 2 through 6.

4. Arch bars are removed at 6–8 weeks depending on occlusal stability and reproducibility.

Complications

1. **Occlusal discrepancy**: Anterior open bite and/or retrognathia can result from inadequately reduced fractures, condylar resorption, avascular necrosis, and/or hardware failure.

2. **Deviation of the chin on opening**: Occurs with comminuted fractures, nonreduced intracapsular fractures, dislocated condylar fractures, condylar resorption, and avascular necrosis.

3. **Facial asymmetry**: Shortening of the ramus due to the loss of vertical height from displaced condylar fractures.

4. **Reduced mandibular mobility**: Often seen with intracapsular fractures and comminuted fractures of the condylar head, and can be an early sign of fibrous ankylosis.

5. **Ankylosis**: Often occurs with intracapsular fractures where the condylar stump is displaced laterally outside of the glenoid fossa, with significant comminution of the condylar head, hemarthrosis, and extended periods of MMF.

6. **Condylar resorption or avascular necrosis**: Can occur from stripping the lateral pterygoid muscle from the condyle. The lateral pterygoid muscle provides significant blood supply to the condylar head.

7. **Chronic pain**: Early pain can be from inadequate repositioning of the articular disc and the retrodiscal tissue into the pre-traumatic position. Late pain is typically from the development of osteoarthritis within the joint complex.

8. **Infection**: Caused by contamination of the surgical field, contamination of the wound, or failed hardware.

9. **Hardware failure**: Occurs from overdrilling screw osteotomies, inadequate irrigation, placement of screws within the line of fracture, and excessive early functioning.

10. **Hematoma and hemarthrosis**: Typically occurs from excessive hemorrhage from the retrodiscal tissue. Prevented by closing the joint space only after hemostasis is achieved. Treated with surgical evacuation of the hematoma.

11. **Frey's syndrome**: Occurs from aberrant innervation of the skin's sympathetic sweat glands by damaged parasympathetic auriculotemporal nerve fibers during the pre-auricular approach. Frey's syndrome is diagnosed by pre-auricular gustatory sweating, flushing, and a positive iodine–starch test, and is treated with botulinum toxin A injections.

12. **Salivary fistula and sialocele**: Occurs from failure to close the parotid capsule appropriately. Treated with the placement of a drain for 3–5 days, antisialogogue agents, and pressure dressings for 7–10 days.

13. **Pseudoarthrosis and failure of osteosynthesis**: Caused by inadequate fracture reduction, hardware failure, mobility at the fracture site, and infection.

14. **Pre-auricular hypoesthesia**: From inadvertent damage to the auriculotemporal nerve during dissection.

References

Aquilina, P., Chamoli, U., Parr, W.C.H., Clausen, P.D. and Wroe, S., 2013. Finite element analysis of three patterns of internal fixation of fractures of the mandibular condyle. *British Journal of Oral and Maxillofacial Surgery*, 51, 326.

Brandt, M.T. and Haug, R.H., 2003. Open versus closed reduction of adult mandibular condyle fractures: a review of the literature regarding the evolution of current thoughts on management. *Journal of Oral and Maxillofacial Surgery*, 61, 1324.

Chan, L.S., Barakate, M.S. and Havas, T.E., 2013. Free fat grafting in superficial parotid surgery to prevent Frey's syndrome and improve aesthetic outcome. *Journal of Laryngology and Otology*, 9, 1.

Ellis, E., McFadden, D., Simon, P. and Throckmorton, G., 2000. Surgical complications with open treatment of mandibular condylar process fractures. *Journal of Oral and Maxillofacial Surgery*, 58, 950.

Forouzanfar, T., Lobbezoo, F., Overgaauw, M., de Groot, A., Kommers, S., van Selms, M. and van den Bergh B., 2013. Long-term results and complication after treatment of bilateral fractures of the mandibular condyle. *British Journal of Oral and Maxillofacial Surgery*, 51(7), 634–8.

Gupta, M., Iyer, N., Das, D. and Nagaraj, J., 2012. Analysis of different treatment protocols for fractures of condylar process of mandible. *Journal of Oral and Maxillofacial Surgery*, 70, 83.

Haug, R.H. and Assael, L.A., 2001. Outcomes of open versus closed treatment of mandibular subcondylar fractures. *Journal of Oral and Maxillofacial Surgery*, 59, 370.

He, D., Yang, C., Chen, M., Bin, J., Zhang, X., Qiu, Y., 2010. Modified preauricular approach and rigid internal fixation for intracapsular condyle fracture of the mandible. *Journal of Oral and Maxillofacial Surgery*, 68, 1578.

Kent, J.N., Neary, J.P., Silvia, C., et al., 1990. Open reduction of mandibular condyle fractures. *Oral and Maxillofacial Surgery Clinics of North America*, 2, 69.

Kim, B.K., Kwon, Y.D., Ohe, J.Y., Choi, Y.H. and Choi, B.J., 2012. Usefulness of the retromandibular transparotid approach for condylar neck fractures and condylar base fractures. *Journal of Craniofacial Surgery*, 23, 712.

Kumaran, S. and Thambiah, L.J., 2012. Analysis of two different surgical approaches for fractures of the mandibular condyle. *Indian Journal of Dental Research*, 23, 463.

Parascandolo, S., Spinzia, A., Parascandolo, S., Piombiro, P. and Califano, L., 2010. Two load sharing plates fixation in mandibular condyle fractures: biomechanical basis. *Journal of Craniofacial Surgery*, 38, 385.

Vesnaver, A., 2008. Open reduction and internal fixation of intra-articular fractures of the mandibular condyle: our first experiences. *Journal of Oral and Maxillofacial Surgery*, 6, 2123.

Yang, M.L., Zhang, B., Zhou, Q., Gao, X.B., Liu, Q. and Lu, L., 2013. Minimally-invasive open reduction of intracapsular condylar fractures with preoperative simulation using computer-aided design. *British Journal of Oral and Maxillofacial Surgery*, 51, e29.

Zide, M.F., 1989. Open reduction of mandibular condyle fractures. *Clinics in Plastic Surgery*, 16, 69.

Zide, M.F. and Kent, J.N., 1983. Indications for open reduction of mandibular condyle fractures. *Journal of Oral and Maxillofacial Surgery*, 41: 89.

Case Reports

Case Report 13.6. A retromandibular approach to an extracapsular condyle fracture. A 46-year-old male status post high-speed motor vehicle accident resulting in a Le Fort III fracture, right comminuted ZMC fracture, right maxilla comminuted fracture, left parasymphysis fracture, and bilateral condylar neck fractures. The patient exhibited a significant decrease in the vertical height of the lower third of the face due to the bilateral displaced condylar neck fractures. The patient was treated with MMF, open reduction of all facial fractures, and removal of her left coronoid process to minimize potential fusion to the right comminuted maxilla. Both condyles were treated with rigid internal fixation in order to allow for early mobilization and to restore the vertical dimension of the lower third of the face. (See Figures 13.34 through 13.40.)

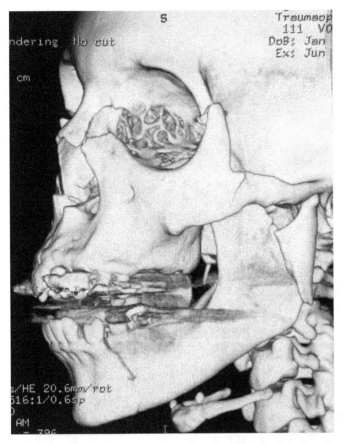

Figure 13.34. 3D reconstruction demonstrating a left displaced condylar neck fracture, a left parasymphysis fracture, and a Le Fort III fracture.

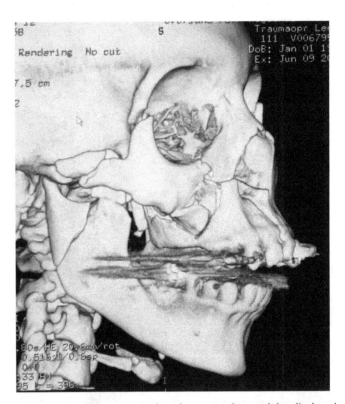

Figure 13.35. 3D reconstruction demonstrating a right displaced condylar neck fracture, a displaced right coronoid process fracture, a comminuted ZMC fracture, a comminuted maxillary fracture, and a Le Fort III fracture.

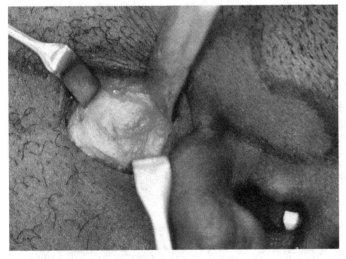

Figure 13.36. Retromandibular approach. The skin incision is placed 5 mm inferior to the lobule of the ear and extends along the posterior border of the ascending ramus. The superficial layer of the deep cervical fascia is exposed.

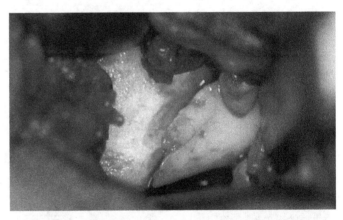

Figure 13.37. The fractured segments are exposed and reduced.

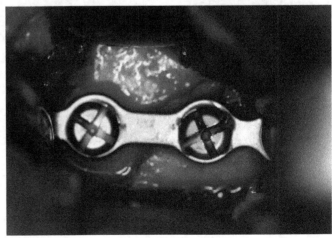

Figure 13.38. A four-hole 2.0 plate is placed to fixate the condylar neck fracture.

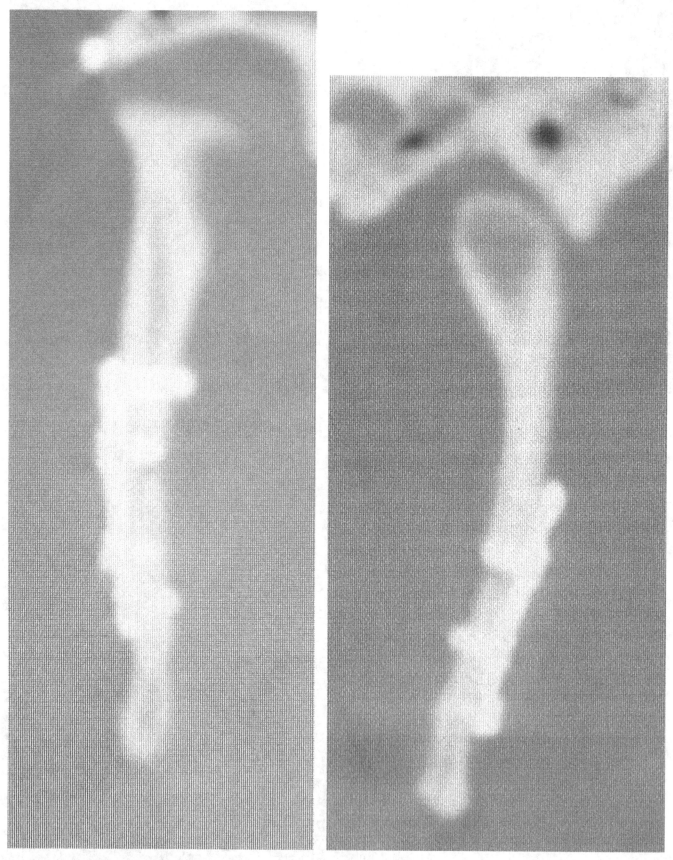

Figure 13.39.   Postoperative computed tomography scan demonstrating anatomical reduction of the bilateral condylar neck fractures and seating of the condylar heads within the glenoid fossa.

Figure 13.40 Postoperative 3D view demonstrating reestablishment of the vertical height of the mandible.

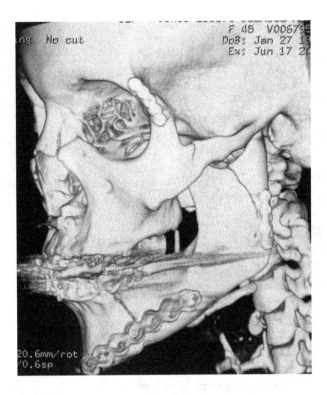

Case Report 13.7. A preauricular approach to an intracapsular condyle fracture. A 34-year-old male involved in an altercation resulting in a knee to the chin.

The patient sustained a grossly displaced right mandibular intracapsular condyle fracture. (See Figures 13.41, 13.42, 13.43, and 13.44.)

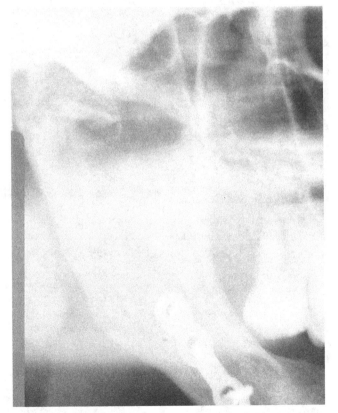

Figure 13.41. Orthopantomogram showing a previously repaired right mandibular angle fracture and a displaced right intracapsular condyle fracture.

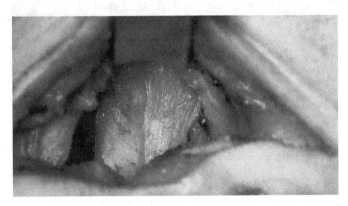

Figure 13.42. Preauricular approach. The eminence and the root of the zygoma are exposed to reveal the lateral capsule of the temporomandibular joint inferior to the arch.

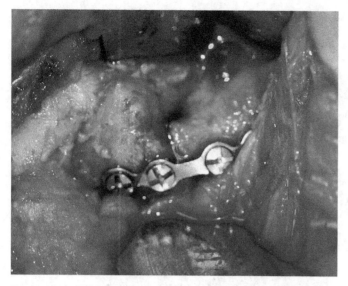

Figure 13.43.   The lateral capsule is opened, and the condylar head is anatomically reduced and fixated with a four-hole 1.0 mm plate.

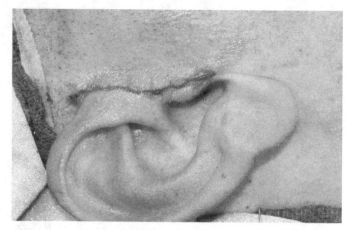

Figure 13.44.   Pre-auricular incision closed and hidden within a natural skin crease anterior to the ear.

Case Report 13.8. An endoscopic approach to an extracapsular condyle fracture. A 58-year-old male presents status post assault resulting in a right condylar neck fracture and a symphysis fracture of the mandible. The patient demonstrated significant malocclusion, deviation to the right on opening, and insufficient occlusion for closed reduction. The patient was treated with endoscopic open reduction and fixation of his right condyle and lag screw fixation of his linear symphysis fracture. (See Figures 13.45, 13.46, and 13.47.)

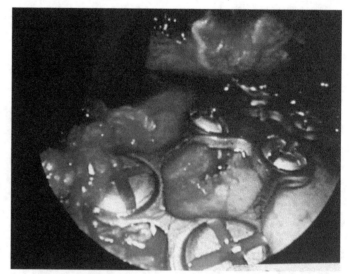

Figure 13.46.   Internal fixation of the right condylar fracture as viewed through the arthroscope.

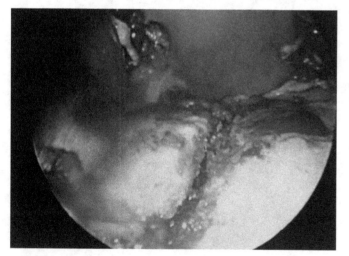

Figure 13.45.   Endoscopic view of the right condylar neck fracture after reduction using a 2.7 mm 30° arthroscope.

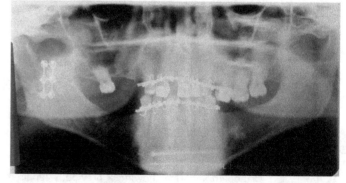

Figure 13.47.   Postoperative orthopantomogram demonstrating anatomical reduction of fractures.

Surgical Management of Atrophic Edentulous Mandibular Fractures

Indications for Open Reduction of Atrophic Edentulous Mandibular Fractures

1. Flail mandible
2. Gross displacement of the fractured segments
3. Infection
4. Non-union or malunion

See Figure 13.48 for a comparison of regions of edentulous mandible fractures.

Contraindications for Open Reduction of Atrophic Edentulous Mandibular Fractures

1. Significant medical comorbidities
2. Unable to tolerate general anesthesia

Transcervical Approach for Open Reduction of Atrophic Edentulous Mandibular Fractures

1. The patient is medically optimized prior to surgery as most patients are elderly and have associated medical comorbidities.
2. Oral intubation is employed if the fractures will be anatomically reduced without the use of the patient's dentures or gunning splints. Nasal intubation is employed if the patient's preexisting dentures/gunning splints and skeletal fixation will be utilized to aid in fracture reduction. Short-acting paralytics are used in order to test for branches of the facial nerve during the transcervical approach.
3. The patient's head is placed within the midline of the table with cervical hyperextension (unless cervical-spine injury or severe degenerative spine disease is present).

Edentulous Fracture Regions (%)

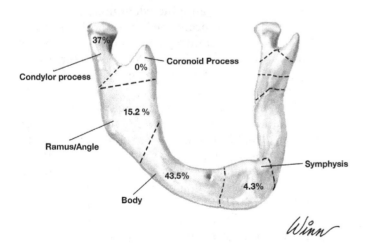

Figure 13.48. Percentage of edentulous mandible fractures by region. Modified from Luyk, NH (1992).

4. The patient is prepped and draped from the orbital rims to the clavicles. The oral cavity is included within the prep.
5. A cervical rhytid is identified that will hide the transcervical incision. A sterile marking pen is utilized to outline the site of the proposed skin incision. Ideally, the facial rhytid is located 1 cm cephalic to the thyroid cartilage (see Figure 13.51 in Case Report 13.9).
6. Local anesthesia containing a vasoconstrictor is infiltrated within a supraplatysmal plane at the site of the proposed incision.
7. A #15 blade is used to transect skin and subcutaneous tissue. The incision should be made in a single, continuous motion and can extend from mastoid process to contralateral mastoid process for bilateral posterior fractures. Needlepoint electrocautery is used to cauterize skin bleeders. The caudal aspect of the incision is undermined 1–2 cm within the subcutaneous tissue plane in order to allow for a tension-free closure at the end of the procedure.
8. The platysma muscle is sharply transected, and the SDCF is identified. A nerve stimulator is used to test for branches of the marginal mandibular and cervical nerves once the SDCF is reached.
9. The anterior border of the SCM muscle is identified. Care is taken to avoid damaging the greater auricular nerve and the external jugular vein along the superficial surface of the SCM.
10. A subplatysmal flap is raised and carried toward the inferior border of the mandible. At a point approximately 1 cm above the hyoid bone, a finger is used to palpate the bilateral submandibular glands. The investing fascia of the submandibular gland is entered at the inferior aspect of the gland. The facial artery and vein are identified, ligated, transected, and reflected superiorly (Hayes–Martin maneuver) along with the investing fascia containing the marginal mandibular nerve. A nerve stimulator is used to identify the marginal mandibular nerve as it courses superficially over the submandibular gland prior to its reflection with the submandibular glands investing fascia.
11. Medially, the anterior digastric tendons and muscles are identified and followed superiorly to the inferior border of the anterior mandible.
12. Once the inferior border of the mandible is reached, a #15 blade or electrocautery is used to transect the pterygomasseteric sling and periosteum.
13. A subperiosteal dissection is employed to expose the fractured segments and the thicker bone of the ramus and symphysis (Figure 13.52, Case Report 13.9). Care is taken to not strip periosteum from the lingual surface or from the alveolar crest so as not to further compromise the vascular supply to the atrophic mandible.
14. The fractured segments are reduced anatomically with digital manipulation. It may aid in the fracture reduction to place a finger on the inside of the

mouth and to place pressure on the lingual surface of the mandible.

15. The fractured segments are initially reduced with 2.0 mini-plates placed at the inferior border of the mandible with 4 mm screws (Figure 13.52, Case Report 13.9). This will allow the placement of a larger reconstruction plate once the fracture or fractures are anatomically reduced.

16. A reconstruction plate is adapted to follow the anatomy of the reduced atrophic mandible (Figure 13.54, Case Report 13.9). The reconstruction plate should be bent passively so as not to distract the condyles from their fossae during rigid plating. Passive plate placement can be optimized by using locking plates and screws.

17. The plate should be fixated with at least three bicortical screws per side. This will allow for greater load sharing and will minimize hardware failure from tension forces. Fixation should be extended to the ramus and symphysis portion of the mandible as this is typically the thickest portion of atrophic edentulous mandibles. Once the reconstruction plate (s) are fixated, the 2.0 mini-plates are removed from the inferior border of the mandible.

18. Immediate bone grafting may or may not be performed depending on the individual case.

19. The site is irrigated, and the incision is closed in a layered fashion with interrupted 4-0 Vicryl sutures used to reapproximate the fascia and platysma muscle, 5-0 Vicryl or Monocryl sutures for the subcutaneous tissue, and a running 5-0 plain gut sutures for the skin edges. Steri-strips are applied over the closed skin incision. Typically, drains and pressure dressings are not necessary.

Postoperative Management

1. Postoperative antibiotic and analgesics are required.
2. Steri-strips are removed after 5 days.
3. The patient is returned to oral function as soon as possible.
4. Future considerations may involve the removal of the reconstruction plate for denture fabrication and dental implants with or without additional grafting.

Complications

1. **Infection**: Early infections are usually caused from failure to follow sterile technique, inadequate closure of incision resulting in hematoma or seroma formation, or infected fracture sites prior to surgery. Late infections are typically from hardware failure, non-ideal fracture reduction, and immunocompromised patients.
2. **Wound dehiscence**: Most commonly seen with transoral approaches. Seen infrequently with transcervical approaches unless the wound is closed under direct tension or if a layered closure is not employed.

3. **Hardware failure**: Hardware failure in the edentulous mandible is often associated with the use of smaller fixation plates. The atrophic edentulous mandible is subjected to different forces than the dentate mandible. As such, the constant forces from the elevator and depressor muscles of the mandible produce constant, multivector tension and torque forces that can lead to fracture displacement and mini-plate failure. A reconstruction plate has the ability to withstand the previously mentioned forces and to provide absolute immobilization of the fractured segments during healing.

4. **Non-union or malunion**: Occur with non-anatomical reduction of atrophic mandible fractures. Can be minimized by obtaining wide surgical access with direct visualization of the fractures, anatomical reduction of fractured segments, minimization of fracture gaps, and the use of rigid fixation in the form of reconstruction plates.

5. **Nerve damage**: In the atrophic mandible, the position of the inferior alveolar nerve can be found along the crest of the alveolar ridge posterior to the mental foramen. Intraoral incisions should be placed within the buccal vestibule and not along the crest of the bone to minimize damage to the inferior alveolar nerve. Damage to the marginal mandibular or cervical nerve is possible from either transcervical or submandibular skin incisions. The incisions should be placed a minimum of 2 cm below the inferior border of the mandible, and a nerve stimulator should be utilized once the platysma muscle is transversed.

Key Points

1. Most patients with atrophic edentulous mandibular fractures have significant medical comorbidities that may influence operative management and postoperative healing. These factors need to be considered when placing the patient under general anesthesia for an extended period of time.

2. There is a direct relationship between the incidence of complications and the degree of bone atrophy when treating atrophic edentulous mandibular fractures. The majority of complications are associated with the inability to adequately reduce the fractured segments and from the poor quality of the dense, sclerotic, poorly vascularized bone. It is paramount to be judicious in the stripping of the periosteum while exposing the fractured segments. Frequently, the periosteum is the only blood supply to the anterior aspect of the atrophic edentulous mandible.

3. Primary healing occurs with accurate anatomical reduction of the fractured segments with the elimination of fracture gaps and immobilization of the fractured segments. This is best achieved with extraoral approaches and rigid fixation with reconstruction plates.

4. The reconstruction plate should fit passively, and locking plates and screws should be utilized. Care is taken to not create a torqueing force that will distract the mandibular condyles from the glenoid fossae.

5. Rigid plating of atrophic edentulous fractures leads to less complications and allows for earlier return to normal function. Rigid plating also eliminates the need for gunning splints and trans-skeletal maxillomandibular fixation, which is often contraindicated in the elderly patient population.

6. Reconstruction plates should be extended to areas of the mandible that are thicker (ramus and symphysis) in order to distribute the tension of the reconstruction plates to stronger segments of bone. Reconstruction plates should be plated with at least three screws on each side of the fracture in order to distribute the load sharing capabilities of the plate.

7. Care should be taken when placing bicortical screws in atrophic sclerotic mandibles in order to minimize damage to the inferior alveolar nerve and overheating the screw osteotomy site, which resultant future hardware failure, and creating additional fractures within the atrophic mandible with non-ideal screw placement.

8. Once plating is completed, a finger should be placed transorally along the lingual plate and the alveolar crest to ensure that the bicortical screws have not penetrated through the lingual plate of bone. Screw overpenetration will create pain, a source of infection, and may limit future prosthetic options for the patient.

9. Immediate bone grafting is advocated when fractured segments cannot be realigned adequately and when a non-union will occur, to add bulk bone to prevent future fractures and for future prosthetic considerations, and to promote revascularization through the transplantation of osteoprogenitor cells. Immediate bone grafting is not necessary in patients for whom prolonged general anesthesia is contraindicated or in patients with near ideal alignment of fractured segments.

10. Gunning splints can be fabricated in patients who are not surgical candidates (Figure 13.49). Gunning splints are skeletally fixated to the upper and lower jaws with trans-skeletal fixation via circum-mandibular wiring, pyriform rim wiring, trans-nasal wiring, or circum-zygomatic wiring. The patient is then placed into MMF by securing the gunning splints together. Gunning splints alone cannot adequately reduce grossly displaced fractures and are not ideal in elderly patients who cannot tolerate MMF due to nutritional deficiencies, COPD, dementia, etc. If gunning splints are fabricated, an opening should be created for nutritional support.

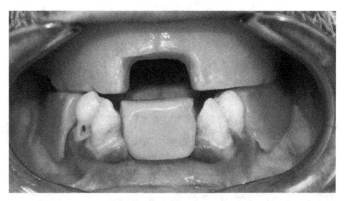

Figure 13.49. An opening is placed within the anterior aspect of the gunning splints to serve as a food port. The above photo is the try-in phase of the gunning splints. Arch bars will be fixated to the splints after the try-in.

References

Aziz, S.R. and Najjar, T., 2009. Management of the edentulous/atrophic mandibular fracture. *Atlas of Oral and Maxillofacial Surgery Clinics of North America*, 17, 75.

Chacon G.E. and Larsen P.E. 2004. Principles of Management of Mandibular Fractures. In: Peterson L.J., Miloro M., Ghali G.E., Larsen P.E. and Waite P.D. Peterson's Principles of oral and maxillofacial surgery. Second Ed. Hamilton, Ontario: BC Decker Inc:, 401–33.

Ellis, E. and Price, C., 2008. Treatment protocol for fractures of the atrophic mandible. *Journal of Oral and Maxillofacial Surgery*, 66, 421.

Landa, L.E., Tartan, B.F., Acartuk, A., Skouteris, C.A., Gordon, C., Sotereanos, G.C., 2003. Transcervical incision for use in oral and maxillofacial surgical procedures. *Journal of Oral and Maxillofacial Surgery*, 61, 343.

Luyk N.H. 1992. Principles of management of fractures of the mandible. In: Peterson L.J., Indresano A.T., Marciani R.D. and Roser S.M. Editors. *Principles of oral and maxillofacial surgery*. Philadelphia, PA: Lippincott-Raven, 381–434.

Luyk, N.H. and Ferguson J.W. 1991. The diagnosis and initial management of the fractured mandible. *Am J Emerg Med*, 9, 352–9.

Madsen, M.J., Haug, R.H., Christensen, B.S. and Aldridge, E., 2009. Management of atrophic mandible fractures. *Oral and Maxillofacial Surgery Clinics of North America*, 21, 175.

Madsen, M.J., Kushner, G.M. and Alpert, B., 2011. Failed fixation in atrophic mandibular fractures: the case against miniplates. *Craniomaxillofacial Trauma Reconstruction*, 4, 145.

Riffat, F., Buchanan, M.A., Mahrous, A.K., Fish, B.M. and Jani, P., 2012. Oncological safety of the Hayes-Martin manoeuvre in neck dissections for node-positive oropharyngeal squamous cell carcinoma. *Journal of Laryngology and Otology*, 126, 1045.

Tiwana, P.S., Abraham, M.S., Kushner, G.M. and Alpert, B., 2009. Management of atrophic edentulous mandibular fractures: the case for primary reconstruction with immediate bone grafting. *Journal of Oral and Maxillofacial Surgery*, 67, 882.

Van Sickles, J.E. and Cunningham, J.L., 2012. Management of atrophic mandible fractures: are bone grafts necessary? *Journal of Oral and Maxillofacial Surgery*, 68, 1392.

Case Report 13.9. A transcervical approach to an atrophic edentulous fracture. A 42-year-old male presents after a construction accident resulting in facial fractures to include the left comminuted zygomaticomax- illary complex (ZMC) fractures, naso-orbital-ethmoid (NOE) complex fractures, bilateral mandibular body fractures, and a left subcondylar fracture. (See Figures 13.50 through 13.56.)

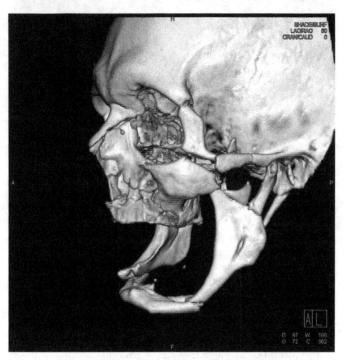

Figure 13.50.   3D reconstruction demonstrating extensive fractures to the lower jaw and midface.

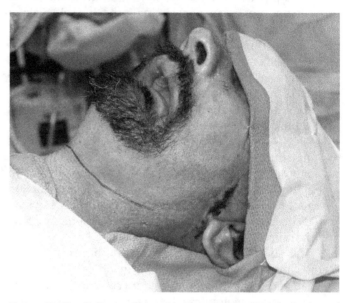

Figure 13.51.   Flail mandible with loss of horizontal projection of the lower third of the face. Marking of planned transcervical apron incision coinciding with a cervical crease approximately 1 cm cephalic to the thyroid cartilage.

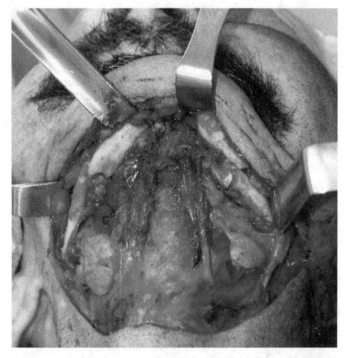

Figure 13.52.   Transcervical apron incision is extended from mastoid process to contralateral mastoid process to allow for wide surgical access of all mandibular fractures.

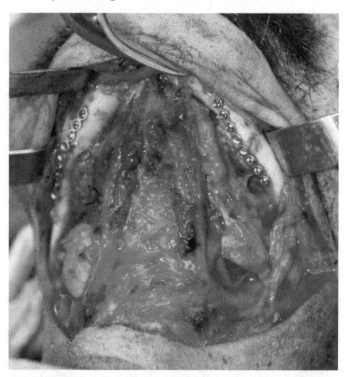

Figure 13.53.   Bilateral body fratures are initially anatomically reduced with 2.0 plates fixated to the inferior border of the mandible.

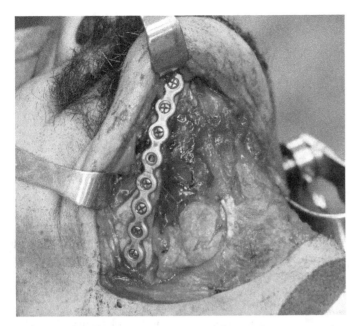

Figure 13.54. The 2.0 plates are removed once the reconstruction plates are secured.

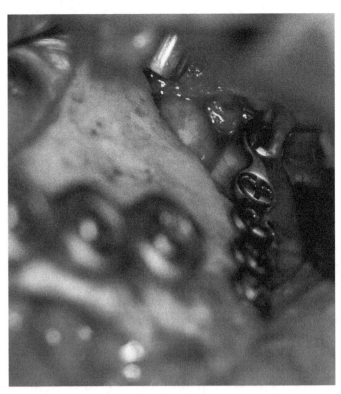

Figure 13.55. The transcervical incision also provides direct access to the left subcondylar fracture.

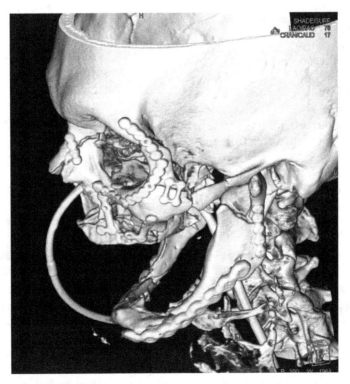

Figure 13.56. Postoperative 3D reconstruction depicting anatomical reduction of the atrophic edentulous mandibular fractures and associated midface fractures.

Surgical Management of Pediatric Mandibular Fractures

Indications for Open Reduction of Pediatric Mandibular Fractures

Displaced noncondylar fractures that cannot be adequately reduced with closed techniques.

Contraindications for Open Reduction of Pediatric Mandibular Fractures

1. Condyle fractures
2. Fractures that can be reduced with closed reduction (external and/or internal skeletal fixation or pediatric splint)
3. Nondisplaced fractures (can be treated with a soft diet) with no or minor changes in occlusion

Pediatric Splint Fabrication and Closed Reduction

1. The patient is placed under general anesthesia via nasal intubation.
2. Weight-appropriate preoperative intravenous antibiotics are administered.
3. A throat pack is placed within the posterior oropharynx. The patient is prepped and draped from the orbits to the clavicles to include the oral cavity.
4. Alginate impressions are taken of both the maxilla and the mandible.
5. The impressions are poured in stone plaster. The mandibular cast is sectioned along the fracture line.
6. The mandibular cast is oriented to the maxillary cast to reestablish the pre-traumatic occlusion. The mandibular cast is looted together with wax and stone plaster. The maxilla and the looted mandibular cast are placed within a single hinged articulator, and an acrylic splint is fabricated with a lingual flange. Holes are placed within the buccal and lingual flange of the splint to facilitate placement of circum-mandibular wires.
7. The splint is inserted and secured to the mandible with 26-gauge circum-mandibular wires (Figure 13.62) placed with an awl. External fixation is applied to the middle one-third of the face via any combination of MMF screws, pyriform aperture screw/wiring, zygomatic arch screws/wiring, infraorbital screws/wiring, or trans-nasal wiring.

Closed Reduction via External Skeletal Fixation (Skeletal Wiring or Drop Wires)

1. The patient is placed under general anesthesia via nasal intubation.
2. Weight-appropriate preoperative intravenous antibiotics are administered.
3. The patient is prepped and draped from the orbits to the clavicles to include the oral cavity.

4. An incision is placed within the maxillary anterior buccal vestibule in order to expose the pediatric pyriform apertures (rims).
5. A fissured bur is used to create an osteotomy at the base of each pyriform aperture. A 25-gauge stainless steel wire is placed through each pyriform aperture and tightened into a loop (Figure 13.59). If additional posterior anchorage is required, circum-zygomatic wires or titanium screws are placed within the zygomatic arch.
6. An awl is used to place circum-mandibular wires (Figures 13.60 and 13.62). The awl is placed from the oral cavity through the skin of the inferior border of the mandible posterior to the mental foramen. The awl is passed in close proximity to the buccal cortex. Once the awl passes through the skin at the inferior border of the mandible, the wire and the awl are redirected through the same percutaneous skin wound and passed along the lingual aspect of the mandible back into the oral cavity. The circum-mandibular wire is then tightened, leaving a loop at its distal end. Care is taken to not over-tighten the circum-mandibular wire as overtightening can transect the thin pediatric mandible. Circum-mandibular wires are placed bilaterally.
7. A final 25-gauge stainless steel wire or heavy elastics are used to place the patient into MMF (Figure 13.61).

Open Reduction with Resorbable Plates and Screws

1. When possible, screw osteotomies (drilling sites) should avoid areas of developing tooth buds. All screw osteotomies that must be placed within areas of developing tooth buds are monocortical in order to minimize the potential for damage to the developing tooth buds.
2. All screw osteotomies are pretapped prior to the insertion of resorbable screws.
3. Resorbable screws have a blunt-ended tip, which aids in preventing damage to developing tooth buds.
4. Fixation plates must be heated in a water bath to aid in plate pliability and adaptation.
5. Resorbable screws are more likely to fracture and do not engage the bone as aggressively as titanium screws.

Postoperative Management

1. The patient is placed on weight-appropriate oral analgesics and antibiotic for 1 week.
2. Patients are placed into MMF for 1 week. After one week, the lingual splint or Risdon cables are left in place and the mouth-opening exercises are initiated. External skeletal fixation is removed after 7–10 days.
3. A soft diet is maintained for a period of 3 weeks.
4. The splint or Risdon cables are removed after 3 weeks provided satisfactory occlusion.

5. Future orthodontic treatment is recommended to correct any occlusal discrepancies that are not corrected by the eruption of the primary dentition.

Complications

1. **Malocclusion**: Can result from numerous causes. Ideally corrected with postoperative orthodontic care.
2. **Dental trauma**: Occurs from placing fixation screws into developing tooth buds. With open reduction techniques, plates and screws should be placed at the inferior border of the mandible to avoid developing tooth buds and the mandibular canal.
3. **Hardware failure**: Due to inappropriate plate placement, resorbable screw fracture or loosening, and patient noncompliance.
4. **Growth abnormalities**: Typically associated with condylar fractures that damage the growth plate.
5. **Ankylosis**: Occurs from prolonged MMF, comminuted condylar fractures, and hemarthrosis.
6. **Paresthesia or anesthesia**: Occurs from damage to the mental nerve or inferior alveolar nerve during tissue dissection or screw placement.
7. **Infection**: Typically from hardware failure or from a foreign body reaction associated with the degradation products of the resorbable hardware. Infections typically resolve after local incision and drainage of the area and the administration of oral antibiotics.

Key Points

1. Mandibular condyle fractures are the most common type of mandibular fractures in the pediatric population.
2. Open treatment of mandibular fractures is typically reserved for older pediatric patients (older than the age of 10).
3. It is difficult to apply traditional Erich arch bars to primary teeth due to their bulbous shape. Risdon cables can be used to apply MMF in patients with primary or mixed dentition (Figure 13.57).
4. When placing MMF screws or other means of skeletal fixation, care is taken to not damage nearby tooth roots or developing permanent teeth.
5. Care is taken when placing circum-mandibular wires to not overtighten the circum-mandibular wires and transect the inferior border of the soft pediatric mandible.
6. It is essential to keep pediatric patients adequately hydrated while MMF is employed.
7. When open reduction is required, the use of monocortical screws is recommended in order to minimize the risk of inadvertent damage to developing tooth buds.

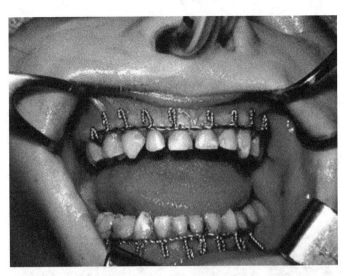

Figure 13.57. Risdon cables. Twenty-four-gauge stainless steel wires are braided and function as arch bar. Each tooth is ligated to the braided arch bar in the standard fashion. Note the low profile of the Risdon cable. (Image courtesy of *Atlas of Oral and Maxillofacial Surgery Clinics of North America.* Kushner, G.M. and Tiwana, P.S., 2009. Fractures of the growing mandible. 17(89), 81.)

8. Resorbable plates should be placed at the inferior border of the mandible to avoid damaging tooth buds and the contents of the mandibular canal. The plates should be fixated with at least two screws on each side of the fracture.

References

Eppley, B.L., 2005. Use of resorbable plates and screws in pediatric facial fractures. *Journal of Oral and Maxillofacial Surgery,* 63, 385.

Lee, H.B., Oh, J.S., Kim, S.G., Kim, H.K., Moon, S.Y., Kim, Y.K., Yun, P.Y. and Son, J.S., 2010. Comparison of titanium and biodegradable miniplates for fixation of mandibular fractures. *Journal of Oral and Maxillofacial Surgery,* 68, 2065.

Srinivasan, I., Kumar, M.V., Kumaran, P.S., Bhandari, A. and Udhya, J., 2013. Management of symphysis fracture of a 3-year-old child prefabricated acrylic splint and circum-mandibular wiring. *Journal of Dentistry for Children,* 80, 36.

Case Reports

Case Report 13.10. Closed reduction via external skeletal fixation. A 7-year-old patient presents after a motor vehicle accident with a displaced mandibular body fracture. The patient was treated with bilateral circum-mandibular wires and bilateral pyriform aperture (rim) wires and closed reduction with heavy elastics for a period of 7 days. (See Figures 13.58, 13.59, 13.60, and 13.61.)

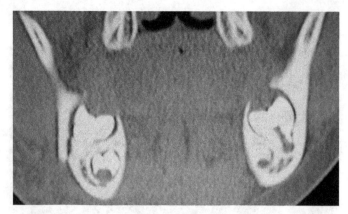

Figure 13.58. Computed tomography scan demonstrating a fracture of the right posterior mandible in an area of developing tooth follicles.

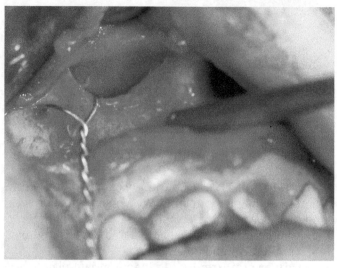

Figure 13.59. Skeletal fixation is employed with 25-gauge wires placed along the bilateral pyriform aperatures well above the roots of the developing canines.

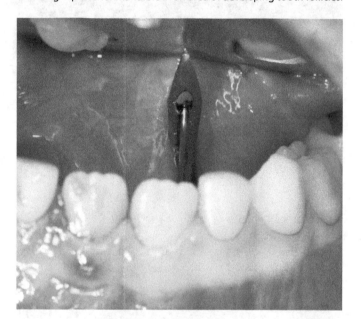

Figure 13.60. Circum-mandibular wires are placed with an awl.

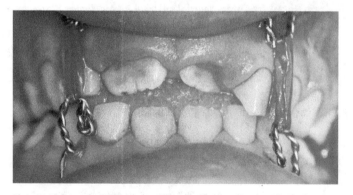

Figure 13.61. Patient in maxillomandibular fixation (MMF) using skeletal fixation and heavy elastics.

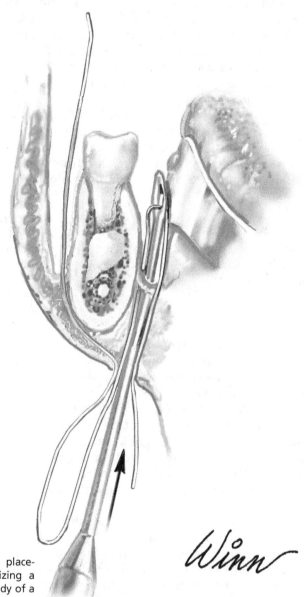

Figure 13.62. Illustration depicting the placement of a circum-mandibular wire utilizing a mandibular awl within the mandibular body of a pediatric patient posterior to the mental foramen.

Case Report 13.11. Open reduction with resorbable plates and screws. A 11-year-old patient presents after an altercation resulting in a displaced symphysis fracture and left mandibular angle fracture through the developing third molar site. Due to the patient's dental development, treatment included the placement of Erich arch bars and resorbable hardware. (See Figures 13.63, and 13.64.)

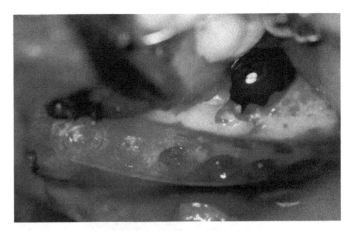

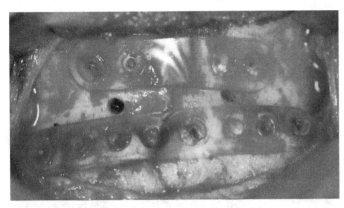

Figure 13.63. The symphysis was treated with superior (monocortical screws) and inferior (bicortical screws) 2.2 mm resorbable plate placement.

Figure 13.64. The developing third molar follicle was removed, and the left angle fracture was reduced and fixated with a 2.2 mm resorbable plate and monocortical resorbable screws.

Surgical Management of Comminuted Mandibular Fractures

Indication for Open Reduction of Comminuted Mandibular Fractures

1. To restore occlusion
2. To restore arch form
3. To restore facial contours
4. To restore function
5. Flail mandible or fractures involving the genial tubercules resulting in posterior displacement of the geniohyoid and genioglossus muscles

Contraindications for Open Reduction of Comminuted Mandibular Fractures

1. Comminuted segments to small to plate
2. When excessive periosteal stripping may lead to severe bone resorption
3. Comminuted fractures with severe tissue loss or tissue avulsion
4. Medical comorbidities that limit or preclude the use of general anesthesia

Postoperative Management

1. Postoperative antibiotics are imperative in open comminuted fractures.
2. The patient is maintained in MMF for 4–6 weeks. If necessary, a feeding tube is placed.
3. Secondary bone grafting may be necessary after hard and soft tissue healing.

Complications

1. **Infection**: Causes include inadequate fracture reduction, teeth within the line of fracture, contaminated wound, failed hardware, and necrotic comminuted bone segments.
2. **Wound dehiscence**: From inadequately vascularized tissue, hematoma or seroma formation, inadequate closure of tissues in a layered fashion, necrotic segments of underlying bone, and closure of tissue under tension.
3. **Non-union or malunion**: Typically from inadequate fracture reduction, fracture mobility, or hardware failure.
4. **Fistula or sialocele development**: Occurs when damage occurs to the parotid or submandibular gland.

Key Points

1. Posterior displacement of the tongue via either a flail mandible or fracture of the genial tubercules should be addressed promptly prior to airway embarrassment (Figure 13.68, Case Report 13.13).
2. Facial lacerations or tissue avulsions allow for excellent exposure to the underlying bones (Figure 13.71, Case Report 13.14).
3. Temporary fixation of comminuted mandibular segments with either wire fixation or mini-plates will allow for the contouring and adaptation of reconstruction plates for permanent rigid fixation of the fractured segments (Figure 13.66, Case Report 13.12).
4. Comminuted fractures should be plated with at least three screws per side of the fracture. Screws should be bicortical when possible and should not be placed in areas of severe comminution (Figure 13.70, Case Report 13.13).
5. Care should be taken to keep periosteal stripping to a minimum in comminuted fractures. The periosteum overlying the lingual aspect of the mandible should be preserved to maintain an adequate blood supply to the fractured and/or comminuted segments.

6. Debridement of nonviable soft and hard tissues, dental fragments, and projectile fragments at the time of surgery will decrease postoperative complications.
7. Always attempt to cover exposed bone when possible. If tissue undermining is inadequate, consider local and regional advancement flaps.

8. Immediate bone grafting of mandibular defects is determined by the size of the defect, the contamination of the wound, and the amount of soft tissue coverage capable of closure without tension.

Case Reports

Case Report 13.12. Grossly comminuted bilateral mandibular fractures. A 24-year-old male presents after a motor vehicle accident with numerous comminuted fractures to his bilateral mandibular angle, body, and anterior mandible. (See Figures 13.65, 13.66, and 13.67).

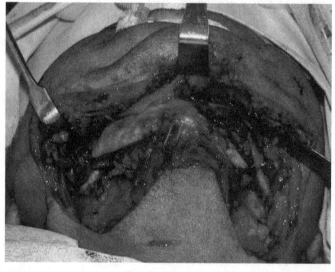

Figure 13.65. A transcervical approach allows for wide surgical access to the comminuted mandibular fractures.

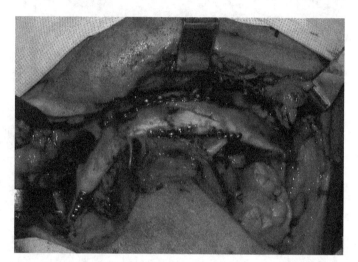

Figure 13.66. Mini-plates are placed at the inferior border of the mandible to temporarily reposition the fractured segments prior to placing a reconstruction plate.

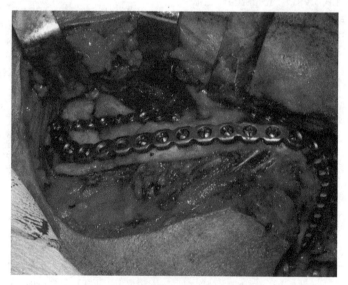

Figure 13.67. Reconstruction plate adapted and fixated to the inferior border of the mandible to provide an inferior tension band and to minimize movement of the fractured segments.

Case Report 13.13. Grossly comminuted anterior mandibular fractures with a flail mandible. A 65-year-old man immediately status post a self-inflicted gunshot wound to the anterior mandible with gross comminution. Upon arrival in the Emergency Department, the man was seated upright and in little distress with a Glasgow Coma Score of 15. After leaving the CT scanner, the patient underwent airway embarrassment from the posterior displacement of his tongue musculature

and sustained an awake tracheotomy in route to the operating room. All mandibular teeth with the exception of #18, #30, and #31 were hopelessly fractured. The three remaining posterior mandibular teeth were utilized to place the patient into MMF via Ivy loops. A 2.8 mm reconstruction plate was used to realign the anterior mandible, and wire fixation was used to secure the lingual plate and reposition the tongue musculature. (See Figures 13.68, 13.69, and 13.70.)

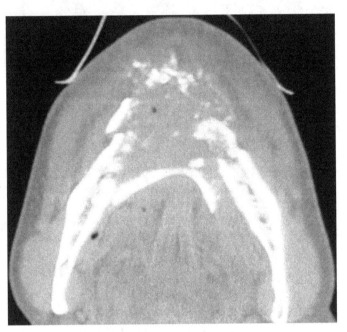

Figure 13.68. Axial CT demonstrating gross displacement of the anterior lingual plate with posterior displacement of the geniohyoid and genioglossus muscles leading to airway embarassment (flail jaw).

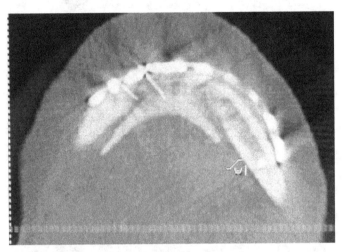

Figure 13.69. Axial postoperative cone beam CT demonstrating the lingual plate and its associated musculature ligated to the reconstruction plate with wire fixation.

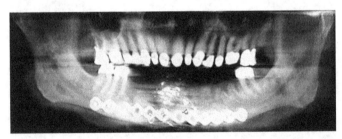

Figure 13.70. The comminuted mandible was treated with a 2.8 mm locking reconstructive plate secured to the mandible with bicortical screws placed inferior to the mandibular canal. All unsalvageable teeth were removed. Retained molar teeth aided in establishing the vertical and anterior-posterior dimension of the mandible.

Case Report 13.14. Comminuted mandibular fractured approached via soft tissue injury. A 36-year-old man sustained a gunshot wound to the left face and mandible, resulting in a comminuted left mandibular body/angle fracture, moderate tissue avulsion, and a stellate, contaminated tissue wound. (See Figures 13.71 and 13.72.)

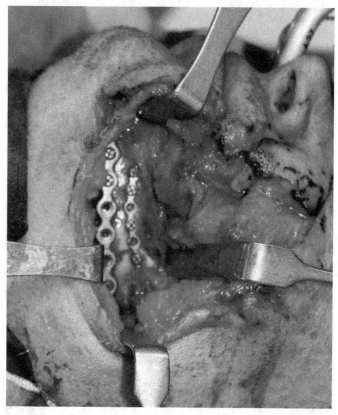

Figure 13.71. Mandible and associated fractures reduced through preexisting tissue avulsion.

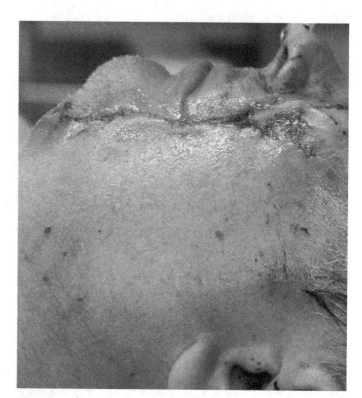

Figure 13.72. Closure of the stellate wound with local flap advancement.

External Fixation of Mandibular Fractures

Indications for External Fixation of Mandibular Fractures

1. Grossly comminuted mandibular fractures where the fractured segments are too small to appropriately plate (bag of bones)
2. Comminuted fractures with severe tissue loss or tissue avulsion
3. Grossly infected fractures
4. Medical comorbidities that limit or preclude the use of general anesthesia

Contraindication for External Fixation of Mandibular Fractures

1. Bone pathology in the area of necessary pin placement

External Fixation Technique

1. Airway patency is secured via either intubation or tracheostomy.
2. The patient is prepped from the orbital rims to the clavicles to include the intraoral cavity.
3. If dentate, all damaged and unsalvageable teeth are removed, and the patient is placed into MMF via arch bars and 24 or 26-gauge stainless steel wires and/or heavy elastics.
4. The fractured segments and the inferior border of the mandible are palpated and mapped with intraoral and extraoral digital manipulation.
5. Stab incisions are placed in the anticipated sites of fixation screw placement.
6. A hemostat is used to dissect to the inferior border of the mandible. Either a trocar or a nasal speculum is used to retract the tissues. The fixation screw is placed within the placement gun, positioned within the trocar or within the nasal speculum, and scrapped along the inferior border of the mandible in order to remove the periosteum and to feel the inferior border of the mandible. The fixation screw is driven through both the buccal and lingual cortical plates. Care is taken to not drive the fixation screw past the lingual plate.
7. At least two fixation screws are placed in each segment of bone. The fixation screws ideally are placed 10 mm from the fracture site and at least 10 mm from adjacent fixation screws.
8. After fixation screw placement, MMF is removed, and a finger is run along the lingual surface of the mandible to check for overpenetration of the fixation

screws within the floor of the mouth. If overpenetration has occurred, the fixation screw is reversed until it is flush with the lingual plate.

9. The connectors/acrylic bar/chest tube is placed 10 mm lateral to the skin surface (Figures 13.74 and 13.75). If acrylic is used, moist sterile gauze is placed over the skin in order to protect against thermal damage from the polymerization of the acrylic.

10. The fixation screws are wrapped in ribbon gauze impregnated with iodoform or antibiotic ointment (Figure 13.74).

Postoperative Management

1. Ribbon gauze impregnated with iodoform or antibiotic ointment wrapped around the fixation pins is changed daily.

2. Postoperative antibiotics are imperative.

3. Fracture adjustments can be made by either adjusting the adjustable connectors or by cutting and refixating the acrylic bar.

4. Fracture healing can be tested by removing connectors or by cutting the acrylic bar to test for mobility.

Complications

1. **Infection**: May be caused from necrosis of bone surrounding the fixator screws, necrotic segments of avulsed bone, tissue trauma or retained unsalvegeable teeth.

2. **Cellulitis around the fixation screws**: Typically from not leaving sufficient space between the connectors/fiber rods/acrylic bar and the skin. 1.0 to 1.5 cm of clearance should be present between the skin and the connectors/fiber rods/acrylic bar. Additional clearance is required in instances where additional facial edema is expected after external fixator placement.

3. **Non-union or malunion**: One the most common complications associated with external fixators. External fixation procedures commonly require a secondary grafting procedure.

4. **Screws becoming detached from the underlying bone**: Typically from not fully engaging the lingual cortex or by placing the connectors/fiber rods/acrylic bar too close to the skin.

5. **Damage to adjacent structures**: Typically to the inferior alveolar nerve, teeth roots, and contents of the floor of the mouth from inappropriate placement of fixation screws.

6. **Percutaneous fistulae formation:** Typically from bone necrosis around the fixator screws.

7. **Damage to the parotid gland or submandibular gland**: Frequently results in sialocele or salivary fistula formation.

8. **Thermal trauma to the underlying skin:** Due to the polymerization of acrylic. Moist gauze should be placed between the skin and the acrylic until the polymerization process is completed.

Key Points

1. There are several types of external fixation systems that range from the use of percutaneous screws (or pins) fixated to an acrylic bar, a chest tube filled with acrylic, and lightweight, adjustable carbon fiber rod systems developed for orthopedic hand and forearm surgery.

2. Percutaneous screws are placed at least 1 cm from the fracture and are placed within thick segments of bone such as the body and symphysis region.

3. Care is taken to avoid placing the percutaneous screws within the fracture, too close to the fracture, within the roots of teeth, within the mandibular canal, or deep to the lingual cortex of the mandible.

4. Percutaneous screws should be placed or angulated far enough apart for the placement of connectors if fiber carbon rod systems are utilized.

5. Connectors and/or the bar should be placed a minimum of 10 mm off of the skin so that, as the tissue swells, the skin will not necrosis.

6. External fixation commonly results in either the nonunion or malunion of fractures and typically requires a secondary grafting procedure.

7. The overall complication rate of the treatment of comminuted mandibular fractures has been reported to be 35% with the use of external pin fixation, 17% with MMF alone, and 10% for patients treated with open reduction with rigid internal fixation. Studies support a higher rate of complications with higher degrees of fracture comminution.

References

Alpert, B., Tiwana, P.S. and Kushner G.M., 2009. Management of comminuted fractures of the mandible. *Oral and Maxillofacial Surgery Clinics of North America*, 21, 185.

Braidy, H.F. and Ziccardi, V.B., 2009. External fixation for mandible fractures. *Atlas of Oral and Maxillofacial Surgery Clinics of North America*, 17, 45.

Ellis, E., Muniz, O. and Anand, K., 2003. Treatment considerations for comminuted mandibular fractures. *Journal of Oral and Maxillofacial Surgery*, 61, 861.

Gibbons, A.J. and Breederveld, M.R.S., 2011. Use of a custom designed external fixator system to treat ballistic injuries to the mandible. *International Journal of Oral and Maxillofacial Surgery*, 40, 103.

Li, Z. and Li, Z.B., 2011. Clinical characteristics and treatment of multiple site comminuted mandible fractures. *Journal of Cranio-Maxillo-Facial Surgery*, 39, 296.

Pereira, C.C., Letícia dos Santos, P., Jardim, E.C., Júnior, I.R., Shinohara, E.H. and Araujo, MM., 2012. The use of 2.4 mm locking plate system in treating comminuted mandibular fracture by firearm. *Craniomaxillofacial Trauma Reconstruction*, 5, 91.

Tucker, D.I., Zachar, M.R., Chan, R.K. and Hale, R.G., 2013. Characterization and management of mandibular fractures: Lessons learned from Iraq and Afghanistan. *Atlas of Oral and Maxillofacial Surgery Clinics of North America*, 21, 61.

Case Report 13.15. Comminuted mandibular fractures with extensive soft tissue injuries reduced via external fixation. A 62-year-old female presents status post motor vehicle accident with an open, comminuted, edentulous mandibular fracture. Due to the

patient's edentulous mandible, significant avulsed bone, and soft tissue injuries, the decision was made to place an external fixation device using fixation screws and a chest tube filled with acrylic resin. (See Figures 13.73 and 13.74.)

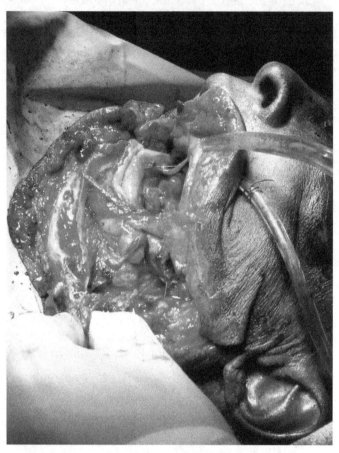

Figure 13.73. Open, comminuted edentulous mandibular fracture with gross hard and soft tissue avulsions.

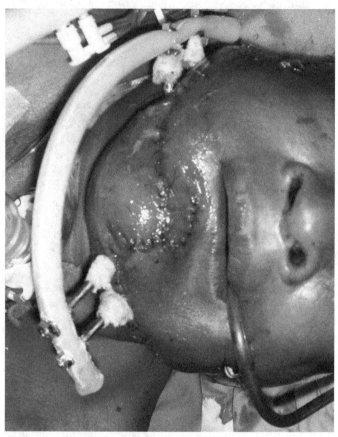

Figure 13.74. External fixation utilizing percutaneous fixation screws and a chest tube filled with acrylic resin. The soft tissue injuries were repaired primarily with local advancement flaps.

Case Report 13.16. Comminuted mandibular fractures reduced via external fixation. A 34-year-old male presents status post a self-inflicted gunshot wound to the symphysis and floor of the mouth with a small-caliber firearm. The patient's anterior mandible was grossly comminuted (bag of bones) and was not amendable to plating. An external fixator with fiber carbon rods and adjustable connectors was utilized to externally fixate the comminuted anterior mandible fracture. (See Figure 13.75.)

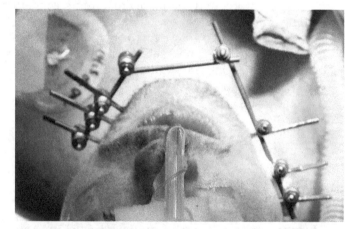

Figure 13.75. The use of a light-weight, adjustable carbon fiber rod external fixation system. The fixation screws are placed 10 mm superficial to the skin in order to prevent tissue swelling into the fixation rods and to minimize the risk of skin cellulitis and pressure necrosis.

Le Fort Fractures

Shahid R. Aziz

Department of Oral and Maxillofacial Surgery, Rutgers University School of Dental Medicine, Camden, New Jersey, USA

Reduction of displaced fractures and restoration of occlusion and facial aesthetics.

Indications for Reduction of Le Fort Fractures

1. Malocclusion
2. Mobility at the fracture site: **Le Fort I** (mobility of the maxilla), **Le Fort II** (mobility of the nasal-maxillary complex), and **Le Fort III** (craniofacial disjunction—mobility of the facial skeleton from the lateral orbital rims to the maxilla)
3. Significant aesthetic deformity

Contraindications

1. Nondisplaced fractures with no malocclusion
2. Contraindications to general anesthesia (medically unstable for treatment)

Anatomy

Le Fort I fracture: Transverse fracture of the maxilla separating the maxillary alveolus from the pterygoid plates, lateral antral wall, lateral nasal wall, and lower third of the septum

Le Fort II fracture: Pyramidal fracture extending from the pterygoid plates superiorly across the lateral antral wall, extending through the infraorbital foramen and medial orbital floor, and posterior to the lacrimal bone, through the nasal bones, and terminating at the nasofrontal suture

Le Fort III fracture: "Craniofacial disjunction"— fracture extending from the pterygoid plates through the zygomaticotemporal and zygomaticofrontal sutures through the lateral orbital wall and posterior orbital wall, and posterior to the lacrimal bone, through the nasal bones, and terminating at the nasofrontal suture

See Figure 14.1 for a comparison of Le Fort fracture patterns.

Le Fort Fracture Signs and Symptoms

Le Fort I fracture: Maxillary mobility, malocclusion, maxillary buccal vestibule and palatal ecchymosis, maxillary crepitus and upper lip and midface edema

Le Fort II fracture: Nasal-maxillary complex mobility, malocclusion, maxillary buccal vestibule and palatal ecchymosis, V2 paresthesia or anesthesia, loss of anterior-posterior dimension of the midface, nasal asymmetry, epistaxis, cerebrospinal fluid (CSF) rhinorrhea, epiphora, subconjunctival hemorrhage, diplopia, enophthalmus, midface and periorbital edema, midface crepitus and ecchymosis

Le Fort III fracture: Complete mobility of the anterior facial skeleton inferior to the zygomaticofrontal suture (craniofacial disjunction), V2 paresthesia or anesthesia, nasal asymmetry, epistaxis, CSF rhinorrhea, epiphora, subconjunctival hemorrhage, traumatic telecanthus, enophthalmus, diplopia, dystopia, increase in the vertical dimension of the face, tenderness and palpation of fractures at the lateral orbital rim, midface and periorbital edema and midface and periorbital crepitus and ecchymosis

Le Fort Reduction Technique

1. Preoperative antibiotics are given to cover sinus flora and wound contamination.
2. The airway is secured via nasal intubation, tracheostomy, or submental intubation.
3. The patient is prepped and draped to include both the oral cavity and the maxillofacial skeleton.
4. Local anesthesia containing a vasoconstrictor is injected into sites of incision placement.
5. Maxillary and mandibular arch bars are placed, and the pre-traumatic occlusion is reestablished. The placement of maxillomandibular fixation (MMF) may be difficult, depending on the displacement of the fractures. For grossly displaced Le Fort fractures, Rowe disimpaction forceps may be used to aid in the mobilization and reduction of the maxilla. When placing the patient into MMF, the fractured maxilla is neutrally set to mandible to ensure proper seating of the condyles.
6. Fractures are typically reduced and fixated with a bottom-to-top rationale. After the establishment of MMF, the mandible is internally fixated prior to fixation of the Le Fort fractures.
7. After the occlusion has been reestablished (and, if necessary, the mandible has been fixated), all facial fractures are exposed. A high maxillary buccal vestibular incision is used in all three types of Le Fort

---

Atlas of Operative Oral and Maxillofacial Surgery, First Edition. Edited by Christopher J. Haggerty and Robert M. Laughlin

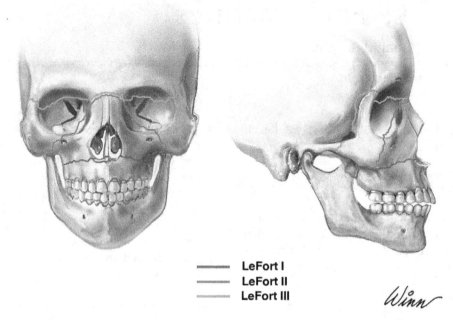

——	**LeFort I**
——	**LeFort II**
——	**LeFort III**

Winn

Figure 14.1.   Le Fort fracture patterns.

fractures (Figure 14.3). Le Fort II and III fractures are approached through a variety of incisions to include subciliary, transconjunctival, superior blepharoplasty, lateral brow, and coronal. Care should be taken to identify and preserve the infraorbital neurovascular bundles.

8. Once all fractures are exposed, manual reduction is employed, and the fractures are stabilized with rigid internal fixation. Fractures are ideally plated along the natural horizontal and vertical buttresses of the face. Depending on the surgeon's preference and the comminution of the fractures, MMF may be utilized for 4–6 weeks without internal fixation. However, from a functional and nutritional standpoint, rigid internal fixation of Le Fort fractures is preferred.

9. Large anterior maxillary wall defects may be repaired with the use of titanium mesh.

10. Once rigid fixation is completed, MMF is released and the occlusion is verified to be stable and reproducible. Light to medium guiding elastics are placed.

11. All incisions are copiously irrigated and closed. Intraoral incisions are closed with 3-0 chromic sutures. Skin incisions are closed in a layered fashion. Transconjunctival incisions are either loosely closed or left open.

Postoperative Management

1. Patients are observed for at least 24 hours postoperatively to ensure airway stability, wound hemostasis, and pain control.

2. Intravenous steroids are tapered and discontinued.

3. Patients are placed on intravenous antibiotics during hospital admission. For patients with an abbreviated hospital course receiving less than 72 hours of intravenous antibiotics, 5 days of oral antibiotics are prescribed.

4. Analgesics are prescribed in either a pill or liquid form depending on whether MMF is employed.

5. Patients are placed on sinus precautions. Sneezing and nose blowing are minimized. Ocean nasal spray and decongestants are recommended.

6. Patients in MMF via light elastics are maintained on a soft mechanical diet for 3–4 weeks. Arch bars are removed at 4–6 weeks post surgery.

Complications

1. **V2 paresthesia or anesthesia**: Minimized with meticulous dissection of the infraorbital nerve.

2. **Enophthalmus**: From inadequately reduced orbital fractures.

3. **Deviated septum or obstructed nasal breathing**: From inadequately reduced fractures of the bony and cartilaginous nasal septum.

4. **Epiphora**: Results from damage of the lacrimal drainage system.

5. **Infection**: Minimized by obtaining sterile operating conditions and pre- and postoperative antibiotic coverage.

6. **Hematoma formation**: Minimized with wound hemostasis prior to wound closure. Large hematomas require surgical exploration and drain placement.

7. **Sinusitis**: Minimized with the use of appropriate antibiotic coverage and nasal decongestants.

8. **Malunion**: Typically occurs due to hardware failure or early, excessive patient functioning.

9. **Malocclusion**: Occurs in up to 20% of cases. Malocclusion may require future orthognathic surgery to correct. Patients typically present with a mild class 3 anterior open bite. Malocclusion is minimized with the use of adequate rigid internal fixation, passive articulation of the maxilla to mandible to prevent condyle malpositioning, the use of Rowe disimpaction forceps to completely mobilize the maxilla, the removal of bony interferences prior to the placement of MMF, and occlusal verification at the end of the procedure.

10. **Exposure of hardware**: Typically occurs from inadequate tissue closure and the inability to obtain a tension-free closure.

Key Points

1. Surgery is often delayed 4–7 days in order to allow for stabilization of the patient (if necessary) and resolution of facial edema.

2. Because MMF will be utilized intraoperatively, oral intubation is contraindicated. Nasal intubation is performed for patients with fractures that do not involve nasal bone comminution, CSF rhinorrhea, or cribriform plate fractures. Submental intubation can be utilized for patients requiring short-term intubation when nasal intubation is contraindicated. Tracheostomy is utilized when nasal intubation is contraindicated, when prolonged ventilation support is required, and in cases of upper airway obstruction (i.e. edema or hematoma formation).

3. The initial step in Le Fort fracture reduction is the restoration of the pre-traumatic occlusion. The occlusion will reestablish the horizontal and vertical dimensions of the face and reduce associated palatal fractures.

4. After establishing MMF, mandible fractures (if present) are repaired prior to the reduction of maxillary and Le Fort fractures.

5. Rigid fixation plates should be strong enough to resist occlusal forces and fracture displacement.

6. Intravenous steroids are used (unless contraindicated) prior to surgery, intraoperatively, and postoperatively to reduce facial edema. Patients requiring long-term steroids require a taper of the medication.

7. Edentulous patients and those with severe maxillary sinus pneumatization may require stabilization with gunning splints or preexisting dentures and skeletal fixation.

References

Fraioli, R.E., Branstetter, B.F. 4th and Deleyiannis, F.W., 2008. Facial fractures: beyond Le Fort. *Otolaryngologic Clinics of North America*, 41(1), 51–76.

Mehta, N., Butala, P. and Bernstein, M.P., 2012. The imaging of maxillofacial trauma and its pertinence to surgical intervention. *Radiologic Clinics of North America*, 50(1), 43–57.

Meslemani, D. and Kellman, R.M., 2012. Recent advances in fixation of the craniomaxillofacial skeleton. *Current Opinion in Otolaryngology and Head and Neck Surgery*, 20(4), 304–9.

Yu, J., Dinsmore, R., Mar, P. and Bhatt, K., 2011. Pediatric maxillary fractures. *Journal of Craniofacial Surgery*, 22(4), 1247–50.

Case Reports

Case Report 14.1. A 53-year-old male presents status post motor vehicle accident with malocclusion, maxillary mobility, and vestibular ecchymosis. (See Figures 14.2, 14.3, 14.4, and 14.5.)

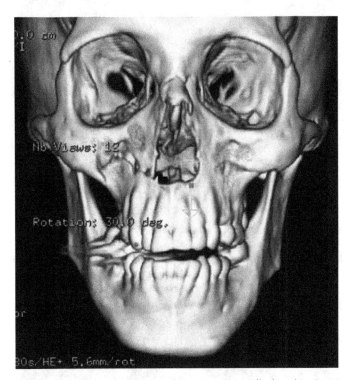

Figure 14.2. 3D reconstruction demonstrating a displaced Le Fort I fracture.

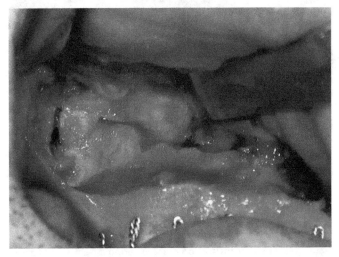

Figure 14.3. Exposure of Le Fort I fracture via maxillary vestibular incision.

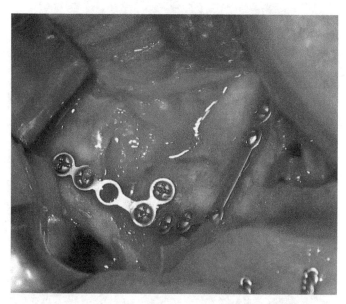

Figure 14.4. Le Fort I fracture reduced with 2.0 plates placed at the pyriform aperture and zygomaticomaxillary buttress.

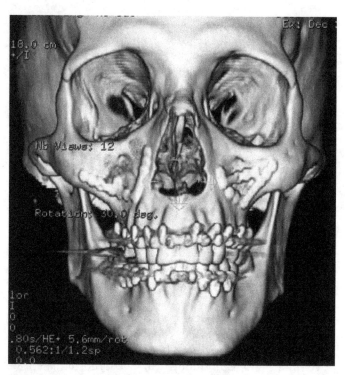

Figure 14.5. Postoperative 3D reconstruction demonstrating maxillomandibular fixation (MMF) and reduction of Le Fort I fractures.

Case Report 14.2. A 20-year-old male presents status post assault with mobility of the nasal-maxillary complex, malocclusion, left side V2 paresthesia, and midface edema and ecchymosis. (See Figures 14.6 and 14.7.)

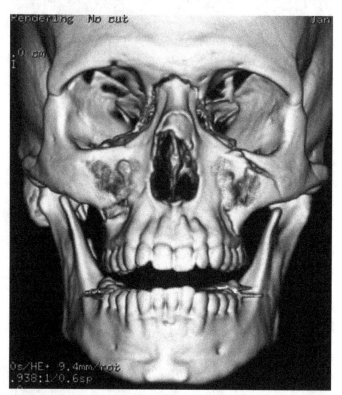

Figure 14.6. 3D reconstruction demonstrating a right-sided Le Fort I fracture and a left-sided Le Fort II fracture.

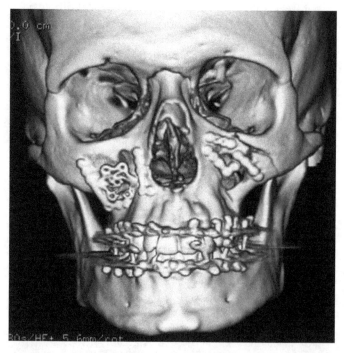

Figure 14.7. Postoperative 3D reconstruction demonstrating maxillomandibular fixation and reduction of the right Le Fort I fracture and the left Le Fort II fracture.

Case Report 14.3. A 38-year-old female presents status post motor vehicle collision with complete craniofacial disjunction, severe facial edema, malocclusion, subconjunctival hemorrhage, and epistaxis. (See Figures 14.8, 14.9, and 14.10.)

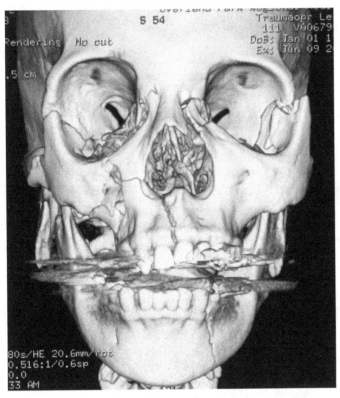

Figure 14.8. 3D reconstruction demonstrating a Le Fort III fracture, right comminuted zygomatic arch fractures, midline palatal fracture, bilateral condyle fractures, and a left parasymphysis fracture of the mandible.

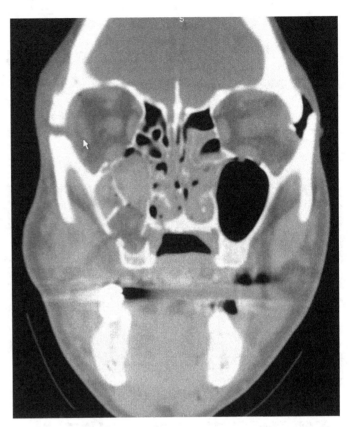

Figure 14.9. Coronal computed tomography (CT) image demonstrating a displaced Le Fort III fracture. Note displacement of the bilateral zygomaticofrontal sutures.

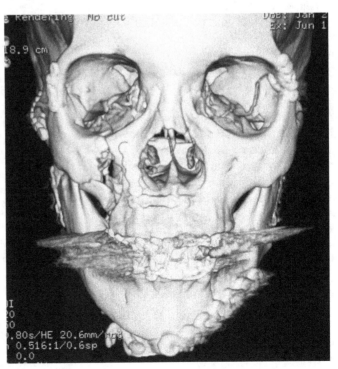

Figure 14.10. Postoperative 3D reconstruction demonstrating maxillomandibular fixation, reduction of Le Fort III, and associated facial fractures.

15 Isolated Zygoma and Zygomaticomaxillary Complex (ZMC) Fractures

Christopher J. Haggerty

Private Practice, Lakewood Oral and Maxillofacial Surgery Specialists, Lees Summit; and Department of Oral and Maxillofacial Surgery, University of Missouri–Kansas City, Kansas City, Missouri, USA

Reduction of Isolated Zygomatic Arch Fractures

Reduction of the zygomatic arch to correct functional and cosmetic deformities.

Indications

1. Loss of arch projection
2. Comminuted arch
3. Entrapment of the coronoid process (limited opening)

Contraindications

1. Fractures over 20 days old; may require osteotomy
2. Minimally displaced fractures with no symptoms
3. Elderly and medically compromised patients

Quinn Approach to the Arch

1. The procedure may be performed with local anesthetic alone, intravenous (IV) sedation, or general anesthesia.
2. Local anesthetic is infiltrated within the tissue overlying the lateral ascending ramus and coronoid process.
3. A #15 blade or electrocautery is used to initiate a 2–3 cm intraoral vestibular incision overlying the ascending ramus. Layers transected include mucosa, subcutaneous tissue, muscle, and periosteum.
4. A periosteal elevator is used to elevate in a subperiosteal plane along the lateral aspect of the vertical ascending ramus and coronoid process.
5. Through the intraoral incision, an instrument (Seldin retractor, urethral sound, and Henahan retractor) is placed between the coronoid process and the zygomatic arch.
6. Lateral pressure is applied to the arch until the medially displaced arch is reduced (Figure 15.1).
7. The oral mucosa is closed with resorbable sutures.
8. An external splint (tongue blade, finger splint, or metal eye patches) may be fixated to the arch if desired.

Gillies Approach to the Arch

1. Preoperative antibiotics are used to cover contamination from skin or scalp flora. Preoperative steroids are administered to decrease postoperative soft tissue edema. General anesthesia is recommended.
2. The patient is placed supine and rotated within a Mayfield headrest.
3. After prepping and draping, the hair is parted, and a sterile marking pen is used to draw a 2–3 cm horizontal temporal line 3 cm inferior to the anterior temporal crest.
4. Local anesthetic containing a vasoconstrictor is injected into the overlying tissue to aid in hemostasis.
5. A skin incision is initiated with a #10 blade to the level of the temporoparietal fascia (superficial temporal fascia). A periosteal elevator or a Henahan retractor is used to dissect through the temporoparietal fascia to the glistening white temporalis fascia (deep temporal fascia) overlying the temporalis muscle.
6. A horizontal incision is made through the temporalis fascia, and the temporalis muscle is exposed.
7. Either a Rowe zygomatic elevator or a urethral sound is inserted between the temporalis muscle medially and the temporalis fascia laterally (Figure 15.2) until it reaches the medial aspect of the zygomatic arch.
8. Lateral pressure is applied to the arch until the medially displaced arch is reduced (Figure 15.3).
9. The incision is closed in a layer fashion.
10. An external splint (tongue blade, finger splint, and metal eye patch) may be fixated to the arch if desired.

Reduction of Zygomaticomaxillary Complex Fractures

Reduction of the bones of the ZMC to reestablish facial projection, orbital volume, and aesthetics.

Indications

1. Limited opening (trismus)
2. Flattening of the malar eminence

Atlas of Operative Oral and Maxillofacial Surgery, First Edition. Edited by Christopher J. Haggerty and Robert M. Laughlin
© 2015 John Wiley & Sons, Inc. Published 2015 by John Wiley & Sons, Inc.

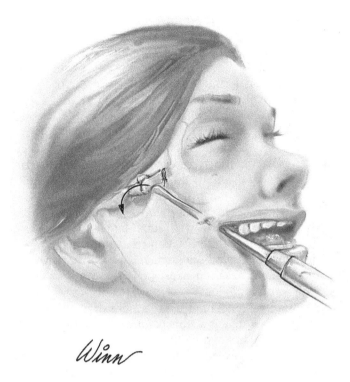

Winn

Figure 15.1. Quinn approach.

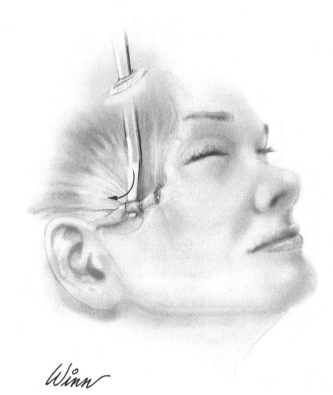

Winn

Figure 15.3. Gillies approach.

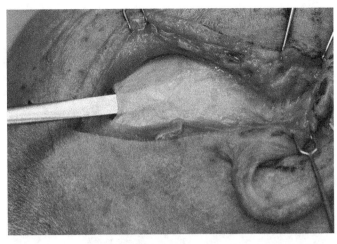

Figure 15.2. Cadaver dissection illustrating the placement of an instrument deep to the temporalis fascia (deep temporal fascia) and superficial to the temporalis muscle.

3. Flattening of the zygomatic arch
4. Antimongoloid slant
5. Enophthalmus
6. Altered globe position
7. Persistent anesthesia or paresthesia
8. Superior orbital fissure (SOF) syndrome
9. Extraocular muscle entrapment

Contraindications

1. Fractures over 20 days old: may require osteotomy
2. Minimally displaced fractures with no symptoms
3. Blindness or open globe injury to the contralateral eye
4. Traumatic hyphema; surgery typically delayed until hyphema resolves
5. Elderly and medically compromised patients

Anatomy

The frontal branch of the facial nerve provides motor innervation to the frontalis, corrugators, and procerus and often to a portion of the orbicularis oculi muscle. Damage to the frontal branch results in the inability to raise the affected eyebrow or wrinkle the affected forehead. The path of the frontal branch can be identified by drawing a line from the tragus to a point 2.0 cm cephalic to the bony superolateral orbital rim. The frontal branch lies within or just deep to the temporoparietal fascia (superficial temporal fascia) and is in close proximity to the periosteum overlying the zygomatic arch (Figure 15.4). The frontal branch is often depicted as being contained within a box 0.8 cm to 3.5 cm (average 2.0 cm) anterior to the anterior extent of the external auditory canal.

Combined Maxillary Vestibular, Lateral Brow, and Transconjunctival Approach

1. Preoperative antibiotics are used to cover contamination from sinus flora.

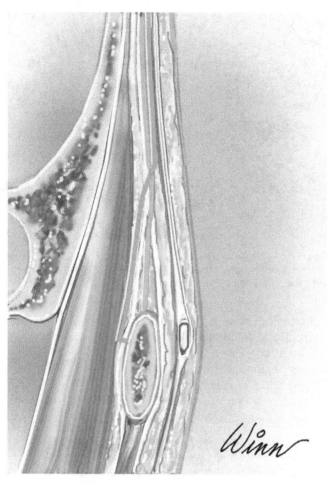

Figure 15.4. The blue line represents the subfascial approach and the green line represents the deep subfascial approach. Modified from Kenkere, D., Srinath, K.S. and Reddy, M., 2013.

2. The patient is placed supine within a Mayfield headrest. Ophthalmic ointment and corneal shields are placed bilaterally.

3. After prepping and draping, local anesthetic containing a vasoconstrictor is infiltrated within the tissue overlying the zygomaticofrontal suture, the zygomaticomaxillary suture, and the inferior orbital rim from a transconjunctival approach.

4. **Maxillary vestibular incision**: A #15 blade or electrocautery is used to initiate the intraoral maxillary vestibular incision (see Figure 15.5 in Case Report 15.1). Layers transected include mucosa, subcutaneous tissue, muscle, and periosteum. A periosteal elevator is used to expose the maxilla from the pterygoid plates laterally and to the pyriform aperture medially. Dissection proceeds cephalically and may include the inferior orbital rim if necessary.

5. **Lateral brow incision**: Palpation over the lateral bony rim will reveal the zygomaticofrontal suture and fracture. An incision with either a blade or a needle-tip Bovie is concealed within the hair bearing portion of the lateral eyebrow and is carried down to peri-

osteum (Figure 15.6, Case Report 15.1). Periosteal dissection continues along the lateral orbital rim and may be connected to the transconjunctival incision if desired, thus allowing access to the entire inferior and lateral orbital rim (Figure 15.8, Case Report 15.1). Alternatively, in females with a high arching lateral brow, a superior blepharoplasty incision may be used.

6. **Transconjunctival incision**: A Bame or Desmarres retractor is placed to evert the lower lid, and a Jaeger or malleable retractor is used to place gentle posterior pressure on the globe itself. A blade is used to create a mucosal incision 2 mm posterior to the orbital septum and lateral to the medial puncta. A malleable retractor is used to retract the orbital fat as the orbital rim is approached. Care is taken to avoid damage to the inferior oblique muscle, which is located between the middle and nasal fat pads. Damage to this structure will result in diplopia and restricted ocular motility.

7. Additional medial orbital wall exposure can be obtained by using a transcaruncular incision. A #15 blade is used to extend the original incision along the entire medial aspect of the orbital rim posterior to the inferior and superior puncta and canilicular system.

8. Exposure of the entire lateral orbital wall can be obtained with a lateral canthotomy. Stevens scissors are inserted within the palpebral fissure deep to the conjunctiva of the lateral-inferior orbital rim. Layers transected include the skin, subcutaneous tissue, orbicularis oculi muscle, orbital septum, inferior limb of the lateral canthal tendon, and conjunctiva.

9. With exposure of the fracture sites, fracture reduction is performed. For grossly displaced fractures or for fractures that are difficult to align, a Carroll–Girard screw can be inserted transorally or transcutaneously to engage the malar eminence. The Carroll–Girard screw provides excellent three dimensions control over the fractured ZMC and aids in the manipulation and reduction of the ZMC fractures.

10. Prior to any plating, the reduced fractures are all visualized to ensure ideal reduction. The zygomaticosphenoid suture should be evaluated along the internal surface of the lateral orbital wall to ensure appropriate fracture reduction prior to employing rigid internal fixation.

11. Displaced ZMC fractures are typically plated in the following sequence: the zygomaticofrontal suture (Figure 15.8, Case Report 15.1), the comminuted zygoma and/or zygomaticotemporal suture, the zygomaticomaxillary suture (Figure 15.7, Case Report 15.1), the orbital rim, and lastly the orbital floor–medial orbital wall (Figure 15.9, Case Report 15.1). Plating sequence variations exist dependent on individual surgeon preferences and the nature/displacement of the fractures.

12. Following fracture plating, extraocular muscle function is evaluated for entrapment while the patient is under general anesthesia with a forced duction test. If

any restrictions in extraocular mobility are detected, the fixation points should be reevaluated and adjustments made accordingly.

13. All incisions are irrigated and closed in layers, and appropriate topical antibiotics and dressings are placed.

14. If a lateral canthotomy was performed, the inferior limb of the lateral canthus is reapproximated, and a meticulous closure of the orbicularis oculi and skin follows. No sutures are required in closing the transconjunctival incision.

Postoperative Management

1. Patients are admitted for 24 hours following ZMC fracture repair in order to evaluate for retrobulbar hematoma formation following surgery.

2. Pain is controlled with either IV or oral analgesics depending on the discourse of the patient.

3. IV or oral antibiotics are utilized postoperatively.

4. Nasal decongestants and sinus precautions are recommended.

Hemicoronal Approach to the Arch

1. Preoperative antibiotics are used to cover contamination from skin and scalp flora. Preoperative steroids are administered to decrease postoperative soft tissue edema.

2. The patient is placed supine within a Mayfield headrest, and a linear band of hair is either shaved or parted in the area of the proposed scalp incision. Ophthalmic ointment and corneal shields are placed.

3. After prepping and draping, either a coronal or a hemicoronal approach is utilized to approach the arch. The scalp and preauricular incision are marked with a sterile marking pen or a 10-gauge needle. Crosshatches can be made with a sterile marking pen or needle to aid in exact reapproximation on closing.

4. A mixture of local anesthetic containing a vasoconstrictor is injected within the subgaleal plane to aid in hemostasis and for hydrodissection of the tissue (Figure 15.11, Case Report 15.2).

5. The skin incision is initiated with a #10 blade and is placed 3 to 5 cm posterior to the patient's hairline (Figure 15.12, Case Report 15.2). The incision either terminates in the midline with a curved anterior release (hemicoronal) or continues to the contralateral side (coronal). A scalloped or stair-stepped incision may be performed in order to break up a potential scar.

6. The scalp incision initially transverses the skin, subcutaneous tissue, and galea. For hemostasis, either Raney clips or a needle-tipped Bovie is utilized. If a full coronal incision is required, it is best to perform the dissection one side at a time in order to minimize blood loss.

7. Blunt dissection begins cephalically within the subgaleal loose areolar connective tissue layer while preserving the attachment of the pericranium to the skull. The dissection proceeds laterally until the superior temporal line (the attachment of the temporalis fascia) is reached.

8. A tunnel is created with either a periosteal elevator or a Henahan retractor from the superior temporal line to the arch. The tunnel is deep to the temporoparietal fascia (superficial temporal fascia) and superficial to the temporalis fascia (deep temporal fascia).

9. A Kelley hemostat is inserted within the tissue tunnel directly superficial to the glistening white temporalis fascia (Figure 15.13, Case Report 15.2). A #10 blade or needle-tip Bovie is used to cut through the remaining scalp directly over the top of the Kelley clamp. Dissection proceeds inferiorly, superficial to the temporalis fascia (Figures 15.14 through 15.16, Case Report 15.2).

10. As the arch is approached, the temporalis fascia will divide into superficial and deep layers. The temporal fat pad will be visualized between the two layers (Figure 15.17, Case Report 15.2). The frontal branch of the facial nerve is located within or along the deep surface of the temporoparietal fascia. In order to avoid damage to the frontal branch, the arch is approached deep to the temporoparietal fascia.

11. The arch may be approached in one of two ways (Figure 15.4, Case Report 15.1). The first approach is referred to as a subfascial approach. This approach involves transecting the superficial layer of the temporalis fascia and dissecting superficial to the temporal fat pad until the superior aspect of the arch is reached. The second approach is referred to as a deep subfascial approach. It involves a dissection deep to the deep layer of the temporalis fascia directly overlying the temporalis muscle until the medial aspect of the arch is reached (Figure 15.18, Case Report 15.2).

12. In order to adequately expose the arch, inferior extension of the preauricular incision is often necessary. By keeping the caudal extent of the preauricular incision within 0.8 cm from the external auditory canal, the frontal branch is avoided. At the level of the arch, a subperiosteal dissection proceeds anteriorly in order to expose the length of the entire zygomatic arch and lateral orbital rim (Figure 15.19, Case Report 15.2).

13. A seldin retractor is used to reduce the arch fracture. Plate fixation is utilized to maintain the arch position (Figure 15.20, Case Report 15.2).

14. If additional displaced fractures are present, additional surgical access can be created with extending the dissection to include the upper midface or orbit and by utilizing additional approaches (Figures 15.21, 15.22, and 15.23, Case Report 15.2).

15. After adequate fracture reduction, all sites are irrigated and closed in a layer fashion with a drain placed superficial to the temporalis fascia.

1. A pressure dressing is applied if a hemicoronal or coronal approach is utilized.
2. Pain is controlled with either IV or oral analgesics depending on the discourse of the patient.
3. IV or oral antibiotics are utilized postoperatively.
4. If placed, the drain is removed at postoperative day 3 or when output is minimal.

Complications

1. **Subcutaneous hematoma or seroma formation**: Minimized with meticulous closure, elimination of dead space, and pressure dressing. If large, will require drainage and drain placement.
2. **Infection**: Minimized with attention to sterile technique, adequate fracture reduction, postoperative antibiotics, and smoking cessation.
3. **Enophthalmus**: Restoring the original orbital volume is necessary to prevent postoperative enophthalmus. Postreduction enophthalmus is caused by an increase in orbital volume from inadequate fracture reduction or from an undiagnosed medial orbital wall or orbital floor fracture.
4. **Diplopia**: Commonly with upward and downward gaze. Usually a result of posttraumatic edema, hematoma formation, muscle contusion, and/or neurogenic causes that typically improves 5 to 10 days post injury. Diplopia caused by muscular entrapment or that does not resolve in 14 days requires exploration and reduction of herniated orbital tissues.
5. **Dystopia**: Inferior globe displacement caused by inadequate reduction of the orbital floor.
6. **Traumatic hyphema**: Bleeding into the anterior chamber of the globe from a ruptured iris or ciliary body vessel. Treatment options include eye protection (rigid shield and eye patch), activity restriction, topical cycloplegics (atropine or scopolamine), systemic or topical corticosteroids, antifibrinolytic agents, analgesics, antiglaucoma medications, beta blockers, and the avoidance of nonsteroidal anti-inflammatory agents. Surgical intervention is rarely indicated.
7. **Retinal detachment**: Symptoms include flashing lights and a field loss described as a curtain or window shade coming over the eye. Urgent surgery is required.
8. **Traumatic optic neuropathy or vascular compromise**: Ranges from mild decrease in visual acuity to loss of vision, diminished color vision, and a relative afferent papillary defect. Due to damage of the optic nerve or central retinal artery.
9. **Superior Orbital Fissure (SOF) syndrome**: The contents of the superior orbital fissure include cranial nerves (CN) III, IV, V1 (the lacrimal, frontal, and nasociliary branches), and VI, and the superior and inferior divisions of the ophthalmic veins. SOF syndrome occurs when hematoma, edema, or displaced fractures compress the contents of the superior orbital fissure. Symptoms include ptosis (CN III), ophthalmoplegia (weakness of the extraoccular muscles from CN III, IV, and VI, often resulting in diplopia), retro-orbital pain, forehead anesthesia (V1), and a fixed dilated pupil (CN III). SOF syndrome is both an indication for open reduction of a ZMC fracture and a potential complication of ZMC reduction. Complete resolution of symptoms often occur after reduction of ZMC fractures; if not, then exploration of the posterior orbital cone is warranted.
10. **Orbital apex syndrome**: Orbital apex syndrome results from fractures that extend through the superior orbital fissure and the optic canal. Involved structures include CN II, III, IV, V1 and VI. Symptoms include SOF syndrome and loss of visual acuity. Treatment is controversial and involves observation alone, high-dose steroids, optic nerve decompression, or a combination of these treatment modalities.
11. **Retrobulbar hematoma**: Caused by hematoma formation with resultant disruption of the retinal circulation which can lead to irreversible ischemia and permanent blindness. Essentially a compartment syndrome with compression of the central retinal artery, which causes ischemia of the optic nerve. Symptoms include severe posterior orbital pain, exophthalmos, globe induration, excessive tension on the eyelids, decreased ocular movement, and decreased visual acuity. Treatment includes orbital decompression with an emergent lateral canthotomy, disinsertion of the orbital septum along the lower lid, evacuation of hematoma, and placement of a drain for 48 hours.
12. **Trismus:** Early trismus results from ZMC fractures that impinge the coronoid process. Late trismus occurs secondarily to fibrous or bony ankylosis of the coronoid process to the arch. Post-operative fibrous or bony ankylosis may be minimized by performing a coronoidectomy at the time of surgical intervention for combined comminuted ZMC fractures and coronoid process fractures (Figures 15.26, 15.27, and 15.28, Case Report 15.3).
13. **Cosmetic deformity**: Cosmetic deformities present as a flattening or concavity of the malar region and/or lateral and inferior orbital rims when ZMC fractures are inappropriately reduced, particularly when viewed from a worm's-eye view. Cosmetic deformities also result from over- or undercorrection of the zygomatic arch.
14. **Facial paralysis**: Damage to the frontal branch of the facial nerve can occur due to significant fracture displacement or during exposure of fractures. Partial paralysis of the frontal branch is treated with observation, and total paralysis is treated with contralateral botox to mask the deinnervation of the frontalis, procerus, and corrugators.

1. Patients with ZMC and orbital fractures should be evaluated by an ophthalmologist prior to surgical intervention for a complete ocular workup and appropriate documentation.
2. All ZMC fractures have an orbital rim component and many have concomitant displaced orbital floor and/or medial wall fractures.
3. Appropriate treatment includes selecting surgical approaches that maximize direct visualization of the fractured ZMC components, minimize morbidity, allow for complete mobilization of the ZMC, and permit rigid internal fixation with fracture immobility.
4. When treating comminuted or significantly displaced ZMC fractures and concomitant panfacial fractures, a coronal approach is suggested. A coronal approach allows the operator exposure to bilateral ZMCs, supraorbital rims, medial orbital rims, lateral orbital rims, nasal bones, and the frontal sinus and will allow for transnasal wiring if indicated. For unilateral comminuted ZMC fractures, a hemicoronal approach is often utilized in combination with transconjunctival and intraoral incisions.
5. Approaching the zygomatic arch in a tissue plane deep to the temporoparietal fascia (superficial temporal fascia) is key to preventing damage to the frontal branch of the facial nerve.
6. A Carroll–Girard screw allows for excellent stabilization and manipulation of the fractured ZMC during plating.
7. The key suture in evaluating the reduction of ZMC fractures is the zygomaticosphenoid suture. The zygomaticosphenoid suture should be evaluated along the internal surface of the lateral orbital wall to ensure appropriate fracture reduction prior to employing rigid internal fixation.
8. ZMC fractures may present with lateral subconjunctival hemorrhage in the shape of a triangle. This is due to the direct oxidation of the red blood cells within the ultrathin subconjuctiva.
9. Signs of ZMC fractures may include intraoral canine fossa pain, intraoral ecchymosis, and trismus.
10. Subciliary and subtarsal incisions have a higher rate of entropion and increased scleral show compared to transconjunctival incisions.
11. Evaluation of the extraocular muscles can be performed with finger tracking. If a restricted range of motion is detected, topical anesthesia is placed within the eye and a forced duction test is performed by grasping the insertion of the rectus muscles at two simultaneous points with two pairs of Adson forceps. The rectus muscles are grasped 7 mm from the limbus, and the globe is manipulated in all directions. A positive forced duction test demonstrates muscular entrapment. A negative forced duction test with restricted extraocular movement indicates muscular hematoma, muscular contusion, or neurogenic causes of muscle paralysis.

Case Report 15.1. A 24-year-old male presents status post an assault resulting in a right displaced ZMC fracture, orbital floor fracture, Le Fort I fracture, and mandible fracture. The patient's symptoms included paresthesia to the cheek, lateral nose, upper lip, and anterior maxillary teeth; diplopia; canine fossa ecchymosis; triangular shaped lateral subconjunctival hemorrhage; and a depressed malar eminence from a worm's-eye view. (See Figures 15.5, 15.6, 15.7, 15.8, and 15.9.)

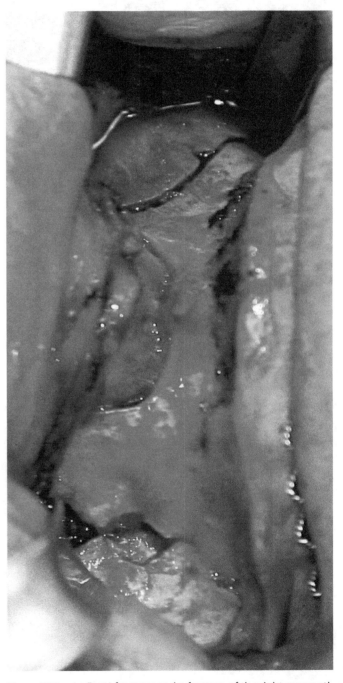

Figure 15.5.   Le Fort I fractures and a fracture of the right zygomaticomaxillary buttress exposed via a maxillary vestibular incision.

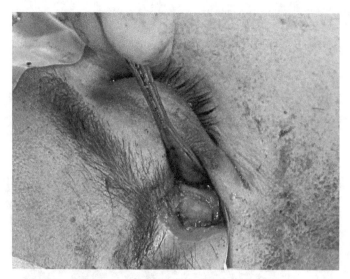

Figure 15.6.   A lateral brow incision is used to expose the zygomatico-frontal suture.

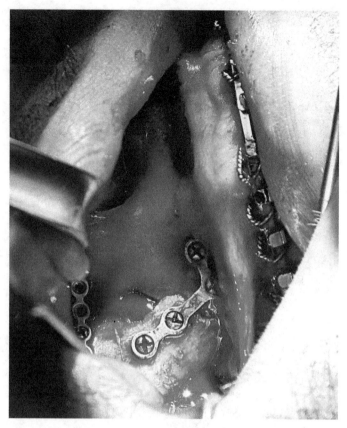

Figure 15.7.   Intraoral plating of the zygomaticomaxillary buttress.

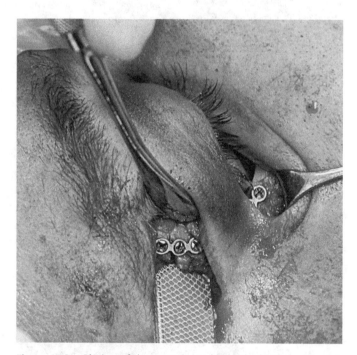

Figure 15.8.   Plating of the comminuted lateral orbital rim. The lateral brow incision can be combined with the transconjuntival incision to allow for wide surgical exposure of the entire lateral orbital rim.

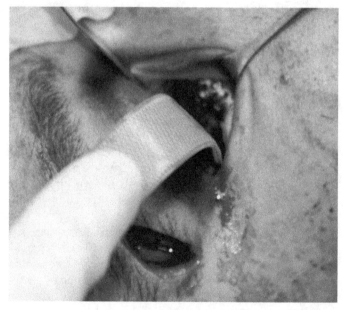

Figure 15.9.   The inferior orbital rim and orbital floor are reconstructed with a combination of a 1.7 mm infraorbital rim plate and a titanium mesh.

Case Report 15.2. A 38-year-old female presents status post an assault resulting in a zygomaticomaxillary complex (ZMC) fracture and a comminuted arch fracture. The patient's symptoms included trismus, paresthesia of the second division of the trigeminal nerve (V2), extraocular muscle entrapment, and significant arch depression. (See Figures 15.10 through 15.25.)

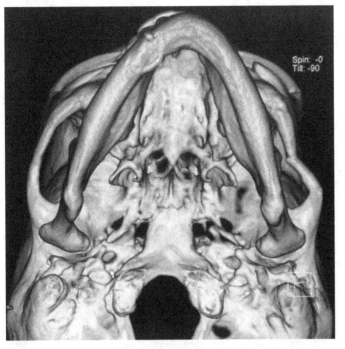

Figure 15.10. 3D reconstruction worm's eye view depicting severe medial displacement of the left zygomatic arch.

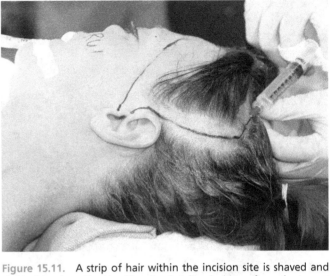

Figure 15.11. A strip of hair within the incision site is shaved and the incision is marked and localized. A line is drawn from the tragus to a point 2 cm superior to the bony superolateral orbital rim to represent the anticipated course of the frontal branch of the facial nerve.

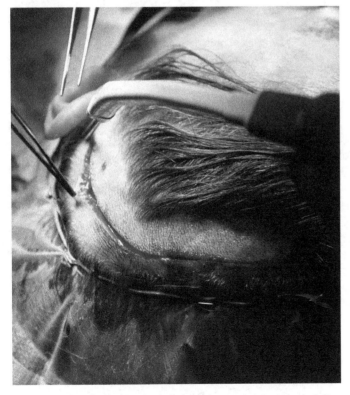

Figure 15.12. The incision is placed 4–5 cm posterior to the hair line with an anterior release or cutback.

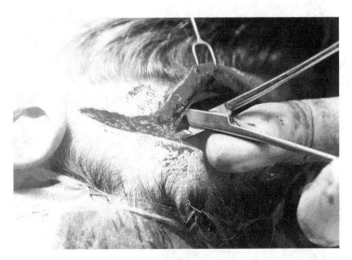

Figure 15.13. A Kelley clamp is used to dissect lateral to the superior temporal line. Dissection proceeds laterally and inferiorly within a tissue plane created between the temporoparietal fascia and the temporalis fascia.

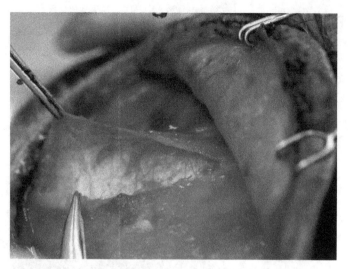

Figure 15.14. The cobweb-like appearance of the temporoparietal fascia within the temporal region.

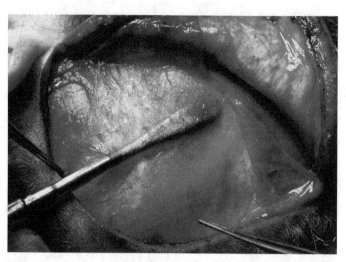

Figure 15.15. A Henahan retractor is used to dissect through the temporoparietal fascia, exposing the glistening white temporalis fascia.

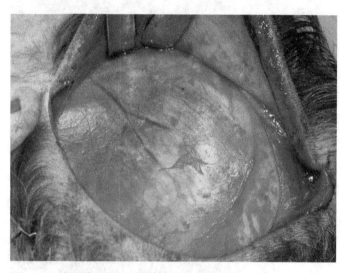

Figure 15.16. The temporalis fascia is exposed.

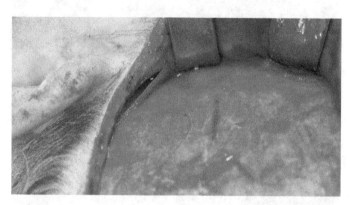

Figure 15.17. The temporal fat pad can be seen between the superficial and deep layers of the temporalis fascia. The frontal branch of the facial nerve lies within or along the deep surface of the temporoparietal fascia.

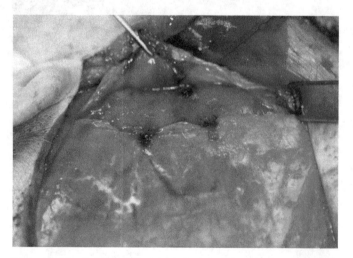

Figure 15.18. A deep subfascial approach is utilized to expose the arch. An incision is created through the deep layer of the temporalis fascia, and the arch is approached just superficial to the temporalis muscle.

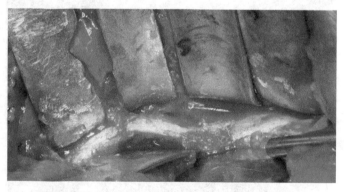

Figure 15.19. Wide surgical access of the entire comminuted zygomatic arch.

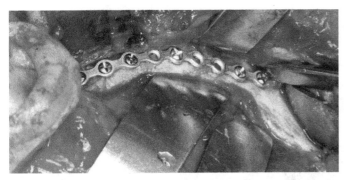

Figure 15.20.   The arch is reduced and plated with a 2.0 mm plate. Care is taken to appropriately reduce the arch and to provide adequate fixation for immobilization of the fractured segments.

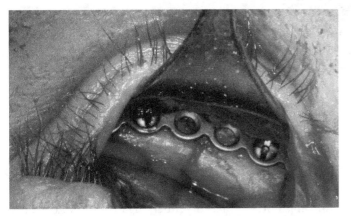

Figure 15.22.   The orbital rim component of the zygomaticomaxillary complex fracture is exposed, reduced, and plated via a retroseptal transconjunctival approach.

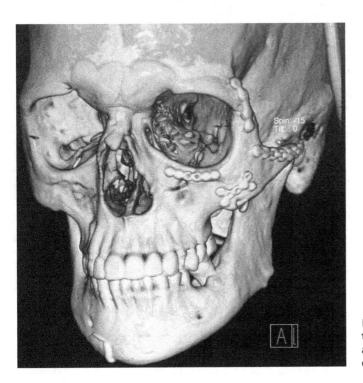

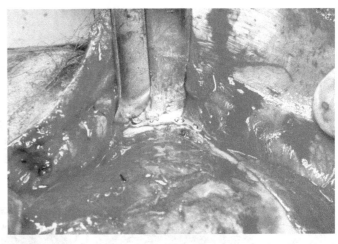

Figure 15.21.   The zygomaticofrontal fracture is exposed, reduced, and plated with a 2.0 mm plate with access from the hemicoronal approach.

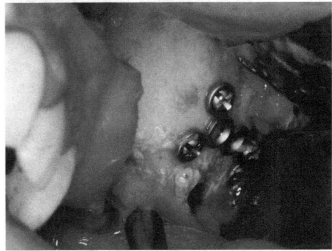

Figure 15.23.   The zygomaticomaxillary buttress fracture is exposed, reduced, and plated via a maxillary buccal vestibular incision.

Figure 15.24.   Postoperative 3D reconstruction demonstrating adequate reduction and plating of the zygomaticomaxillary complex and arch fractures.

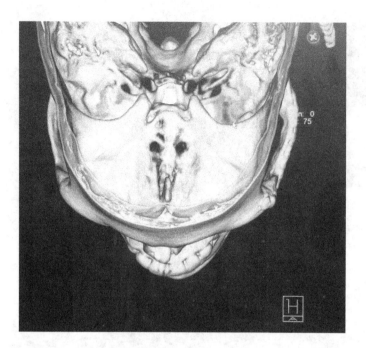

Figure 15.25.   Bird's-eye view demonstrating appropriate reduction of the left arch fracture.

Case Report 15.3. A 24-year-old presents 8 weeks status post a gunshot wound to the right cheek. The patient sustained a grossly displaced ZMC fracture, a comminuted right posterior maxilla, and a medially displaced coronoid process fracture. The patient was treated at another facility without surgical intervention. The patient subsequently developed ankylosis of the right infratemporal fossa and has a maximum vertical opening of 1 cm. This case illustrates the importance of early surgical intervention, appropriate fracture reduction, and early and aggressive physical therapy. The author routinely performs coronoidectomies in situations where both the coronoid process and the ZMC are fractured and displaced. (See Figures 15.26, 15.27, and 15.28.)

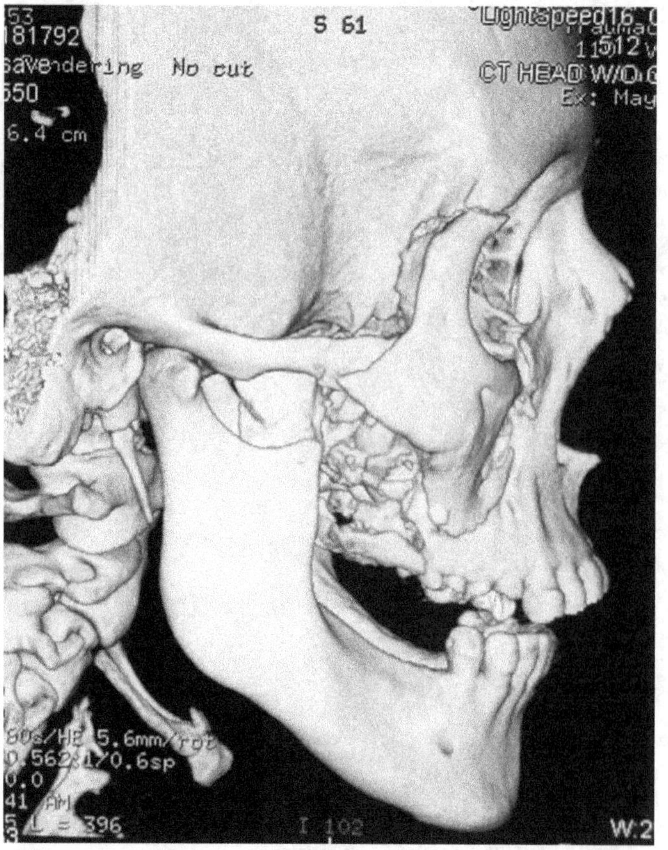

Figure 15.26.   3D reconstruction illustrating a displaced right zygomaticomaxillary complex fracture, a comminuted posterior maxilla, and a medially displaced coronoid process fracture.

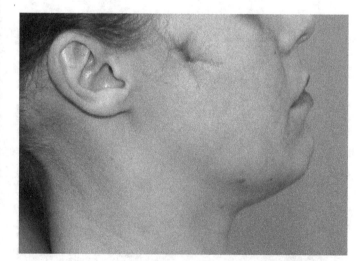

Figure 15.27.   Gunshot entry wound to the right cheek.

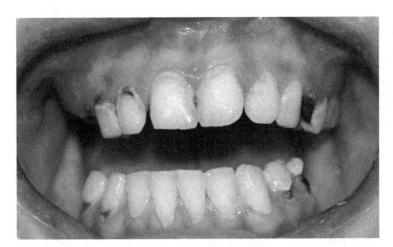

Figure 15.28. Patient's maximum vertical opening (less than 1 cm) 8 weeks after injury. The patient exhibits significant impingement/ankylosis of the right coronoid process from the unrepaired ipsilateral fractures.

References

Abubaker, A.O., 1998. The coronal approach. *Oral and Maxillofacial Surgery Update*, 2, 61–79.

Bailey, J.S. and Goldwasser, M.S., 2004. Management of zygomatic complex fractures. In *Peterson's principles of oral and maxillofacial surgery*. Hamilton, ON: BC Decker Inc. Pp.445–62.

Blanchaert, R.H., 1995. Naso-orbital-ethmoidal fractures: anatomic correlation. *Oral and Maxillofacial Surgery Knowledge Update*, 1(2), 109–24.

Boyd, S.B., 1995. Naso-orbital-ethmoidal fractures: primary treatment. *Oral and Maxillofacial Surgery Knowledge Update*, 1(2), 125–36.

Chang, E.L., Hatton, M.P., Bernardino, C.R. and Rubin, P.A., 2005. Simplified repair of zygomatic fractures through a transconjunctival approach. *Ophthalmology*, 112, 1302.

Chotkowski, G., Eggleston, T.I. and Buchbinder, D., 1997. Lag screw fixation of a nonstable zygomatic complex fracture: a case report. *Oral and Maxillofacial Surgery*, 55, 183.

Ellis, E. and Kittidumkerng, W., 1996. Analysis of treatment for isolated zygomaticomaxillary complex fractures. *Journal of Oral and Maxillofacial Surgery*, 54, 386.

Ellis, E. and Zide, M.F., 2006. Transconjunctival approaches. *Surgical Approaches to the Facial Skeleton*, 41–64.

Haggerty, C., Demain, N. and Marchena, J., 2012. Zygomaticomaxillary complex fractures. In *Current therapy in oral and maxillofacial surgery*. Amsterdam: Elsevier. Pp.324–33.

Heiland, M., Schulze, D., Blake, F. and Schmelzle, R., 2005. Intraoperative imaging of zygomaticomaxillary complex fractures using a 3D C-arm system. *International Journal of Oral and Maxillofacial Surgery*, 34, 369.

Hoelzle, F., Klein, M., Schwerdtner, O., Lueth, T., Albrecht, J., Hosten, N., Felix, R. and Bier, J., 2001. Intraoperative computed tomography with the mobile CT Tomoscan M during surgical treatment of orbital fractures. *International Journal of Oral and Maxillofacial Surgery*, 30, 26.

Hollier, L.H., Thornton, J., Pazmino, P. and Stal, S., 2003. The management of orbitozygomatic fractures. *Plastic and Reconstructive Surgery*, 111, 2386.

Kenkere, D., Srinath, K.S. and Reddy, M., 2013. Deep subfascial approach to the temporal area. *Journal of Oral and Maxillofacial Surgery*, 71, 382.

Kushner, G.M., 2006. Surgical approaches to the infraorbital rim and orbital floor: the case for the transconjunctival approach. *Journal of Oral and Maxillofacial Surgery*, 64, 108.

Lieblich, S.E. and Piecuch, J.F., 1995. Orbital-zygomatic trauma. *Oral and Maxillofacial Surgery Knowledge Update*, 1(2), 165–76.

Ochs, M.W. and Johns, F.R., 1998. Evaluation and management of periorbital and ocular injuries. *Oral and Maxillofacial Surgery Knowledge Update*, 2, 45–60.

Stanley, R., 1999. Use of intraoperative computed tomography during repair of orbitozygomatic fractures. *Archives of Facial Plastic Surgery*, 1, 19.

Walton, W., Von Hagen, S., Grigirian, R. and Zarbin, M., 2002. Management of traumatic hyphema. *Survey Ophthalmology*, 47, 297.

CHAPTER

16

Orbital Fractures

Eric Nordstrom,[1] Michael R. Markiewicz,[2] and R. Bryan Bell[3]

[1]*Department of Oral and Maxillofacial Surgery, Oregon Health and Science University; and Head and Neck Surgical Associates, Portland, Oregon, USA; Department of Oral and Maxillofacial Surgery, Anchorage Oral and Maxillofacial Surgery, Anchorage, Alaska, USA*

[2] *Department of Oral and Maxillofacial Surgery, Oregon Health and Science University, Portland, Oregon, USA*

[3] *Providence Cancer Center; Trauma Service/Oral and Maxillofacial Surgery Service, Legacy Emanuel Medical Center; Oregon Health and Science University; and Head and Neck Surgical Associates, Portland, Oregon, USA*

Reconstruction of traumatic orbital defects and restoration of pre-traumatic orbital volume.

Indications for Reduction of Orbital Fractures

1. Entrapment demonstrated with a positive forced duction test
2. Significant increase in orbital volume
3. Dystopia (vertical or horizontal)
4. Enophthalmos
5. Binocular diplopia that lasts longer than 10–14 days
6. Foreign body
7. Hard and/or soft tissue loss: orbital floor defect of greater than 1 cm or greater than half of the orbital floor surface area

Contraindications

1. Medically unstable
2. Edema significant enough to limit clinical exam (relative contraindication)
3. Globe rupture or hyphema, or other forms of ocular trauma
4. Active infection

Anatomy

Bones composing the orbit (7): Maxilla, palatine, sphenoid (greater and lesser), zygomatic, frontal, ethmoidal, and lacrimal. The superior orbital fissure separates the greater and the lesser wings of the sphenoid bone

Contents of the superior orbital fissure: CN III, IV, V1 (nasociliary, frontal and lacrimal branches of the ophthalmic nerve), and VI; sympathetic fibers from the cavernous plexus and the inferior and superior ophthalmic veins

Contents of the inferior orbital fissure: CN V2 (maxillary nerve), zygomatic nerve, infraorbital nerve, parasympathetic fibers from the pterygopalatine (Meckel's) ganglion, the infraorbital vessels and emissary veins connecting the inferior ophthalmic vein to the pterygoid venous pl

Contents of optic canal: Optic nerve, meninges, sympathetic fibers, and the ophthalmic artery.

Important orbital wall landmarks

1. The optic nerve is located 42 mm, on average, from an intact adult infraorbital (inferior orbital) rim
2. The anterior ethmoidal foramen-artery is located 24 mm posterior to the infraorbital rim and anterior lacrimal crest
3. The posterior ethmoidal foramen-artery is located 36 mm posterior to the infraorbital rim and anterior lacrimal crest

Transconjunctival (Retro-Septal) Approach

1. The patient is placed under general anesthesia with either oral or nasal intubation depending on the nature of the associated facial fractures and the need for maxillomandibular fixation (MMF).
2. The patient is positioned within a Mayfield headrest to allow for manipulation of the head during the procedure.
3. The patient is prepped with ophthalmic betadine solution (betadine scrub is not recommended for mucous membranes application) and draped. Lacrilube and corneal shields are placed.
4. Local anesthesia containing a vasoconstrictor is injected at the sites of the proposed incisions. A higher concentration of local anesthetic should be utilized to decrease the volume injected and minimize distortion of the soft tissue architecture.
5. The lower lid is retracted anteriorly with a Desmarres lid retractor (see Figure 16.9 in Case Report 16.1). A malleable retractor is used in conjunction with the corneal shield to retract the globe posterosuperiorly. Care is taken to avoid excessive globe pressure. Additionally, the anesthesiologist should be informed that there will be pressure on the globe to alert him or her of the possibility of decreased pulse rate (oculocardiac reflex).
6. The transconjunctival incision is initiated lateral to the medial puncta and 5 mm anterior to the scleral-conjunctival interface with a protected needle tip or Colorado tip bovie. The incision transects mucosa directly

Atlas of Operative Oral and Maxillofacial Surgery, First Edition. Edited by Christopher J. Haggerty and Robert M. Laughlin
© 2015 John Wiley & Sons, Inc. Published 2015 by John Wiley & Sons, Inc.

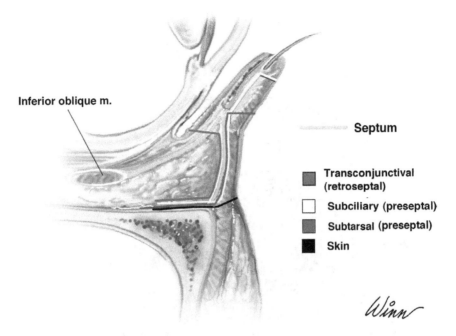

Inferior oblique m.

Septum

- ■ **Transconjunctival (retroseptal)**
- □ **Subciliary (preseptal)**
- ■ **Subtarsal (preseptal)**
- ■ **Skin**

Winn

Figure 16.1. Approaches to the infraorbital (inferior orbital) rim and floor. Note that the subciliary and the subtarsal approaches access the rim by creating a stair-step incision through the orbicularis oculi muscle at any point along the dissection.

overlying the infraorbital rim. Once the mucosa is transected, the postseptal approach (Figure 16.1) results in herniation of peri-orbital fat within the incision site. Herniated fat is retracted posteriorly with an orbital or malleable retractor. Dissection proceeds toward the periosteum overlying the infraorbital rim. The periosteum is transected and reflected to expose the infraorbital rim/floor of the orbit. Care is taken to not transect the inferior oblique muscle as it passes between the nasal (medial) and central fad pads.

7. All displaced fractures (rim and floor) are exposed. Subperiosteal dissection is performed anterior to the transconjunctival incision to expose the infraorbital rim (Figure 16.10, Case Report 16.1) and posteriorly to expose any defects within the orbital floor. The transconjunctival incision may be extended laterally (Figure 16.2) to the zygomaticofrontal suture if additional exposure of the lateral orbital rim is necessary. A lateral canthotomy may be employed if sufficient exposure of the lateral rim cannot be achieved without stretching the lateral orbital tissues excessively.

8. If additional exposure of the medial orbital wall is necessary, the transconjunctival incision may be extended medially (Figure 16.2), posterior to the caruncle (transcaruncular incision), and extended along the medial orbital wall. The transcaruncular incision is placed along the conjunctival groove just posterior to the lacrimal sac and semilunar fold. The incision can be extended along the medial orbital rim for approximately 12 mm. A subperiosteal tissue

dissection is utilized to expose the medial orbital rim and orbital wall.

9. All orbital rim fractures should be exposed to include adjacent uninvolved bone for adequate fixation. All orbital floor fractures should ideally have an area of intact bone circumferentially surrounding the defect.

10. All areas of tissue entrapment are carefully freed from the orbital floor defect with a blunt-tipped elevator (Cottle or freer elevator) prior to the placement of any orbital fixation devices (Figure 16.3).

11. Orbital fixation devices include orbital rim plates, stock titanium orbital meshes, stock preformed titanium orbital reconstruction plates, and custom, prefabricated implants. Orbital rims are typically fixated prior to orbital floors. Orbital rim plates are adapted to the orbital rim and fixated to the uninvolved adjacent orbital rim bone once reduction is obtained. Orbital floor devices are placed, ensuring that all edges of the orbital floor device are positioned on solid bone and with no entrapment of orbital tissues beneath the device (Figure 16.3; see also Figure 16.11, Case Report 16.1). The posterior ledge of an orbital floor device requires a minimum of a 2–3 mm purchase. The orbital floor device is evaluated for adequate antral bulge reconstruction, orbital volume restoration, and intact bone along the periphery of the device prior to fixation.

12. The orbital floor device can be fixated with self-drilling 4 mm screws along the infraorbital rim (provided the rim is intact). If an orbital floor device cannot be placed without entrapment of tissues, a molded piece of

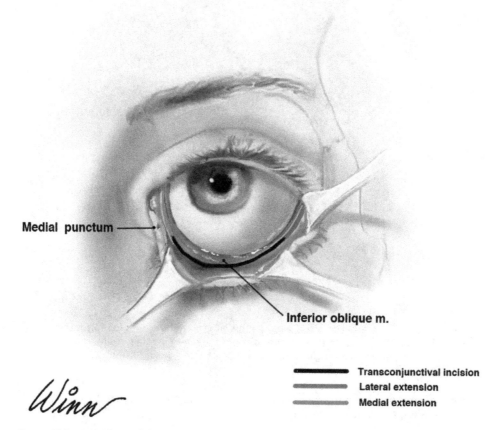

Medial punctum

Inferior oblique m.

━━━ Transconjunctival incision
━━━ Lateral extension
━━━ Medial extension

Figure 16.2.   Locations of the transconjunctival incision with medial and lateral extensions.

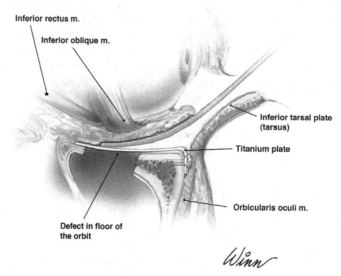

Inferior rectus m.

Inferior oblique m.

Inferior tarsal plate (tarsus)

Titanium plate

Orbicularis oculi m.

Defect in floor of the orbit

Figure 16.3.   Transconjunctival approach depicting appropriate reconstruction of an orbital floor defect with elevation of herniated contents from the maxillary sinus and the posterior aspect of the orbital floor device resting on solid bone.

smooth alloplastic material can be utilized if the defect is not excessively large to accept the material without distortion. Once materials have been fixated, the orbital soft tissue around the margins of the device are reevaluated to ensure no tissue entrapment, and a final forced duction test is performed.

13. Once anatomic reduction has been verified, additional fixation screws are placed. Complete closure of the transconjunctival incision is not recommended as excessive suturing can contribute to shortening of conjunctival tissues. For large incisions, 2-4, 6-0 plain gut sutures may be placed in an interrupted fashion to loosely reapproximate the conjunctiva.

Upper Eyelid (Superior Blepharoplasty, Supratarsal Fold) Incision Approach

1. Steps 1–4 of the above transconjunctival approach are followed.
2. An incision is made parallel to the superior palpebral sulcus within a naturally occurring skin crease (Figure 16.4) or, if edema is present, 10 mm above the upper eyelid. The involved upper eyelid may be compared to the contralateral side to ensure appropriate incision placement. The incision may be extended laterally into the crow's feet area for additional exposure, staying 6 mm superior to the lateral canthus to avoid the frontal branch of the facial nerve.
3. The incision transverses skin, subcutaneous tissue, and the orbicularis oculi. A skin-muscle flap is developed, staying superficial to the orbital septum–levator aponeurosis (Figure 16.5). The dissection is directed superiorly and laterally toward the zygomaticofrontal suture or supraorbital rim. While retracting the skin-muscle flap superiorly with a double-ended skin hook, a periosteal incision is made over the rim (Figure 16.4). The trochlea and superior oblique muscle may be dissected from the trochlear fossa for added exposure of the orbital rim. Fractures are exposed, reduced, and fixated with orbital rim plates (Figure 16.4) and/or mesh.

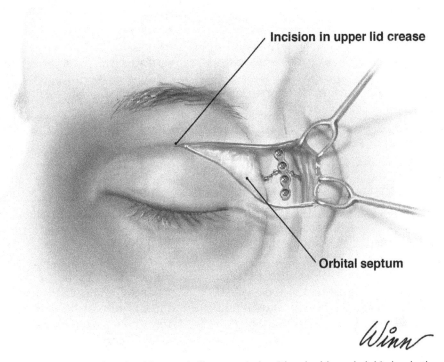

Incision in upper lid crease

Orbital septum

Winn

Figure 16.4. While retracting the skin-muscle flap superiorly with a double-ended skin hook, the periosteum is incised and the orbital rim fractures are exposed, reduced, and fixated.

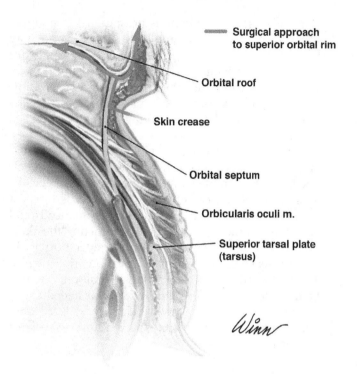

Surgical approach to superior orbital rim

Orbital roof

Skin crease

Orbital septum

Orbicularis oculi m.

Superior tarsal plate (tarsus)

Winn

Figure 16.5. A superior blepharoplasty approach is initiated with a skin incision made parallel to the superior palpebral sulcus within a naturally occurring skin crease. The dissection remains superficial to the orbital septum.

4. After appropriate supraorbital rim reconstruction and orbital volume restoration, closure of the upper eyelid incision is performed in a layered fashion with 4-0 Vicryl sutures to close the periosteum and running 6-0 fast-absorbing gut sutures to close skin. Avoid excessive bites of skin as this can contribute to shortening of the upper lid and increase scleral show.

Postoperative Management

1. Immediate postoperative visual acuity and extraocular muscle movement tests are performed. Evaluation is ideally performed within the post-anesthesia care unit (PACU) so that deficits amenable to surgical intervention may be performed as soon as possible. Basic salt solution (BSS) irrigant should be used if there is suspicion that eye lubricants could be interfering with visual exams. Except in the setting of true entrapment with significant inflammation, extraocular movement should not cause pain postoperatively.
2. Patients are typically admitted for 23-hour observation following extensive orbital surgery.
3. If intraoperative computed tomography (CT) scanning is not readily available, a postoperative CT scan should be performed to evaluate the position of the orbital fixation device and to identify any areas of potential entrapment.

4. A course of steroids and antibiotics in the perioperative period is recommended.
5. Head-of-bed elevation is recommended during the immediate postoperative period.
6. Ice is applied to the affected periorbital region for the first 48 hours.
7. Sinus precautions are used preoperatively and for 2 weeks after orbital repair.
8. Oxymetazoline nasal spray is recommended for symptomatic relief in the immediate postoperative period for 2–3 days only.
9. Pseudoephedrine hydrochloride is recommended for symptomatic relief in the immediate postoperative period and is scheduled for 5 days.
10. Lacrilube may be used in the setting of severe chemosis.
11. Ophthalmic eye drops are not routinely prescribed, but they may be used for lagopthalmos with transconjunctival incisions for 5–7 days.

Complications

Early Complications

1. Optic neuropathy resulting in partial or complete vision loss
2. Entrapment of the extraocular muscles, esotropia, or disorders of ocular motility
3. Corneal abrasion or other globe injury

Late Complications

1. Volume-associated changes resulting from inadequate reduction of orbital contents: enophthalmos, lateral or vertical dystopia, or hypoglobus
2. Ectropion or entropion with or without lower lid retraction and increased scleral show

Key Points

1. Pre-septal approaches are prone to ectropion, which is particularly true when combined with a lateral canthotomy. When performing lateral canthotomies, care should be taken to resuspend the periorbital musculature and to perform an accurate lateral canthopexy upon closure. When wide access is required to expose the infraorbital rim, particularly in a posttraumatic patient where edema persists, an infraorbital (mid-lid) incision (Figure 16.6) is a predictable means of obtaining wide surgical exposure of the infraorbital rim and orbital floor without the need for a lateral canthotomy. The infraorbital incision provides acceptable cosmesis, while minimizing the risk of ectropion and increased scleral show.
2. In the author's experience, a transconjunctival incision combined with a lateral canthotomy for disarticulation of the lower lid often results in an

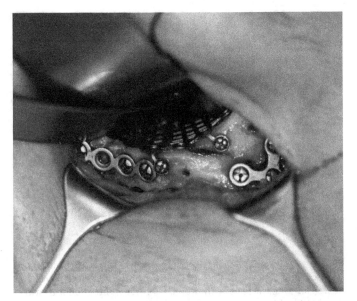

Figure 16.6. Infraorbital (mid-lid) or subtarsal incisions allow for wide surgical exposure of the infraorbital rim and floor without the need for a lateral canthotomy when repairing complex orbital fractures and/or in cases of significant periorbital edema.

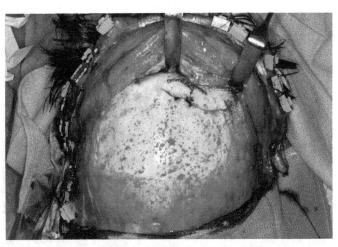

Figure 16.7. Grossly comminuted or displaced fractures of the supraorbital roof, combined neurosurgical intervention or orbital fractures combined with additional facial fractures are best managed with wide surgical access via a coronal approach with or without additional approaches.

unnatural appearance of the lateral periorbita. An isolated postseptal transconjunctival approach combined with an upper lid blepharoplasty approach typically provides adequate access to the orbit for most applications and results in better postoperative cosmesis. For grossly comminuted or displaced fractures of the supraorbital rim, combined neurosurgical intervention or orbital fractures combined with additional facial fractures, a coronal approach provides direct access to the upper half of the orbit and supraorbital roof (Figure 16.7).

3. The key to successful orbital reconstruction is to reestablish pre-traumatic orbital volume through restoration of the critical orbital bulges located postero-inferiorly (antral bulge) and postero-medially (ethmoidal bulge). The typical error is that the surgeon places the orbital implant flush with the anterior portion of the orbit, and it extends directly back to the posterior wall of the maxillary sinus. A similar error is made along the medial orbital wall by inaccurately positioning the orbital implant into the ethmoidal labyrinth.

4. In the author's experience, titanium plates are the most predictable and versatile implant materials due to the rapid bending of the devices to the anatomical contours of orbital floor and medial orbital wall fractures without the need for a second surgical site. For larger fractures, preformed titanium orbital reconstruction plates (Synthes, Paoli PA) allow for rapid and accurate

restoration of orbital volume. Care must be taken to avoid "yaw" inaccuracies during device placement, which result in unfavorable positioning of the implant within the posterior-medial orbit with resultant postoperative enophthalmos.

5. Once the orbital device is secured, a forced duction should be performed to verify free ocular mobility. Projection, globe position, and eyelid anatomy should also be evaluated prior to extubation.

6. Intraoperative CT scanners provide immediate quality control and allow for intraoperative revision of inaccurately positioned orbital devices. A radiolucent and carbon-fiber Mayfield headrest is required, and preoperative consent for the possibility of multiple CT scans is advisable. Modern mobile CT scanners can be linked to navigation systems to provide real-time assistance in accurate implant placement.

7. Recently, preoperative computer-assisted planning with virtual correction and construction of stereolithographic models has been combined with intraoperative navigation in an attempt to more accurately reconstruct the bony orbit and optimize treatment outcomes. Surgical procedures are preplanned with virtual correction by mirroring an individually defined 3D segment of the unaffected side into the deformed side, creating an ideal unilateral reconstruction. These computer models are used intraoperatively as a virtual template to navigate the preplanned bony contours and globe projection.

Case Report

Case Report 16.1. A 27-year-old male presents status post motor vehicle accident resulting in a large step defect to the right orbital floor with herniation of the orbital contents into the maxillary sinus. (See Figures 16.8 through 16.12.)

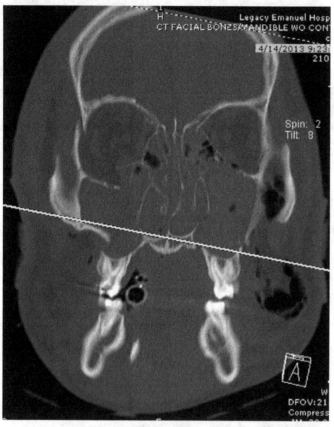

Figure 16.8.   Coronal computed tomography scan demonstrating a right orbital floor fracture, a significant change in right orbital volume, and fluid within the bilateral maxillary sinuses.

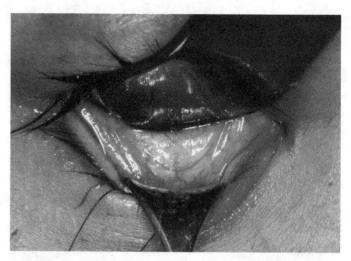

Figure 16.9.   A malleable retractor is used to retract the globe posterosuperiorly, and a Desmarres lid retractor is utilized to retract the lower lid anteroinferiorly in preparation for a retroseptal transconjunctival incision.

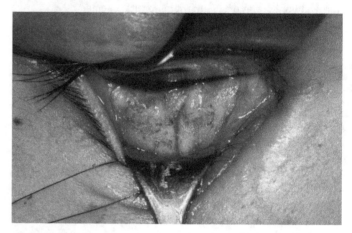

Figure 16.10.   The orbital rim and orbital floor are exposed.

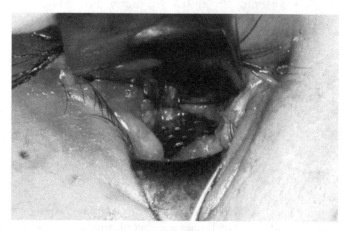

Figure 16.11.   A titanium mesh is bent to reestablish pre-traumatic orbital volume, to elevate herniated tissue from the sinus, and to bridge any continuity defects located within the fractured orbital floor.

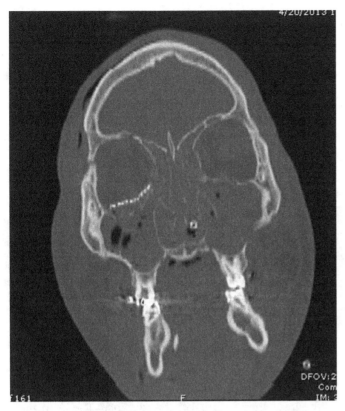

Figure 16.12. Postoperative coronal computed tomography scan demonstrating appropriate reconstruction of the orbital floor defect and reestablishment of pre-traumatic orbital volume.

References

Baumann, A. and Ewers, R., 2000. Transcaruncular approach for reconstruction of medial orbital wall fracture. *International Journal of Oral and Maxillofacial Surgery*, 29(4), 264–7.

Bell, R.B. and Al Bustani, S., 2012. Management of orbital fractures. In: S.C. Bagheri, R.B. Bell and H.A. Kahn, eds. *Current therapy in oral and maxillofacial surgery*. Philadelphia: Elsevier.

Bell, R.B. and Markiewicz M.R., 2009. Computer assisted planning, stereolithographic modeling and intraoperative navigation for complex orbital reconstruction: a descriptive study on a preliminary cohort. *Journal of Oral and Maxillofacial Surgery*, 67(12), 2559–70.

Converse, J.M., Firmin, F., Wood-Smith, D. and Friedland, J.A., 1973. The conjunctival approach in orbital fractures. *Plastic and Reconstructive Surgery*, 52(6), 656–7.

Ducic, Y. and Verret, D.J., 2009. Endoscopic transantral repair of orbital floor fractures. *Otolaryngology—Head Neck Surgery*, 140(6), 849–54.

Markiewicz, M.R., Dierks, E.J. and Bell, R.B., 2012. Does intraoperative navigation restore orbital dimensions in traumatic and post-ablative defects? *Journal of Craniomaxillofacial Surgery*, 40(2), 142–8.

Markiewicz, M.R., Dierks, E.J., Potter, B.E. and Bell, R.B., 2011. Reliability of intraoperative navigation in restoring normal orbital dimensions. *Journal of Oral and Maxillofacial Surgery*, 69(11), 2833–40.

Shorr, N., Baylis, H.I., Goldberg, R.A. and Perry, J.D., 2000. Transcaruncular approach to the medial orbit and orbital apex. *Ophthalmology*, 107(8), 1459–63.

Tessier, P., 1969. Surgical widening of the orbit. *Annales de Chirurgie Plastique et Esthétique*, 14(3), 207–14.

Tessier, P., 1973. The conjunctival approach to the orbital floor and maxilla in congenital malformation and trauma. *Journal of Maxillofacial Surgery*, 1(1), 3–8.

Walter, W.L., 1972. Early surgical repair of blowout fracture of the orbital floor by using the transantral approach. *Southern Medical Journal*, 65(10), 1229–43.

17

Nasal Fractures

Hani F. Braidy and Vincent B. Ziccardi

Department of Oral and Maxillofacial Surgery, New Jersey Dental School, University of Medicine and Dentistry of New Jersey, Newark, New Jersey, USA

Reduction of displaced nasal bones and associated nasal structures.

Indications for Closed Reduction of Nasoseptal Fractures

1. Displaced fractures with cosmetic deformity
2. Fractures with resulting nasal obstruction
3. Severely comminuted fractures

Indications for Open Reduction of Nasoseptal Fractures

1. Severely displaced fractures
2. Severe displacement of the nasal cartilage complex
3. Concomitant extensive lacerations
4. Remaining deformity after closed reduction

Contraindications

1. Cerebrospinal fluid (CSF) rhinorrhea
2. Old fractures (>4 weeks)

Anatomy

1. The pyramidal-shaped nasal bone complex includes the paired nasal bones that articulate with the nasal processes of the frontal bone and the maxilla.
2. The nasal septum consists of the following structures: crest of the maxillary and palatine bone, perpendicular plate of the ethmoid, vomer, and quadrangular cartilage.
3. The nose has an extensive blood supply derived from the internal carotid (anterior ethmoidal artery and branches) and external carotid (greater palatine, superior labial, sphenopalatine, and angular arteries) artery.
4. Anterior epistaxis typically involves a complex of vessels known as Little's area or Kiesselbach's plexus (the confluence of the anterior ethmoidal, greater palatine, superior labial, and sphenopalatine arteries).

Closed Nasoseptal Reduction Technique

1. Depending on the degree of displacement, patients are treated with local, intravenous, or general anesthesia. With general anesthesia, the patient is orally intubated, and the nasal cavities and maxillofacial skeleton are prepped and draped.
2. The nasal complex is anesthetized with local anesthetic containing a vasoconstrictor injected along the nasal floor, lateral nasal walls, septum, turbinates, and nasal bridge. Infraorbital, infratrochlear, and supratrochlear bilateral blocks are performed as well.
3. Intranasal packings containing oxymetazolin (or 4% cocaine) are placed within the bilateral nasal cavities (see Figure 17.4 in Case Report 17.1).
4. A sterile marking pen is used to mark the location of the medial canthal tendons (MCT) and the midline.
5. The distance between the nostril and the bridge of the nose (nasofrontal suture) is estimated by placing the Goldman elevator against the external surface of the nose with its tip next to the medial canthus (Figure 17.5, Case Report 17.1). A fingertip from the dominant hand is placed on the instrument to "mark" that distance. The instrument is introduced into the nose and directed superiorly and laterally to reduce the displaced nasal bones, while the fingers of the nondominant hand provide counterpressure externally and aid in molding the nasal bones (Figure 17.1; and see Figure 17.6, Case Report 17.1).
6. An Asch forceps is then used to reduce the nasal septum over the maxillary crest (Figure 17.7, Case Report 17.1). If the nasal septum cannot be reduced with the Asch forceps alone, a septoplasty can be performed with a Killian or hemi-transfixion incision with mucoperichondrial flap elevation.
7. The nose is reexamined with a nasal speculum to view the position of the septum and to evaluate the nasal passages for obstruction and septal hematoma formation. Doyle splints are placed if septal hematoma evacuation has been performed or if tears are present within the nasal mucosa to minimize synechiae formation (Figure 17.9, Case Report 17.1). Doyle splits are impregnated with triple antibiotic ointment, placed within the nasal passages, and secured to the membranous septum with a 3-0 silk suture (Figure 17.10, Case Report 17.1).
8. Steri-strips are placed over the nasal bridge (Figure 17.11, Case Report 17.1), and an Aquaplast thermoplastic nasal splint is heated, trimmed, and applied to the nasal dorsum (Figure 17.12, Case Report 17.1).

Atlas of Operative Oral and Maxillofacial Surgery, First Edition. Edited by Christopher J. Haggerty and Robert M. Laughlin.
© 2015 John Wiley & Sons, Inc. Published 2015 by John Wiley & Sons, Inc.

Open Nasoseptal Reduction Technique

1. General anesthesia is utilized. Patient prepping, draping, local anesthetic placement, and intranasal packings are placed in a similar fashion to the closed nasoseptal reduction technique.
2. Open exposure of the nasal complex is performed using any combination of skin lacerations, lynch incisions, open-sky ("H") incisions (Figures 17.14 and 17.16, Case Report 17.2), open rhinoplasty, and septoplasty incisions.
3. Conservative exposure of the cartilage and bony fragments is recommended to minimize the risk of devitalization. Care is taken to not strip the media canthal tendons from their insertions.
4. Mini-plates and screws are used to stabilize the displaced fragments (Figure 17.14, Case Report 17.2). In avulsive injuries or when extreme comminution is present, a split calvarial bone graft or other autogenous or alloplastic implant may be required to reconstruct the nasal bridge.
5. Cartilage is sutured in place with slow resorbing sutures. Doyle splints will provide additional support for comminuted segments.
6. Skin and intranasal incisions are closed with resorbable sutures.
7. If nasal dorsal sutures are placed, Aquaplast thermoplastic nasal splints are typically not placed as they will interfere with wound care.

Postoperative Management

1. The patient is instructed to apply ice to the face and keep the head elevated for 48 hours.
2. The patient is instructed to avoid nose blowing, sneezing, and strenuous activity to avoid rebleeding or fracture displacement.
3. Analgesics, decongestants, and broad-spectrum antibiotics are prescribed.
4. Intranasal packing (iodoform gauze) is removed 3–5 days postoperatively to prevent toxic shock syndrome and sinusitis. If additional internal support is required, a new intranasal packing can be placed. Doyle splints can be left in place for several weeks. External nasal splints are removed 7–10 days postoperatively.

Complications

Early Complications

1. **Epistaxis**: Minor bleeding may be controlled by elevation of the head and external pressure. More persistent nasal bleeding may require placing an intranasal pack.

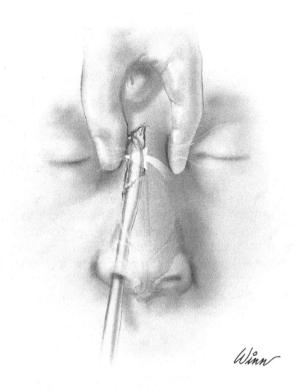

Figure 17.1. The nasal fracture is reduced with a lateral and superior rotation of the reduction forcep.

2. **Septal hematoma**: Immediate drainage of the hematoma and placement of an intranasal pressure packing is paramount to prevent cartilage necrosis, septal perforations, and saddle nose deformity.
3. **Nasolacrimal duct injury**: A consultation with an ophthalmologist is necessary if epiphora does not improve within a few weeks after resolution of edema.
4. **CSF rhinorrhea**: Typically present with fractures of the cribriform plate. Diagnosed with B2 transferrin (preferred method), ring test, or CSF glucose analysis.

Late Complications

1. **Nasal deformity, septal deformity, or saddle nose deformity**: Secondary rhinoplasty may be needed to address this late complication.
2. **Nasal obstruction**: Typically results from a deviated septum, this complication can be addressed by secondary septorhinoplasty.
3. **Septal perforation**: Typically results from unrecognized septal hematoma. Treatment involves local flap advancements.
4. **Synechiae**: Synechiae result from damage to the nasal mucosa resulting in scar tissue formation, commonly

between the turbinate and the septum. Synechiae formation results in nasal obstruction. Treatment requires secondary release.

1. Thorough clinical and radiographic examinations are performed in order to evaluate for cribriform plate fractures, septal hematoma, and CSF rhinorrhea.
2. If extensive facial edema is present, reduction is delayed 5–7 days until the majority of the edema has resolved.
3. Most causes of nasal epistaxis are effectively treated with an anterior nasal pack. One-fourth-inch Vaseline iodoform gauze is packed in a layered fashion starting at the nasal floor. Alternatively, commercially prepared nasal packs such as a Merocel pack (Medtronic, Jacksonville, FL, USA) or a Rapid Rhino (ArthroCare ENT, Austin, TX, USA) act as nasal tampons to stop anterior nasal bleeds. In the event that hemostasis is not achieved with the placement of an anterior nasal pack, a posterior nasal bleed is suspected. A pediatric Foley catheter is lubricated with an antibiotic ointment, introduced into the nostril, and inserted posteriorly until its tip can be visualized in the posterior pharynx. The balloon is inflated with 7–10 cc of normal saline and pulled against the nasopharynx, and tightly secured by clamping a hemostat adjacent to the nostril. To prevent alar necrosis, the nostril is padded with gauze. The anterior nasal cavity is then packed with iodoform gauze or other commercial nasal packs. Alternatively, an Epistat nasal catheter (Medtronic) (Figure 17.2) can be introduced into the nasal passage, and pressure may be applied to an anterior bleed, posterior bleed, or both. For persistent epistaxis that is refractory to treatment, interventional radiology may be required to embolize the offending vessel.

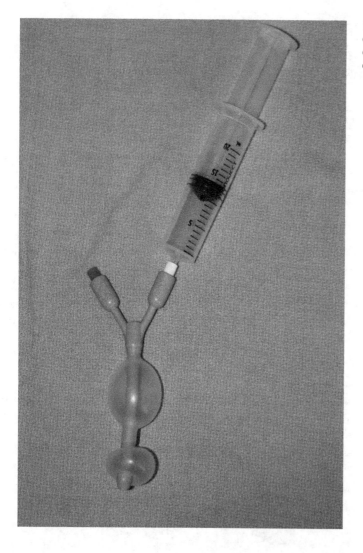

Figure 17.2. Epistat nasal catheter capable of placing anterior, posterior, or combined nasal pressure to arrest epistaxis.

Case Reports

Case Report 17.1. A 58-year-old female presents after a fall resulting in grossly displaced nasal bone fractures. On presentation, a nasal speculum examination was performed that identified a large septal hematoma and gross septal deviation. The septal hematoma was promptly drained in the emergency department and an intranasal pressure packing consisting of 1/4 inch ribbon gauze impregnated with antibiotic ointment was placed. The patient was taken to the operating room for closed reduction of her septal and nasal fractures. (See Figures 17.3 through 17.12.)

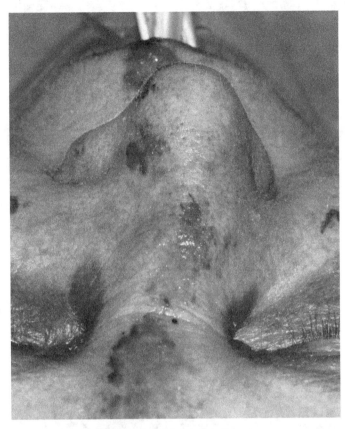

Figure 17.3. Gross nasal and septal deformity.

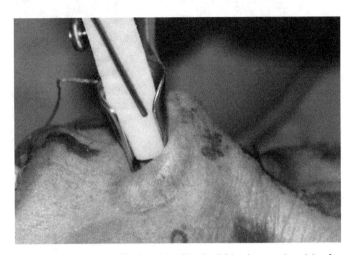

Figure 17.4. Oxymetazolin pads placed within the nasal cavities for hemostasis.

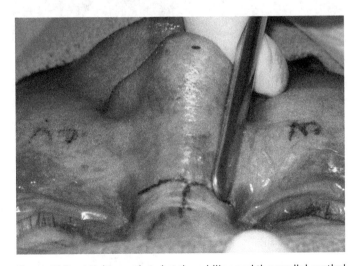

Figure 17.5. Marks are placed at the midline and the medial canthal tendons (MCT). The distance from the nostril to the MCT is estimated with a Goldman elevator.

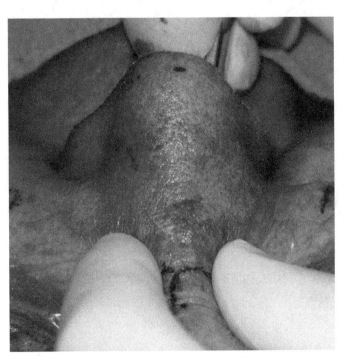

Figure 17.6. A Goldman elevator is used to reduce the displaced nasal fractures. The nondominant hand is used to apply counterpressure and to mold the fractured nasal bones.

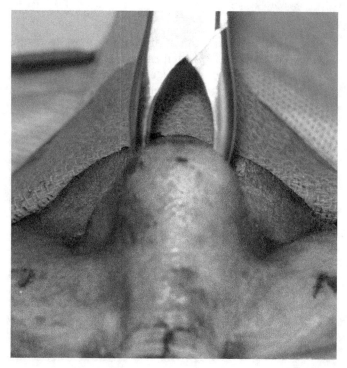

Figure 17.7. Asch forceps used to reduce the septal fracture and position the septum midline.

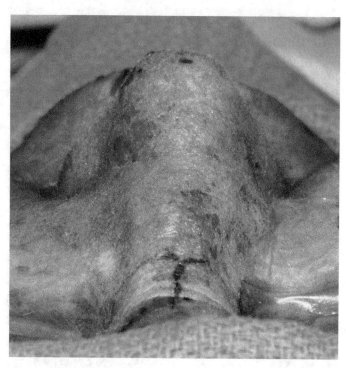

Figure 17.8. Postreduction view. Nasal tip, septum, and nasal bones are midline.

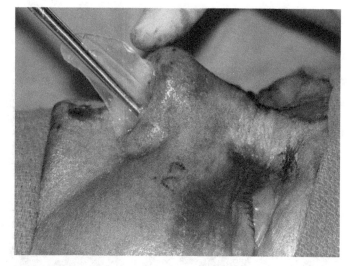

Figure 17.9. Doyle splints impregnated with antibiotic ointment are placed.

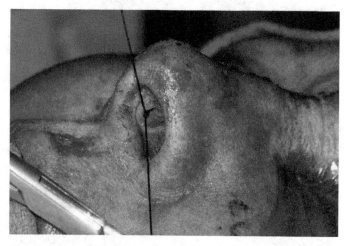

Figure 17.10. Doyle splints are secured to the membranous septum with silk sutures.

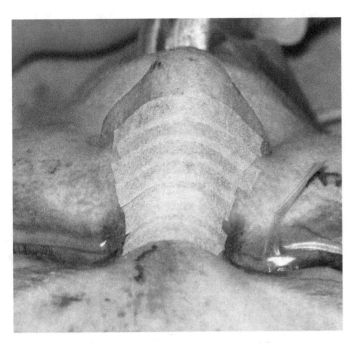

Figure 17.11. Steri-strips are placed over the nasal dorsum.

Figure 17.12. Aquaplast thermogenic splint in place.

Case Report 17.2. A 41-year-old male presents status post an assault resulting in extensive midface fractures. Due to the extent of his injuries and significant facial edema, the patient was taken to the operating room 10 days later, allowing for swelling to subside. An open approach to the nasal bone complex was performed utilizing an open-sky incision with the application of low-profile titanium plates and screws. (See Figures 17.13, 17.14, 17.15, and 17.16.)

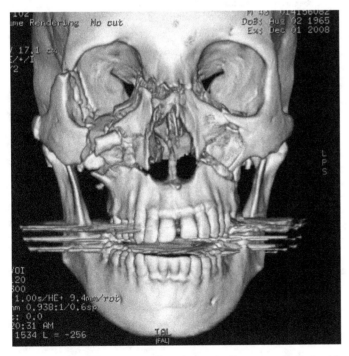

Figure 17.13. 3D reconstruction demonstrating comminuted midface and nasal fractures.

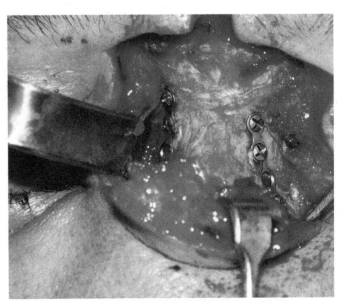

Figure 17.14. Open-sky ("H") incision is utilized to gain access to the comminuted nasal fractures.

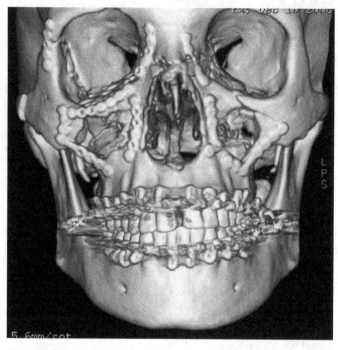

Figure 17.15. Postoperative 3D reconstruction demonstrating reduction of comminuted nasal fractures and associated facial fractures.

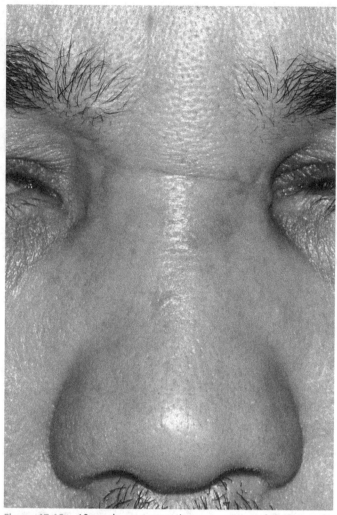

Figure 17.16. 10 weeks postoperative appearance of the open-sky ("H") approach.

References

Bartkiw, T.P., Pynn, B.R. and Brown, D.H., 1995. Diagnosis and management of nasal fractures. *International Journal of Trauma Nursing*, 1(1), 11–18.

Fattahi, T., Steinberg, B., Fernandes, R., Mohan, M. and Reitter, E., 2006. Repair of nasal complex fractures and the need for secondary septo-rhinoplasty. *Journal of Oral and Maxillofacial Surgery*, 64(12), 1785–9.

Indresano, T., 2005. Nasal fractures. In: R. Fonseca, ed. *Oral and maxillofacial trauma*. Vol. 2. 3rd ed. St. Louis, MO: Elsevier Saunders. Pp. 737–50.

Kucik, C.J. and Clenney, T., 2005. Management of epistaxis. *American Family Physician*, 71(2), 305–11.

Mondin, V., Rinaldo, A. and Ferlito, A., 2005. Management of nasal bone fractures. *American Journal of Otolaryngology*, 26(3), 181–5.

Powers, M.P., 2005. Management of soft tissue injuries. In: R. Fonseca, ed. *Oral and maxillofacial trauma*. Vol. 2. 3rd ed. St. Louis MO: Elsevier Saunders. Pp. 791–800.

Ziccardi, V.B. and Braidy, H., 2009. Management of nasal fractures. *Oral and Maxillofacial Surgery Clinics of North America*, 221(2), 203–8, vi.

CHAPTER 18

Frontal Sinus Fractures

Gabriel C. Tender,[1] Arnett Klugh III,[2] Min S. Park,[2] Robert M. Laughlin,[3] and Christopher J. Haggerty[4]

[1]Department of Neurosurgery, Louisiana State University Health Sciences Center, New Orleans, Louisiana, USA

[2]Department of Neurosurgery, Naval Medical Center San Diego, San Diego, California, USA

[3]Department of Oral and Maxillofacial Surgery, Naval Medical Center San Diego, San Diego, California, USA

[4]Private Practice, Lakewood Oral and Maxillofacial Surgery Specialists, Lees Summit; and Department of Oral and Maxillofacial Surgery, University of Missouri–Kansas City, Kansas City, Missouri, USA

A method of correcting cosmetic and functional defects of the frontal sinus via obliterating nonfunctional nasofrontal ducts (NFDs) and reconstructing the anatomy of the anterior table. A method of prophylactically minimizing the formation of mucoceles and pyoceles by removing respiratory mucosa from the frontal sinus. A method of removing displaced posterior table segments via craniotomy and cranialization.

Indications to Frontal Sinus Obliteration

1. Significant anterior table displacement
2. Significant anterior table comminution
3. Foreign body within the frontal sinus, contaminated site
4. Potential injury to NFDs
5. Cosmetic deformity

Indication for Frontal Sinus Cranialization

1. Significant posterior table displacement
2. Significant posterior table comminution
3. Penetrating injury
4. Foreign body within the anterior cranial fossa
5. Cerebrospinal fluid (CSF) leak with extensive dural tears
6. Frontal lobe damage or need for craniotomy access

Contraindications for Surgical Management of Anterior Table Frontal Sinus Fractures

1. No evidence of NFD damage on computed tomography (CT) scanning, and minimal cosmetic defect
2. Medically unstable

Contraindications for Surgical Management of Posterior Table Frontal Sinus Fractures

1. Nondisplaced posterior table fractures
2. Medically unstable

Anatomy

The frontal sinus begins to develop at age 6 and is completely developed by age 12–16. The floor of the frontal sinus is formed medially by the ethmoid bones and laterally by the supraorbital roof. The entire frontal sinus is lined with pseudostratified ciliated respiratory epithelium. The cilia beat backward and medial to lateral as they push mucus into the NFDs, which drain below the middle meatus, anterior to the ethmoid infundibulum.

Coronal Incision Layers

1. Skin
2. Subcutaneous connective tissue
3. Galea aponeurotica
4. Loose areolar subgaleal connective tissue
5. Pericranium

Surgical Management of Anterior Table Frontal Sinus Fractures

1. The patient is positioned in 30° reverse Trendelenburg. The head is placed within a Mayfield headrest (with or without three-pin skull fixation), and the head is positioned in 15–20° extension. The scalp is prepped and draped in a sterile fashion.
2. Triple-antibiotic ointment and a comb may be utilized to create a horizontal part within the patient's hairline approximately 5 cm posterior to the patient's hairline. Alternatively, a strip of hair may be shaved within the site of the proposed coronal incision. For patients with signs of male pattern baldness, it is acceptable to place the incision more posteriorly in order to minimize the potential for a noticeable scar (Figure 18.4 [all figures cited in this chapter appear in the Case Reports]).
3. Local anesthesia containing epinephrine is injected along the incision line, and tumescent solution is deposited within the loose areolar subgaleal connective

Atlas of Operative Oral and Maxillofacial Surgery, First Edition. Edited by Christopher J. Haggerty and Robert M. Laughlin

© 2015 John Wiley & Sons, Inc. Published 2015 by John Wiley & Sons, Inc.

173

tissue in order to further aid in hemostasis and to hydrodissect this layer from the underlying pericranium (Figure 18.6).

4. A scalloped coronal incision (Figure 18.4) is created from preauricular region to preauricular region. The inferior extent of the incision is determined by the amount of exposure required. The forehead and supraorbital regions can be accessed by limiting the inferior incision to the level of the auricular helix. Access to the zygomatic arch requires a preauricular extension to the level of the ear lobe (Figure 18.5).

5. Scalp bleeding is controlled with either Raney clips or needle-tipped cautery.

6. Elevation of the coronal flap occurs within the subgaleal loose areolar connective tissue just superficial to the pericrainum (Figure 18.7). The temporal and preauricular plane of dissection is superficial to the temporalis fascia (Figure 18.8). Care is taken during coronal flap design and reflection to preserve pericranial attachments for the use of a pedicled, vascularized pericranial flap (Figure 18.18).

7. The anterior table of the frontal sinus is removed in order to allow for wide surgical access of the frontal sinus. The peripheral margins of the frontal sinus can be identified with instrumentation (Figure 18.10) and/or a fiber-optic light source (Figures 18.9, 18.31, and 18.32). The anterior table may be removed with any combination of saws, burs (Figure 18.11), chisels, and/or ronguers. The use of saws and burs will frequently allow for the anatomical repositioning of the removed segments at the completion of the frontal sinus exploration or obliteration.

8. Once all bony fragments from the anterior table have been removed, the NFDs are evaluated for trauma and patency. Patency is determined by placing a sterile medium within the frontal sinus (propofol, methylene blue, or sterile water) and observing for drainage from the nasal cavity or posterior oral pharynx. Frontal sinuses with patent NFDs are repaired by anatomically reconstructing the anterior table. If damage to the NFDs is suspected, a curette and/or handpiece is utilized to remove bony septi and mucosa from within the NFDs and from the entire frontal sinus (Figures 18.13, 18.14, 18.15, 18.16, and 18.17).

9. The NFDs are obliterated with temporalis muscle and fibrin sealant (Figures 18.20 and 18.21). A pedicled pericranial flap is laid within the frontal sinus (Figure 18.22). In cases where the pericranial flap does not completely fill the frontal sinus defect, either abdominal fat (Figure 18.23) or a synthetic filler may be utilized to obliterate the frontal sinus defect.

10. Depending on the comminution of the anterior table, the original segments of the anterior table are anatomically repositioned (Figure 18.24) and secured with rigid fixation (Figure 18.25), or a titanium mesh is placed.

11. The coronal incision is closed in a three-layered fashion: 2-0 interrupted Vicryl sutures to reapproximate the galea, 3-0 Vicryl sutures to reapproximate the subcutaneous tissue, and 3-0 nylon sutures or skin staples to close the skin. If a pre-auricular extension was required, the subcutaneous tissues are closed with 4-0 Monocryl sutures, and 5-0 plain gut sutures are used to close the skin (Figure 18.26).

12. A thin layer of triple-antibiotic ointment, an overlying telfa dressing, and a light pressure dressing are placed over the incisions. Drains are typically not required with adequate closure.

Surgical Management of Posterior Table Frontal Sinus Fractures

1. Steps 1–6 of the surgical management of anterior table frontal sinus fractures are performed. It is recommended that three-pin Mayfield skull fixation is utilized to prevent movement of the head during craniotomy.

2. A perforator drill and craniotome are utilized to perform an anterior craniotomy (Figure 18.33) to remove both the anterior and the posterior table of the frontal sinus and to provide access to the anterior cranial fossa. Care is taken to not penetrate the superior sagittal sinus posterior to its origin at the foramen cecum of the frontal bone.

3. A blunt-ended Penfield elevator is utilized to separate the dura from the overlying calvarium prior to elevating and removing the craniotomy segment (Figure 18.34). For noncomminuted fractures, the anterior and posterior tables of the frontal sinus are removed en bloc. For comminuted table fractures, the bone fragments are removed, providing wide surgical access to the anterior cranial fossa.

4. All respiratory mucosa and septi are removed on the back table (Figure 18.35).

5. The posterior table is removed in order to allow forward herniation (cranialization) of the frontal lobes into the frontal sinus.

6. The anterior cranial fossa is inspected, and appropriate neurosurgical intervention is performed. Bone shards and foreign bodies are removed. The dura is inspected for tears, and repairs are made as needed (Figure 18.36). If the anterior frontal dura mater is disrupted, direct watertight repair can be difficult because the dura is thin and

the working space under the frontal lobes is limited. In order to minimize postoperative CSF fistula formation through the cribriform plate, a pedicled galea rotational flap can be inserted between the dura and the cribriform plate, with or without an additional layer of dural substitutes (e.g., Duragen or Duraform).

7. Respiratory mucosa is removed from the NFDs, and the NFDs are obliterated.
8. The anterior table is anatomically repositioned provided sufficient segment size exists (Figure 18.37). Reinforced mesh (Figure 18.38) or custom implants are placed based on the severity of the injury, the ability to reposition the anterior table segments, and the reconstruction of potential cosmetic defects to the anterior calvarium.
9. Steps 11–12 of the surgical management of anterior table frontal sinus fractures are performed.

Postoperative Management

1. Intravenous analgesics and anti-emetics are administered based on symptoms.
2. A short course of intravenous steroids is administered.
3. Postoperative antibiotics are given based on the contamination of the wound and serial examinations during the postoperative period.
4. Incisions are cared for with meticulous incision management and the application of triple-antibiotic ointment for 5–7 days.
5. Drains and pressure dressings are typically removed at 48–72 hours postoperatively.
6. Follow-up CT scans are performed at 6 months, 12 months, 24 months, 5 years, and 10 years postoperatively in order to identify mucoceles, pyoceles, abscess formation, and osteomyelitis.

Complications of Frontal Sinus Fractures

1. **CSF rhinorrhea**: Results from fractures of the posterior table and/or cribriform plate. CSF rhinorrhea is detected via B2 transferrin testing (most accurate), ring testing, and glucose concentration testing of nasal secretions.
2. **Neurologic disorders**: From damage to the underlying frontal lobe and associated structures.
3. **Meningitis**: May develop from either CSF leak or traumatic blockage of the NFDs.
4. **Osteomyelitis**: May result after surgery. More commonly results from long-term infections of the frontal sinus from nonsurgical treatment at the time of initial injury.
5. **Mucoceles and pyoceles**: Mucoceles are the most common chronic complication associated with operated and non-operated frontal sinus fractures.

Treatment consists of exploration of the frontal sinus and curettage or ostectomy of mucoceles, pyoceles, and surrounding involved bone.
6. Brain abscess
7. Cavernous sinus thrombosis
8. **Anosmia**: Results from damage to the cribriform plate.
9. Chronic headache
10. **Cosmetic defect and contour deformities**: Corrected with the anatomical repositioning of noncomminuted anterior table segments and/or the use of titanium mesh. Postoperative defects are treated with bone grafts, custom implants, and fillers.

Key Points

1. The goal of frontal sinus surgery is to create a "safe sinus." When the NFDs are damaged/non-patent, all respiratory mucosa must be removed in order to minimize the formation of mucoceles and pyoceles.
2. NFDs must be evaluated and their patency determined. This is accomplished by placing an angiocatheter into the NFDs, introducing a sterile liquid medium (propofol, normal saline, sterile infant milk, methylene blue, or flourescein), and watching for the emergence of the liquid from beneath the middle meatus within the nose or its collection within the posterior oral pharynx.
3. Nondisplaced frontal sinus fractures without evidence of NFD damage are managed nonsurgically.
4. Anterior (outer) table fractures with damage to the NFDs are managed with exploration of the frontal sinus, the removal of all respiratory mucosa from the frontal sinus, obliteration of the NFDs and frontal sinus, and the reconstruction of the anterior table (frontal sinus obliteration).
5. Posterior (inner) table fractures are managed with exploration of the frontal sinus and anterior cranial fossa, the removal of all respiratory mucosa from the frontal sinus, obliteration of the NFDs, and the reconstruction of the anterior table (frontal sinus cranialization).
6. Cranialization involves the removal of the entire posterior table through a formal craniotomy and allowing the frontal lobe to herniate forward into the frontal sinus.
7. NFDs are obliterated in all cranialization procedures in order to prevent nasal contaminants from entering the anterior cranial fossa. When the posterior table is intact and the NFDs are patent, there is no need to obliterate the frontal sinus or the NFDs.
8. It is recommended that abdominal fat grafts be taken from the lower left quadrant as scars to the right upper quadrant may mimic cholecystectomy incisions and scars to the right lower quadrant may mimic appendectomy incisions.

Case Report 18.1. Obliteration (isolated anterior table fractures). A 28-year-old male presents status post an all-terrain vehicle rollover in which he sustained multiple facial fractures, including an anterior table frontal sinus fracture, Le Fort III fractures, Le Fort II fractures, Le Fort I fractures, and bilateral orbital floor and zygomatico-maxillary complex fractures. On review of the head and maxillofacial CT scans, there were no signs of intracranial injury, no damage to the posterior table of the frontal sinus, and significant radiographic evidence of damage to the bilateral NFDs. The patient was taken to the operating room and submentally intubated. Access to the facial fractures was obtained through a coronal approach with inferior extension to the ear lobes, subtarsal approaches to the orbits, and intraoral incisions. The patency of the NFDs were assessed intraoperatively with the application of sterile propofol placed within the frontal sinus and the failure of the propofol to drain from the nasal cavity. The associated facial fractures were repaired, the frontal sinus and the NFDs were obliterated, and the outer table was repositioned into an anatomical and cosmetic position. (See Figures 18.1 through 18.27.)

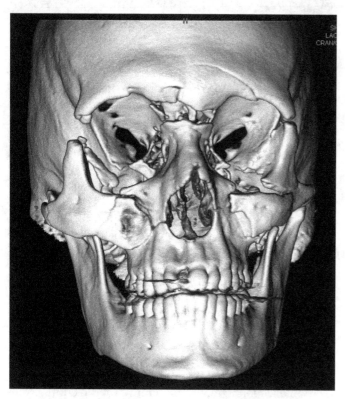

Figure 18.1. 3D reconstruction demonstrating frontal sinus fractures with associated facial fractures.

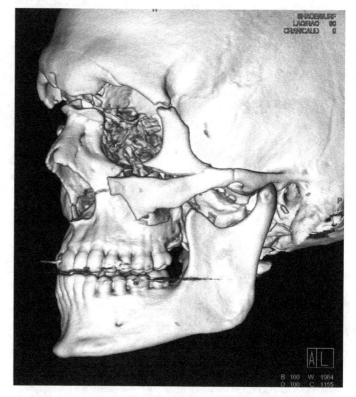

Figure 18.2. Lateral 3D reconstruction demonstrating displaced fractures of the frontal sinus and gross comminution of the bones comprising the nasofrontal ducts.

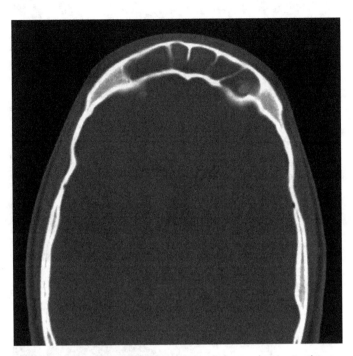

Figure 18.3.   Axial computed tomography scan demonstrating an intact posterior table with no evidence of intracranial injuries, fluid within the frontal sinus, and multiple frontal sinus septi.

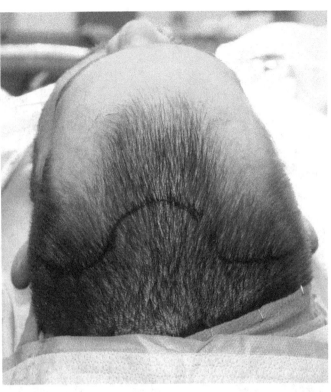

Figure 18.4.   A scalloped marking is made posterior to the hairline at the site of the proposed coronal incision.

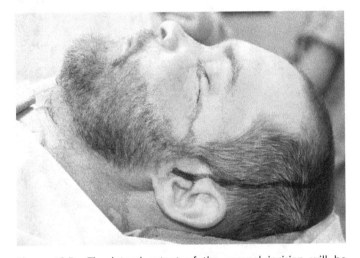

Figure 18.5.   The lateral extent of the coronal incision will be extended to the level of the ear lobe to allow for exposure of the frontal sinus and other associated facial fractures.

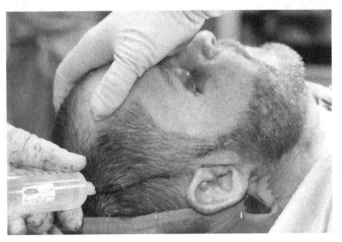

Figure 18.6.   Tumescent solution is injected within the subgaleal connective tissue plane to aid in hemostasis and to hydrodissect this layer from the underlying pericranium.

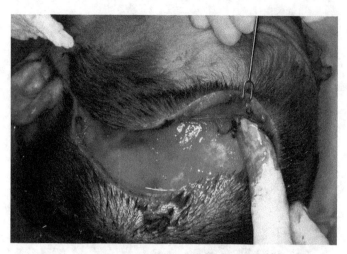

Figure 18.7.   Reflection of the coronal flap with gentle traction and finger dissection within the loose areolar subgaleal plane. The pericranium is left attached to the calvarian to serve as a vascularized tissue flap to line the frontal sinus.

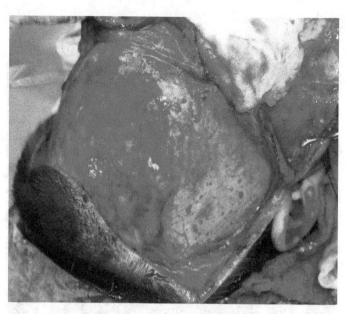

Figure 18.8.   Lateral elevation of the coronal flap superficial to the temporalis fascia.

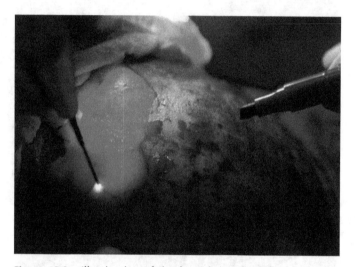

Figure 18.9.   Illumination of the frontal sinus is performed with a sterile light source. The boundaries of the frontal sinus are outlined with either a sterile marking pen or electrocautery.

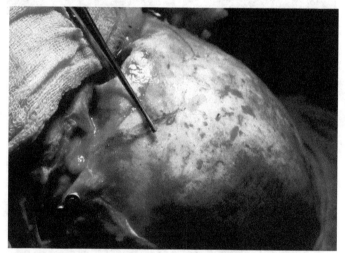

Figure 18.10.   A pair of pickups may be used to confirm the dimensions of the frontal sinus; however, this technique is ineffective for frontal sinuses with septi.

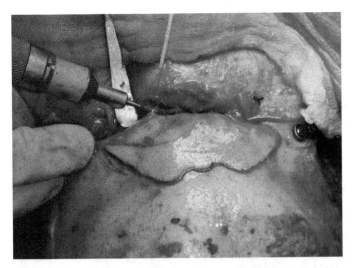

Figure 18.11. A fissured bur with copious irrigation is used to perform a peripheral ostectomy of the anterior table. Wide surgical exposure is necessary to provide access to the NFDs and entire frontal sinus.

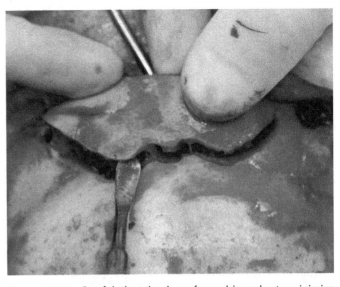

Figure 18.12. Careful elevation is performed in order to minimize damage to the anterior table.

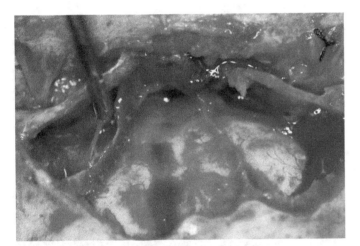

Figure 18.13. Bony septi and mucosa within the frontal sinus.

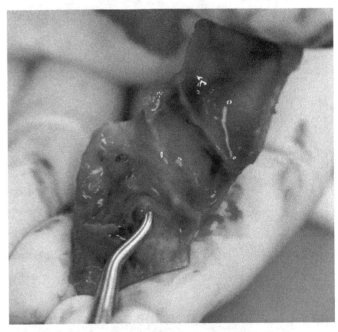

Figure 18.14. Septi and mucosa on the undersurface of the removed anterior table is excised with either a curette (above) or with a bur with copious irrigation.

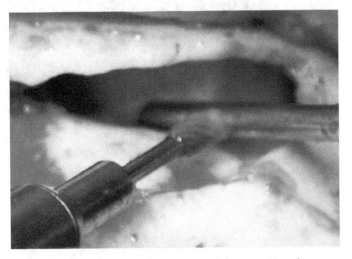

Figure 18.15. A bur is used to remove all bony septi and mucosa from the frontal sinus.

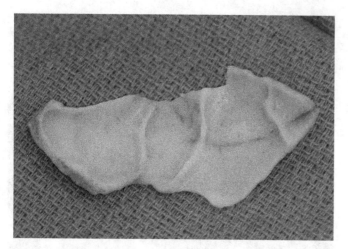

Figure 18.16. All mucosa has been removed from the undersurface of the anterior table.

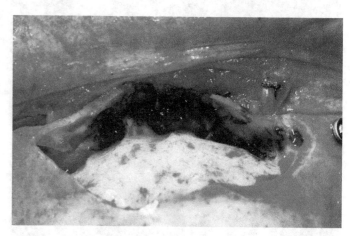

Figure 18.17. The frontal sinus is fully exposed, all peripheral margins have been unroofed, all mucosa from within the frontal sinus and nasofrontal ducts have been removed, and all septi have been eliminated.

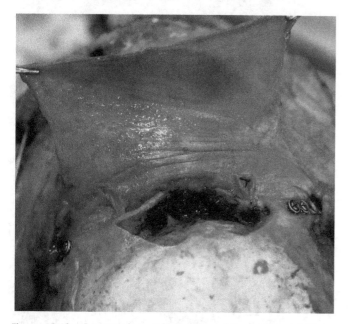

Figure 18.18. Preservation and elevation of the pericranial flap to line the frontal sinus.

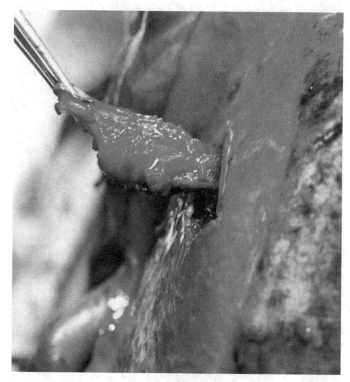

Figure 18.19. A small segment of the temporalis muscle is harvested.

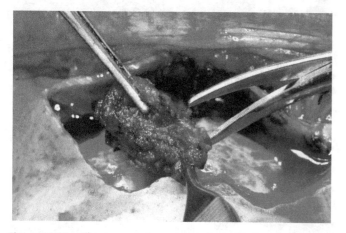

Figure 18.20. The temporalis muscle is transected and utilized to obliterate the nasofrontal ducts.

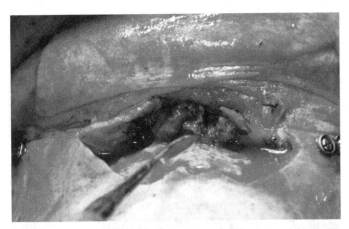

Figure 18.21. The damaged nasofrontal ducts are obliterated with fibrin sealant and temporalis muscle.

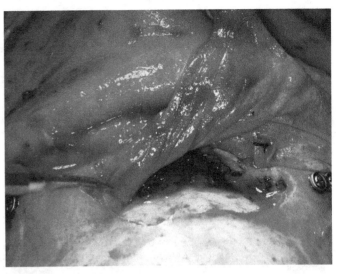

Figure 18.22. The pedicled pericranial flap is trimmed and laid within the frontal sinus.

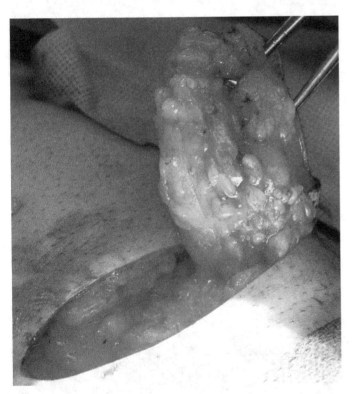

Figure 18.23. Abdominal fat may be harvested and placed over the pericranial flap in large frontal sinus defects.

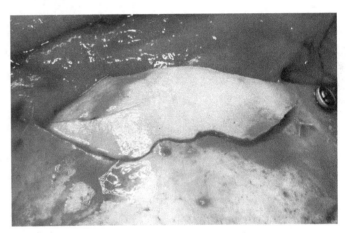

Figure 18.24. The anterior table bone segment is anatomically positioned.

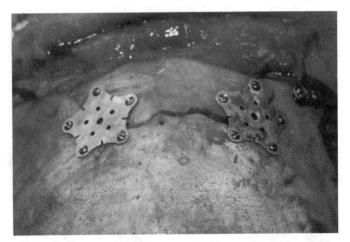

Figure 18.25. The anterior table bone segment is fixated with two low-profile mesh micro-bur hole covers. For large defects, mesh reconstruction is applicable.

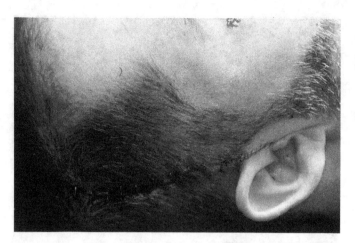

Figure 18.26.   After the placement of all deep sutures, the scalp is reapproximated with either Vicryl sutures or staples, and the skin is reapproximated with 5-0 plain gut sutures.

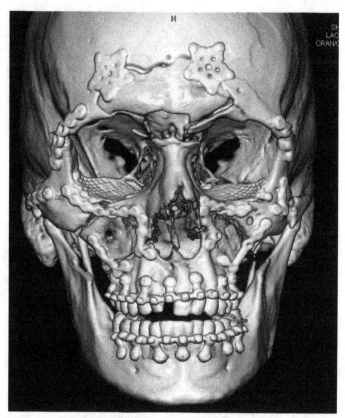

Figure 18.27.   Postoperative 3D reconstruction depicting an anatomically repositioned anterior table of the frontal sinus and repair of associated facial fractures.

Case Report 18.2. Cranialization (posterior table involvement). A 42-year-old male status post motor vehicle accident resulting in anterior and posterior table frontal sinus comminution with posterior table displacement, cribriform plate fracture, CSF rhinorrhea and damage to the NFDs. (Please see Figures 18.28 through 18.38.)

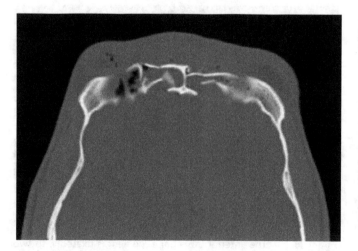

Figure 18.28.   Axial computed tomography scan demonstrating comminuted anterior and posterior table frontal sinus fractures.

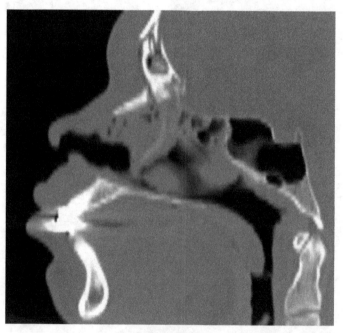

Figure 18.29.   Sagittal computed tomography scan demonstrating anterior and posterior table fractures.

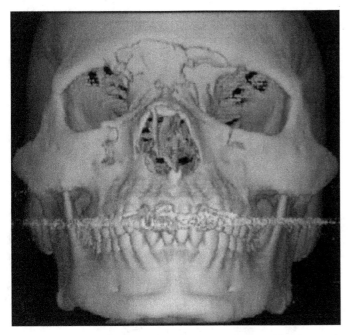

Figure 18.30. 3D reconstruction demonstrating combined comminuted anterior table and naso-orbito-ethmoidal fracture.

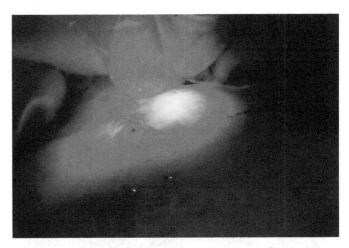

Figure 18.31. A fiber-optic light source is used to identify frontal sinus dimensions.

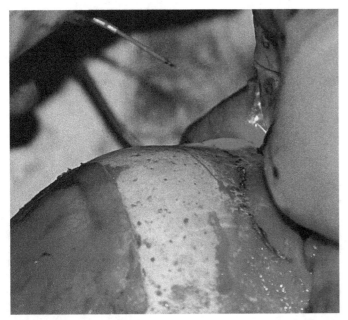

Figure 18.32. The margins of the frontal sinus are outlined with needle tip cautery prior to anterior craniotomy.

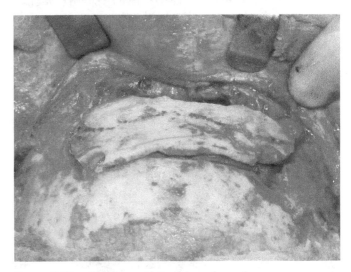

Figure 18.33. Anterior craniotomy is performed.

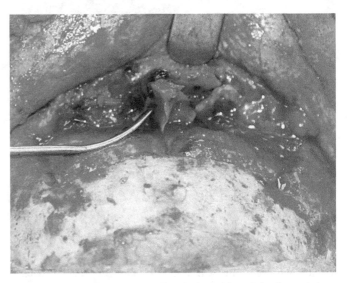

Figure 18.34. The anterior and posterior tables of the frontal sinus are removed, exposing the underlying frontal lobe. Note the disarticulation of the cribriform plate.

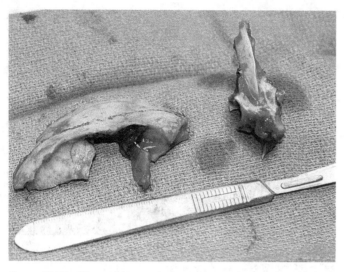

Figure 18.35. The en bloc craniotomy segment is placed on the back table, where all respiratory mucosa and septi are removed and the anterior table is reconstructed.

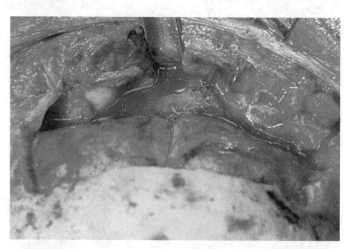

Figure 18.36. The dura was inspected for lacerations, respiratory mucosa was removed from the frontal sinus, the naso-orbito-ethmoidal fractures were reduced, and the nasofrontal ducts were obliterated with temporalis muscle and fibrin sealant.

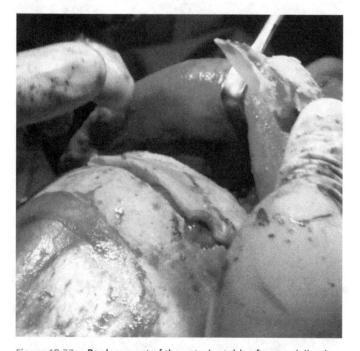

Figure 18.37. Replacement of the anterior table after cranialization.

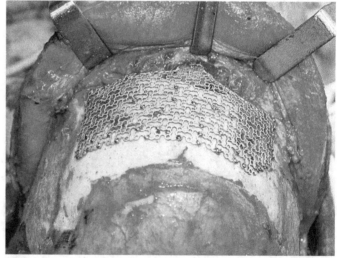

Figure 18.38. Placement of titanium mesh to reinforce the anterior table.

References

Bell, R.B., Dierks, E.J., Brar, P., Potter, J.K. and Potter, B.E., 2007. A protocol for the management of frontal sinus fractures emphasizing sinus preservation. *Journal of Oral and Maxillofacial Surgery*, 65, 825.

Gonty, A.A., Marciani, R.D. and Adornato, D.C., 1999. Management of frontal sinus fractures: a review of 33 cases. *Journal of Oral and Maxillofacial Surgery*, 57, 372.

Sivori, L.A., de Leeuw, R., Morgan, I. and Cunningham, L.I., 2010. Complications of frontal sinus fractures with emphasis on chronic craniofacial pain and its treatment: a review of 43 cases. *Journal of Oral and Maxillofacial Surgery*, 68, 2041.

Tiwari, P., Higuera, S., Thronton, J. and Hollier, L.H., 2005. The management of frontal sinus fractures. *Journal of Oral and Maxillofacial Surgery*, 63, 1354.

19 Panfacial and Naso-Orbito-Ethmoid (NOE) Fractures

Celso F. Palmieri, Jr. and Andrew T. Meram
Department of Oral and Maxillofacial Surgery, Louisiana State University Health Sciences Center, Shreveport, Louisiana, USA

Reduction and reconstruction of hard and soft tissue injures of the facial skeleton to allow for early and total restoration of facial form, symmetry, and function.

Indications for Reduction of Panfacial and NOE Fractures

1. To establish airway security in the presence of unstable fractures, expanding hematoma, and foreign body aspiration
2. Extensive soft tissue injury requiring debridement with primary closure
3. Profuse blood loss from facial injuries
4. Large, open, contaminated compound wounds
5. Concomitant systemic injuries requiring immediate operative intervention by another surgical subspecialty
6. Restoration of pre-injury facial aesthetics and function
7. Prevention of latent cosmetic and functional deficits

Contraindications

1. Patients with severe, compromising, concomitant systemic trauma, rendering them unstable for open reduction with internal fixation (ORIF)
2. Unstable patients requiring correction of blood volume, electrolyte, and nutritional deficits
3. Significant facial edema in stabilized patients that interferes with the ability to obtain an accurate clinical evaluation, obscures maxillofacial anatomy or surgical landmarks, and makes the surgical procedure itself more difficult
4. Increased intracranial pressure (>15 mm Hg) in patients with concomitant head injuries

Anatomy

The facial skeleton receives support and stability from a series of transverse and vertical facial buttresses. Facial buttresses represent areas of thick bone that support the surrounding thinner facial bones, sustain masticatory forces, and protect vital structures. Restoration of facial width, height, and projection is achieved by reducing and reconstructing the facial buttresses.

Transverse (Horizontal) Facial Buttresses

1. **Superior transverse facial buttress (frontal bar)**: Orbital plate of the frontal bone and the cribriform plate of the ethmoid
2. **Middle transverse facial buttress**: Temporal bone, zygomatic arch, infraorbital rim and orbital floor, frontal process of the maxilla, and nasal bones. Crosses the zygomaticotemporal, zygomaticomaxillary, and nasofrontal sutures
3. **Inferior transverse facial buttress**: Hard palate and maxillary alveolus
4. **Superior transverse mandibular buttress**: Inferior alveolar ridge of the mandible
5. **Inferior transverse mandibular buttress**: Inferior border of the mandible from angle to angle

Vertical Facial Buttresses

1. **Central nasoethmoidal buttress**: Ethmoid and vomer bones
2. **Nasomaxillary buttresses**: Frontal process of maxilla, nasal bones, nasion and medial walls of maxillary sinuses, and orbits
3. **Zygomaticomaxillary buttress**: Posterior maxillary molars vertically through zygomaticomaxillary sutures, zygomatic bodies, and lateral orbital walls into the frontal bones
4. **Pterygomaxillary buttresses**: Pterygoid processes of sphenoid bone and posterolateral and posteromedial walls of maxillary sinuses
5. **Posterior mandibular buttress**: Ascending ramus and condyle

Figure 19.1 shows horizontal and vertical facial buttresses.

Naso-orbital-ethmoidal (NOE) complex: often divided into two components: the interorbital space and the medial orbital wall

a. Interorbital space: two ethmoidal labyrinths, superior and middle turbinates, and perpendicular plate of ethmoid

---

Atlas of Operative Oral and Maxillofacial Surgery, First Edition. Edited by Christopher J. Haggerty and Robert M. Laughlin
© 2015 John Wiley & Sons, Inc. Published 2015 by John Wiley & Sons, Inc.

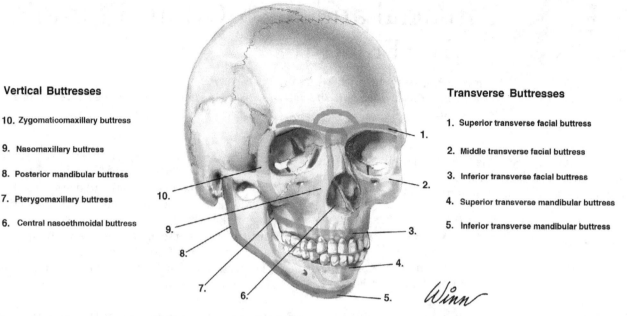

Figure 19.1.   Transverse and vertical buttresses of the facial skeleton.

b. Medial orbital wall: anteriorly—lacrimal bone, lacrimal apparatus, and lamina papyracea; posteriorly—body of sphenoid and medial canthal tendon

c. Signs of NOE fractures include a lack of skeletal support on palpation of the nose, a wide and depressed nasal radix (flat nose), an upturned nasal tip, lacrimal dysfunction, a swollen medial canthal area, traumatic telecanthus, a shortened palpebral fissure, enophthalmos, ocular dystopia, cerebrospinal fluid (CSF) rhinorrhea, and a positive eyelid traction test.

Medial canthal tendon (MCT): The MCT is formed from fibrous bands that originate from the tarsal plates of the upper and lower lids and insert at the frontal process of the maxilla (anterior limb) and at the posterior and superior aspect of the lacrimal bone (posterior limb). The segment of bone that the MCT attaches to is often called the central fragment.

Markowitz NOE Classification System: Based on the fracture patterns of the central fragment and associated MCT attachment

Markowitz Type I: A large central fragment of bone without avulsion of the MCT

Markowitz Type II: Comminution of the central fragment without avulsion of the MCT

Markowitz Type III: Comminution of the central fragment with avulsion of the MCT

Panfacial fracture and NOE reduction technique

1. The patient is positioned supine on the operating room table, the cervical spine (if involved) is stabilized and the airway are secured.

2. Corneal shields are lined with LacriLube ointment and placed over the corneas.

3. The patient's posterior oropharynx is suctioned, and a moistened Ray-Tec gauze is placed within the posterior oropharynx to serve as a throatpack.

4. The patient's oral cavity is cleaned with Chlorhexidine Gluconate 0.12% mouth rinse and a toothbrush. Care is taken to scrub the existing dentition, gingiva, and tongue thoroughly.

5. The patient is prepped and draped to allow for visualization of all involved structures and normal adjacent anatomy.

6. All planned incision sites are marked and subsequently injected with local anesthesia containing a vasoconstrictor.

7. Avulsive and contaminated soft tissue injuries are irrigated and debrided to remove all foreign bodies and debris, often with pulsatile lavage. Soft tissue injuries are assessed for use as possible areas of surgical access.

8. Maxillary and mandibular arch bars are placed in order to reestablish the patient's pre-trauma occlusion and to serve as a stable base for the repair of mandibular and facial bone fractures.

9. If mandibular fractures are present, attention is first turned toward the reduction of the mandibular fractures based on the patient's occlusion and known anatomical landmarks. Mandibular fractures are exposed using the standard intraoral or extraoral incisions, reduced, and internally fixated (Figure 19.5, Case Report 19.1). In cases with bilateral subcondylar fractures, at least one condyle

is opened, reduced, and rigidly fixated in order to establish proper vertical height (Figure 19.4, Case Report 19.1).

10. Once the mandible is repaired, attention is directed toward midface fractures.

11. All remaining facial fractures are exposed through a combination of approaches. Existing lacerations can be utilized as well. Specific techniques are discussed in detail in preceding chapters.

12. NOE fractures are reduced and fixated by reconstructing the nasomaxillary vertical facial buttresses and the superior and middle transverse facial buttresses. Often, calvarian and columellar strut grafting and concomitant medial canthal tendon (MCT) resuspension is required.

13. Markowitz type I and mild type II fractures are repaired with repositioning of the central segment with bone plates. Markowitz III and grossly comminuted type II fractures are repaired with a combination of bone plates and transnasal wiring in order to reposition the displaced or avulsed MCT.

14. The avulsed MCT or small bone segment containing the MCT (central fragment) is identified. For unilateral Markowitz type II/III fractures, a 28- or 30-gauge wire (with or without a barb) is used to pass twice through the MCT or central fragment. The wire is passed through the nasal cavity posterior and superior to the lacrimal bone with either a bone awl or a spinal needle. A small fixation plate (anchor plate) is secured to the contralateral side within solid bone along the medial orbital wall or reconstructed nasal bridge. The wire is secured to the anchor plate to restore the intercanthal distance. For bilateral Markowitz type II/III fractures, transnasal wiring of the bilateral MCT or central fragment is performed and secured to the anchor plate to correct the intercanthal distance. In either situation, a slight overcorrection is performed.

15. After reduction and fixation of all facial fractures, maxillomandibular fixation (MMF) is released, and the occlusion is checked to ensure adequate stability. If the occlusion is non-ideal, the patient is placed back into MMF, the facial fractures are reevaluated, and adjustments are made.

16. All incisions are irrigated with copious normal saline and closed. Large, avulsive tissue injuries may require debridement and closure with either local or regional flap elevation.

17. At the completion of the procedure, the patient's oropharynx is suctioned, and the throat pack is removed and MMF is typically reapplied with either elastics or stainless steel wires.

18. The corneal shields are removed, and the eyes are flushed with balanced salt solution. All blood and prep are removed from the patient's skin with a wet and a dry lap.

19. Steri-strips and pressure dressings are applied. If indicated, a rigid c-collar is placed.

Postoperative Management

1. Multidisciplinary management is necessary during the immediate postoperative period. This includes coordination with any and all consult teams (i.e., trauma, oral and maxillofacial surgery, plastic surgery, otolaryngology, neurosurgery, orthopedic surgery, ophthalmology, hospitalist, nutritionist, physical therapy, and occupational therapy).

2. A noncontrast computed tomography (CT) scan of the face with 3D reconstruction should be obtained immediately postoperatively to assess for proper fracture reduction and fixation. Importance should be paid to 2D views (axial, coronal, and sagittal) in particular because they may show levels of detail that are unavailable in 3D images. In cases involving the frontal sinus, additional CT scans of the head and face should be obtained at periods of 3–6 months postoperatively for the first year and then yearly for the next 5 years to ensure proper pneumatization of the sinuses, to rule out mucocele formation, and to assess for proper stability of the fracture segments.

3. A vision exam is necessary immediately upon awakening in the operating room (if applicable) and daily thereafter as indicated by ophthalmology.

4. Immediate postoperative medications include analgesics, decongestants, corticosteroids, and antibiotics. Triple-antibiotic ointment may be applied liberally to all skin wounds, and oral disinfectant mouth rinses such as 0.12% chlorhexidine gluconate (Peridex) may be used.

5. If drains have been placed, they are removed when output is less than 20–30 mL's in a 24-hour period.

6. In cases where the nasal bones are involved, hemostatic packings placed perioperatively are removed 24–48 hours postoperatively. Doyle splints are removed in 7 days. External nasal splints are left in place for 1–2 weeks postoperatively.

7. Ice packs are beneficial for the first 24–48 hours postoperatively to minimize edema.

8. Nonresorbable sutures are removed from the skin in 5–7 days. Staples are removed in 10–14 days. Patients are advised to avoid sun exposure and to apply sunscreen and/or Kelo–Cote ointment to the wounds for a period of 6 months.

9. Sinus precautions are necessary for a minimum of 3 weeks to avoid possible periorbital subcutaneous emphysema and/or oroantral fistula formation.

This requires that the patient not perform nose blowing and that they sneeze with their mouths open to decrease sinus pressure. Postoperative decongestants, oxymetazoline nasal spray, and nasal saline sprays are taken as needed to minimize congestion.

10. In cases where the patient is placed into MMF, the duration of MMF is highly variable and dependent on several factors, including the degree and type of fractures involved, the type of fixation applied, the age of the patient, and the stability of the patient's occlusion. Arch bars are cleaned daily with disinfectant mouth rinses utilizing a soft toothbrush, with care made to avoid the intraoral incisions. Wax can be applied to the wires to minimize trauma to the labial mucosa.

11. In cases where MMF is utilized, the patient is kept on tube feeding immediately postoperatively until the patient has stabilized and is able to tolerate full liquids. At that time, the patient is maintained on a full liquid diet until the MMF has been released. After MMF is released, and in cases not requiring MMF, patients are limited to a soft, nonchew diet for a minimum of 6 weeks to minimize masticatory forces on the healing facial bones.

12. In cases involving mandible fractures, physiotherapy is utilized to prevent and/or address postoperative trismus and ankylosis of the condyles. The goal should be made to achieve a maximal incisal opening of 40 mm within 4 weeks postoperatively.

Complications

Complications are specific to the bones and structures involved as panfacial and NOE-type fractures involve numerous facial regions.

Early Complications

1. **Decrease in posterior facial height**: Occurs with significant continuity defects to the vertical buttresses of the face and with unreduced bilateral mandibular condyle fractures (typically presents as an anterior open bite). Treatment involves osteotomizing the fractures and/or orthognathic surgery.

2. **Increase in facial width**: Often results from nonreduced or poorly reduced palatal fractures. Also occurs when combined mandibular symphysis fractures and bilateral condylar neck fractures are not adequately reduced or fixated. Results from a tendency of the midface and mandible to splay open with or without concomitant malocclusion, when anatomical reduction is not achieved. Treatment

involves osteotomizing the fractures and/or orthognathic surgery.

3. **Decrease in anterior-posterior facial projection**: Can occur with any fracture that increases the facial width and NOE fractures. Treatment involves osteotomizing the fractures and/or orthognathic surgery.

4. **Traumatic telecanthus**: Normal intercanthal distance in males is 33–34 mm, in females 32–33 mm, or an interpupillary distance of 60–62 mm. Traumatic telecanthus should be repaired early with transnasal wiring or late with canthopexy.

5. Infections and brain abscess

6. Hydrocephalus

7. Meningitis

8. Neurologic deficits, including motor and sensory (anesthesia and paresthesia) deficits

9. Nasal obstruction and/or deformities

10. CSF leak

11. Anosmia

12. Blindness

13. Subcutaneous emphysema

14. Hematoma

15. Malocclusion

Late Complications

1. Posttraumatic seizures
2. Mucocele and mucopyocele of the frontal sinus
3. Osteomyelitis
4. Contour deformities
5. Chronic headaches and/or neurological deficits
6. Scarring
7. Malunion
8. Nonunion
9. Diplopia
10. Enophthalmos
11. Entropion or ectropion
12. Upper eyelid ptosis
13. Lower eyelid retraction
14. Epiphora
15. Hardware failure
16. Temporomandibular joint dysfunction
17. Ankylosis
18. Dental problems
19. Fistula formation (oro-antral, oro-nasal, or orocutaneous)

Key Points

1. Facial trauma repair is typically performed from a bottom-top (beginning with the mandible) and inside-out sequencing (repair of deep structures first and superficial structures last).

2. Often, cervical spine stabilization is required. Cervical spine stabilization involves leaving the patient within a c-collar, stabilization with a three-pronged Mayfield head clamp, or sand bags placed lateral to the neck (least preferred method). Regardless of the technique, cervical spine mobilization should be minimal.

3. Important anatomical landmarks include knowledge of the correct horizontal and vertical buttresses of the craniomaxillofacial skeleton.

4. Panfacial trauma is often associated with severe concomitant systemic injuries, and therefore necessitates a multidisciplinary team approach to management.

5. Panfacial fractures can result in widening of the facial complex with concomitant loss of the facial projection. Emphasis must be placed on anatomical reduction of the bones and restoration of the maxillomandibular arch form.

6. With sagittal palatal fractures, or in situations with a mandibular symphysis fracture associated with bilateral condylar neck fractures where anatomical reduction is not achieved, there is a tendency for the midface and mandible to splay open with possible concomitant malocclusion.

7. Traumatic telecanthus with an intercanthal distance of greater than 40 mm is nearly pathognomonic of an NOE fracture. Traumatic telecanthus is due to disruption of the MCT or the central fragment of bone that serves as an attachment for the MCT.

8. Transnasal wiring is necessary with displaced NOE fractures that involve central fragments too small to plate (some Markowitz type II fractures) and with grossly comminuted central fragments with complete avulsion of the insertion of the MCT (Markowitz type III).

9. Goals of NOE repair include anatomical reduction of all fractures, correcting traumatic telecanthus, obtaining a midline position of the nasal septum, reconstruction of dorsal nasal deformities (calvarian strut grafts and columellar strut grafts), anatomical positioning of the lower lateral cartilages, and the correction of enophthamlos, ocular dystopia, and lacrimal dysfunction.

10. Lateral midface width and projection are dependent on the anatomical repositioning of the ZMC, with the reduction of the sphenozygomatic suture being of utmost importance.

Case Report

Case Report 19.1. A 40-year-old male reports to the emergency department after a high-speed all-terrain vehicle accident. On arrival, a cricothyrotomy was emergently performed due to upper airway obstruction. Once the patient was stabilized, a CT scan was obtained that demonstrated panfacial fractures involving all facial bones with the exception of the frontal bone. Fractures included an NOE-type I fracture, a LeFort II fracture, bilateral zygomaticomaxillary complex (ZMC) fractures, bilateral infraorbital rim and orbital floor fractures, a midline palatal fracture, bilateral subcondylar fractures, and a symphysis fracture. In addition to his extensive facial injuries, the patient also sustained a cervical spine fracture and was stabilized in a c-collar. With the airway and cervical spine secured, the patient was taken to the operating room, and the urgent cricothyrotomy was converted to an open tracheotomy. The facial fractures were reduced and fixated utilizing a bottom-up, inside-out sequence. (See Figures 19.2 through 19.14.)

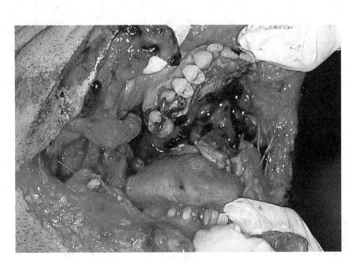

Figure 19.2. Patient presents with extensive hard and soft tissue facial injuries.

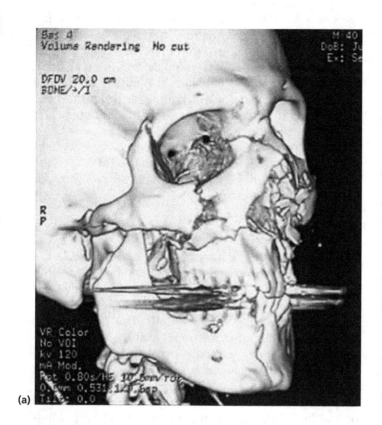

(a)

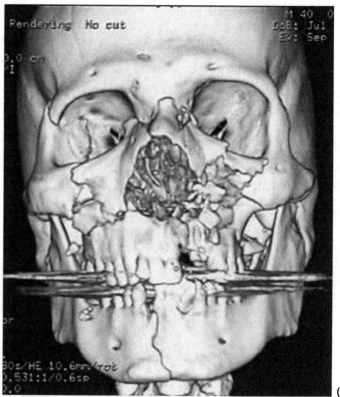

(b)

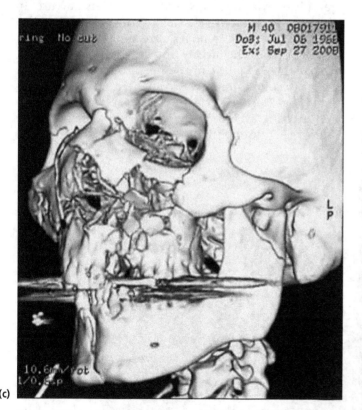

(c)

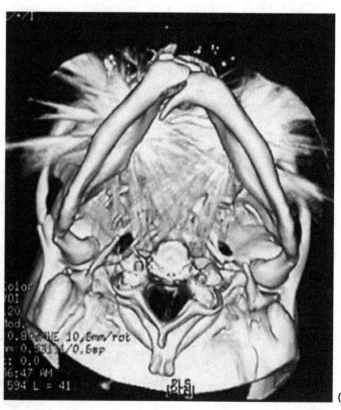

(d)

Figure 19.3. (a–d) Selected preoperative 3D reconstruction computed tomography images of the facial fractures demonstrating bilateral mandibular condyle fractures, an anterior mandibular fracture, a Le Fort II fracture, bilateral zygomaticomaxillary complex fractures, comminuted nasal fractures, bilateral infraorbital rim and floor fractures, a palatal fracture, bilateral comminuted antral wall fractures, and a type I naso-orbito-ethmoidal (NOE) fracture.

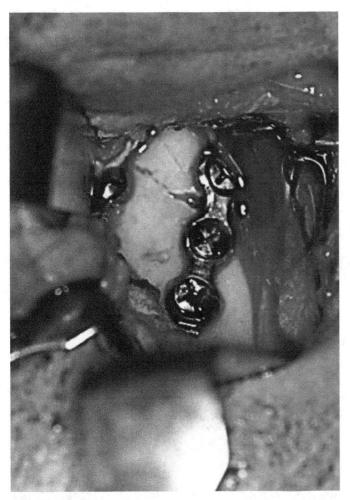

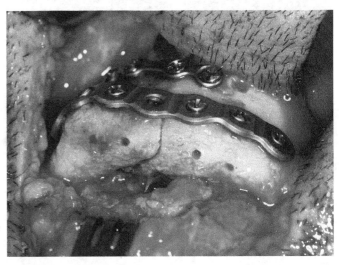

Figure 19.5. Open reduction with internal fixation of the symphysis fracture using the two-plate technique through an existing laceration. Note anatomic reduction of the lingual aspect of the symphysis.

Figure 19.4. Open reduction with internal fixation of the left subcondylar fracture using the two-plate technique through a retromandibular incision.

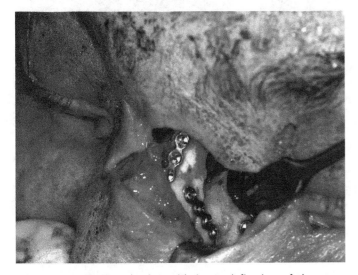

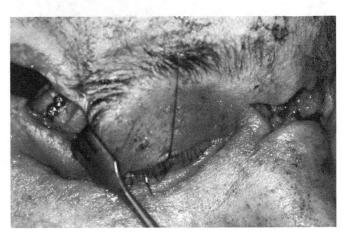

Figure 19.6. Open reduction with internal fixation of the naso-orbito-ethmoidal and nasal bone fractures using an open-sky ("H") incision.

Figure 19.7. Open reduction with internal fixation of the left zygomaticofrontal suture through a lateral brow incision.

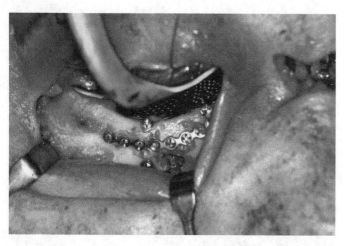

Figure 19.8. Open reduction with internal fixation of the right infraorbital rim and orbital floor through a subciliary incision.

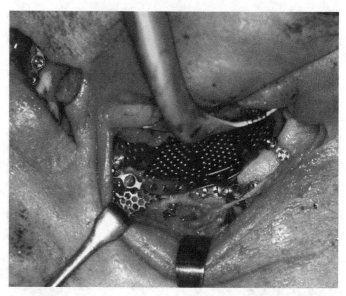

Figure 19.9. Open reduction with internal fixation of the left infraorbital rim and orbital floor through a subciliary incision.

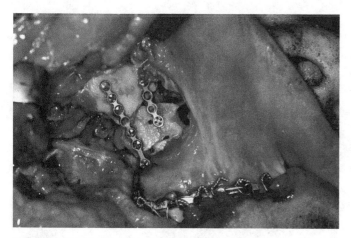

Figure 19.10. Open reduction with internal fixation of the right zygomaticomaxillary and nasomaxillary buttresses.

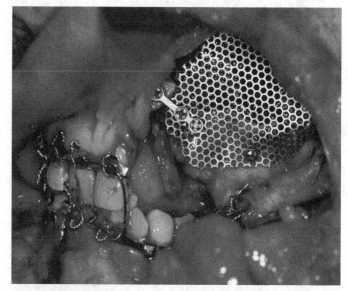

Figure 19.11. Open reduction with internal fixation of the left nasomaxillary buttress and titanium mesh reconstruction of a large anterior maxillary sinus wall defect.

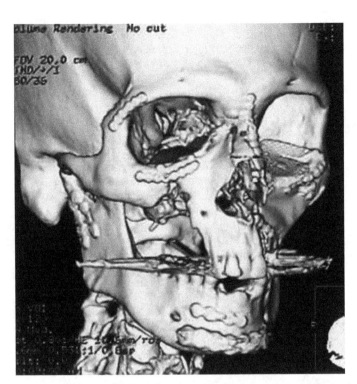 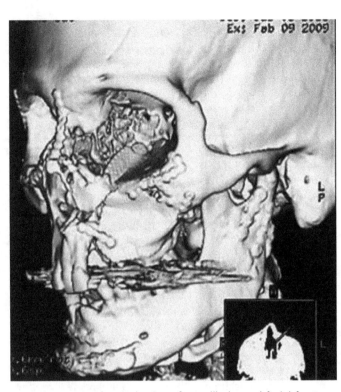

Figures 19.12. and 19.13.   Postoperative 3D reconstruction images demonstrating appropriate reduction of mandibular and facial fractures with restoration of facial height, width and projection.

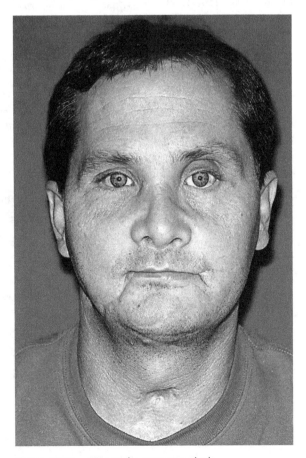

Figure 19.14.   15 months postoperatively.

References

Bluebond-Langner, R. and Rodriguez, E.D., 209. Application of skeletal buttress analogy in composite facial reconstruction. *Craniomaxillofacial Trauma and Reconstruction*, 2, 19–25.

Cohen, S.R. and Kawamoto, H., 1992. Analysis and results of treatment of established posttraumatic facial deformities. *Plastic and Reconstructive Surgery*, 90, 574–84.

Gasparini, G., Brunelli, A., Rivaroli, A., Lattanzi, A. and DePonte, F.S., 2002. Maxillofacial traumas. *Journal of Craniofacial Surgery*, 13, 645–9.

Girotto, J.A., MacKenzie, E., Fowler, C., Redett, R., Robertson, B. and Manson, P.N., 2001. Long-term physical impairment and functional outcomes after complex facial fractures. *Plastic and Reconstructive Surgery*, 108, 312–27.

Gruss, J.S., 1995. Advances in craniofacial fracture repair. *Scandinavian Journal of Plastic and Reconstructive Surgery and Hand Surgery* (Suppl. 27), 67–81.

Gruss, J.S., 1995. Craniofacial osteotomies and rigid fixation in the correction of post-traumatic craniofacial deformities. *Scandinavian Journal of Plastic and Reconstructive Surgery and Hand Surgery* (Suppl. 27), 83–95.

Gruss, J.S., Bubak, P.J. and Egbert, M., 1992. Craniofacial fractures: an algorithm to optimize results. *Clinics in Plastic Surgery*, 19, 195–206.

Gruss, J.S. and Mackinnon, S.E., 1986. Complex maxillary fractures: role of buttress reconstruction and immediate bone grafts. *Plastic and Reconstructive Surgery*, 78, 9–22.

Hopper, R.A. and Gruss, J.S., 2012. Maxillofacial trauma. In: M.W. Mulholland, K.D. Lillemoe, G.M. Doherty, R.V. Maier, D.M. Simeone and G.R. Upchurch, Jr., eds. *Greenfield's surgery: scientific principles & practice*. 5th ed. Philadelphia: Lippincott Williams & Wilkins.

Hopper, R.A., Salemy, S. and Sze, R.W., 2006. Diagnosis of midface fractures with CT: what the surgeon needs to know. *Radiographics*, 26, 783–93.

Kelley, P., Crawford, M., Higuera, S. and Hollier, L.H., 2005. Two hundred ninety-four consecutive facial fractures in an urban trauma center: lessons learned. *Plastic and Reconstructive Surgery*, 116, 42e–49e.

Kelly, K.J., Manson, P.N., Van der Kolk, C.A., Markowitz, B.L., Dunham, C.M., Rumley, T.O. and Crawley, W.A., 1990. Sequencing Le Fort fracture treatment. *Journal of Craniofacial Surgery*, 1, 168–78.

Luce, E.A., 1992. Developing concepts and treatment of complex maxillary fractures. *Clinics in Plastic Surgery*, 19, 125–31.

Manson, P.N., Clark, N., Robertson, B. and Crawley, W.A., 1995. Comprehensive management of pan-facial fractures. *Journal of Craniofacial Trauma*, 1, 43–56.

Manson, P.N., Clark, N., Robertson, B., Slezak, S., Wheatly, M. and Van der Kolk, C.A., 1999. Subunit principles in midface fractures: the importance of sagittal buttresses, soft-tissue reductions, and sequencing treatment of segmental fractures. *Plastic and Reconstructive Surgery*, 103, 1287–306.

Markowitz, B.L. and Manson, P.N., 1989. Panfacial fractures: organization of treatment. *Clinics in Plastic Surgery*, 16, 105–14.

Markowitz, B.L., Manson, P.N., Sargent, L., Vander Kolk, C. A., Yaremchuk, M., Glassman, D. and Crawley, W. A., 1991. Management of the medial canthal tendon in nasoethmoid orbital fractures: the importance of the central fragment in classification and treatment. *Plastic and Reconstructive Surgery*, 87, 843–53.

McDonald, W.S. and Thaller, S.R., 2000. Priorities in the treatment of facial fractures for the millennium. *Journal of Craniofacial Surgery*, 11, 97–105.

Rohrich, R.J. and Shewmake, K.B., 1992. Evolving concepts of craniomaxillofacial trauma management. *Clinics in Plastic Surgery*, 19, 1–10.

Romeo, A., Pinto, A., Cappabianca, S., Scaglione, M. and Brunese, L., 2009. Role of multidetector row computed tomography in the management of mandibular traumatic lesions. *Seminars in Ultrasound CT MR*, 30, 174–80.

Stanley, R.B., 1984. Reconstruction of midface vertical dimension following Lefort fracture treatment. *Archives of Otolaryngology*, 110, 571–5.

Stanley, R.B., 1989. The zygomatic arch as a guide to reconstruction of comminuted malar fractures. *Archives of Otolaryngology*, 115, 1459–62.

Tang, W., Feng, F., Long, J., Lin, Y., Wang, H., Liu, L. and Tian, W., 2009. Sequential surgical treatment for panfacial fractures and significance of biological osteosynthesis. *Dental Traumatology*, 25, 171–75.

Tessier, P., 1986. Complications of facial trauma: principles of late reconstruction. *Annals of Plastic Surgery*, 17, 411–20.

Tullio, A. and Sesenna, E., 2000. Role of surgical reduction of condylar fractures in the management of panfacial fractures. *British Journal of Oral and Maxillofacial Surgery*, 38, 472–6.

20 Soft Tissue Injuries

Jason Jamali, Antonia Kolokythas, and Michael Miloro
Department of Oral and Maxillofacial Surgery, College of Dentistry, University of Illinois Chicago, Chicago, Illinois, USA

Stensen's Duct Repair

A means of reestablishing parotid salivary flow through a damaged or severed Stensen's duct (parotid duct).

Indication

1. Traumatic transection of Stensen's duct

Contraindications

1. Partial transaction with adequate salivary flow through the orifice of Stensen's duct
2. Intervention may be delayed in the medically compromised or unstable patient.

Anatomy

Parotid duct (Stensen's duct): The anticipated course of the parotid duct is predicted by drawing a line from the tragus of the ear to the mid-portion of the upper lip. Stensen's duct originates from the anterior portion of the parotid gland and continues anteriorly toward the anterior border of the masseter muscle. At the level of the masseter muscle, the duct courses medially piercing through the buccal fat pad and buccinator muscle before terminating at its papilla orifice within the buccal mucosa adjacent to the maxillary second molar. The length of the duct is approximately 7.0 cm. Both the zygomatic and buccal branches of the facial nerve may cross the path of Stensen's duct.

Parotid Duct Repair Technique

1. A thorough clinical examination is performed to evaluate facial nerve function as parotid duct injuries frequently occur in conjunction with facial nerve injuries.
2. The patient is placed under general anesthesia within an operating room. Short-acting paralytics are used to allow for further facial nerve stimulation with a nerve stimulator during the procedure. The patient is prepped intraorally and extraorally and draped to allow for full exposure of the facial wounds.
3. The facial wounds are debrided and irrigated with light pressure. Pulsatile irrigation is deferred in cases where the facial nerve is exposed or damaged.
4. Exploration of the wound is commonly performed with magnification (loupe vs. operating microscope).
5. The duct is cannulated intraorally via the orifice of Stensen's duct with an IV angiocatheter (Figure 20.5, Case Report 20.2), or a 16-gauge epidural catheter. Lacrimal probe dilation is typically necessary to enlarge the duct to accommodate a catheter (Figure 20.2, Case Report 20.1 and Figure 20.4, Case Report 20.2).
6. Saline or propofol (TEVA Pharmaceuticals, North Wales, PA, USA) is injected through the cannula while the wound is observed for leakage. Toluidine blue has been used in the past, but typically it obscures the remainder of the field for repair.
7. If present, the location of transection is confirmed, and an attempt is made to identify and cannulate the proximal end of the duct over the same cannula placed transorally, obturating the distal portion of the duct. A blue background may be placed for visual enhancement of the surgical field.
8. Primary anastomosis is performed over the cannulated ends of the duct using nonresorbable nylon (9-0, 10-0) or silk (7-0, 8-0) sutures.
9. For large segmental defects of the duct, microsurgical repair with interposition grafting may be considered. Donor veins include the facial vein, the saphenous vein, and veins from the forearm.
10. Distal ductal injuries may be treated through a fistulization procedure where the cannulated duct proximal to the injury is diverted intraorally and sutured to the buccal mucosa, creating a new orifice.
11. Proximal injuries closer to the duct and those with extensive parenchymal damage may be treated with ligation of the proximal stump. Salivary flow may be decreased using anticholinergic medications or low-dose radiation to the gland.
12. After definitive treatment of ductal discontinuity, the parotid capsule is closed in order to minimize sialocele

---

Atlas of Operative Oral and Maxillofacial Surgery, First Edition. Edited by Christopher J. Haggerty and Robert M. Laughlin.
© 2015 John Wiley & Sons, Inc. Published 2015 by John Wiley & Sons, Inc.

formation. If extensive parenchymal damage is present, a drain is placed and sewed to the anterior skin edge of the wound.

13. The wound is irrigated and closed in layers, and a pressure dressing is applied for 48 hours.

Postoperative Management

1. Pressure dressings are removed after 48 hours.
2. If present, drains are removed after 1 week.
3. The intraoral stent or catheter is removed after 2 weeks.

Complications

1. **Sialocele and salivary fistula formation**: May result from unidentified or incompletely repaired ductal injury, extensive parenchymal gland damage, or failure to adequately close the parotid capsule. Early management involves opening the anterior aspect of the wound and placing a drain, pressure dressings, repeat aspirations, anti-sialagogues, and anti-cholinergic medications. Late management includes botulinum toxin injections, tympanic neurectomy, parotidectomy, and low-dose radiation therapy.
2. **Salivary gland hypofunction**: In the event that parotid injury or ductal repair results in decreased salivary flow, artificial salivary substitutes, sialogogues, or cholinergic medications may be used to augment saliva production.
3. **Facial nerve deficits**: These should be followed with neurosensory testing in cases in which facial nerve function has been demonstrated to be intact, and only transient deficits are expected (neurapraxia and axontotmesis). With transaction injuries of the facial nerve (neurotmesis), repair is indicated.

Key Points

1. All deep facial lacerations involving the parotid gland should have the parotid duct cannulated in order to evaluate the integrity of Stensen's duct (Figure 20.2, Case Report 20.1).
2. Ductal injuries overlying the masseter muscle are most amenable to repair, whereas intraparenchymal ductal injuries are difficult to identify and repair.

Distal ductal injuries may be treated with fistulization or redirection of the duct intraorally within the buccal mucosa.

3. The choice of ductal repair is dependent upon the location of injury and the ability to identify both proximal and distal ends of the parotid duct.
4. Delayed repairs may be complicated by sialocele formation and scar formation. Immediate primary repair is preferred.
5. Sialography may be used preoperatively to diagnose ductal injury. Sialography may also be used postoperatively to evaluate and monitor the status of the repair and function of the parotid gland.
6. Damage to the facial nerve must be ruled out with penetrating injuries to the parotid region.
7. All hard and soft tissue injuries require meticulous debridement and closure, with special emphasis placed on aligning the vermilion border of the lip if involved.

References

Demian, N. and Curtis, W., 2008. A simple technique for cannulation of the parotid duct. *Journal of Oral and Maxillofacial Surgery*, 66, 1532–3.

Lewkowicz, A.A., 2002. Traumatic injuries to the parotid gland and duct. *Journal of Oral and Maxillofacial Surgery*, 60, 676–80.

Liang, C., 2004. Reconstruction of traumatic stensen duct defect using a vein graft as a conduit: two case reports. *Annals of Plastic Surgery*, 52, 102–4.

Lim, Y.C., 2008. Treatment of an acute salivary fistula after parotid surgery: botulinum toxin type A injection as primary treatment. *European Archives of Otorhinolaryngology*, 265, 243–5.

Steinberg, M.J., 2005. Management of parotid duct injuries. *Oral Surgery, Oral Medicine, Oral Pathology, Oral Radiology, and Endodontology*, 99, 136–41.

Sujeeth, S., 2011. Parotid duct repair using an epidural catheter. *International Journal of Oral and Maxillofacial Surgery*, 40, 747–8.

Van Sickels, J.E., 2009 Management of parotid gland and duct injuries. *Oral and Maxillofacial Surgery Clinics of North America*, 21, 243–6.

Von Lindern, J.J., 2002. New prosepects in the treatment of traumatic and postoperative parotid fistulas with type A Botulinum toxin. *Plastic and Reconstructive Surgery*, 109, 2443–5.

Case Report 20.1. A 27-year-old female presents status post assault with a kitchen knife resulting in a deep laceration involving the parotid gland and surrounding structures. (See Figures 20.1 and 20.2.)

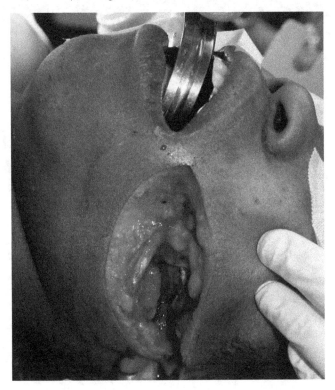

Figure 20.1.   Deep facial laceration involving the parenchyma of the parotid gland.

Case Report 20.2. A 29-year-old man presents status post gunshot wound injury to the left face. The patient was intubated on arrival due to airway concerns. The patient sustained hard and soft tissue damage, including the parotid gland and surrounding structures. (See Figures 20.3, 20.4, 20.5, 20.6, and 20.7.)

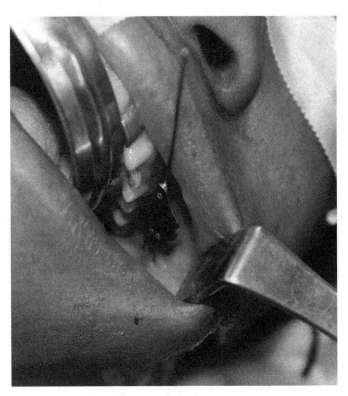

Figure 20.2.   Complete cannulation of the parotid duct with a lacrimal probe confirmed no involvement of the parotid duct in this injury.

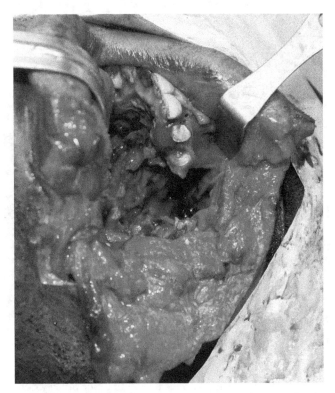

Figure 20.3.   Extensive hard and soft tissue injuries to the parotid region.

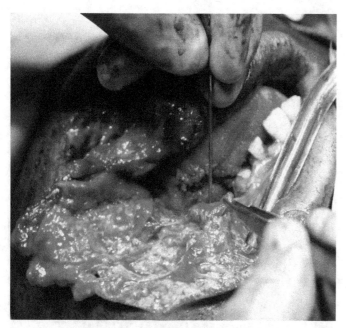

Figure 20.4.   Lacrimal probe used to identify and dilate the proximal aspect of the parotid duct.

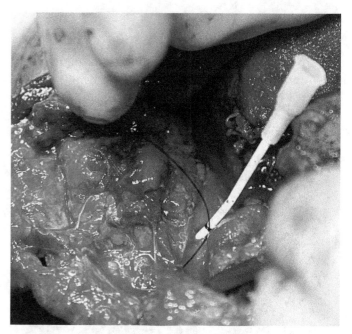

Figure 20.5.   The proximal end of the duct is cannulated with an angiocatheter. The distal end of the parotid duct could not be located due to the extensive soft tissue injuries. The catheter was sewn into the intraoral buccal mucosa to create a new orifice.

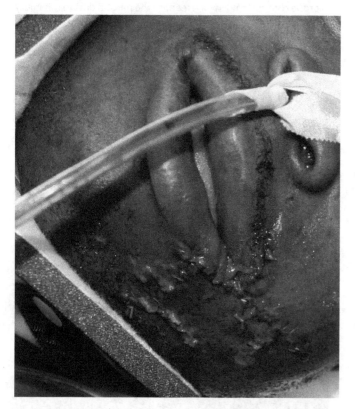

Figure 20.6.   Patient immediately after repair of hard and soft tissue injuries to the oral cavity, parotid duct stenting, and primary closure of the stellate wound.

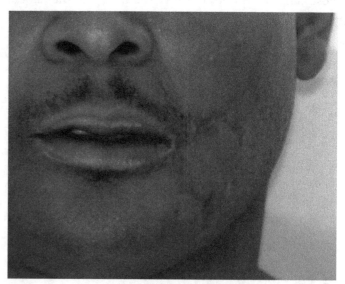

Figure 20.7.   Patient 12 months after injury with adequate saliva flow, a properly aligned vermillion border, and a well-healed scar.

Complex Facial Laceration Repair

The repair of complex soft tissue trauma with debridement, irrigation, exploration, repair of involved structures, and layered closure techniques.

Indications

1. Closure of soft tissue lacerations and defects following traumatic injury
2. Limit scar contracture and soft tissue deformity
3. Minimize adverse aesthetic outcomes

Contraindications

1. Wound contamination
2. Medically compromised or unstable patients
3. Definitive closure may be delayed until associated fractures have been addressed

Anatomy

1. **Scalp**: Layers from superficial to deep include the skin, subcutaneous tissue, galea aponeurotica, loose areolar tissue, and pericranium.
2. **Periorbital region**: The lacrimal gland is located within the anterior aspect of the superior lateral orbit. Lacrimal secretions drain into the upper and lower lid medial puncta, which drain into the lacrimal canaliculi. The lacrimal canaliculi travel 2.0 mm vertically before coursing medially 6.0 mm toward the lacrimal sac. The lacrimal sac drains into the nasolacrimal duct before emptying into the inferior meatus of the nose, inferior to the inferior turbinate.

Technique

1. The patient is positioned for best access and visualization.
2. The wound is irrigated, prepped, and draped in a sterile fashion.
3. Local anesthesia containing a vasoconstrictor is injected within areas of tissue trauma. In areas of avulsive defects where local flaps will be utilized, lidocaine without epinephrine should be considered. Nerve blocks are used where possible (mental, infraorbital, and supraorbital or supratrochlear). Injection along the wound edges may help with hemostasis; however, care must be taken not to distort wound edges during closure.
4. The tissue injury is meticulously irrigated with sterile saline, and complete wound exploration and debridement is performed. Pulsatile pressure irrigation should be utilized for wound debridement unless facial nerve injury is suspected.
5. Vital structures are examined for damage and repaired accordingly (nasolacrimal duct, parotid duct, facial nerve, underlying fractures, and hematomas adjacent to cartilage).
6. Areas of obvious nonvital necrotic tissue are debrided to healthy bleeding tissue.
7. Large, avulsive defects require repair with local and regional flaps and/or tissue-grafting procedures.
8. Closure is performed in a layered fashion. The deeper layers are closed using buried resorbable sutures. A layered closure minimizes potential dead space and hematoma formation. Superficial layers are closed with eversion of the skin edges. The closure should avoid excess tension and strangulation of the tissues as evidenced by blanching of the wound edges. Care is taken to properly align important anatomic landmarks such as the vermillion border, the gray line of the eyelid, and the nasal sill.
9. Ointments and dressings may be applied after closure. Bolsters may be used following repair of ear lacerations to prevent hematoma formation.

Postoperative Management

1. Antibiotic coverage and tetanus prophylaxis may be necessary (dog and human bites).
2. Drains are removed after 48–72 hours or when drainage is minimal. Nonresorbable sutures are removed at 5–7 days after repair, followed by application of steri-strips if necessary. Scalp staples are removed 10–14 days after repair.
3. Avoidance of sun exposure and sunblock is recommended to avoid hyperpigmentation.
4. Scar massage and/or steroid injections will minimize hypertrophic scarring.

Complications

1. **Hypertrophic scars**: Hypertrophic scars are limited to the original scar borders. Treatment involves silicone sheeting, steroid injections, and/or dermabrasion (elevated scars). Scar revisions are performed 6–12 weeks after repair during maximum collagen remodeling. Small scars may be excised (after 6 months), while larger scars may require various soft tissue rearrangements such as Z-plasty, broken-line closure (W-plasty or geometric design repair), and local flaps (advancement, transposition, and rotation).
2. **Keloid formation**: Keloids extend beyond the original scar borders into the adjacent tissues. The incidence of keloids is increased in Fitzpatrick skin types III–VII (darker skin). Any excision or debulking of a keloid must be combined with other modalities to prevent recurrence. Steroid (triamcinolone) injections and silicone sheets may be used for this purpose.
3. **Dyschromias**: Minimized with avoidance of direct sunlight.

4. **Depressed scars**: Minimized with proper eversion of the wound edges during initial tissue reapproximation. Fat atrophy may contribute to the depression of scar tissues. Various implants and aesthetic skin fillers have been used, including alloderm, collagen, fat, and hyaluronic acid.

Key Points

1. All wounds are considered contaminated and must be thoroughly and meticulously irrigated and debrided. Foreign bodies (dirt, glass, and asphalt) not debrided will lead to wound infection, wound dehiscence, and flap necrosis.
2. All complex soft tissue lacerations should be explored to rule out injury to underlying vital structures (neural, vascular, canalicular, and/or ductal injury) prior to closure.
3. The scalp is highly vascularized and can be associated with significant blood loss over a short period

of time (Figure 20.8). The scalp should be closed in a layered fashion to eliminate potential dead space (Figure 20.9).

4. Signs of lacrimal system dysfunction include persistent epiphora, conjunctivitis, and dacryocystitis. Lacrimal system damage is tested for by utilizing a dacryocystogram and a Jones I/Jones II test. The lacrimal drainage system can be repaired by establishing a new drainage system via a dacryocystorhinostomy. (See Figures 20.10 and 20.11.)
5. Avulsive injuries to the eyelids up to 25% can be closed primarily. Avulsive injuries to the eyelids of 25% or greater are repaired with tissue grafts (postauricular tissue) or local flaps.
6. An intranasal examination is performed in order to identify septal hematoma formation or avulsion with exposure of the underlying cartilage. Nasal hematomas present as reddish-bluish elevations of the nasal septal soft tissue and should be drained immediately with an incision parallel to the nasal floor. Packings, Doyle

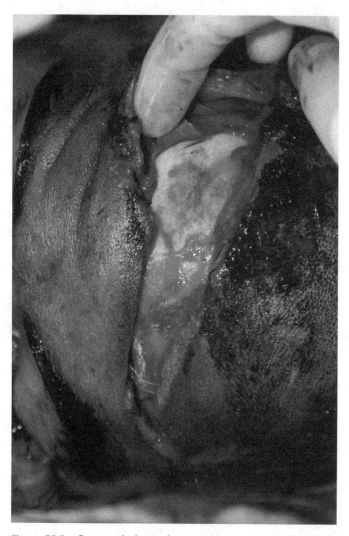

Figure 20.8. Deep scalp lacerations can be associated with significant blood loss.

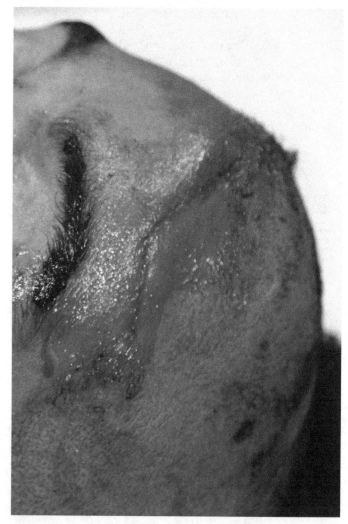

Figure 20.9. Scalp laceration closed primarily after establishing hemostasis and gross debridement.

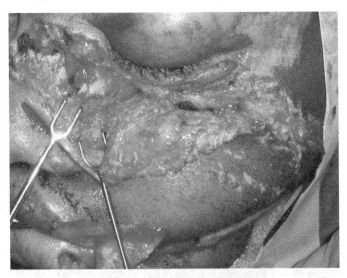

Figure 20.10.   Nasal and periorbital lacerations are evaluated for lacrimal system damage.

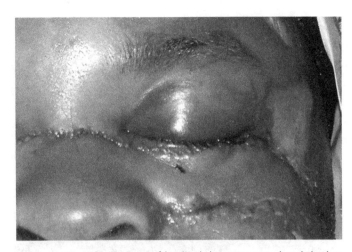

Figure 20.11.   The patency of lacrimal duct was tested and the lacerations were closed in a layered fashion.

splints, or mattress sutures may be used after drainage to prevent the reformation of the hematoma.

7. All ear lacerations should have a complete otoscopic examination to evaluate the tympanic membranes (rupture and hematotympanum), lacerations involving the external auditory canal, and foreign bodies. External ear hematomas should be drained, and a pressure dressing placed. The ear has a tremendous vascular supply and can remain perfused with a small pedicle. Small areas of exposed cartilage are managed with antibiotic impregnated dressings. Large areas of exposed cartilage are managed with skin grafts.

8. The reestablishment of the vermillion border is the key step in repairing lip lacerations (see Figure 20.6, Case Report 20.1; Figures 20.12 and 20.13; and 20.18, Case Report 20.3). The closure of full-thickness lip lacerations begins from the inside (mucosa) out (skin). Avulsive injuries to the lips of up to 25% can be primarily closed. Defects greater than 25% will require local flaps to minimize microstomia.

9. Neck wounds are divided into three zones. Unstable patients require urgent explorations with general anesthesia. Stable patients require CT angiogram and

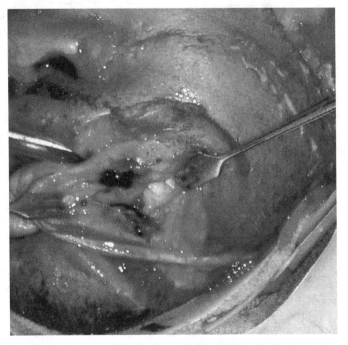

Figure 20.12.   Complex facial lacerations involving the left oral commissure and vermilion border.

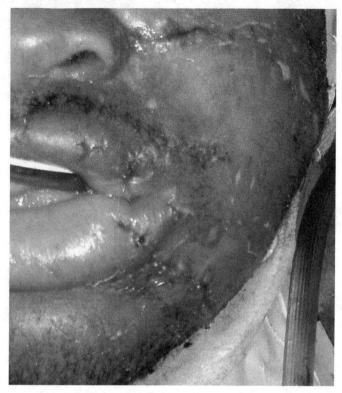

Figure 20.13.   The initial step in the closure of complex lip lacerations is the reapproximation of the vermillion border, followed by an inside-out closure with reapproximation of the orbicularis oris.

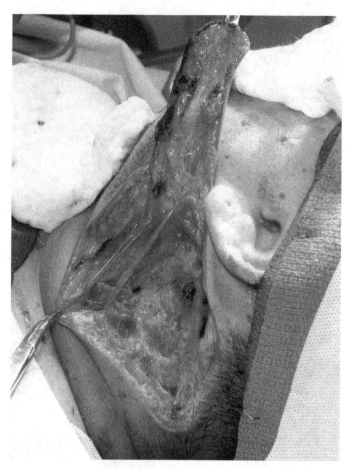

Figure 20.14.   Neck wounds in stable patients are explored, debrided, and closed after a computed tomography angiogram.

possible esophagography depending on the zone and depth of injury (Figure 20.14).

References

Janfaza, P., 2011. *Surgical anatomy of the head and neck.* Cambridge, MA: Harvard University Press.

Persing, J.A., 2007. *Soft tissue surgery of the craniofacial region.* London: Informa Health Care USA.

Facial Nerve Injury Repair

A means of repairing traumatic injuries (complete transection) of the facial nerve with direct anastomosis or interposition grafting.

Indications

1. Traumatic injuries of the facial nerve along its extratemporal course associated with facial weakness or paralysis
2. Traumatic neurotmetic (transaction) injuries of the facial nerve
3. Facial nerve injuries proximal to a vertical line dropped from the lateral canthus are amenable to surgical repair. Distal nerve injuries are typically not repairable due to extensive nerve arborization and adjacent nerve recruitment

Contraindications

1. Intratemporal nerve damage
2. Neuropraxic or axonotmetic facial nerve injuries, with temporary paresthesia
3. Injuries >1 year old (due to muscle atrophy)
4. Bell's palsy or viral-related facial nerve weakness

Anatomy

Following its exit from the stylomastoid foramen, the main trunk of the facial nerve may be localized in relation to the following landmarks:

1. Tragal pointer (the nerve is located 1.0 cm deep and slightly anterior and inferior to the tragal pointer)
2. Attachment of posterior digastric muscle (the nerve is located superior to the medial attachment of the posterior belly of the digastric muscle)
3. Tympanomastoid suture (the nerve is located 5–10 mm caudal to the anterior aspect of the tympanomastoid suture)
4. Styloid process (trunk begins posterior before coursing lateral to the styloid process).

After coursing in an anterior-superior direction for 14.0 mm on average, the pes anserinus gives rise to the five branches of the facial nerve (temporal, zygomatic, buccal, mandibular, and cervical).

Technique

1. Under general anesthesia, the patient is positioned in a supine position with the head turned to the contralateral side. The neck is slightly extended.
2. The patient is prepped and draped in normal sterile fashion.
3. For immediate repair, access is obtained through the existing laceration. In cases of delayed repair, a modified Blair incision is utilized that combines a pre-auricular incision with a submandibular lazy "S" extension for complete exposure. After developing a sub-SMAS (superficial musculoaponeurotioc system) skin flap anteriorly, the main trunk of the facial nerve is located using the landmarks discussed in this chapter.
4. The tragal pointer is identified through a subperichondral dissection along the medial aspect of the tragal cartilage. After anterior-inferior blunt dissection, the nerve will be found 1.0 cm deep to the tragal pointer.
5. Alternatively, the trunk may be approached inferiorly. Retraction of the sternocleidomastoid muscle exposes the posterior belly of the digastric muscle, which is followed toward the digastric groove. The trunk will be found within this location at the depth of this plane superiorly.
6. Mobilization of the superficial aspect of the parotid gland will allow identification of the facial nerve proximally along its terminal branches. Additionally, a superficial parotidectomy may alleviate tension applied to the facial nerve across larger gaps of traumatic discontinuity.
7. The wound is explored, and the proximal and distal facial nerve ends are identified (Figure 20.16, Case Report 20.3). Damage to the parotid gland or Stensen's duct should be identified because sialocele formation may compromise the facial nerve repair.
8. With the aid of microscopy and a colored background (Figures 20.16 and 20.17, Case Report 20.3), adhesions are removed and the proximal nerve is interrogated with electrical stimulation. If no response is elicited, a neurotomy is performed. The Victor–Meyer neurotomy instrument is used to remove the damaged or scarred regions until a normal appearance of the nerve ends and fascicular pattern is encountered.
9. An end-to-end anastomosis is performed if the gap of discontinuity is small enough to allow for a tension-free nerve repair (Figure 20.17, Case Report 20.3).

If significant tension is encountered, cable grafting (sural and greater auricular), jump grafts, crossover facial nerve grafting, allogeneic nerve grafts (AxoGen, Alachua, FL, USA), or nerve conduits (autogenous or alloplastic) may be considered.

10. The fascicular pattern of the facial nerve should be identified; epineurial suturing with nonresorbable sutures is sufficient in regions that have a monofascicular (one-fascicle) or oligofascicular (fewer than 10 fascicles) pattern.
11. Align and orient the nerve fascicles as best as possible (coaptation). If a fascicular or perineurial repair is chosen, the epineurium should be removed at the ends (~5.0 mm), and any protruding axons are trimmed.
12. With the epineurial repair, 8-0 nylon sutures are preferred. A tension-free repair is mandatory.
13. Confirm that the nerve fascicles remain properly oriented. This is easier in more proximal locations of the nerve where the diameter is greater. Begin with the placement of two sutures at 180° around the nerve periphery. Approximation is preferred over strangulation because overtightening of the sutures may result in twisting of the fascicles. Leave the initial suture ends long enough to allow manipulation of the nerve stumps during the remainder of the nerve repair.
14. The nerve is rotated to allow for suturing of the remainder of the epineurium. The number of sutures depends upon the diameter of the nerve; however, four sutures are typically sufficient.
15. The knots of the nonresorbable suture should be trimmed (1.0–2.0 mm).
16. The wound is closed in a layered fashion following wound irrigation.

Postoperative Management

1. An intensive postoperative regimen of aggressive physiotherapy with daily exercises is necessary to ensure proper motor reeducation.
2. Supportive eye care may be necessary (tear substitutes, lid taping, and gold weight placement).

Complications

1. **Synkinesis**: Defined as involuntary muscular movements occurring simultaneously with voluntary movements. Physiotherapy and biofeedback are started immediately. Botulinum toxin injections may be considered.
2. **Exposure eye keratopathy**: Treated with supportive eye care.
3. **Sialocele**: Treated with drainage and pressure dressings.

1. Facial nerve injuries medial (distal) to a vertical line dropped from the lateral canthus do not require repair.
2. Immediate repair should be performed whenever possible. If, after confirmation of complete nerve transaction, a delayed repair is planned, the identified nerve ends should be appropriately tagged with nonresorbable suture to facilitate identification later.
3. Electrophysiologic (EP) testing (electromyogram [EMG]) is used to determine the prognosis of recovery in instances where nerve transection has not been verified. Accurate results from EMG may not be useful until up to 10–21 days post injury when fibrillation potentials appear.

References

Blanchaert, R.H., 2001. Surgical management of facial nerve injuries. *Atlas of the Oral and Maxillofacial Surgery Clinics of North America*, 9, 43–58.

Coker, N.J., 1991. Management of traumatic injuries to the facial nerve. *Otolaryngologic Clinics of North America*, 24, 215–27.

Davis, R.E., 1995. Traumatic facial nerve injuries: review of diagnosis and treatment. *Journal of Cranio-Maxillofacial Trauma*, 1, 30–41.

Janfaza, P., 2011. *Surgical anatomy of the head and neck*. Cambridge, MA: Harvard University Press.

Pather, N., 2006. Landmarks of the facial nerve: implications for parotidectomy. *Surgical and Radiologic Anatomy*, 28, 170–75.

Rovak, J.M., 2004. Surgical management of facial nerve injury. *Seminars in Plastic Surgery*, 18, 23–29.

Case Report

Case Report 20.3. A 32-year-old male status post motor vehicle accident with extensive soft tissue injuries to the maxillofacial complex. On examination, evidence of a facial nerve deficit was identified via left facial muscle weakness. The patient was taken urgently to the operating room, and the through-and-through soft tissue injuries were explored under general anesthesia. The facial wounds were debrided, explored, and irrigated. The transected facial nerve branches were identified and repaired under magnification. At the completion of the neural anastomosis, the wounds were irrigated, and the complex soft tissue lacerations were closed in a layered fashion. (See Figures 20.15, 20.16, 20.17, and 20.18.)

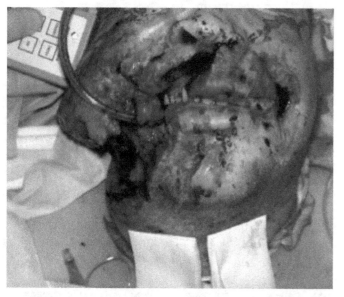

Figure 20.15.   Initial presentation demonstrating severe soft tissue injuries.

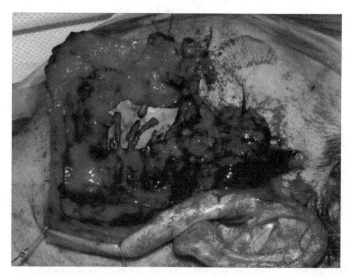

Figure 20.16.   Proximal and distal end of the severed facial nerve are identified. Colored backgrounds aid in visualization during the anastomosis procedures.

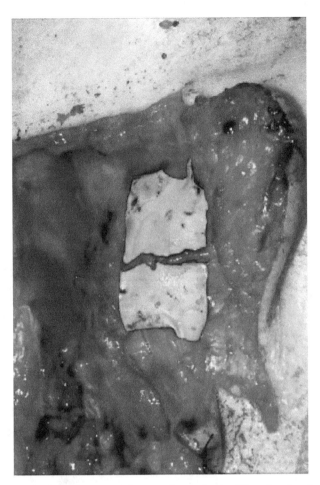

Figure 20.17.   The severed nerve is repaired with a tension-free anastomosis using microscopy.

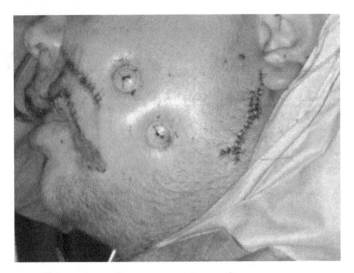

Figure 20.18.   Immediate postoperative result.

PART FOUR

ORTHOGNATHIC AND CRANIOFACIAL SURGERY

CHAPTER
21

Maxillary Surgery

Christopher Choi,[1] Brian B. Farrell,[2] and Myron R. Tucker[2]
[1]Inland Empire Oral and Maxillofacial Surgeons, Rancho Cucamonga, California, USA
[2]Private Practice, Carolinas Center for Oral and Facial Surgery, Charlotte, North Carolina, Department of Oral and Maxillofacial Surgery, Louisiana State University Health Science Center, New Orleans, Louisiana, USA

Le Fort 1 Osteotomy (Single Piece)

A means of repositioning an intact maxilla to correct congenital and acquired dentofacial deformities.

Indications

1. Correction of maxillary dentofacial deformities in all three planes of space
2. Access to pathologic lesions located within the maxillary sinus, nasal cavity, and/or skull base
3. Interpositional bone grafting for the atrophic, edentulous maxilla

Contraindications

1. Surgery performed prior to the complete eruption of the maxillary permanent dentition
2. Medical conditions prohibiting surgery

Surgical Anatomy

The vasculature supply of the maxilla is abundant and is supplied via the terminal branches of the maxillary (posterior superior alveolar, infraorbital, descending palatine, and sphenopalatine arteries), the ascending pharyngeal (branch of external carotid artery), and the ascending palatine (branch of facial artery) arteries via the soft palate.

The maxilla is composed of three vertical buttresses: the zygomaticomaxillary, nasomaxillary, and pterygomaxillary buttresses. The zygomaticomaxillary buttress laterally and the nasomaxillary buttress (piriform rim) medially form the periphery of the maxillary sinus and serve as areas for fixation after Le Fort procedures. The pterygoid plates comprise the pterygomaxillary buttress located just posterior to the maxilla.

The infraorbital nerve is the terminal branch of the second division (V2) of the trigeminal nerve. The infraorbital nerve supplies sensation to the lower eyelid, lateral aspect of nose, and upper lip and is encountered during subperiosteal elevation of the lateral wall of the maxilla.

Technique

1. The patient is placed supine on the operating room table and nasally intubated. The anesthesia tube is secured, all extremities are padded, and a urinary catheter is placed for procedures exceeding 150 minutes. Lacrilube is placed within the orbits, and opsites are placed to protect the periorbital regions during the procedure. A throat pack is placed within the posterior oropharynx, and the oral cavity is prepped with betadine solution and/or chlorhexidine gluconate 0.12% oral rinse and a toothbrush to include all teeth, the gingiva, the tongue, and the palate. The maxillofacial skeleton is prepped with betadine scrub from the hairline to the clavicles, and the patient is draped in a sterile fashion to allow for exposure of and access to the oral cavity, nasal bridge, and orbits.
2. Local anesthesia containing a vasoconstrictor is placed circumferentially within the maxillary vestibule. Additionally, the nasal floor, nasal septum, and inferior turbinates are injected to assist in hemostasis.
3. A Kirschner wire may be inserted within the nasofrontal suture (Figure 21.1 [all figures cited in this section appear in Case Report 21.1, unless otherwise noted]) to establish a vertical reference for the maxilla. A Boley gauge is utilized to measure from the Kirschner wire to an anterior maxillary reference point (the anterior maxillary orthodontic arch wire, the orthodontic brackets of teeth #8 and #9, or the incisive edges of teeth #8 and 9), and the measurement is recorded.
4. In select cases, enameloplasty is performed with a large diamond bur and copious irrigation on selected tooth surfaces that are determined preoperatively.
5. A maxillary vestibular incision is initiated through mucosa from the maxillary premolar to the midline (Figure 21.2). The incision is positioned 10 mm cephalic to the mucogingival junction and parallels the mucogingival junction. A mucosal releasing incision may be incorporated at the first molars to allow for increased flap elevation. The incision is extended through subcutaneous tissue, muscle, and periosteum.
6. A subperiosteal dissection exposes the lateral maxillary wall, the zygomaticomaxillary and nasomaxillary buttresses, and the piriform aperture (Figure 21.3). The identical incision and dissection is performed on the contralateral side.
7. Sharp, subperiosteal dissection is used to enter the nasal cavity and to elevate the nasal mucosa from

Atlas of Operative Oral and Maxillofacial Surgery, First Edition. Edited by Christopher J. Haggerty and Robert M. Laughlin
© 2015 John Wiley & Sons, Inc. Published 2015 by John Wiley & Sons, Inc.

the piriform aperture. A periosteal elevator is used to elevate the nasal mucosa from the lateral nasal walls and the nasal floor. Careful elevation and reflection of the nasal mucosa will minimize nasal mucosal tears during downfracture of the maxilla.

8. A retractor is placed posterior to the maxilla to expose the pterygomaxillary junction (the junction of the maxillary tuberosity and the pterygoid plates) and to reflect the overlying tissue. An elevator is placed along the lateral nasal wall of the nasal cavity within the submucosal plane to protect the nasal mucosa during the osteotomy (Figure 21.3). ·

9. A reciprocating saw is utilized to create a horizontal osteotomy from a point just posterior to the maxillary tuberosity to a point just superior to the nasal floor (Figure 21.4). The osteotomy is placed superior to the apices of the maxillary teeth. The osteotomy is mirrored on the opposite side.

10. A double guarded vomer osteotome is used to separate the nasal septum and vomer bone from the nasal crest of the maxilla (Figure 21.5).

11. A curved pterygoid osteotome is used to divide the pterygomaxillary junction. The osteotome is placed between the maxillary tuberosity and the pterygoid plates and is directed medially and inferiorly, away from the pterygoid plexus and internal maxillary artery (Figure 21.6). A finger can be placed on the palate at the hamular notch region to palpate the separation.

12. A single guarded osteotome is used to separate the lateral nasal wall (Figure 21.7). A change in sound is audible posteriorly as the thicker, perpendicular plate of the palatine bone is engaged. Partial sectioning of the palatine bone minimizes unfavorable fracture patterns during downfracture, which may cause disruption of the orbits and/or cranial base.

13. After the completion of all maxillary osteotomies, the downfracture of the maxilla is performed with digital pressure. Tessier mobilizers are placed posterior to the maxillary tuberosities (Figure 21.8) in order to distract the maxilla forward and laterally to complete the bony separation and to stretch the posterior soft tissue pedicle. The maxilla should be capable of mobilization of 1.5 cm in all directions.

14. The greater palatine arteries should be identified and preserved or ligated (surgeon's preference).

15. Interferences within the areas of the nasal crest of the maxilla, the lateral nasal wall, and the posterior and lateral aspects of the maxillary sinus are removed (Figure 21.9).

16. The anterior nasal spine may be reduced, especially in cases of maxillary advancement and superior repositioning.

17. The field is irrigated, and all debris is suctioned.

18. Inferior turbinectomies and inferior septoplasty are adjunctive procedures that may be indicated in cases of significant superior repositioning or when nasal obstruction is apparent. A vertical incision is made through the nasal mucosa overlying the inferior turbinates, and the inferior turbinates are identified. A Kelley or Allis clamp is used to grasp the inferior turbinate at its base, and electrocautery or heavy scissors are used to transect the turbinate. The nasal mucosa is closed using chromic gut sutures.

19. In cases of superior maxillary repositioning, the inferior portion of the cartilaginous nasal septum is resected to prevent septal deviation against the superiorly repositioned and fixated maxilla.

20. The patient is placed in maxillomandibular fixation (MMF) with the use of a surgical splint. The maxillomandibular complex is rotated into position, ensuring that the condyles are seated ideally within the glenoid fossa. Any interferences are removed to achieve even passive contacts and the appropriate preplanned vertical dimension of the maxilla. For surgery designed to alter the vertical dimension of the maxilla, the prerecorded measurements from the Kirschner wire are used to determine the amount of maxillary repositioning based on the presurgical workup.

21. Fixation is applied to the zygomaticomaxillary buttress and the nasomaxillary buttress (piriform rim) bilaterally (Figure 21.10; see also Figure 21.17, Case Report 21.2). Bone grafts may be placed within the osteotomy gaps for large advancements or inferior repositioning (Figure 21.11).

22. After the application of rigid fixation, the patient is removed from MMF to assess occlusion, mandibular movements, and overall facial symmetries. Any occlusal or midline discrepancies, jaw movement asymmetries, nasal deviations, or areas of excessive bleeding should be corrected with the release of fixation and ensuring the removal of all bony interferences, complete condylar seating, the correction of septal deviation and achieving tissue hemostasis.

23. An alar cinch suture is placed to minimize unaesthetic widening of the alar base.

24. Mucosal closure is initiated with a V–Y closure (Figure 21.12) to avoid thinning of the upper lip. A single-prong skin hook is used to form the vertical leg of the closure, and is closed with several passes of chromic gut in a running fashion. The vertical leg is connected to the gingiva and closure is completed in a continuous, horizontal mattress fashion with chromic sutures (Figure 21.13).

25. Prior to extubation, an orogastric tube is passed to empty contents of the stomach.

26. The patient is placed into guiding elastics to help guide the jaw into occlusion.

Postoperative Management

1. A pressure dressing and ice packs are utilized to minimize edema and hematoma formation.

2. Humidified oxygen and head-of-bed elevations are recommended for 24 hours.
3. A Yankauer suction is placed bedside for persistent intraoral secretions.
4. Scissors or wire cutters should be on the patient at all times if heavy maxillomandibular fixation is applied.
5. Antibiotics, analgesics, anti-emetics, and steroids are recommended.
6. The septum should be evaluated postoperatively to identify septal hematoma formation.
7. Nasal congestion may be treated with nasal suctioning, nasal rinses, and decongestants.
8. Epistaxis may be minimized with head-of-bed elevations, pressure dressings, oxymetazoline sprays, and posterior packings for severe cases.

Complications

1. **Deviated nasal septum**: Results from inadequate inferior septoplasty during superior maxillary positioning. Managed postoperatively with adjunctive septoplasty.
2. **Hardware failure**: Exposed hardware, hardware fracture, palpable fixation, and loose screws. Treatment involves hardware removal with or without replacement depending on the amount of bone union.
3. **Damage to apices of teeth**: The horizontal osteotomy should be placed at least 5 mm superior to the anticipated apices of the maxillary dentition.
4. **Malunion and non-union**: Inadequate fixation or failed fixation.
5. **Unfavorable aesthetic result**: From poor treatment planning or unrealistic patient expectations.
6. **Hemorrhage**: Common sources include the greater palatine artery and pterygoid plexus. Also consider atriovenous malformations and undiagnosed bleeding disorders.
7. **Infection**: Rare. Treated with antibiotics with or without drain placement and suspect hardware removal.

Key Points

1. The ascending pharyngeal and ascending palatine arteries maintain perfusion to the downfractured maxilla.
2. Impacted wisdom teeth may be removed at the time of Le Fort surgery. Care is taken to place the curved pterygoid osteotome posterior to the impacted teeth.
3. Posterior bony interferences may result in condylar displacement or distraction, asymmetrical jaw movements (deviations), malocclusion, and aberrant maxillary position.
4. Insufficient mobilization of the maxilla prior to fixation may hinder optimal advancements.
5. The zygomaticomaxillary and nasomaxillary buttresses contain thicker areas of bone and are ideal for securing fixation.

Reference

Perciaccante, V.J. and Bays, R.A., 2004. Maxillary orthognathic surgery. In: M. Miloro, ed. *Peterson's principles of oral and maxillofacial surgery*. 2nd ed. London: BC Decker. Pp. 1179–204.

Case Report

Case Report 21.1. Le Fort I osteotomy: single piece. This procedure is shown in Figures 21.1 through 21.13.

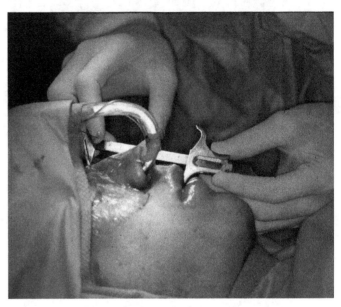

Figure 21.1. Patient prepped and draped. A midline vertical measurement is taken from a Kirschner wire placed within the nasofrontal suture to an anterior maxillary reference point (orthodontic brackets or incisal edges of the central incisors or the maxillary arch wire).

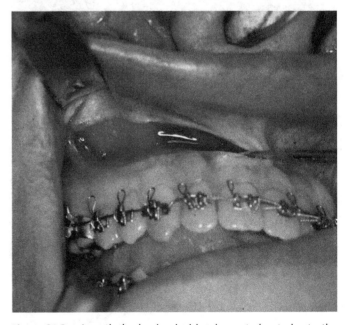

Figure 21.2. A vertical releasing incision is created anterior to the zygomaticomaxillary buttress in the area of the premolars and the incision is carried anteriorly to the midline.

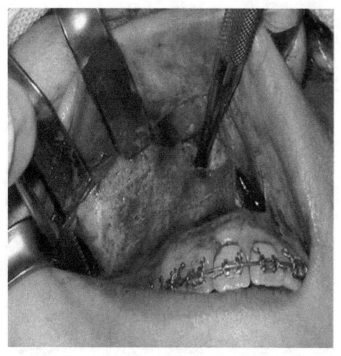

Figure 21.3. Subperiosteal elevation and exposure of the lateral wall of the maxilla. A subperiosteal pocket is made posteriorly to the pterygoid plates and along the lateral nasal wall. An elevator is placed to protect the nasal mucosa during the osteotomy.

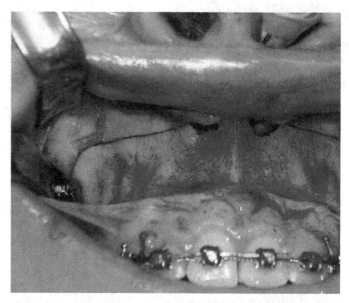

Figure 21.4. A reciprocating saw is used to create an osteotomy from the zygomaticomaxillary buttress to the lateral nasal wall at a point just superior to the nasal floor.

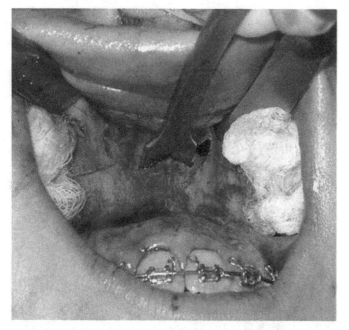

Figure 21.5. A vomer osteotome is used to separate the nasal septum and vomer from the nasal crest of the maxilla.

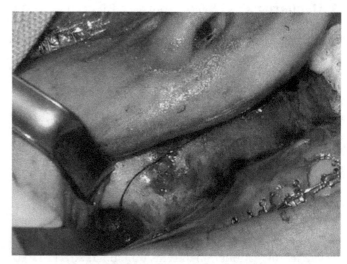

Figure 21.6. A curved pterygoid osteotome is directed medially and inferiorly to separate the pterygoid plates from the posterior maxilla.

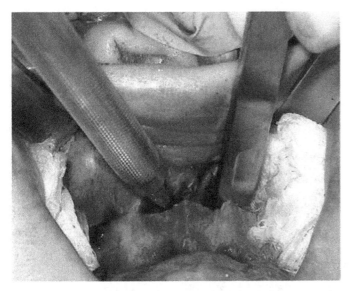

Figure 21.7. A single guarded osteotome is used to separate the lateral nasal walls. A #9 periosteal elevator is used to reflect nasal mucosa to visualize the lateral nasal walls.

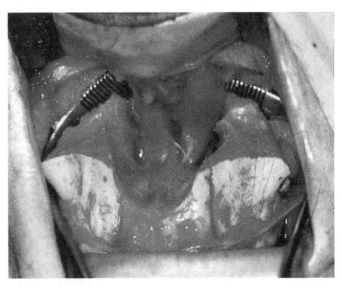

Figure 21.8. Downfracture of the maxilla followed by mobilization with Tessier mobilizers.

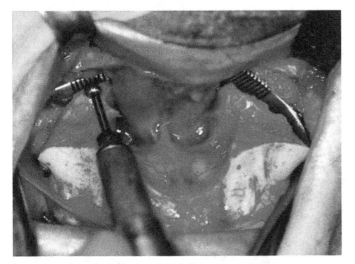

Figure 21.9. Bony interferences are removed with ronguers and/or rotary instruments.

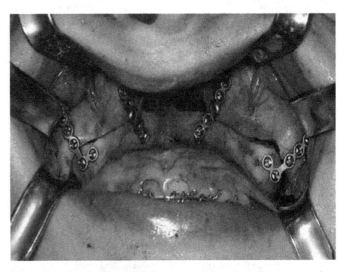

Figure 21.10. Fixation utilizing plates placed at the zygomatico-maxillary and nasomaxillary buttresses.

Figure 21.11. Alternatively, screw fixation can be utilized for telescoped segments of bone and for bone-grafting procedures during maxillary surgery.

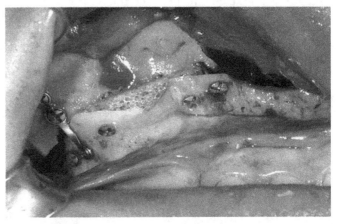

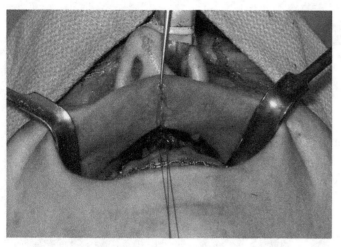

Figure 21.12.   A V–Y closure followed by approximation of the circumvestibular incision.

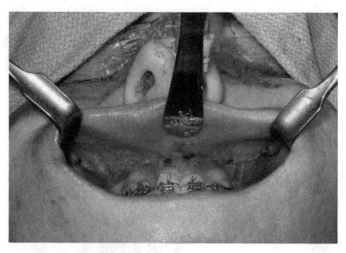

Figure 21.13.   The circumvestibular incision is closed with chromic sutures in a continuous, horizontal mattress fashion.

Segmental Maxillary Osteotomy (Two or Three Pieces)

A means of correcting maxillary transverse discrepancies (deficiency or excess) and/or multiple planes of occlusion.

Indications

1. The two-piece osteotomy corrects transverse discrepancies
2. The three-piece osteotomy corrects vertical and transverse discrepancies

Contraindication

1. Inadequate space for interdental osteotomies

Segmental Osteotomy Technique

1. Procedure follows LeFort I single-piece osteotomy steps 1 through 12.
2. The orthodontic arch wire is sectioned within the area of the proposed interdental osteotomies.

   a. For a two-piece maxilla, the interdental osteotomy can be made within the midline between the central incisors. If the transverse discrepancy is unilateral, the interdental osteotomy can be made between the first premolar and canine or between the canine and lateral incisor on the involved side.
   b. For a three-piece maxilla, the interdental osteotomies are made bilaterally between the first premolar and canine or between the canine and lateral incisor. Ideally, the canine should be kept within the anterior segment.

3. The interdental osteotomies are initiated prior to downfracture for better stability and control of the osteotomies (Figure 21.14 [all figures cited in this section appear in Case Report 21.2]). The gingiva is retracted inferiorly within the area of the interdental osteotomy to the level of the alveolar ridge in a subperiosteal plane. The prominences of teeth roots are visualized. Care is taken to fashion the osteotomy parallel to the tooth roots, perpendicular to the alveolar bone, and between the roots. A sagittal saw is used to initiate the interdental osteotomy. The osteotomy is taken through the palatal plate without penetrating the palatal mucosa. A finger may be placed on the palate to palpate for blade penetration through the palatal cortex. The osteotomy should extend from the horizontal Le Fort osteotomy inferiorly and interdentally.

4. After downfracture and mobilization of the maxilla, the vertical osteotomies are extended posteriorly within the palate utilizing a reciprocating saw (Figure 21.15). The palatal osteotomies are placed lateral to the midline due to the increased mucosal tissue thickness and minimal bone thickness of the parasagittal region. Care must be taken to ensure the palatal mucosa is not violated. The parasagittal osteotomies may be beveled in a tangential fashion so that if the palatal mucosa tears, there is bony overlap.

   a. For a two-piece maxilla, the parasagittal cut is connected to the interdental osteotomy based on the presurgical workup. The interdental osteotomy associated with a two-piece osteotomy is typically located lateral to the canine or within the dental midline.
   b. For a three-piece maxilla, the parasagittal cuts are connected to the interdental osteotomies based on the presurgical workup. A variety of palatal osteotomy designs are available depending on the amount of maxillary expansion and movement of the anterior segment. Interdental osteotomies are typically placed lateral to the canines; however, they may be placed lateral to the lateral incisors with caution.

5. After downfracture, the interdental osteotomies are completed with saws, burs, and/or thin chisels. Osteotomes may be used to separate the segments. All segments are manually mobilized in the horizontal and vertical dimensions to ensure appropriate separation. Interdental bony interferences are removed with small chisels and/or burs (Figure 21.16). The palate is visually inspected for tears.
6. The maxillary splint is wired to the maxillary dentition, and the individual segments are positioned within the splint. A wire can be passed through the molar bands to serve as a handle to assist in widening the maxilla. Interferences should be removed to allow for passive positioning of the segments within the surgical splint. A palatal strap or lingual flange should be incorporated into the splint to add rigidity.
7. Interpositional bone grafts may be placed within the osteotomy sites to aid in stability and provide a construct for new bone growth.
8. Refer to Le Fort 1 single-piece osteotomy from step 15 onward for the remainder of the procedure.

Postoperative Management

1. Guiding elastics are utilized to aid in the positioning of the mandibular dentition within the guide.
2. Maxillary splints should remain in place for 4–6 weeks to allow for complete osseous healing.
3. The removal of the splint needs to be coordinated with the treating orthodontist so that a transpalatal arch wire may be placed immediately after splint removal to minimize transverse relapse.

Segmental Osteotomy Complications

1. **Palatal tears**: Result from excessive expansion and/or mechanical perforation.
2. **Vascular insult and ischemia to maxillary gingiva**: May progress to avascular necrosis of the segment.
3. Fistula formation: Oroantral fistulas typically develop from the extraction of erupted or partially erupted third molars in conjunction with Le Fort I osteotomies. Oroantral and oronasal fistulas may also occur due to non-healing palatal tears.
4. Gingival recession and/or periodontal defects at the interdental osteotomy site.
5. Tooth damage or loss at the interdental osteotomy site.
6. Relapse in the transverse dimension.

Key Points

1. The transverse expansion of the maxilla should be limited to 10 mm or less at the second molars to prevent nonunion, relapse, and palatal tension necrosis.
2. Each individual maxillary segment must be completely free and mobile from adjacent segments to allow for passive seating within the surgical splint. Failure of

passive segment positioning within the surgical guide may result in the deformation of the surgical splint and occlusal discrepancies.

Reference

Perciaccante, V.J. and Bays, R.A., 2004. Maxillary orthognathic surgery. In: M. Miloro, ed. *Peterson's principles of oral and maxillofacial surgery*. 2nd ed. London: BC Decker. Pp. 1179–204.

Case Report

Case Report 21.2. Le Fort I osteotomy: segmental. (See Figures 21.14, 21.15, 21.16, and 21.17.)

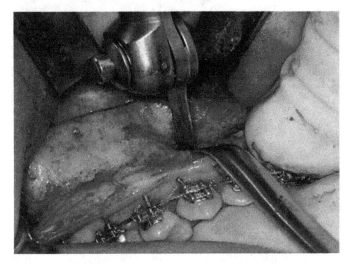

Figure 21.14.   The interdental osteotomies are initiated with a sagittal saw prior to the downfracture of the maxilla.

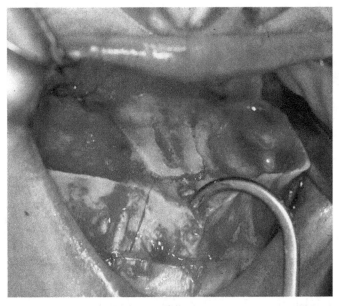

Figure 21.15.   A bone hook is used to inferiorly distract the maxilla, and all bony interferences are removed. A reciprocating saw is used to perform the parasagittal osteotomies within the maxilla.

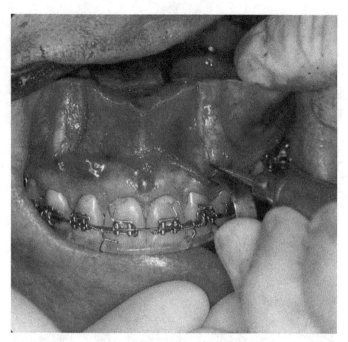

Figure 21.16. A 701 bur can be used to relieve interferences within the interdental osteotomy sites.

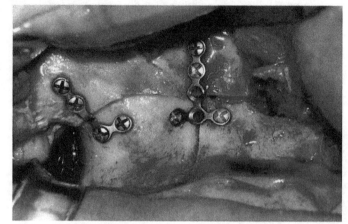

Figure 21.17. Bone plates may be positioned to span interdental osteotomy sites to add rigidity to the maxilla.

Surgically Assisted Rapid Palatal Expansion (SARPE)

A combined means of orthodontic-surgical expansion of the maxillary arch in cases of transverse maxillary deficiency in patients in whom the palatal suture is completely fused.

Indications

1. Maxillary transverse deficiency
   a. Stand-alone procedure for an isolated maxillary transverse deformity
   b. Preliminary procedure prior to definitive orthognathic surgery
2. Arch length and tooth mass discrepancy (crowding)
3. To expand the arch in cases of maxillary hypoplasia associated with clefts of the palate
4. To overcome the resistance of the midpalatal suture when orthodontic palatal expanders have failed
5. Skeletally mature patient: The age at which surgical intervention is required to assist with palatal expansion is controversial and ranges from 14 to 25 years

Contraindications

1. Noncompliant patient: The patient or guardian must activate the palatal device daily in the postoperative period
2. Patients with significant periodontal disease

3. Patients who have not reached skeletal maturity (prior to skelatal maturity, an orthodontic palatal expander is recommended)
4. Medical condition prohibiting surgical intervention

Anatomy

The hard palate consists of two palatal processes of the maxilla and two horizontal plates of the palatine bones that form the palatine sutures. The midpalatal suture extends from the incisive foramen to the posterior aspect of the palate. The midpalatal suture is perpendicular to the palatomaxillary suture, which joins the horizontal process of the palatine bones and the palatal process of the maxilla.

The midpalatal suture remains patent until late adolescence. The process of palatal fusion is characterized by progressive sutural interdigitation and ossification that is typically completed within the third decade of life.

Technique

1. Prior to the start of the case, verify that the palatal expander is in place and secure, and that the device key to activate the appliance is present (Figure 21.20 [all figures cited in this section appear in Case Report 21.3]).
2. This procedure follows Le Fort I single-piece osteotomy steps 1 through 12. The maxilla is *not* downfractured (Figures 21.21).
3. The osteotomies at the zygomaticomaxillary buttresses are relieved to allow for clearance during separation (Figure 21.22).

4. The gingiva is elevated in the area between the central incisors to expose the alveolus. A sagittal saw is used to make the midline osteotomy from the piriform rim to the alveolus (Figure 21.23). Chisels are used to complete the osteotomy along the midpalatal suture.
5. The palatal appliance is activated within the operating room to ensure equal separation of the two halves, and clearance at the zygomaticomaxillary buttresses is confirmed (Figure 21.24).
6. Refer to Le Fort 1 single-piece osteotomy from step 23 onward for the remainder of the procedure.

Postoperative Management

1. The palatal appliance is activated on postoperative day 3 by utilizing the distraction frequency as determined by the orthodontist.

Complications

1. **Intraoperative or immediate postoperative bleeding**: Arterial bleeding from the descending palatine arteries may be controlled by downfracturing the maxilla and ligating the vessel(s), or through interventional radiology.
2. **Failure to expand or unilateral expansion only postoperatively**: Reoperation is indicated.
3. Relapse: Minimized with the placement of a transpalatal bar following the removal of the palatal expansion device.
4. Oronasal fistula development.
5. Palatal tissue irritation from the appliance.
6. Appliance loosening or breakage.

Key Points

1. SARPE procedures are primarily for V-shaped arches where the anterior expansion required is greater than or equal to the posterior expansion.
2. The patient's models can be hand articulated to visualize the transverse discrepancy. An arch width analysis can be conducted between teeth across the arch and compared to the opposite arch. The buccal-lingual inclination of the teeth should also be taken into account. Orthodontics alone cannot mask a skeletal transverse discrepancy of greater than 5 mm.

3. A segmental Le Fort expansion greater than 7 mm is considered the upper limit of expansion. In cases where significant maxillary expansion is required, a SARPE procedure is considered more stable. Future maxillary segmental surgery may need to be performed based on skeletal growth, relapse, and dysgnathia; however, the movements will be more stable after SARPE expansion.
4. Radiographs of the central incisors should be taken to ensure sufficient room for interdental osteotomy.
5. All osteotomies completed during a Le Fort I osteotomy are completed for the SARPE procedure; however, the maxilla is not downfractured. Separation of pterygoid plates is based on the surgeon's preference and the amount of posterior expansion required.
6. The area of the greatest resistance to maxillary expansion is the zygomaticomaxillary buttresses. The palatal appliance should be activated within the operating room to ensure symmetrical bilateral expansion of the maxilla with no interferences.
7. Transverse maxillary expansion is the most unstable maxillary movement. Overcorrection is recommended to allow for relapse.
8. A tooth-borne (Haas and Hyrax appliance) or bone-borne palatal appliance can be used. The tooth-borne appliances are less invasive and hygienic, and thus allow for better patient compliance. Tooth-borne appliances also create an occlusal tipping effect at the level of the alveolar bone and teeth. This tipping effect can be minimized with tooth-borne appliances that engage at least three posterior teeth. A bone-borne appliance has more control over orthopedic (versus teeth) movements at the level of the palate, but it is more invasive and requires a steep palatal vault for anchorage.

References

Spalding, P.M., 2004. Craniofacial growth and development: current understanding and clinical considerations. In: M. Miloro, ed. *Peterson's principles of oral and maxillofacial surgery.* 2nd ed. London: BC Decker. Pp. 1051–86.

Suri, L. and Taneja, P., 2008. Surgically assisted rapid palatal expansion: a literature review. *American Journal of Orthodontics and Dentofacial Orthopedics*, 133, 290–302.

Case Report

Case Report 21.3. A surgically assisted rapid palatal expansion (SARPE) procedure is shown in Figures 21.18 through 21.28.

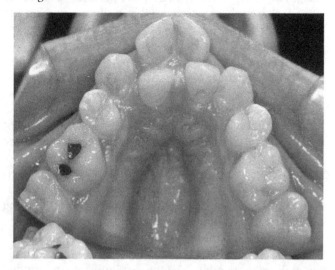

Figure 21.18. Occlusal view of a patient with a V-shaped arch, inadequate arch space, severe anterior crowding, and transverse discrepancy.

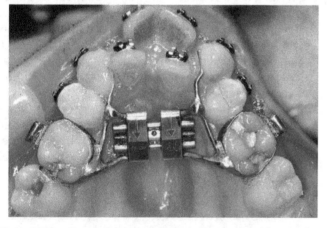

Figure 21.20. Hyrax palatal expander and orthodontic brackets in place.

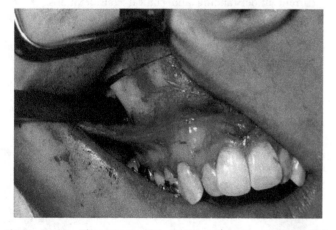

Figure 21.22. The osteotomies at the zygomaticomaxillary buttresses are relieved to allow for clearance during separation.

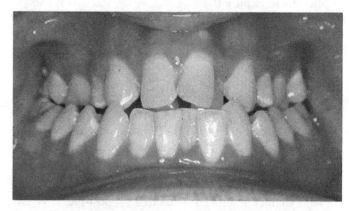

Figure 21.19. Anterior-posterior view of the patient in Figure 21.18 demonstrating significant maxillary transverse discrepancy.

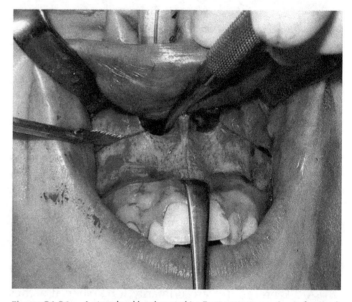

Figure 21.21. A standard horizontal Le Fort osteotomy is performed.

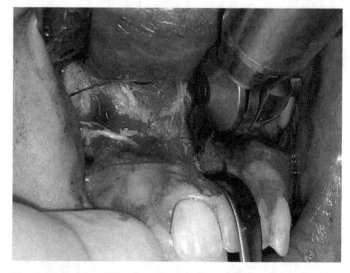

Figure 21.23. A midline interdental osteotomy is performed with a sagittal saw.

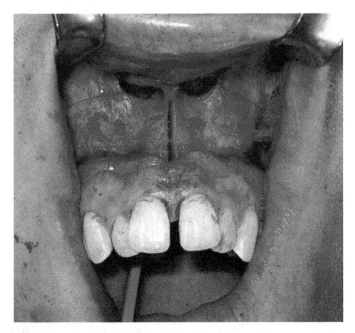

Figure 21.24.   The palatal expander is activated to ensure passive symmetrical separation of segments.

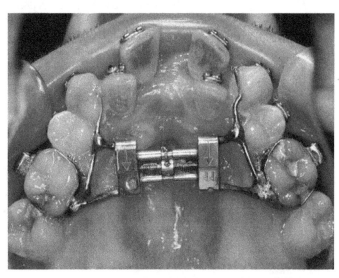

Figure 21.25.   Post-expansion occlusal view demonstrating midline diastema.

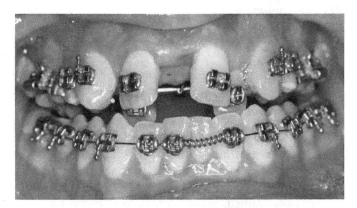

Figure 21.26.   Post-expansion anterior-posterior view demonstrating overcorrection of maxillary transverse discrepancy.

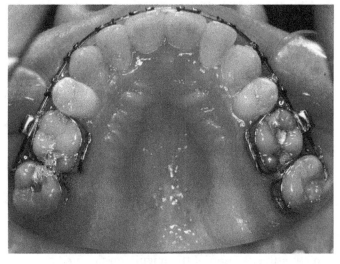

Figure 21.27.   Occlusal view demonstrating a U-shaped arch form with resolution of transverse discrepancy.

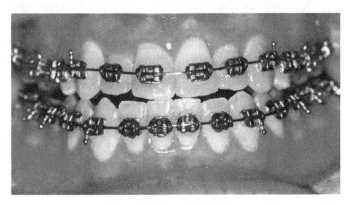

Figure 21.28.   Anterior-posterior view demonstrating correction of a transverse maxillary discrepancy with anterior open bite. The patient will require future mandibular surgery.

22 Mandibular Osteotomies

Brian B. Farrell and Myron R. Tucker

Private Practice, Carolinas Center for Oral and Facial Surgery, Charlotte, North Carolina, USA; and Department of Oral and Maxillofacial Surgery, Louisiana State University Health Science Center, New Orleans, Louisiana, USA

Sagittal Ramus Osteotomy (Bilateral Sagittal Split Osteotomy)

A means of surgically repositioning the lower jaw through mandibular osteotomies.

Indications

1. The correction of congenital dentofacial deformities, including mandibular deficiency, hyperplasia, asymmetry, and dysgnathia
2. The correction of acquired dentofacial deformities resulting from facial trauma, tumor ablative surgery, and temporomandibular joint asymmetries and deformities

Contraindications

1. Distorted ramus anatomy (thin or abnormal shape)
2. Excessive counterclockwise rotation (greater than 2 cm apertognathia requires two-jaw surgery)
3. Mandibular advancements greater than 12 mm
4. Neurosensory concerns
5. Previous head and neck radiation

Anatomy

Retrolingual depression: A depression located on the lingual aspect of the mandible between the lingula and the posterior border of the mandible.

Lingula: Entrance of the neurovascular bundle into the mandibular canal. The sagittal ramus osteotomy is initiated superior to the lingula.

Antelingula: Prominence along the lateral ramus predicting the position of the lingula on the medial aspect of the ramus.

Inferior alveolar nerve: Neurovascular bundle which enters the mandibular canal adjacent to the lingual, and exits the mandible anteriorly at the mental foramen.

Sagittal Ramus Osteotomy

Technique

1. The patient is nasally intubated, and the tube is secured. A throat pack is positioned at the level of the hypopharynx.
2. Local anesthetic containing a vasoconstrictor is injected along the external oblique ridge, retromolar trigone, and posterior buccal vestibule.
3. The patient is prepped and draped in the standard sterile fashion to include the oral cavity and maxillofacial skeleton.
4. Preplanned enameloplasty is performed, and a posterior bite block is placed.
5. A #15 blade is used to initiate an incision through mucosa only, positioned 2–3 cm lateral to the external oblique ridge (Figure 22.5, Case Report 22.1). The soft tissue is reflected medial over the external oblique ridge exposing the underlying muscle (Figure 22.6, Case Report 22.1). A sharp dissection proceeds to the lateral ramus transecting muscle and periosteum.
6. A periosteal elevator is used to dissect within a subperiosteal plane to expose the lateral mandible anteriorly to the Dalpont prominence adjacent to the molars. The dissection continues posteriorly to expose the external oblique ridge and the superior portion of the ascending ramus. A sigmoid notch retractor is positioned to elevate and retract the temporalis attachment from the ascending ramus. Subperiosteal dissection continues on the medial surface of the mandible, creating a subperiosteal pocket superior to the lingula. The inferior alveolar neurovascular bundle is identified. Identification can be accomplished by direct visualization or by palpation of the lingula with a nerve probe.
7. A Seldin retractor is placed within the lingual subperiosteal pocket and rotated 45° to protect the inferior alveolar neurovascular bundle and to create a space for the insertion of the reciprocating saw (Figure 22.7, Case Report 22.1).
8. A reciprocating saw initiates the horizontal osteotomy of the medial cortex at a 45° angle (the cut may be more vertical if the ramus is thin) (Figure 22.8, Case Report 22.1). The tip of the saw should extend into the retrolingular depression with the blade at full depth to score the osteotomy superior to the neurovascular bundle (Figure 22.1; see also Figure 22.2).

Atlas of Operative Oral and Maxillofacial Surgery, First Edition. Edited by Christopher J. Haggerty and Robert M. Laughlin.

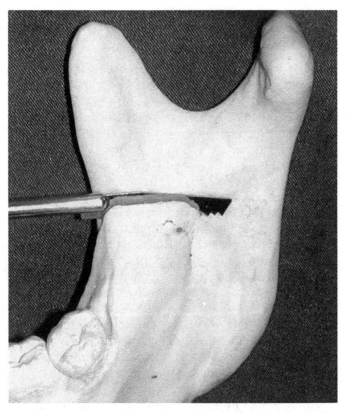

Figure 22.1. The Hunsuck modification involves splitting the mandible anterior to the posterior border by placing the reciprocating saw within the retrolingual depression superior to the insertion of the inferior alveolar nerve and lingula.

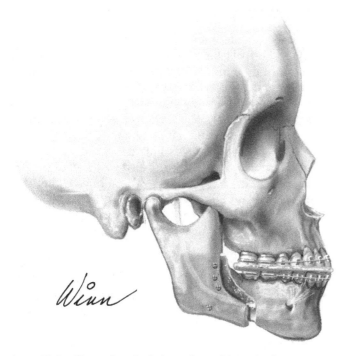

Figure 22.2. Illustration depicting a favorable sagittal ramus osteotomy split (Hunsuck modification), mandibular advancement, and fixation with positional screws.

9. The osteotomy is extended anteriorly through the cortical bone medial to the external oblique ridge and lateral to the dentition. The osteotomy is extended to the bony prominence located along the buccal aspect of the molar region (Dalpont prominence) (Figure 22.9, Case Report 22.1).

10. The bite block is removed. A channel retractor is placed along the inferior border of the mandible along the anterior aspect of the Dalpont prominence. The channel retractor is rotated 45° to expose the inferior border of the mandible, allowing for the insertion of the reciprocating saw.

11. The vertical osteotomy is initiated at the anterior aspect of the Dalpont prominence at the inferior border and transects both the buccal and lingual cortical plates inferior to the mandibular canal. The osteotomy continues vertically as a tangential cut through the lateral cortex only to connect the osteotomy along the external oblique ridge (Figure 22.10, Case Report 22.1).

12. The bite block is returned to stabilize the mandible during the separation of the mandible into proximal and distal segments. During separation (splitting) of the sagittal ramus osteotomy, the osteotomy should be visualized along its entire length to ensure equal separation throughout.

13. Osteotomes are used to facilitate the initial separation of the osteotomy (Figure 22.11, Case Report 22.1). Care is taken to avoid using the osteotomes as a fulcrum posterior to the dentition to prevent the development of a lingual plate fracture within the distal segment.

14. After initial separation, larger osteotomes or spreaders are used within the osteotomy to provide equal separation and to complete the split. Care is taken to ensure that the inferior border is associated with the proximal segment (Figure 22.12, Case Report 22.1). The inferior border of the mandible provides structural integrity to the proximal segment, aiding in avoiding unfavorable fractures.

15. The neurovascular bundle is identified early to ensure proper positioning and to avoid further iatrogenic injury with instrumentation between the osteotomy.

16. The nerve typically will course within the distal segment and require minimal manipulation (Figure 22.13, Case Report 22.1). Occasionally, the nerve will remain encased within the mandibular canal in the proximal segment and requires release by removal of the overlying bone. Elevators and/or osteotomes may be used to free the nerve and allow positioning within the confines of the distal segment.

17. The muscular and tendinous attachments of the medial pterygoid muscle are released with a J stripper

from the inferior and medial aspect of the distal segment to ensure passive repositioning of the mandible. Mandibular setback surgery will require release of soft tissue from the medial aspect of the proximal segment to create a pocket for the repositioned distal segment.

18. Maxillomandibular fixation (MMF) is established using the prefabricated occlusal splint with 24- or 26-gauge stainless steel wires.

19. Passive positioning of the proximal and distal segments is confirmed. Bony interferences are removed with saws, burs, and rasps to improve bone contact (Figure 22.14, Case Report 22.1).

20. The inferior borders of the mandible are aligned, and the condyles are seated with firm pressure in a posterior-superior vector.

21. Fixation can be applied using percutaneous (Figure 22.15, Case Report 22.1) or transoral access. Trocar positioning is determined by passing a local anesthetic needle through the skin followed by a stab incision with a #15 blade. The trocar allows placement of rigid internal fixation perpendicular to the cortex.

22. Fixation options include positional screws placed in a line at the superior border (Figure 22.15, Case Report 22.1, and Figure 22.24, Case Report 22.2) or in an inverted L pattern (Figure 22.2). Stability of the osteotomy is improved with spacing of the positional screws over the span of the osteotomy. Plates with monocortical fixation may be placed on the lateral border of the mandible. A combination of bicortical positional screw(s) and plates may be used if there is inadequate bone available in the distal segment for isolated screw fixation (concomitant third molar removal) (Figure 22.21, Case Report 22.2) or in cases of long advancements with limited bony overlap (Figure 22.16, Case Report 22.1).

23. At the completion of fixation, MMF is released and the occlusion is verified. Deviation of the occlusion to one side may indicate failure to seat the condyle and requires removal of fixation on the affected side with repositioning of the proximal segment.

24. The trocar incision is closed with a single interrupted suture. The intraoral incisions are closed with resorbable sutures (Figure 22.17, Case Report 22.1).

25. The throat pack is removed, and the surgical splint is removed. Guiding elastics may be utilized to facilitate neuromuscular guidance and reprogramming. A pressure dressing is applied to aid in control of postoperative edema.

Intraoral Vertical Ramus Osteotomy (IVRO)

Technique

1. An incision is placed through mucosa positioned lateral to the external oblique ridge similar to that performed for a sagittal ramus osteotomy. The incision length is ample enough to allow appropriate access (4–5 cm) to the ramus.

2. A subperiosteal dissection is performed to expose the lateral aspect of the mandible. The elevator is carried over the lingual aspect of the mandible immediately posterior to the dentition to ensure adequate soft tissue reflection to prevent tears when the notch retractor is used to strip the temporalis tendon from the ascending ramus. The dissection should expose the entire ramus from the posterior border to the anterior border and from the sigmoid notch superiorly to the antegonial notch inferiorly (Figure 22.27, Case Report 22.3).

3. A channel retractor is placed into the sigmoid notch on the medial aspect of the mandible. A reciprocating saw is used to separate the coronoid process to improve visibility and eliminate the pull of the temporalis muscle. The coronoid can be removed completely through reflection of the tendinous attachment.

4. The lateral aspect of the mandible is exposed with the placement of Bauer retractors into the sigmoid and antegonial notches, respectively. Additional retraction is accomplished with a large right-angle toe-out retractor positioned at the posterior border (a LeVasseur retractor is also frequently used). The soft tissue dissection and osteotomy of the coronoid are performed with the use of a bite block. The mouth is closed during the creation of the vertical ramus osteotomy for accessibility to the posterior border.

5. The orientation of the vertical ramus osteotomy is established by paralleling the posterior border of the mandible utilizing an oscillating saw (105°). The orientation of the osteotomy is important to avoid carrying the osteotomy into the condylar neck or off of the posterior border. The osteotomy is positioned posterior to the lingula and entrance of the inferior alveolar nerve into the mandibular canal, and typically establishes a proximal segment measuring 8–10 mm from the posterior border.

6. Rotation of the oscillating saw creates the initial osteotomy mid-ramus. With orientation of the osteotomy confirmed, the oscillating saw is "walked" superiorly into the sigmoid notch cutting on the outstroke as the shaft is positioned against the ramus (Figure 22.28, Case Report 22.3). The saw is then returned to the

mid-ramus area and redirected inferior into the antegonial notch in a similar fashion.

7. After the vertical ramus osteotomy is completed, the proximal segment is stabilized with a kochar clamp while the muscular and periosteal attachment from the inferior medial aspect of the segment is released. The soft tissue release establishes a pocket for telescoping of the posteriorly repositioned distal segment.

8. Maxillomandibular fixation is established utilizing the prefabricated occlusal splint and ensuring that the proximal segment remains lateral to the distal segment (Figure 22.29, Case Report 22.3). Failure to do so may result in loss of the proximal segment medially, requiring a release of MMF to locate and lateralize the proximal segment.

9. The proximal segment is adapted to passively and evenly contact the distal segment. Bony interferences (usually superior toward the sigmoid notch) are reduced with a recontouring bur or rasp from either segment to ensure passive overlap. Seating of the condyle is subtle (contrary to firm seating with class II corrections).

10. Application of rigid internal fixation requires percutaneous access via trocar placement. Stabilization of the vertical ramus osteotomy is generally performed via three positional screws oriented in a vertical fashion (Figure 22.3; and see 22.30, Case Report 22.3).

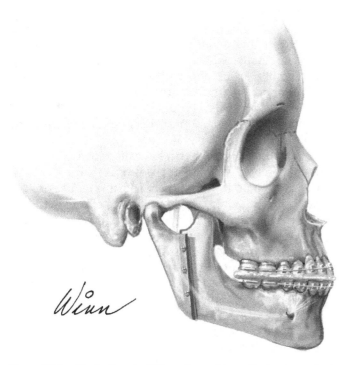

Figure 22.3.   Illustration depicting a favorable vertical ramus osteotomy split, mandibular setback, and fixation with vertically oriented positional screws.

Surgeons may elect to complete a period of maxillomandibular fixation with or without wire osteosynthesis stabilizing the segments should rigid fixation not be utilized.

11. The inferior portion of the proximal segment may be reduced if excessive lateral or inferior projection is noted as creating a palpable bony elevation externally. The intraoral and percutaneous wounds are closed in a similar fashion to the sagittal ramus osteotomy noted in this chapter.

Technique

1. Access to the ramus may be achieved through either a transoral or a transcutaneous submandibular-risdon approach. With extra oral approaches, the avoidance of paralytics should be reviewed with the anesthesia team preoperatively to allow for testing of the facial nerve (CN VII) during soft tissue dissection with a nerve stimulator.

2. Sharp and blunt dissection of the tissue layers is completed to the angle of the mandible. The subperiosteal dissection of the ramus is completed superiorly from the angle of the mandible to expose the sigmoid notch between the base of the coronoid process and condylar neck.

3. The planned bony osteotomy (vertical ramus osteotomy, inverted L osteotomy or C osteotomy) is completed under direct visualization once the soft tissues have been adequately reflected from the surgical field. After separation of the mandible into proximal and distal segments, the prefabricated occlusal splint is used to place the patient into MMF and the mandible is repositioned based on the presurgical plan. The proximal and distal segments are rigidly fixated utilizing positional screws and/or plates.

4. Closure of the wound is completed in a layered fashion with special care to ensure that the marginal mandibular nerve is not impinged or damaged. The skin may be closed with a nonresorbable or resorbable suture.

Note: Correction of severe mandibular deficiency with a large counterclockwise movement requires bone grafting within the osteotomy to ensure maintenance of continuity and bone union.

1. Nonsteroidal anti-inflammatory drugs, antibiotics and analgesics are prescribed. Liquid medications are prescribed for patients in MMF.

2. Meticulous oral hygiene is reinforced.

3. Oral or intravenous steroids may be used to lessen postoperative edema.
4. Ice is applied for the first 24–48 hours. Warm moist heat with gentle massage may be applied after the initial 48 hours.
5. Facial pressure dressings may be removed at 48 hours if applicable.
6. Nausea and vomiting are minimized with the use of an in-and-out orogastric tube placement at the conclusion of the procedure prior to extubation. Prophylactic anti-emetics are recommended (transdermal or rectal for patients in MMF) during the immediate postoperative period.
7. Adequate oral intake is necessary to maintain hydration. Initial intake is generally in the form of clear liquids with a conversion to a soft nonchew diet over the first week. The consistency of the diet increases gradually over the following weeks as discomfort and edema subside and as range of motion and activity return.
8. Guiding elastics are applied early in the postoperative period to facilitate neuromuscular reprogramming. The pattern frequently follows the skeletal correction; class II vector (upper 2s to lower 3s) after mandibular advancement for hypoplasia or class III pull (upper 3s to lower 2s) following maxillary advancement or mandibular setback for a class III skeletal discrepancy. The elastics are worn routinely over the first week with removal for isolated intervals for intake and hygiene.

Complications

Intraoperative Complications

1. **Transection of the inferior alveolar nerve**: May occur during the vertical anterior (inferior border) osteotomy or during the osteotomy of the lateral cortex. The exposure of the transected distal stump may require the creation of a buccal window within the mandible to allow reapproximation. A tension-free reapproximation is performed utilizing 2–3 epineural sutures.
2. **Injury to the lingual nerve or chordae tympani**: May be injured with excessive tissue manipulation, overpenetration of positional screws, and/or damage from the reciprocating saw during the osteotomy.
3. **Bleeding**: Excessive intraoperative bleeding with mandibular surgery is not common with proper surgical technique. Vascular injuries may result from aggressive retraction and/or disruption of the periosteum along the lingual surface of the mandible. Instrument misdirection within the osteotomy may injure the neurovascular bundle. The internal maxillary or masseteric

artery may be encountered with osteotomies extending into the sigmoid notch (IVRO). The facial artery may be injured with overextension of instrumentation at the inferior aspect of the vertical ramus osteotomy. Management of intraoperative bleeding includes hypotensive anesthesia, gauze packing, electrocautery, vasoconstrictor injection, and resorbable hemostatic agents.
4. **Unfavorable fractures**: Occur due to incomplete osteotomies, the presence of third molars, excessive force during separation of osteotomies, and patients with little or no marrow space. The goals for management of unfavorable fractures include completing the osteotomy so that segments can be adequately repositioned, reestablishing continuity of the fractured segments (consolidating the pieces), repositioning the mandible based on the presurgical plan, providing adequate fixation of the segments to prevent movement at the osteotomy, and ensuring bony continuity between segments to allow union.
5. **Damage to the facial nerve**: Traditionally, this is seen with transcutaneous approaches, but it may occur as a result of damage or penetration to the periosteum during intraoral procedures.

Postoperative Complications

1. **Infection**: The incidence of an infection after a mandibular osteotomy is low (2–7%) and typically occurs within the first month after surgery. Superficial infections are managed with incision and drainage through the vestibular incision with evacuation of the collection (hematoma/purulence) and antibiotic coverage. Late infections may be the result of loose hardware and require exploration of the surgical site with possible screw/plate removal.
2. **Malocclusion**: Subtle occlusal discrepancies are frequently noted early in the postoperative period secondary to muscle influence and posturing. The occlusal deviation is addressed with guidance elastics and continued neuromuscular reprogramming. Deviation of the mandibular midline creating asymmetry may be the result of improper proximal segment positioning via torqueing of the condyle or condylar sag. Minor discrepancies are addressed with early and aggressive orthodontic therapy. Pronounced deviation may require revision surgery to provide improved positioning of the segments.
3. **Fixation failure or nonunion**: Signs of fixation failure include palpable mobility of the segments, persistent infection, an open bite tendency, a class III occlusion on the affected side, a midline shift toward the opposite side, and premature contact on the affected side. Early surgical management may be required to

reinforce the fixation and stabilize the osteotomy. A delayed return to the operating room to address a non-union is more complicated, and management is similar to that for a non-union after traumatic mandibular fracture.

Key Points

1. The sagittal ramus osteotomy is the preferred surgical technique to address mandibular hyperplasia when the pattern of ramus divergence is U shaped. The anatomic consideration for mandibular setback can be best determined on plain films through a submental vertex or 3D imaging (cone beam computed tomography). Completion of a sagittal ramus osteotomy on a divergent V-shaped mandible will create a bony gap within the osteotomy between the proximal and distal segments upon repositioning. An appreciation of this anatomic relationship will prevent the overtightening of fixation that may torque the condyle and create medial displacement of the condyle.
2. A divergent ramus pattern (V shaped) is frequently best managed with an intraoral (IVRO) or transoral (TOVRO) vertical ramus osteotomy. The completion of the osteotomy will create telescoping of the divergent mandible upon setback. Performing a vertical ramus osteotomy on a parallel U-shaped mandible will create bony interferences that will require aggressive recontouring to prevent lateral displacement of the proximal segment to accommodate the distal segment movement posterior.
3. The completion of the sagittal ramus osteotomy into the retrolingual depression is vital for mandibular setback procedures. The Hunsuck modification (Figure 22.1) allows the distal segment to move posteriorly without impingement on the pterygomasseteric sling, maximizing the skeletal stability of the movement.
4. Lingual segment fractures may be associated with the simultaneous removal of third molars during the mandibular osteotomy or excessive instrumentation of the osteotomy posterior to the dentition. The early removal of wisdom teeth (9 to 12 months prior to osteotomy) to allow sufficient healing of the site and careful separation of the superior portion of the osteotomy will decrease the chance of a lingual segment fracture.
5. The osteotomy through the inferior border is the most technique-sensitive aspect of the sagittal ramus osteotomy. Maintaining the inferior border of the mandible's association with the proximal segment provides structural integrity that aids in the avoidance of unfavorable fracture.
6. Complications that arise intraoperatively are typically a result of deviation from the standard techniques of osteotomy completion, separation, or fixation.

7. Mandibular setback surgery positions the superior border of the distal mandible posterior and inferior to that of the proximal segment when the inferior borders are aligned. The proximal segment on mandibular setback procedures using a sagittal ramus osteotomy requires recontouring of the anterior and superior aspect (Figures 22.22, 22.23, and 22.24, Case Report 22.2) for visibility, to avoid periodontal issues, and to prevent over-rotation of the segment. If not sufficiently reduced, the prominence of the proximal segment will elevate the soft tissues, creating irritation and challenges with hygiene that lead to periodontal issues. The improper alignment of the superior borders results in the over-rotation of the proximal segment with violation of the pterygomasseteric sling, leading to concerns regarding stability.
8. In osteotomies completed in young patients with "green stick" mandibles (low modulus of elasticity), the angle and posterior border frequently will remain intact, requiring additional efforts to complete the separation into proximal and distal segments. The identification of the inferior alveolar nerve within the osteotomy will allow for positioning of an osteotome or saw to redirect the osteotomy medial into the retrolingual depression and prevent the development of a proximal segment fracture should it extend laterally.

Case Reports

Case Report 22.1. Sagittal Ramus Osteotomy: Mandibular Advancement. A 28-year-old female with class II deep bite malocclusion as a result of mandibular hypoplasia. (See Figures 22.4 through 22.19.)

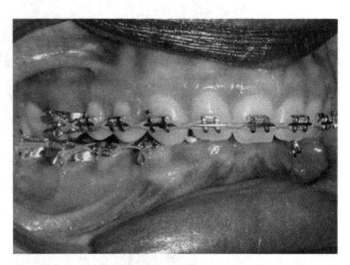

Figure 22.4. Preoperative image depicting a class II deep bite malocclusion and mandibular retrognathia.

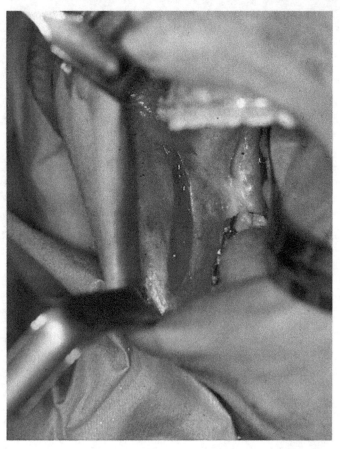

Figure 22.5.   Incision initiated through mucosa only positioned 2–3 cm lateral to the external oblique ridge.

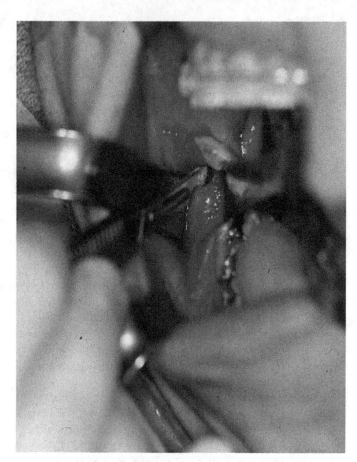

Figure 22.6.   The soft tissue is reflected medially over the external oblique ridge exposing the underlying muscle. A #15 blade is used to transect the overlying muscle and periosteum to expose the lateral ramus.

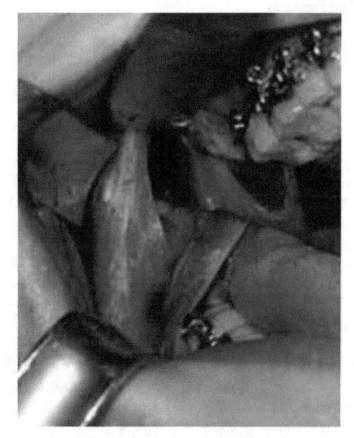

Figure 22.7.   A subperiosteal tissue pocket is created along the retrolingual depression to visualize the inferior alveolar nerve and for the insertion of the reciprocating saw.

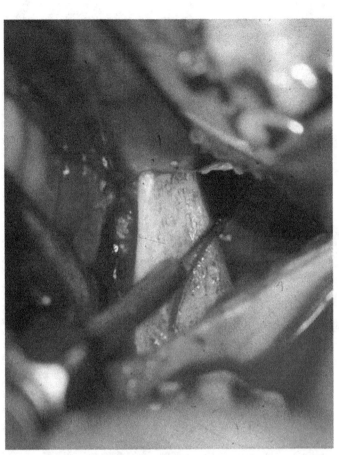

Figure 22.8.   A modified Hunsuck osteotomy is created with a reciprocating saw. A 45° angle is ideal to minimize unfavorable splits. More vertical osteotomies may be necessary in thin mandibles.

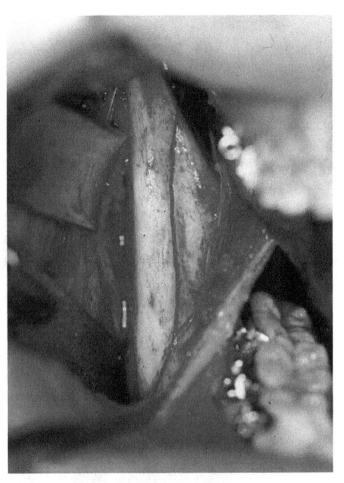

Figure 22.9.   The osteotomy is extended to the bony prominence located along the buccal aspect of the molar region (Dalpont prominence).

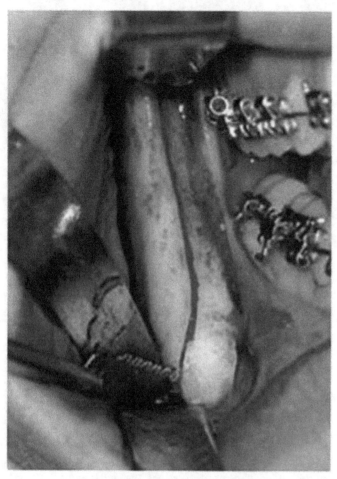

Figure 22.10. The osteotomy continues vertically as a tangential cut through the lateral cortex to connect the osteotomy along the external oblique ridge, and an inferior border osteotomy is performed.

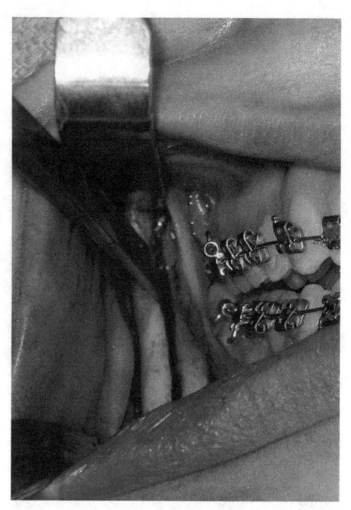

Figure 22.11. Osteotomes are used to propagate the split of the proximal and distal segments of the mandible.

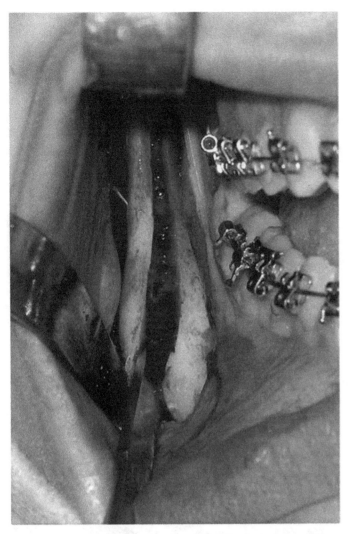

Figure 22.12. The inferior border is mobilized. Care is taken to ensure that all segments of the split are separated evenly to prevent unfavorable fractures.

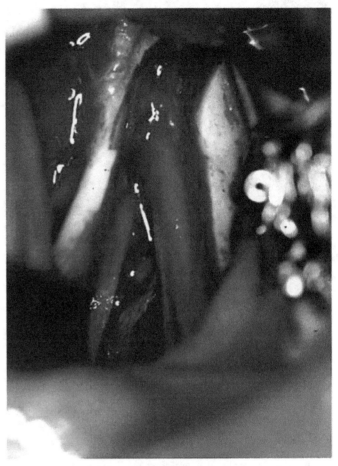

Figure 22.13. The inferior alveolar nerve is visualize immediately after the propagation of the split. Care is taken to preserve the nerve within the distal segment of the mandible.

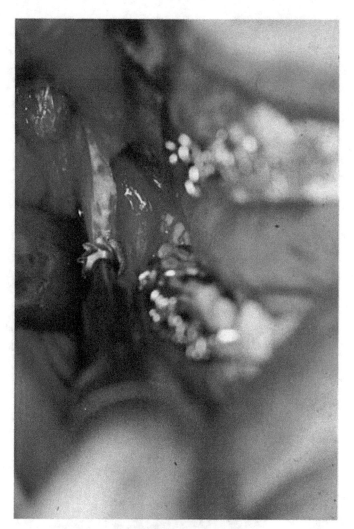

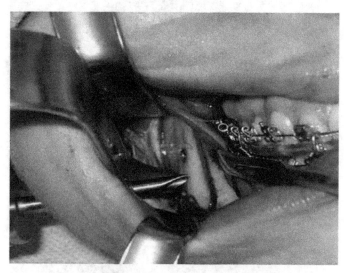

Figure 22.15. The condyles are seated within the glenoid fossa, and fixation is applied via percutanous access.

Figure 22.14. After detachment of the medial pterygoid muscle and confirmation of passive movement of the proximal and distal segments of the mandible, all bony interferences are removed.

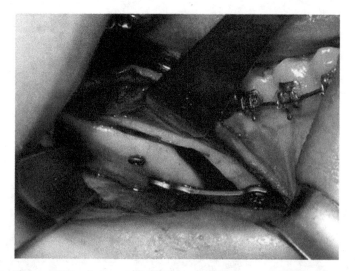

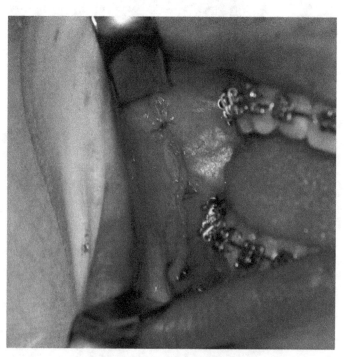

Figure 22.16. For mandibular advancements, monocortical plates may be used with or without positional screws for added rigidity.

Figure 22.17. Mucosal incisions are closed primarily with chromic sutures in a continuous horizontal mattress fashion.

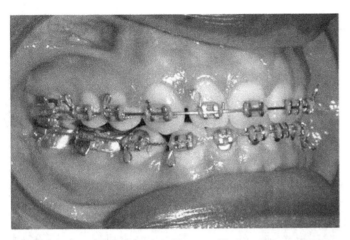

Figure 22.18. Patient 6 weeks after mandibular advancement surgery and orthodontic movement.

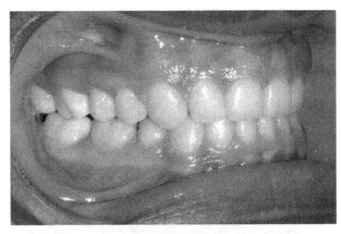

Figure 22.19. Final patient mandible position and occlusion.

Case Report 22.2. Sagittal Ramus Osteotomy: Mandibular Setback. An 18-year-old female with class III malocclusion as a result of asymmetrical mandibular hyperplasia. (See Figures 22.20 through 22.26.)

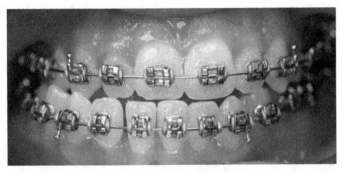

Figure 22.20. Preoperative image depicting a class III malocclusion and asymmetric mandibular prognathism.

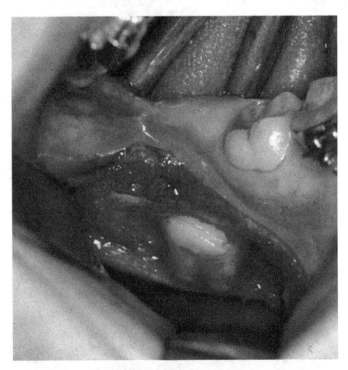

Figure 22.21. Developing wisdom tooth and inferior alveolar nerve visualized after sagittal split osteotomy.

231

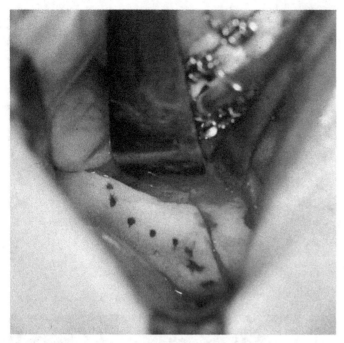

Figure 22.22.   The proximal segment on mandibular setback procedures using a sagittal ramus osteotomy requires recontouring for visibility, the avoidance of periodontal issues, and prevention of overrotation of the segment.

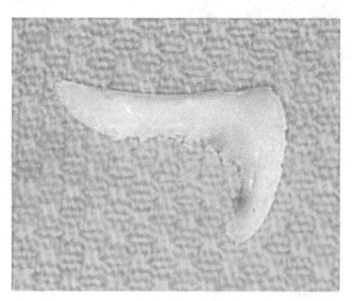

Figure 22.23.   Resected piece of the anterior and superior border of the proximal segment.

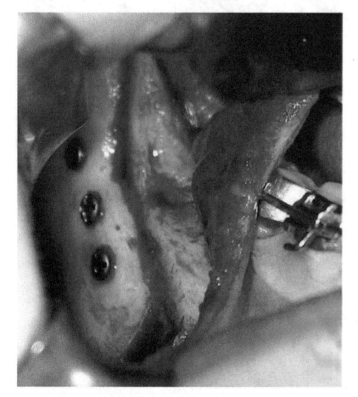

Figure 22.24.   Proximal and distal segments stabilized with superior border positional screw fixation after recontouring of the proximal segment.

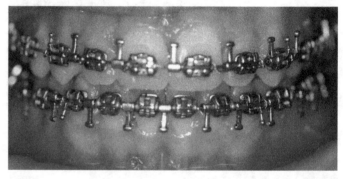

Figure 22.25.   Patient 4 weeks after mandibular setback surgery and orthodontic movement.

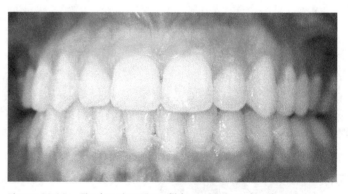

Figure 22.26.   Final patient mandible position and occlusion.

Case Report 22.3. Intraoral Vertical Ramus Osteotomy (IVRO). A 21-year-old male with class III malocclusion as a result of mandibular hyperplasia. (See Figures 22.27, 22.28, 22.29, and 22.30.)

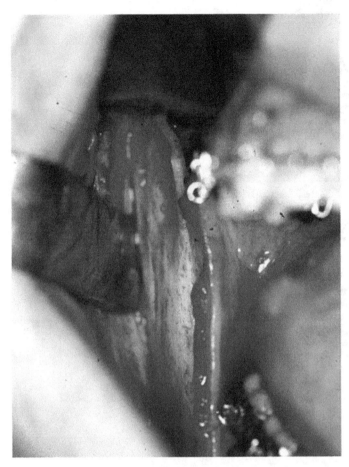

Figure 22.27.   The lateral ramus is exposed from the sigmoid notch superiorly to the antegonial notch inferiorly. The coronoid process has been removed to improve visibility and to eliminate the pull of the temporalis muscle.

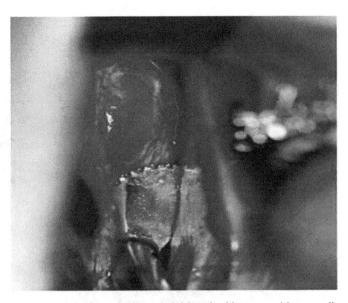

Figure 22.28.   The osteotomy is initiated mid-ramus with an oscillating saw and is "walked" superiorly into the sigmoid notch and inferior to the antegonial notch.

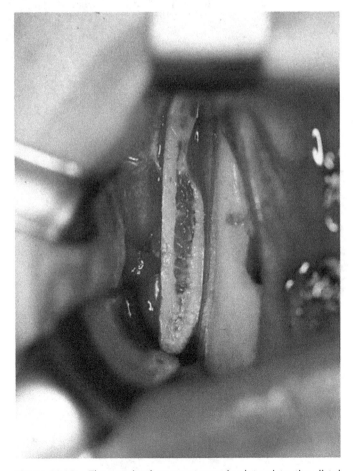

Figure 22.29.   The proximal segment remains lateral to the distal segment when maxillomandibular fixation is applied.

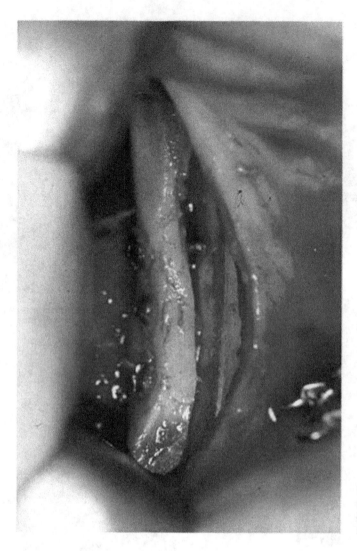

Figure 22.30.   Stabilization of the vertical ramus osteotomy is performed via vertically oriented positional screws (a minimum of three) placed percutaneously.

Genioplasty (Anterior Sliding Osteotomy)

Bart C. Farrell, Brian B. Farrell, and Myron R. Tucker

Private Practice, Carolinas Center for Oral and Facial Surgery, Charlotte, North Carolina, USA; and Department of Oral and Maxillofacial Surgery, Louisiana State University Health Science Center, New Orleans, Louisiana, USA

A means of augmentation or reduction of the anterior mandible.

Indications

1. Correction of skeletal deformities, including mild retrognathia, macrogenia, microgenia, and genial asymmetry
2. Enlargement of the posterior airway space for treatment of obstructive sleep apnea

Contraindications

1. Retrognathia with normal genial development
2. Difficult or distorted anatomy
3. Short mandibular symphysis
4. Neurosensory concerns

Anatomy

Mental nerve and foramen: The genu of the mental nerve may course anteriorly 1-5 mm before exiting the mental foramen at the apices of the premolar teeth.

Mentalis muscle: A midline muscular band that originates from the incisive fossa of the mandible and inserts along the skin of the lower lip. Functions to protrude the lower lip.

Genioglossus muscle: A paired extrinsic tongue muscle that originates from the superior genial tubercle and inserts into the body of the tongue. Functions to protract and depress the tongue.

Technique

1. The patient is prepped and draped to include the oral cavity and maxillofacial region. The patient is nasally intubated, and the tube is secured. A throat pack is positioned at the level of the hypopharynx.
2. Local anesthetic containing a vasoconstrictor is injected within the anterior mandibular vestibule from mental foramen to mental foramen with direct injection within the mentalis muscles.
3. An incision is created within the anterior mandibular vestibule, 1 cm anterior to the depth of the vestibule (Figure 23.1, Case Report 23.1). An anteriorly placed incision will conserve both attached and unattached tissue for closure. An incision placed too close to the attached tissue will cause recession due to scar contracture and could compromise the incisor teeth. Once through the mucosa, the small branches of the mental nerve coursing superficially into the lower lip are identified and reflected laterally from the surgical field. The dissection is carried sharply through the mentalis muscle with a heavy scissor (Metzenbaum). Caution should be taken to minimize dissection toward the skin to avoid iatrogenic perforation of the lower lip.
4. The symphysis is exposed anteriorly in a subperiosteal manner to the inferior border (Figure 23.2, Case Report 23.1). Minimal dissection is required superiorly to avoid unnecessary striping of the attached tissue over the mandibular incisor teeth and preserve the superior portion of the mentalis muscle for closure.
5. The dissection is carried posteriorly to locate the mental foramen (Figure 23.3, Case Report 23.1). Subperiosteal dissection is carried inferior and posterior to the mental foramen to expose the inferior border of the body of the mandible.
6. A sagittal saw is used to score a vertical line marking the skeletal midline to serve as a reference during manipulation of the anterior segment (Figure 23.4, Case Report 23.1, and Figure 23.10, Case Report 23.2). The planned osteotomy should be placed at least 5 mm inferiorly to the visualized mental foramen and apices of the anterior teeth. The horizontal osteotomy should extend as far posteriorly as possible within the body of the mandible without encroaching on the mandibular canal.
7. A reciprocating saw is used to score the facial cortex for the planned osteotomy bilaterally (Figure 23.10, Case Report 23.2).
8. Once satisfied with the osteotomy design, the saw is held upright while cutting through both the facial and lingual cortices from the inferior border to the midline. The osteotomy is then duplicated on the contralateral side. Once the osteotomy is complete, the inferior border is downfractured and mobilized.

Atlas of Operative Oral and Maxillofacial Surgery, First Edition. Edited by Christopher J. Haggerty and Robert M. Laughlin
© 2015 John Wiley & Sons, Inc. Published 2015 by John Wiley & Sons, Inc.

9. The free segment can be stabilized with a towel clamp or wire. A wire-passing bur may be used to create an opening through the facial cortex for a 26-gauge wire. The wire or towel clamp can be used to control the free segment in preparation for fixation (Figure 23.4, Case Report 23.1).

10. The segment is repositioned according to the treatment plan and inspected to ensure appropriate positioning and symmetry. Calipers can be used to determine the extent of skeletal change to aid in transferring the presurgical plan to the surgery. Jigs may be fabricated from virtual planning when the chin possesses a pronounced deformity (asymmetry) to aid in the establishment of skeletal symmetry and projection (Figures 23.12 and 23.13, Case Report 23.3).

11. Plate or positional screw fixation may be used to stabilize the anterior segment (Figure 23.5, Case Report 23.1, and Figure 23.11, Case Report 23.2). Visualization of the fixated anterior segment and extraoral palpation of the osteotomy "wings" are performed to ensure symmetry and correct positioning of the anterior segment.

12. Soft tissue closure is accomplished in a layered fashion beginning with reapproximation of the periosteum and mentalis muscle with interrupted resorbable sutures. Adequate resuspension of the mentalis muscle (Figure 23.6, Case Report 23.1) is imperative to prevent ptosis of the soft tissue drape. A single midline mucosal suture is placed to aid in orientation of the mucosal closure. Primary closure of the mucosa is completed with a continuous resorbable suture.

13. A dressing may be placed over the chin to facilitate redraping the overlying soft tissue. The dressing is applied over the anterior mandible and submental area to support the soft tissue and to apply pressure to the surgical site in an effort to minimize edema.

Postoperative Management

1. Antibiotics coverage is recommended for one week postoperatively.
2. Analgesics and anti-emetics are prescribed.
3. Facial dressings are removed at 5–7 days postoperatively.
4. Meticulous oral hygiene is reinforced.

Complications

1. **Sublingual hematoma formation**: Bleeding may occur if vessels are severed or if the soft tissue is excessively traumatized. Failure to diligently address hemostasis may result in the development of a sublingual hematoma. An expanding hematoma may elevate the tongue, requiring exploration and evacuation of the extravisated blood to avoid potential airway compromise.
2. **"Witches chin"**: Occurs from failure to resuspend the mentalis muscle and/or wound dehiscence. Results in ptosis of the soft tissue envelope. Corrected via resuspension of the mentalis musculature and appropriate wound closure.
3. **Pointed chin**: Occurs from a short osteotomy between the parasymphysis regions. The chin will appear narrow and pointed. Treatment includes anterior mandibular osteotomy to include the body of the mandible.
4. **Asymmetric chin**: Due to poor treatment planning and/or inappropriate segment placement.

Key Points

1. It is imperative that the facial and lingual cortices are transected at the same level in order to prevent a decrease in the vertical height of the chin as it is advanced.
2. For patients with obstructive sleep apnea, cone beam computed tomography can demarcate the anatomic boundaries of the posterior airway space and allows for the identification of areas that may be the etiology of soft tissue collapse. The base of the tongue is frequently the etiology of a narrow posterior airway. Advancing the genioglossus attachment at the genial tubercles via an anterior segmental osteotomy can increase the airway space and address the anatomic source of obstructive sleep apnea.
3. Bone-grafting materials may be used within the anterior segmental osteotomy to eliminate or soften the step expected at the osteotomy site after large advancements. Grafting may aid in creating a subtle bony transition and provide more aesthetic soft tissue contours within the lower face.
4. In situations where the skeletal midline is deviated from the dental midline, traditional orthognathic surgery to correct a malocclusion may not achieve facial symmetry. Adjunctive osteotomies on the inferior border of the mandible or chin may be required to correct underlying skeletal deformities.
5. The establishment of symmetry within an anterior mandible that possesses vertical distortion of the inferior border will often generate an unequal osteotomy gap necessitating shims and/or grafting when the segment is repositioned.
6. Virtual planning improves the accuracy when correcting an asymmetrical dentofacial deformity. Virtual planning provides insight prior to the operation about the skeletal deformity and the movements necessary to reposition the chin symmetrically. Cutting templates can be fabricated in addition to jigs that are attached to a stable reference (occlusal arch) that transfers the virtual plan and accurately repositions the anterior segment.
7. Chin implants can be used for augmentation or to improve the contour of the anterior mandible. Stock or custom implants can be used to achieve the desired projection and contour. The advantages of chin implants compared to anterior segment osteotomies include a less invasive procedure with decreased potential neurosensory

change. Disadvantages include potential bone remodeling or resorption if not adequately stabilized, infection, displacement, development of a fibrous capsule, foreign body reaction, and inability to affect the airway space.

Case Reports

Case Report 23.1. Symmetrical genial advancement. (See Figures 23.1 through 23.8.)

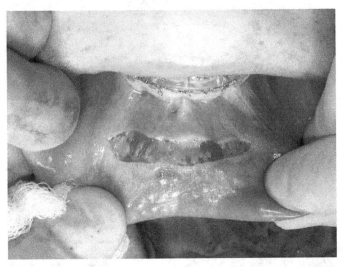

Figure 23.1. An incision through mucosa is created within the anterior mandibular vestibule.

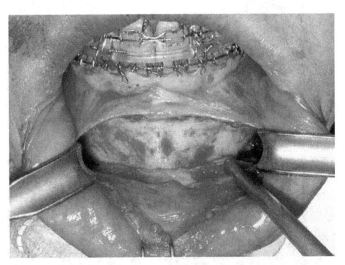

Figure 23.2. The symphysis and inferior border of the mandible are exposed.

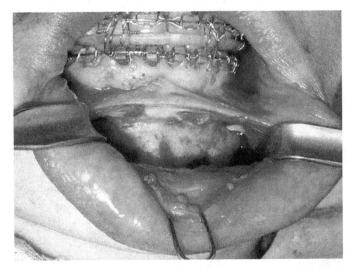

Figure 23.3. The bilateral mental foramen are identified. Lateral dissection proceeds posteriorly and inferiorly to the mental foramen.

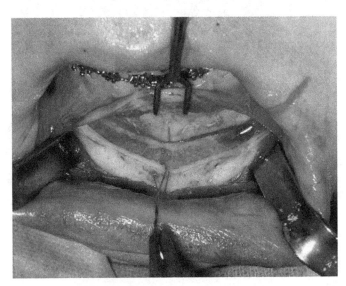

Figure 23.4. The midline is marked, the osteotomy is completed, and a guide wire is placed to allow for control of the free segment during repositioning and fixation.

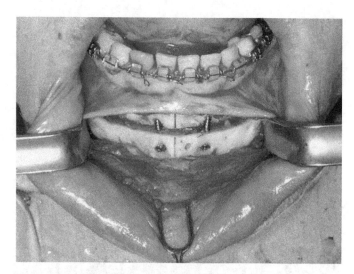

Figure 23.5. Fixation is accomplished with positional screws once the desired amount of augmentation has been achieved.

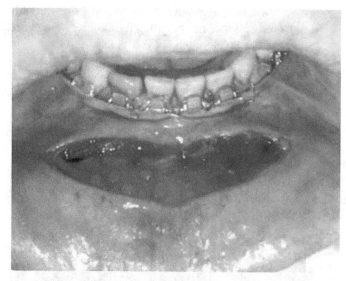

Figure 23.6. The mentalis muscle is resuspended.

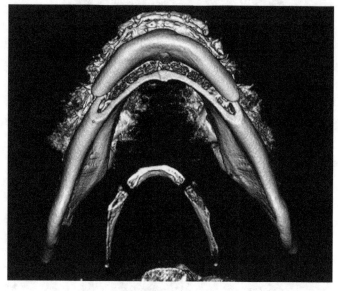

Figure 23.7. Postoperative 3D axial computed tomography image demonstrating symmetrical advancement of the anterior segmental osteotomy.

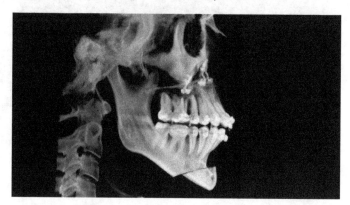

Figure 23.8. Postoperative 3D reconstruction demonstrating symmetrical advancement of the anterior segmental osteotomy.

Case Report 23.2. Symmetrical genial setback. (See Figures 23.9, 23.10, and 23.11.)

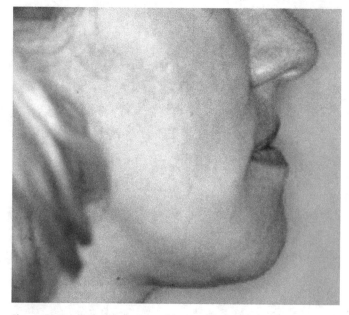

Figure 23.9. Patient presents with mandibular hyperplasia and symmetrical macrogenia.

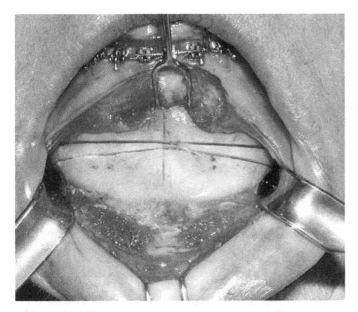

Figure 23.10. The vertical midline and the osteotomy sites are marked. A symmetrical wedge of bone will be removed to correct the patient's symmetrical macrogenia.

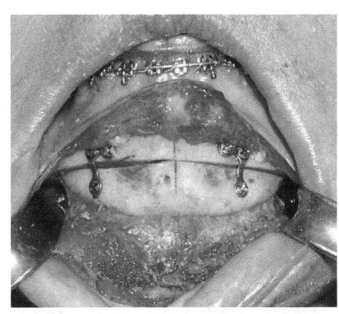

Figure 23.11. The anterior segment is repositioned posteriorly and fixated.

Case Report 23.3. Asymmetrical genial movements. (See Figures 23.12 and 23.13.)

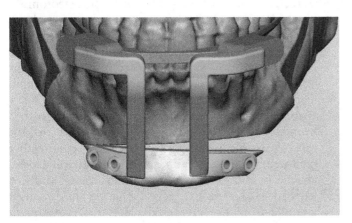

Figure 23.12. Virtual surgical planning and the fabrication of custom guides are recommended for the correction of severe genial asymmetries.

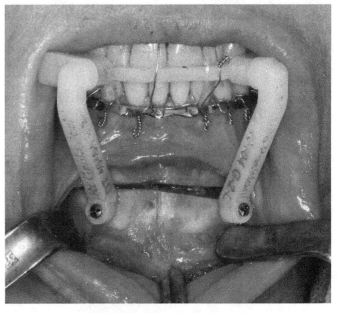

Figure 23.13. The osteotomy is completed, and the anterior segment's positioning guide is in place.

Reference

Tucker, M.R., 1995. Orthognathic surgery versus orthodontic camouflage in the treatment of mandibular deficiency. *Journal of Oral and Maxillofacial Surgery*, 53, 572–8.

24 Maxillary Distraction Using Le Fort I Osteotomy and a RED 2 External Fixator

Lester Machado

Division of Oral and Maxillofacial Surgery, Rady Children's Hospital of San Diego, San Diego, California, USA

A method of obtaining significant advancement of the maxilla and midface with the use of distractors.

Indications

1. Maxillary advancement in noncleft patients of greater than 8 mm
2. Maxillary advancement in cleft patients of greater than 5 mm
3. Maxillary downgrafting where stability is in question
4. Maxillary advancement and/or downgrafting movements where stability using rigid fixation would be impossible to achieve

Contraindications

1. Incomplete development of the skull
2. Developmental delay that compromises comprehension and cooperation
3. Seizure history
4. Psychological instability: severe depression, anxiety, or schizophrenia
5. Uncooperative patient

Technique

1. After oral endotracheal intubation, the tube is secured and corneal shields with ophthalmic ointment are placed bilaterally (Figure 24.1 [all figures cited in this chapter appear in Case Report 24.1]). The face, scalp, and oral cavity are prepped in a sterile fashion. A half sheet with two towels is placed under the patient's head, and the inner towel is clamped to expose the frontal and temporal areas bilaterally down to the upper neck. A split sheet is then applied to cover the rest of the body. The area where the halo will be attached must be in the field.
2. Local anesthesia is injected within the maxillary vestibule and into the greater palatine canals. The fixation device is assembled on the back table of the sterile field. The vertical bars are joined to the halo.
3. Eight fixation screws are lightly lubricated with ointment and inserted partially into the desired positions within the anterior cortex of the skull. It should be noted that the manufacturer recommends six screws in the halo, but eight screws enhance stability.
4. Two horizontal bars are attached to the vertical bar for four-point fixation of the maxilla. Four-point fixation allows for complete control of the movement of the maxilla in all dimensions.
5. A maxillary vestibular incision is utilized to expose the anterior and lateral walls of the maxilla as in the Le Fort 1 osteotomy procedure. The mucosa is elevated from the anterior nasal spine extending posterior to the nasal tuberosity area in a tunnel fashion. The nasal mucosa is elevated from the floor of the nose, the lateral nasal walls, and the nasal septum. Care is taken to minimize tears within the nasal mucosa.
6. A reciprocating saw is used to create the osteotomy at the Le Fort I level. The horizontal osteotomy is placed 5–6 mm above the roots of the longest maxillary teeth and superior to the junction of the nasal floor and the pyriform rim. Sufficient space is required on the maxilla for placement of the fixation plates without compromising the teeth roots.
7. The bone attachments are released similarly to a standard Le Fort I osteotomy. The nasal crest of the maxilla is released from the septum–vomer with a guarded vomer osteotome. A single guarded osteotome is used to separate the lateral nasal walls. A curved osteotome is used to separate the posterior maxilla from the pterygoid plates just anterior to the pterygomaxillary junction or within the posterior part of the tuberosity bilaterally. The maxilla is gently downfractured. Any tethering of the nasal mucosa to the palatal mucosa in the cleft case is identified and carefully divided. Holding the maxilla down, the nasal mucosa is checked for full release from the maxilla.
8. Ronguers are used to remove any remaining posterior attachments of the lateral nasal walls. The maxilla is mobilized without tearing the mucosal attachments. Full mobility of the maxilla is essential, yet care must be taken to retain all of the soft

Atlas of Operative Oral and Maxillofacial Surgery, First Edition. Edited by Christopher J. Haggerty and Robert M. Laughlin.
© 2015 John Wiley & Sons, Inc. Published 2015 by John Wiley & Sons, Inc.

tissue attachments for blood supply. You may not start placement of the distractor unless full mobility of the maxilla is achieved.

9. Two L-shaped plates are secured to the anterior superior edge on each side of the maxilla. Four or five screws are used to attach each plate, and one screw hole is left empty in the short arm of the L for a full-length 25-gauge stainless steel wire (Figure 24.2). The long wire is passed through the most anterior hole on the plate and then bent away from the field and tagged with a hemostat.

10. A long 25-gauge wire is passed through the orthodontic tube on the upper first molar on each side. The wire is bent on itself when passed halfway. The two free ends are tagged to each other with a hemostat on each side. Four points of fixation are established on the maxilla to control maxillary movement in all directions.

11. A 15# blade is used to create a tiny nick in the nasolabial fold at the very base of the nose a few millimeters lateral to the philtrum bilaterally. Each pair of the two pairs of wires attached to the maxillary plates are passed through the ipsilateral skin openings using a fine-tipped hemostat, externalizing the maxillary wires (Figure 24.2). Alternatively, the wire may be passed with a Keith needle. The dental wires are passed through the oral cavity (Figure 24.3).

12. Before attaching the fixation device, ensure that it is properly assembled and that all of the assembly screws are fully tightened. To attach the halo requires two people. The surgeon holds the halo in the ideal position as the assistant surgeon tightens the screws by hand. If the screws were to be tightened using the screwdriver, a temporal bone fracture could occur.

13. The screws are tightened from front to back and on both sides at the same time. The goal is to engage the point of the screw in firm contact with the outer cortex of the skull. The vertical bars of the fixator remain midline (Figure 24.4).

14. The halo device is positioned 2–3 cm above the supraorbital rim parallel to the Frankfurt horizontal plane. All of the fixation screws should be within the hairline. At least four fixation screws are used on each side, for a total of eight. All fixation screws are finger tightened as tight as possible without undue pressure on the temporal bones. Stability of the external fixation device is confirmed by gently moving the device and observing the head move.

15. The maxilla is attached to the two short horizontal bars of the fixator (Figure 24.5). If vertical movement is desired, the horizontal bar attached to the vertical screw must be configured to drive the maxilla in the desired direction as it is activated. The two wires attached to the maxillary plates are attached to the upper horizontal bars. The two wires attached to the first molars are covered with a sterile urinary catheter to protect the lips, and they are attached to the lower horizontal bar.

16. An alar cinch suture is placed to minimize alar widening during advancement. The mucosal incision is closed with a resorbable suture. Final adjustments are made to the distractor, and the fixation screws are gently hand tightened one more time before the patient is awakened from anesthesia.

17. The screwdrivers for the fixation device and wire cutters are given to the anesthesiologist and labeled with the patient's name. The anesthesiologist is taught how to remove the vertical bar in case of an airway emergency during emergence by cutting the four wires and removing the upper screw that secures the vertical bars (Figure 24.6). Emergency removal of the vertical bar in the case of an airway crisis is also reviewed with the recovery room staff. The patient can only be extubated when fully awake (Figure 24.7).

Postoperative Management

1. The patient is placed on a full liquid diet following the procedure.

2. Meticulous oral and appliance hygiene is enforced.

3. A latency period of 3–7 days is observed prior to activation of the device.

4. A distraction rate of 1 mm per day is typically observed. The device is activated by turning the four screws on the horizontal bars at a rate of 0.5 mm twice each day.

5. Patients are monitored closely during distraction. At each visit, the fixator screws are manually tightened to prevent migration of the halo.

6. After the ideal position of the maxilla is achieved, the last turn of the distractor is completed and the consolidation phase begins. The consolidation phase continues for a minimum of 8 weeks. Early release of the fixation has been linked with significant relapse. Bone healing can be monitored with cephalometric head films.

7. At the time of appliance removal, the four wires are cut and the device is carefully removed by unscrewing the eight fixation screws. The two intraoral wires are removed from the first molar. The final two wires connected to the maxillary plates can be removed with local anesthesia or with intravenous sedation.

8. After removal of the appliance, there is a short period of time when the regenerated bone can be molded with elastic therapy to achieve an ideal occlusal result. Each case will require a differing level of force to close the bite, but it can usually be accomplished with elastic bands to the orthodontic hooks.

Complications

1. Migration of the halo inferiorly toward the brow from incomplete mobilization of the maxilla
2. Relapse
3. Hardware failure
4. Temporoparietal skull fracture as a result of overtightening halo screws
5. Unequal distraction in one or more planes

Key Points

1. Surgical distraction should be delayed until skeletal maturity is completed, preventing the need for repeat procedures.
2. Most cleft cases have already undergone multiple surgical procedures within the maxilla, and greater care must be taken to ensure adequate blood supply to the maxilla. The soft tissue attachments of the soft palate must be retained. If the greater palatine arteries can be preserved, then the blood supply to the regenerate is enhanced. Keeping the vestibular incision from second bicuspid to second bicuspid is another maneuver to enhance blood supply to the maxilla.
3. The maxilla must be released from all of its bone attachments for full mobilization. Failure to fully mobilize the maxilla and remove potential bony interferences will result in incomplete and/or asymmetrical distraction. The bone attachments to be cut are identical to those in a Le Fort I osteotomy.
4. The posterior osteotomies may be initiated between the maxilla and the pytergoid plates or in the posterior part of the tuberosity. By having the posterior osteotomy within the posterior part of the tuberosity and crossing across the hard palate, you can minimize velopharyngeal insufficiency.
5. The maxillary artery and vein are located just posterior to the posterior wall of the maxilla. Both structures can lead to significant bleeding if inadvertently cut.
6. The nasal mucosa is adherent to the floor of the nose and is elevated carefully. Where the nasal crest of the maxilla connects to the cartilage of the septum, the mucosal attachment is adherent and is more challenging to disarticulate without tearing the mucosa. Mucosal tears result in increased postoperative bleeding and discomfort. In cleft cases without an intact hard palate, the nasal mucosa will be bound to the palatal mucosa within a band of scar tissue. This presentation is more difficult. Tearing can be avoided by creating the bone cuts and carefully starting the downfracture. As the maxilla is slowly lowered, electrocautery can be used to divide the nasal mucosa away from the palatal mucosa, working from anterior to posterior.

Case Report

Case Report 24.1. An 18-year-old patient born with orbital hypertelorism and bilateral cleft lip and palate after cleft lip repair (age 2 months), cleft palate repair (age 18 months), sphincteroplasty (age 3 years), facial bipartition and orbital repositioning (age 6 years), and dentoalveolar cleft grafting (age 8 years) with severe maxillary hypoplasia and dysgnathia. (See Figures 24.1 through 24.8.)

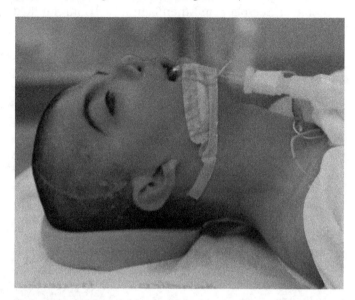

Figure 24.1.   The patient is positioned supine on the table, corneal shields are put in place, and the oral endotracheal tube is secured in an inferior vector.

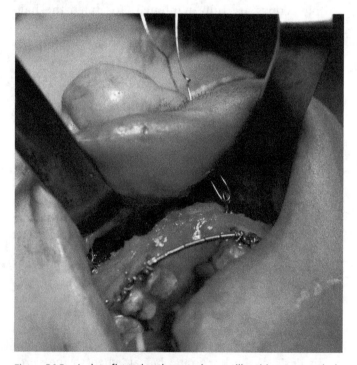

Figure 24.2.   L plate fixated to the anterior maxilla with one screw hole left empty for the placement of a 25-gauge stainless steel wire. The piriform wires are placed transcutaneously at the level of the nasal sill.

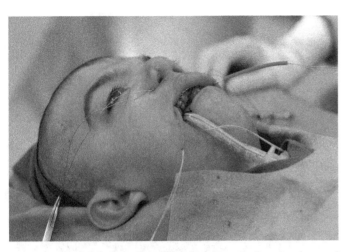

Figure 24.3. The dental wires secured to the molar bands are passed through the oral cavity.

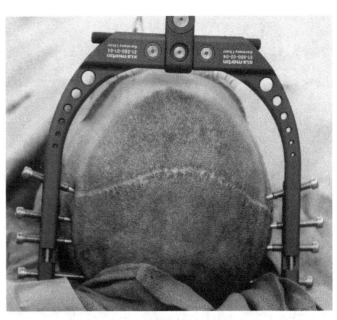

Figure 24.4. Fixation screws are in place within the anterior cortex of the skull, the halo device is positioned 2–3 cm above the supraorbital rim parallel to the Frankfurt horizontal plane, and the vertical bars of the fixator remain midline.

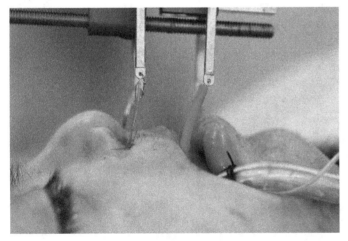

Figure 24.5. The maxilla is attached to the two short horizontal bars of the fixator.

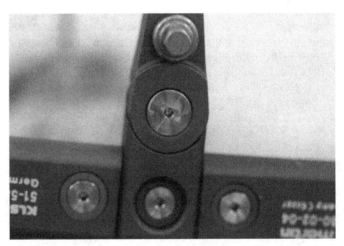

Figure 24.6. The upper screw used to remove the vertical bar and to change the vertical dimension of the distraction.

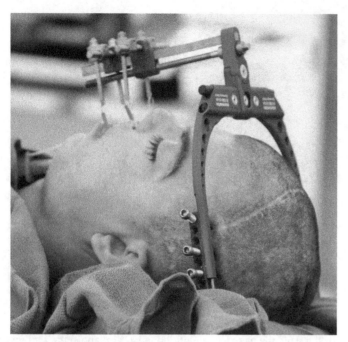

Figure 24.7.   The halo device secured to the skull in the appropriate position. The patient is allowed to fully awaken prior to extubation.

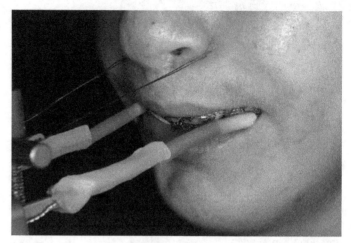

Figure 24.8.   Patient during the distraction process. The position of the maxilla can be altered by making adjustments within the distractor connections. The two wires attached to the first molars are covered with a catheter to protect the lips over the course of treatment.

References

Nout, E., Wolvius, E.B., van Adrichem, L.N.A., Ongkosuwito, E.M. and van der Wal, K.G.H., 2006. Complications in maxillary distraction using the RED-2 device: a retrospective analysis of 21 patients. *International Journal of Oral and Maxillofacial Surgery*, 35, 897–902.

Polley, J. and Figueroa, A., 1997. Management of severe maxillary deficiency in childhood and adolescence through distraction osteogenesis with an external rigid distraction device. *Journal of Craniofacial Surgery*, 8, 181–5.

Polley, J.W. and Figueroa, A.A., 1998. Rigid external distraction: its application in cleft maxillary deformities. *Plastic Reconstructive Surgery*, 102, 1360–72.

CHAPTER 25

Dentoalveolar Cleft Repair

Jeremiah Jason Parker[1] and Christopher T. Vogel[2]
[1]*Private Practice, Montgomery, Alabama, USA*
[2]*Department of Oral and Maxillofacial Surgery, University of Missouri–Kansas City, Kansas City, Missouri, USA*

The reconstruction of congenital anterior maxillary alveolus and maxilla defects, and the closure of associated oronasal fistulae.

Indications

1. To provide a stable osseous medium for the eruption and orthodontic movement of teeth within a region of a maxillary cleft
2. Closure of oronasal fistulae
3. Improvement of facial aesthetics by providing osseous support to the nasal base and continuity to the dentoalveolar arches
4. To establish proper periodontal support for neighboring dentition
5. To provide an osseous medium for the eventual placement of endosteal implants
6. To provide a stable and intact maxillary arch for future orthognathic procedures

Contraindications

1. Active infection
2. Poor patient compliance concerning oral hygiene
3. Collapsed cleft with plans for future orthodontic expansion. The palate is expanded in order to widen the cleft to the desired arch shape prior to grafting. The expanded cleft permits greater visualization and instrumentation of the cleft. Additionally, it is exceptionally difficult to orthodontically widen the cleft space once the graft has consolidated (refer to Key Point 1, this chapter)

Technique

1. The patient is positioned supine and orally intubated with an oral RAE tube.
2. The neck is hyperextended for better visualization of the palate and alveolar process. A throat pack is placed within the posterior oropharynx. The patient is prepped to include the oral cavity, the nasal passages, the surrounding maxillofacial skeleton, and, if present, the oronasal fistula. The patient is draped to allow for exposure of the oral cavity and nasal passages.
3. Local anesthesia containing a vasoconstrictor is injected along the palate, nasal floor, maxillary vestibule, and attached and unattached tissue of the anterior maxilla or cleft. The local anesthesia needle is used as a probe and allows the operator to determine the extent of the cleft and the position of the bone prior to making an incision. In cases involving a complete bilateral cleft with a mobile anterior segment, injection of the anterior segment with a vasoconstrictor is contraindicated due to the tenuous blood supply to the segment.
4. An incision is initiated along the lateral aspect of the cleft (Figure 25.1). A #15 blade is utilized to create a full-thickness mucoperiosteal incision along the lateral aspect of the cleft overlying sound bone. The anterior aspect of the incision extends to the height of the maxillary vestibule, and the posterior aspect of the incision extends along the posterior border of the cleft within the hard palate. The incision should divide the oral and nasal mucosa.
5. The incision is extended laterally utilizing buccal and palatal intrasulcular incisions. The lateral extent of the incision extends to the distal aspect of the last molar and terminates with a buccal posterior and superior releasing incision (Figure 25.2).
6. The medial incision extends in an intrasulcular fashion along the buccal and palatal surfaces of the teeth and terminates at the contralateral canine or first molar for unilateral clefts (Figure 25.2). The medial incision terminates at the midline for bilateral clefts.
7. A subperiosteal dissection is utilized to expose the piriform aperture, the anterior nasal spine, and the floor of the nose. Supernumerary or malformed teeth are extracted at this time. Care is taken to avoid exposure of the crown of developing impacted canine teeth. If the crown of an impacted canine tooth is exposed during the cleft dissection, strong consideration for the extraction of the tooth should be made. Grafting procedures adjacent to the crown of an exposed tooth significantly decrease the overall success rate of the graft.
8. In cases where a fistula is present, a subperiosteal, full-thickness tissue dissection is initiated along the internal aspect of the cleft and is extended superiorly along the lateral walls of the cleft to the floor of the nose and the

Atlas of Operative Oral and Maxillofacial Surgery, First Edition. Edited by Christopher J. Haggerty and Robert M. Laughlin
© 2015 John Wiley & Sons, Inc. Published 2015 by John Wiley & Sons, Inc.

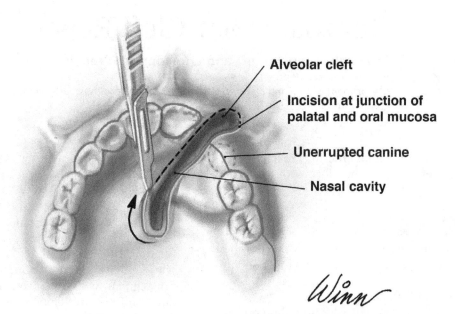

Figure 25.1.   An incision is initiated along the lateral aspect of the cleft overlying sound bone within the keratinized tissue lateral to the cleft. The anterior aspect of the incision extends to the height of the maxillary vestibule, and the posterior aspect of the incision extends along the posterior border of the cleft within the hard palate.

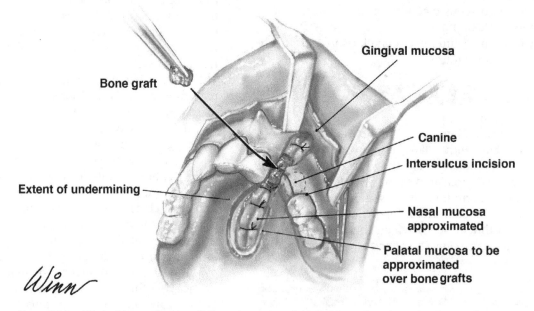

Figure 25.2.   The incision extends medially to the canine and laterally to the tuberosity. The nasal mucosa is inverted and closed, and grafting material is placed within the cleft defect.

cartilaginous nasal septum. The tissue reflected from the internal aspect of the cleft is carefully elevated, inverted, and sutured together to form a new nasal barrier. The tissue edges are sutured together using 5-0 Vicryl buried sutures in a horizontal mattress fashion, resulting in the tissue edges being inverted within the nasal cavity (Figure 25.3). A biological collagen membrane is trimmed and adapted to the nasal floor.

9. Periosteal releasing incisions are made within the full-thickness mucoperiosteal tissue reflections, and

the labial mucosa is advanced until the tissue can easily be approximated over the cleft defect without tension.

10. Grafting material is placed within the cleft defect and compacted to eliminate dead space. The authors prefer to use either bone marrow from the anterior hip or a mixture of mineralized and demineralized human cadaveric bone depending on the size and nature of the cleft. The grafted area should extend from the nasal floor to the alveolar crest.

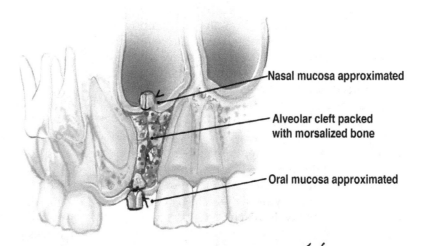

Nasal mucosa approximated

Alveolar cleft packed with morsalized bone

Oral mucosa approximated

Winn

Figure 25.3. Particulate bone is compacted within the cleft defect to eliminate dead space.

11. A second biological collagen membrane is trimmed and adapted to contain the graft material within the cleft defect. The mucoperiosteal tissue elevations are closed over the grafted defect and membrane in a tension-free manner. Additional releasing incisions, subperiosteal dissection, and/or periosteal scoring is accomplished in order to obtain a tension-free primary closure (Figure 25.4).

12. In the case of a bilateral cleft, the procedure described in Steps 1 through 12 would be performed on the largest cleft side first. The contralateral cleft is repaired

in a similar fashion after a healing period of at least 6 months.

Postoperative Management

1. Meticulous oral hygiene is mandatory to minimize the risk of infection.
2. Nasal decongestants are prescribed.
3. Patients with unilateral cleft repair remain on a pureed diet for 3–4 weeks, while 6 weeks is recommended for patients with bilateral cleft repair.
4. Physical activity depends on the graft donor site, with 4–6 weeks of restricted activity recommended for patients with hip grafts.
5. Nonsteroidal anti-inflammatory drugs and narcotics are utilized for pain control.
6. Antibiotics are continued for 10 days postoperatively.

Complications

1. **Infection**: Infections are rare and typically result from inadequate oral hygiene in the immediate postoperative period or from the exposure of a retained impacted tooth. Infections may result in loss of the graft and the creation of larger oronasal fistulae.
2. **Failure of spontaneous eruption**: Although rare, canines that fail to erupt through the grafted alveolar segment may be surgically exposed following graft consolidation in a manner no different from that seen in noncleft patients.
3. **Graft loss**: Common reasons for graft loss include infection and inadequate soft tissue coverage. Meticulous attention is paid to achieving a tension-free closure of the overlying mucosal flaps. A small intraoral dehiscence may be effectively treated with local debridement and typically will not result in complete

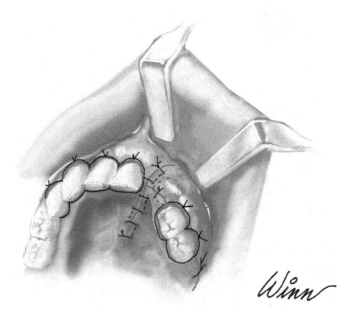

Winn

Figure 25.4. The oral mucosa advancement flaps are primarily closed in a tension-free manner.

graft loss. Some graft size reduction is expected after all grafting procedures (especially in compromised areas) and is not considered a complication. Overgrafting is recommended provided sufficient soft tissue coverage.

4. **Maxillary growth restriction**: Maxillary growth restrictions are frequently associated with primary grafting procedures and present as asymmetric maxillary hypoplasia resulting from scar tissue formation from the initial grafting procedure. This is not to be mistaken for symmetric maxillary hypoplasia that is often present in cleft patients regardless of surgical correction. Definitive treatment involves widening the palate and maxillary advancement surgery via orthognathic surgery or distraction osteogenesis once skeletal maturity is reached (14–18 years of age).

Key Points

1. Bone grafting within the maxilla may be classified as either primary or secondary depending on the timing of surgical intervention. Primary grafting, however, has been associated with adverse effects on maxillary skeletal growth, and, as a result, secondary grafting procedures are preferred.

2. Secondary bone grafting of maxillary dentoalveolar clefts is typically performed during the mixed-dentition stage prior to the eruption of the involved canine, ideally between the ages of 7 and 11 years. Higher success rates are achieved when grafting is performed when the canine root is approximately two-thirds formed and the clinical crown is completely encased in bone.

3. Bilateral maxillary clefts require grafting in a two-stage procedure to minimize compromising the blood supply to the anterior segment.

4. Incisions are ideally placed within areas that will allow for the eruption of impacted teeth through keratinized tissue in order to ensure optimal periodontal support. However, this is not always possible due to the relative lack of keratinized tissue in the cleft area.

5. Both autogenous (donor sites include the hip, calvaria, tibia, mandible, and rib) and alloplastic grafting material have been used with success to reconstruct dentoalveolar clefts. High success rates have been achieved using recombinant bone morphogenic protein-2 (BMP-2) with demineralized bone matrix as an off-label substitute for autogenous grafts in both initial and salvage procedures.

6. Supernumerary or malformed teeth are removed at the time of graft placement. Exposed canines within the cleft contribute to the failure of grafting procedures. Care should be taken to minimize clinical crown exposure, and if significant exposure occurs, consideration should be made to extracting the exposed canine.

7. Membranes may or may not be placed depending on the surgeon's preference, the size of the cleft, and the ability to achieve primary closure of the mucoperiosteal tissue flaps. Alloderm may be used when there is an inability to close the mucoperiosteal tissue elevation in a tension-free manner.

8. Avoid extensive reflection of the labial mucosa covering the premaxillary segment in patients with bilateral clefts to avoid compromising its vascular supply.

9. Immobilization of the premaxillary segment in patients with bilateral clefts is crucial to minimize the potential for non-union. Splints may be utilized to provide stability and are typically left in place for 4–8 weeks postoperatively.

10. Orthodontic treatment should resume 6 weeks after the closure of oronasal fistulae and successful graft placement. Passive orthodontics remain in place during this period to aid in stability across the segment.

11. Significant lip and nose changes are expected with bilateral cleft reconstruction. As such, delayed lip–nose revisions are recommended over simultaneous procedures with grafting.

12. Secondary bone-grafting procedures are often needed prior to endosteal implant placement to provide sufficient osseous volume. However, even with sufficient hard tissue volume, due to the unnatural morphology and soft tissue topography within the grafted cleft sites, implants frequently must be placed in less than ideal orientations and angulations. Additionally, there is often a lack of keratinized tissue present within the edentulous site, which leads to non-ideal periodontium and increased risk of future implant failure. Therefore, it is imperative that the restoring dentist is actively involved with the treatment planning of these patients prior to their grafting procedure. Careful consideration should be made when comparing implants versus fixed prosthodontics. Appropriately positioned and axially loaded dental implants have the advantage of stimulating graft retention, whereas a fixed prosthesis will add stability across the grafted segment.

Case Reports

Case Report 25.1. An 8-year-old patient presents after closure of a left complete cleft lip and palate. The patient also has a right-sided minor incomplete cleft and is congenitally missing teeth #7 and #10. Early grafting was performed to allow the palatally malpositioned impacted canine bone and mucosa to erupt through. (See Figures 25.5, 25.6, 25.7, 25.8, and 25.9.)

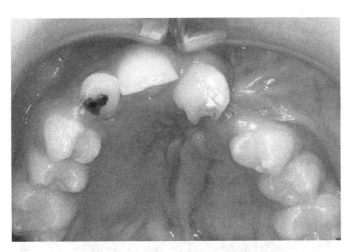

Figure 25.5.   An 8-year-old patient 6 months after left-sided dentoal-veolar cleft repair. The patient exhibits a transverse maxillary defi-ciency, dysgnathia, and maxillary hypoplasia. There has been some collapse of the grafted space. The left central incisor is malformed.

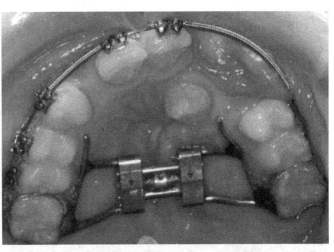

Figure 25.6.   At age 10, the patient with significant arch expansion (orthodontic maxillary expander in place), improved occlusion, and a palatally erupting canine. Note that the left central incisor has been altered to give the appearance of a normal central. The canine has erupted palatally as predicted and can now be moved into the arch where space has been made. An additional graft to the alveolar cleft will be performed in order to give the orthodontist enough alveolar bone to move the canine into position.

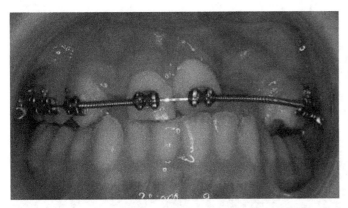

Figure 25.7.   At age 10, the maxilla demonstrates maxillary hypo-plasia and hypoplastic tissue. Now that room has been made, the canine can be moved into position.

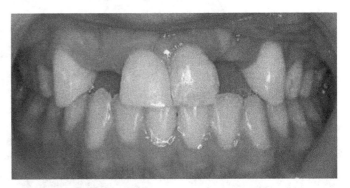

Figure 25.8.   At age 14, the maxillary arch is fully expanded, the dentition is aligned, and space is created for either implant place-ment or a bridge.

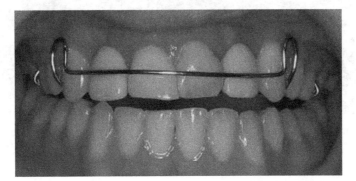

Figure 25.9.   At age 16, the orthodontics are completed, and the patient is placed within a retainer that incorporates the missing lat-eral incisors. Once the patient has reached skeletal maturity, these teeth can be replaced with either implants or bridges.

Case Report 25.2. A 14-year-old patient presents after closure of a left complete cleft lip and palate. The left-sided dentoalveolar cleft was repaired at age 9. Tooth #10 was extracted at the time of dentoalveolar cleft grafting because it was malformed and erupted high into the cleft. (See Figures 25.10, 25.11, and 25.12.)

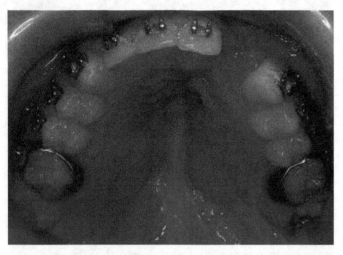

Figure 25.10.   There is healthy attached tissue, but a slight deficiency in the ridge remains. A decision is made to perform an additional graft to the ridge and place an implant to replace the missing lateral.

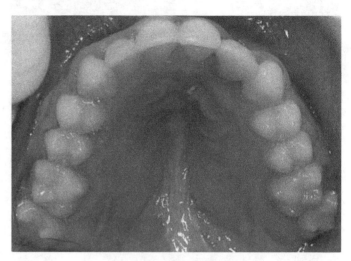

Figure 25.12.   Restored dentition and reconstructed maxillary alveolus. There is a slight indentation within the buccal alveolus in the area of the original cleft.

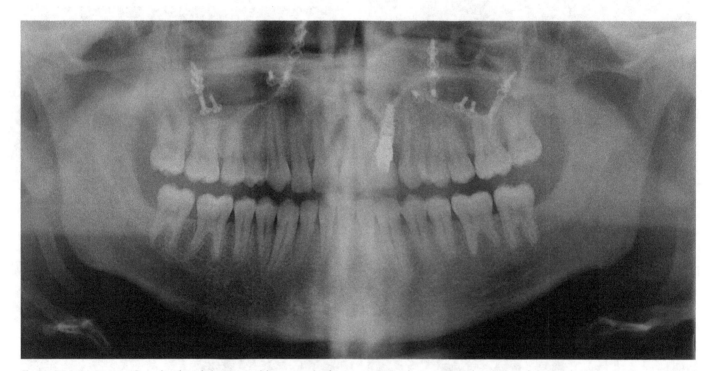

Figure 25.11.   At age 18, an implant is in place with a ceramic abutment. Note the superior placement of the implant due to the scarcity of bone and the presence of thick scar tissue.

References

Bruce, E.N., 2000. Alveolar-anterior maxillary cleft repair. *Atlas of Oral and Maxillofacial Surgery Clinics of North America*, 17, 167–73.

Cho-Lee, G.Y., Garcia-Diez, E.M., Nunes, R.A., Martí-Pagès, C., Sieira-Gil, R. and Rivera-Baró, A., 2013. Review of secondary alveolar cleft repair. *Annals of Maxillofacial Surgery*, 3, 46–50.

Deodatta, B.V. and Ferdinand, O.A., 2002. Rhinoplasty in adolescent cleft patients. *Oral and Maxillofacial Surgery Clinics of North America*, 14, 453–61.

Epker, B.N., 2009. Alveolar-anterior maxillary cleft repair. *Atlas of Oral and Maxillofacial Surgery Clinics of North America*, 17, 167–73.

Francis, C.S., Mobin, S.N. and Lypka, M.A., 2013. rhBMP-2 with a demineralized bone matrix scaffold versus autologous iliac crest bone graft for alveolar cleft reconstruction. *Plastic and Reconstructive Surgery*, 131, 1107–15.

Kaban, L.B. and Troulis, M.J., 2004. *Pediatric oral and maxillofacial surgery*. Philadelphia: W.B. Saunders.

Kazemi, A., Stearns, J.W. and Fonseca, R.J., 2002. Secondary grafting in the alveolar cleft patient. *Oral and Maxillofacial Surgery Clinics of North America*, 14, 477–90.

Koh, K.S., Kim, H., Oh, T.S., Kwon, S.M. and Choi, J.W., 2013. Treatment algorithm for bilateral alveolar cleft based on the position of the premaxilla and width of the alveolar gap. *Journal of Plastic, Reconstructive and Aesthetic Surgery*, 66(9), 1212–8.

Larsen, P.E., 2004. Reconstruction of the alveolar cleft. In M. Miloro, ed. *Peterson's principles of oral and maxillofacial surgery*. London: B.C. Decker. Pp. 859–70.

Matsa, S., Murugan, S. and Kannadasan, K., 2012. Evaluation of morbidity associated with iliac crest harvest for alveolar cleft bone grafting. *Journal of Oral and Maxillofacial Surgery*, 11, 91–5.

Meyer, S. and Molsted, K., 2013. Long-term outcome of secondary alveolar bone grafting in cleft lip and palate patients: a 10-year follow-up cohort study. *Journal of Plastic Surgery and Hand Surgery*, 47(6), 503–8.

Miloro, M., Ghali, G.E. and Larsen, P.E., 2004. *Peterson's principles of oral and maxillofacial surgery*. 3rd ed. London: B.C. Decker.

Posnick, J.C., 2000. Cleft lip and palate: bone grafting and management of residual oronasal fistula. In J.C. Posnick, ed. *Craniofacial and maxillofacial surgery in children and young adults*. Philadelphia: W.B. Saunders. Pp. 827–59.

Posnick, J.C., 2000. *Craniofacial and maxillofacial surgery in children and young adults*. Philadelphia: W.B. Saunders.

Toscano, D., Baciliero, U. and Gracco, A., et al., 2012. Long-term stability of alveolar bone grafts in cleft palate patients. *American Journal of Orthodontics and Dentofacial Orthopedics*, 142, 289–99.

26 Cleft Palate Repair

Bart Nierzwicki[1] and Thaer Daifallah[2]
[1]*Private Practice, Millennium Surgical, Chicago, Illinois, USA*
[2]*Department of Oral and Maxillofacial Surgery, University of Missouri–Kansas City, Kansas City, Missouri, USA*

A means of repairing congenital palatal defects utilizing nasal and oral mucoperiosteal flaps to achieve complete palate closure and velopharyngeal competence with minimal impact of maxillary growth.

Indication

1. Hard and soft tissue defects of the palate

Contraindications

1. No absolute contraindications
2. Relative contraindications include medical comorbidities which preclude the use of general anesthesia

Anatomy

Muscles of soft palate:
1. Levator palatini
2. Tensor palatini
3. Palatopharyngeus
4. Palatoglossus
5. Musculus uvulae

Bardach Two-Flap Palatoplasty Technique

1. The patient is placed supine on the operating table and orally intubated with a RAE endotracheal tube.
2. The neck is carefully hyperextended for better visualization of the palate and alveolar process.
3. The oral cavity and face are prepped with povidone–iodine and draped.
4. A Dingman or similar retractor is inserted to allow complete exposure of the palate from the uvula to the anterior maxillary alveolus.
5. Methylene blue on a 30G needle tip is used to mark the proposed incision sites adjacent to the cleft defect.
6. Local anesthetic containing a vasoconstrictor is infiltrated into the upper lip vestibule, alveolar cleft, hard palate, soft palate, and vomer mucoperiosteum.
7. Nasal cavities are packed with oxymetazoline-soaked cottonoids.
8. Incisions are initiated with a #15c blade immediately adjacent to the cleft at the junction of the nasal and oral mucosal lining within the soft and hard palate bilaterally.

The incisions originate at the posterior aspect of the cleft and extend anteriorly to the junction of the palatal and alveolar mucosa (Figure 26.1, Case Report 26.1). A second incision is initiated at the junction of the hard palate and the maxillary alveolus. This incision originates at the termination of the first incision and extends posteriorly around the maxillary tuberosities bilaterally.

9. Along the entire length of the cleft, a cottle elevator is used to elevate a full-thickness mucoperiosteal flap separating the nasal mucosa from the oral mucosa. Care is taken to preserve the greater palatine vascular pedicle.
10. Once elevated, the oral mucosal flaps are retracted laterally with 4-0 silk sutures (Figure 26.2, Case Report 26.1). Fibrous attachments around the vascular pedicle are freed, and the abnormal attachments of the levator palatini and tensor palatini muscle area are released bilaterally from the palatine bones.
11. The nasal lining is freed from the palatine bone, and the levator palatini muscle is freed from the nasal and oral lining. Judicious use of bipolar cautery is utilized for hemostasis.
12. A vomer flap is elevated to allow for a tension-free closure of the nasal mucosa. The vomer mucoperiosteum is split asymmetrically, and it is elevated from the anterior edge of the cleft and extends to the junction of the hard and soft palate.
13. The hard palate extent of the cleft is repaired with a two-layer closure. The soft palate extent of the cleft is repaired with a three-layer closure. The nasal lining of the hard palate and soft palate is primarily closed using 5-0 Monocryl interrupted and running sutures (Figure 26.3, Case Report 26.1). For wide clefts where primary closure of the nasal mucosa cannot be achieved, acellular dermis (AlloDerm Lifecell, Bridgewater, NJ, USA) can be sewn to the nasal lining of the hard and soft palate to minimize the risk of fistula formation. Alternatively, a dermal graft can be used from the groin area. Because the autologous dermis is elastic in nature, it is easier to suture than AlloDerm.
14. Intravelar veloplasty is performed. The velum musculature is detached and repositioned posteriorly and toward the midline. The uvula is split, and excess mucosal tissue is excised. The uvula is reconstructed using 5-0 Monocryl interrupted horizontal mattress sutures.

Atlas of Operative Oral and Maxillofacial Surgery, First Edition. Edited by Christopher J. Haggerty and Robert M. Laughlin
© 2015 John Wiley & Sons, Inc. Published 2015 by John Wiley & Sons, Inc.

15. The 4-0 silk retraction sutures are removed, and the oral mucosa is primarily closed from the uvula to the anterior extent of the incision with 5-0 Monocryl interrupted horizontal mattress sutures (Figure 26.4, Case Report 26.1). Nasal and oral lining are sutured together with 5-0 Monocryl to obliterate dead space between nasal and oral linings. Additional sutures are placed between the hard palate mucoperiosteum and the attached gingiva anteriorly and laterally using 4-0 Monocryl interrupted sutures. Exposed alveolar bone is covered with the vomer flap from the noncleft side and the lip vestibular mucosal flap.

Postoperative Management

1. The airway is closely monitored within the first 24–48 hours for concerns related to postoperative edema.
2. Flap checks are performed within the first 48 hours to evaluate blood flow within the palatal mucosal flaps.
3. Postoperative nutrition is aimed at preventing suction-generated stress on the palate repair. A full liquid diet is maintained for the first week.
4. Adequate oral hygiene for patients with teeth.
5. Five days of postoperative antibiotics based on the patient's weight in kilograms is recommended.

Complications

1. **Flap necrosis**: Due to severance of the greater palatine vascular pedicle.
2. **Velopharyngeal insufficiency (VPI)**: VPI results from improper muscle repositioning and/or insufficient soft palate length. Symptoms of VPI include hypernasality and nasal air emissions. VPI can be treated with secondary palatal lengthening, a superiorly based pharyngeal flap, or sphincter (lateral) pharyngoplasty.
3. **Oronasal fistula**: Results from the inability to achieve complete, tension-free closure of all flaps or from flap necrosis due to loss of blood supply. Symptoms include nasal air escape and regurgitation of oral fluids. Its incidence is related to the surgeon's experience (the most significant variable) and the patient's age at the time of repair. Less often related is the type of repair or the severity of the cleft deformity. This can be corrected with re-elevation of palatal flaps as in the original repair, local pedicled flaps (the tongue flap, musculo-mucosal flap, temporalis flap, and local palatal mucoperiosteal flap), dermis grafts, or a vascularized pedicle flap such as the facial artery musculo-mucosal flap (FAMM flap).
4. **Maxillary growth restriction**: Restricted maxillary growth frequently occurs when repairs are attempted before 9 months of age. Twenty-five percent of patients repaired between 9 and 18 months of age show some maxillary growth restriction. Maxillary growth restrictions are initially managed with orthodontics, including maxillary expansion and face mask protraction

appliances, and later with orthognathic surgery once skeletal maturity is reached.

Key Points

1. Regardless of the technique utilized, the goals of cleft palate surgery include establishing an intact palate along the entire course of the palatal defect, avoiding oro-nasal fistulae, and minimizing the risk of VPI through the creation of a dynamic soft palate that allows for natural phonation.
2. Although not always possible, especially with wide clefts, exposure of the palatal bone should be minimized in order to prevent the formation of palatal scar tissue resulting in restricted maxillary growth.
3. Advantages of the Bardach two-flap palatoplasty technique include the complete closure of the entire palate in a one-stage procedure, the creation of a more physiologic soft palate muscle sling, and a layered closure technique. The hard palate is closed in two layers (nasal mucosa and oral mucosa). The soft palate is closed in three layers (nasal mucosa, soft palate musculature, and oral mucosa).
4. Speech outcomes are better when soft and hard palate repair is completed before speech development (9–12 months of age).

Case Report

Case Report 26.1. Bardach two-flap palatoplasty. (See Figures 26.1, 26.2, 26.3, and 26.4.)

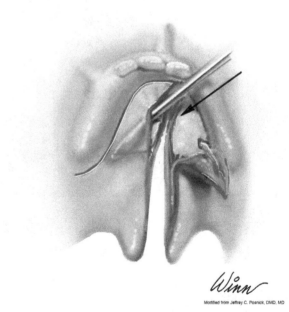

Figure 26.1.   An incision separating the oral and nasal mucosa is initiated. The incision originates at the uvula and extends anteriorly to the junction of the palatal and alveolar mucosa. A second incision is initiated at the junction of the hard palate and the maxillary alveolus. This incision originates at the termination of the first incision and extends posteriorly around the maxillary tuberosities bilaterally. (Image modified with permission from Dr. Jeffrey C. Posnick.)

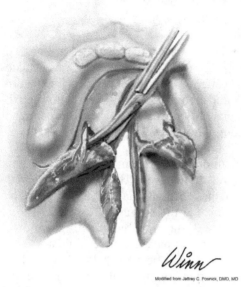

Figure 26.2.   Along the entire length of the cleft, a cottle elevator is used to elevate a full-thickness mucoperiosteal flap separating the nasal mucosa from the oral mucosa. Care is taken to preserve the greater palatine vascular pedicle. (Image modified with permission from Dr. Jeffrey C. Posnick.)

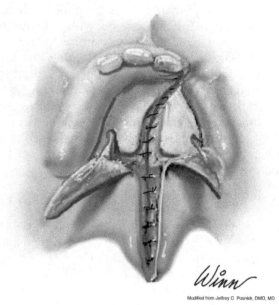

Figure 26.3.   The nasal lining of the hard palate and soft palate is primarily closed using 5-0 Monocryl interrupted and running sutures. (Image modified with permission from Dr. Jeffrey C. Posnick.)

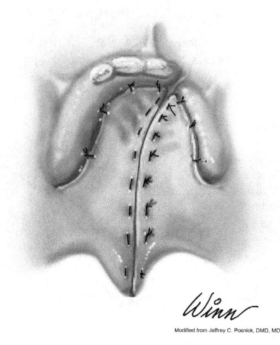

Figure 26.4.   The oral mucosa is closed from the uvula to the anterior extent of the incision. Additional sutures are placed between the hard palate mucoperiosteum and the attached gingiva anteriorly and laterally. (Image modified with permission from Dr. Jeffrey C. Posnick.)

References

Katzel, E.B., Basile, P., Koltz, P.F., Marcus, J.R. and Girotto, J.A., 2009. Current surgical practices in cleft care: cleft palate repair techniques and postoperative management. *Plastic and Reconstructive Surgery*, 124, 899–906.

Losken, H.W., van Aalst, J.A., Teotia, S.S., Dean, S.B., Hultman, S. and Uhrich, K.S., 2011. Achieving low cleft palate fistula rates: surgical results and techniques. *Cleft Palate-Craniofacial Journal*, 48, 312–20.

Padwa, B.L. and Mulliken, J.B., 2003. Complications associated with cleft lip and palate repair. *Oral and Maxillofacial Surgery Clinics of North America*, 15, 285–96.

Salyer, K.E., Sng, K.W. and Sperry, E.E., 2006. Two-flap palatoplasty: 20-year experience and evolution of surgical technique. *Plastic and Reconstructive Surgery*, 118, 193–204.

27 Cleft Lip Repair

Bart Nierzwicki[1] and Thaer Daifallah[2]
[1]*Private Practice, Millennium Surgical, Chicago, Illinois, USA*
[2]*Department of Oral and Maxillofacial Surgery, University of Missouri–Kansas City, Kansas City, Missouri, USA*

A technique of repairing congenital lip defects utilizing a three-layer closure of skin, muscle, and mucosa to achieve nasal and labial symmetry and normal lip function with minimal visible scarring.

Indication

1. Unilateral or bilateral, complete or incomplete cleft lip deformity

Contraindications

1. No absolute contraindications
2. Adequate patient's age, weight, and hemoglobin ("rule of 10s")

Anatomy

1. Orbicularis oris muscle
2. Columella
3. Philtral ridges and tubercle (procheilon)
4. White skin roll (epidermis–vermilion junction line)
5. Red line (vermilion–mucosa junction line)
6. Alar cartilage
7. Lower lateral cartilage
8. Nasal septum
9. Anterior nasal spine

Modified Millard's Rotation-Advancement Flap Technique

1. The patient is placed supine on the operating table and orally intubated with a RAE endotracheal tube.
2. The oral cavity and face are prepped with povidone–iodine and draped.
3. A sterile marking pen or methylene blue on a 30G needle tip are used to mark the rotational flap (M flap), advancement flap (L flap), columella flap (C flap), and turbinate flap. Points of the Cupid's bow are marked on the epidermis–vermilion junction line (the white skin roll), and the vermilion–mucosa junction line (the red line) is also marked (Figure 27.1; see also Figure 27.3 in Case Report 27.1). Important landmarks in marking order:

   - Landmark 2 is the top of the Cupid's bow on the noncleft side.
   - Landmark 3 is the end of the white roll on the non-cleft side.
   - Landmark 1 represents the middle of the Cupid's bow.
   - Landmark 3' is the end of the white roll on the cleft side.
   - Landmark 4 is the noncleft-side labial commissure.
   - Landmark 5 is the cleft-side labial commissure.
   - Landmark 6 is the center of the columella.
   - Landmark 7 is the base of the columella on the noncleft side.
   - Landmark 8 is the base of the columella on the cleft side.
   - Ideally, the distance from 4 to 2 should be equal to that from 5 to 3'; however, it is not always possible.
   - The distance from 2 to 7 must equal that from 3 (and 3') to 8.

4. Local anesthetic containing a vasoconstrictor is infiltrated into above flaps (weight-based dosage).
5. The nasal cavities are packed with oxymetazoline-soaked cottonoids.
6. Incisions are made with a #15c scalpel blade around the rotation flap and C flap, extending across the white roll into the vermilion.
7. Elevation of mucosal flaps in the submucosal plane; all abnormal orbicularis oris attachments are removed from the premaxilla.
8. The M flap is elevated in the submucosal plane, and the C flap in the subdermal plane.
9. The orbicularis oris muscle is elevated from the overlying skin and mucosa within the rotation flap and completely detached from the nasal floor and anterior nasal spine for downward rotation.
10. An incision from the C flap is extended into the caudal nasal septal base through the mucosa and partially through the mucoperichondrium with sharp dissection to perform septoplasty.
11. A ligamentous attachment anterior to the caudal septum is detached, and submucoperichondrial dissection allows separation of the cartilaginous septum from the mucoperichondrium.
12. Separation of the septum from the vomer and reduction into the midline position.

Atlas of Operative Oral and Maxillofacial Surgery, First Edition. Edited by Christopher J. Haggerty and Robert M. Laughlin
© 2015 John Wiley & Sons, Inc. Published 2015 by John Wiley & Sons, Inc.

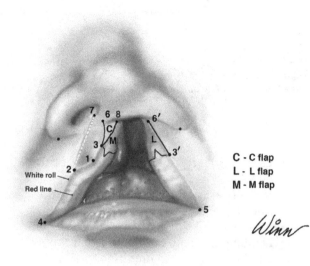

Figure 27.1. A pen and a 30G needle tip mark the rotational flap (M flap), advancement flap (L flap), columella flap (C flap), and turbinate flap of a cleft lip.

C - C flap
L - L flap
M - M flap

White roll
Red line

13. The M flap is rotated to deepen the vestibule and sutured with 5-0 Monocryl.
14. L flap elevation and orbicularis oris dissection.
15. Attachment of the L flap to the inferior edge of the caudal septal mucoperichondrial incision with 5-0 Monocryl to create the nasal floor on the cleft side.
16. Elevation of the inferior turbinate flap from the lateral nasal wall by incising in all areas except attachment to the anterior lateral nasal wall. This flap is then rotated from lateral to medial, and it is repaired to the superior edge of the caudal septal mucoperichondrial incision with 5-0 Monocryl to create the top layer of the nasal floor on the cleft side.
17. Reconstruction of orbicularis oris continuity with 5-0 polydiaxanone horizontal mattress sutures.
18. Insertion of the C flap into the nasal floor.
19. Suturing of mucosal and skin incisions (Figure 27.5, Case Report 27.1), and the placement of Dermabond along the skin incision edges.
20. Insertion of lubricated nasal stents.

Postoperative Management

1. Local wound care and topical antibiotic ointment to prevent crusting or drying.
2. Arm restrains for 7–10 days to prevent accidental trauma to the lip; restraints can be removed when the infant is under supervision.
3. Feeding utilizing a Brecht feeder (syringe with a small tube) for the first 2 days. Use of pacifiers are discouraged for a minimum of 2 days.

4. Upper lip massaging with silicone creams (Scarzone) beginning 3 weeks postop.
5. Nasal stents are removed after 1 week and then used for 12 hours in each 24-hour period for 3–6 months.

Complications

1. **Wound infection**: Rare but can have devastating outcomes, resulting in contraction of tissue and scarring that makes revision more challenging.
2. **Excess scaring**: Due to infection or closure under tension. Hypertrophic scars are managed by massaging the area and using topical steroids. Possible surgical revision or laser treatment after age 5.
3. **Wound dehiscence**: Rare, but may result from trauma to the flap postoperatively and/or failure to achieve layered closure. More commonly seen with inexperienced surgeons.
4. **Poor cosmetic outcomes**: Related to surgical planning, improper techniques, and the level of the surgeon's skill and experience.

Key Points

1. Rule of 10s to qualify infant for early surgical repair. The infant should be at least 10 weeks old and 10 lbs. in weight, with a hemoglobin of at least 10 g/100 ml.
2. Goals of repair: Continuity of the orbicularis oris muscle, and symmetry of the nasal ala, nostrils, philtral ridges, and Cupid's bow. Also, adequate nasal tip projection and fullness to the philtral tubercle.
3. The surgeon should ensure that the distance between the nasal alar base and the vermillion white roll is equal between cleft and noncleft sides.
4. The release of the periosteum covering the piriform aperture on the cleft side will allow elevation and superior placement of the nasal alar base on the cleft side for appropriate symmetry.

Case Report

Case Report 27.1. A 4-month-old male born with a complete unilateral cleft lip involving the left side. The vertical lip height deficiency is approximately 3 mm. Due to the severely deviated nasal septum (to the right) and the enlarged left inferior turbinate causing nasal airway obstruction, a septoplasty and inferior turbinectomy were planned utilizing the turbinate mucosal flap to reconstruct the nasal floor on the cleft side. (See Figures 27.2, 27.3, 27.4, 27.5, and 27.6.)

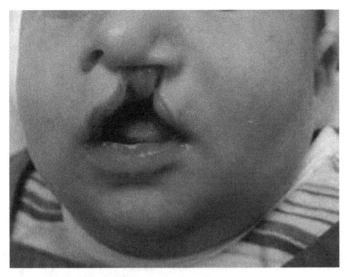

Figure 27.2.   Complete left cleft lip at 4 months of age.

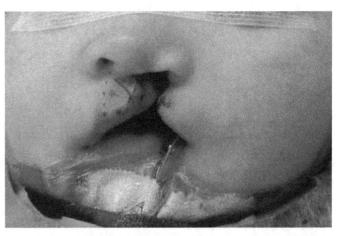

Figure 27.3.   Preoperative markings. Note the interrupted line depicting the distance from the noncleft-side columellar base to the noncleft-side Cupid's bow peak. Landmarks 1, 2, 3, and 3' are tattooed with methylene blue on a 30G needle tip.

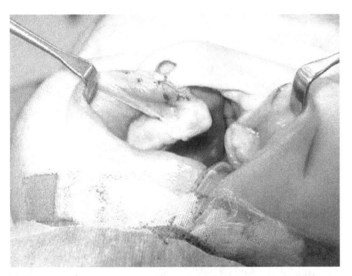

Figure 27.4.   Mucosal flaps: the rotational M (medial; noncleft side) flap and advancement L flap (lateral; cleft side).

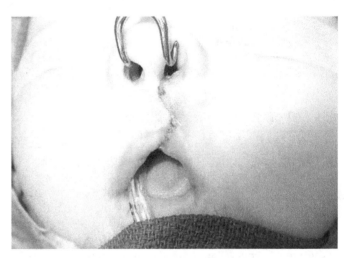

Figure 27.5.   Immediate post-cheiloplasty: note alignment of the vermilion border, white skin roll, and red lines.

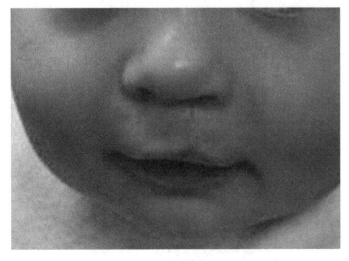

Figure 27.6.   One year postoperatively.

References

Millard, D.R., 1976. *Cleft craft. The evolution of its surgery. I: the unilateral deformity*. Boston: Little, Brown. P. 251.

Millard, D.R., 1960. Complete unilateral clefts of the lip. *Plastic and Reconstructive Surgery*, 25, 595–605.

Millard, D.R., 1964. Refinements in rotation advancement cleft lip technique. *Plastic and Reconstructive Surgery*, 33, 26–38.

Nordoff, M.S., 1984. Reconstruction of vermillion in unilateral and bilateral cleft lips. *Plastic and Reconstructive Surgery*, 73(1), 52–61.

Stal, S., Brown, R.H., Higuera, S., Hollier, L.H., Jr., Byrd, H.S., Cutting, C.B. and Mulliken, J.B., 2009. Fifty years of the Millard rotation-advancement: looking back and moving forward. *Plastic and Reconstructive Surgery*, 123, 1364–77.

CHAPTER

28

Orthognathic Surgery in the Cleft Patient: Le Fort I Osteotomy

Shahid R. Aziz
Rutgers University School of Dental Medicine, Camden, New Jersey, USA

A means of establishing maxillary form and function in the dentoalveolar cleft patient.

Indications

1. Restore facial symmetry
2. Establishment of a class 1 dental occlusion
3. Place the components of the craniofacial skeleton in an ideal aesthetic position
4. Provide stability to the clefted maxilla

Contraindications

1. Class 1 occlusion
2. Dental malocclusion not associated with dentofacial deformities
3. Medical contraindication to general anesthesia
4. Psychological instability

Technique: Modifications to Le Fort I Osteotomies for Unrepaired and Repaired Alveolar Clefts

1. In addition to the standard vestibular incision for a Le Fort osteotomy, extensions are made vertically along the alveolar cleft and oronasal fistula to the palatal aspect of the fistula, thus separating the oral and nasal mucosa. The palatal aspect of these incisions must be undermined to provide for a tension-free closure. However, the palatal mucosa must remain intact to avoid any interruption of blood flow.
2. Osteotomies and bony separation are completed in the same manner as in a traditional Le Fort I osteotomy. However, with an unrepaired unilateral alveolar cleft, once the Le Fort I osteotomy is completed, the maxilla is in two pieces.
3. Downfracture is done by hand with gentle digital pressure. Tessier retractors are placed posterior to the tuberosities, the maxillary soft tissue pedicle is carefully stretched, and the segments are mobilized. Tessier retractors are preferred over Rowe forceps in order to minimize potential trauma to the palatal mucosa.
4. The deviated nasal septum and vomer are trimmed. Bony interferences are removed.

5. The alveolar dental defect is closed by moving the two segments of the maxilla together with the aid of the surgical splint.
6. Cancellous bone grafting may be utilized to fill any residual defects within the alveolus and nasal floor. Cortico-cancellous blocks can be utilized to fill voids within the Le Fort osteotomy.
7. The incisions are primarily closed with care to completely close the oronasal fistula in a watertight, tension-free fashion.
8. If there is a significant degree of bone grafting, some authors advocate keeping the patient in maxillomandibular fixation (MMF) for 4–6 weeks to minimize graft loss.

Technique: Modifications to Le Fort I Osteotomies for Bilateral Clefts

Bilateral cleft patients typically exhibit severe maxillary dysplasia with hypoplastic lateral segments. The premaxillary segment is frequently mobile, malpositioned, and associated with residual oronasal fistulae, bony defects, significant soft tissue scarring, and a tenuous vascular supply. Due to these circumstances, the following surgical modifications are recommended:

1. Vestibular incisions extend from the zygomatic buttress region to the alveolar defects. Within the region of the alveolar cleft, the incision is continued along the mesial line angles of the canine defects.
2. The premaxillary segment incisions are placed adjacent to the distal line angle of the incisor tooth on each side and connected palatally.
3. The nasal and oral mucosa are separated. Care must be taken to maintain the labial vestibule of the premaxillary segment.
4. Osteotomies are completed as normal. However, with an unrepaired bilateral alveolar cleft, once the Le Fort osteotomy is completed, the maxilla is in three pieces.
5. Downfracture is done by hand with gentle digital pressure. Tessier retractors are placed posterior to the tuberosities, the maxillary soft tissue pedicle is carefully stretched and the segments are mobilized. Tessier

---

Atlas of Operative Oral and Maxillofacial Surgery, First Edition. Edited by Christopher J. Haggerty and Robert M. Laughlin
© 2015 John Wiley & Sons, Inc. Published 2015 by John Wiley & Sons, Inc.

retractors are preferred over Rowe forceps in order to minimize potential trauma to the palatal mucosa.

6. The deviated nasal septum and vomer are trimmed. Bony interferences are removed.
7. The premaxillary segment is osteotomized from a palatal approach with an osteotome, with concomitant removal of the vomer bone.
8. The lateral segments are brought into contact with the premaxillary segment utilizing a prefabricated splint. This will close the alveolar cleft defects.
9. Cancellous bone is placed into any voids within the alveolus.
10. Cortico-cancellous blocks are interposed in areas of bony voids along the Le Fort osteotomy.
11. Primary closure of all incisions is performed.
12. MMF may be considered to stabilize the grafted areas.

Postoperative Management

1. Airway security in the immediate postoperative phase is essential.
2. Adequate pain control, antibiotic coverage, and the use of prophylactic steroids is indicated.
3. Frequent monitoring of the gingival perfusion of the anterior maxilla via assessing capillary refill (perfusion) is imperative in bilateral clefts patients status post orthognathic surgery.
4. Patients must maintain adequate oral fluid intake to avoid dehydration.
5. Meticulous oral hygiene is necessary to minimize postoperative infection.
6. Caloric intake and adequate nutrition are essential. A nutritional plan should be created based on the patient's caloric needs to ensure proper nutrition during the initial 2–3 weeks of the postoperative period until masticatory function returns.
7. For patients requiring MMF, MMF is typically released 3–4 weeks postoperatively. Light elastics are used to maintain or reprogram occlusion, and passive mouth-opening exercises are initiated.
8. Orthodontic therapy typically resumes 6–8 weeks post surgery.

Complications

1. **Relapse**: Cleft orthognathic patients typically exhibit a higher degree of surgical relapse than noncleft orthognathic patients. This is due to a much tighter and less forgiving soft tissue envelope found within cleft patients. Relapse often requires a second orthognathic procedure to correct.
2. **Velopharyngeal dysfunction after maxillary advancement**: Consultation with a speech pathologist may be sufficient for mild to moderate cases. Severe cases may require additional pharyngeal surgery.
3. **Alar base widening**: May be minimized postoperatively with the placement of an alar cinch suture.
4. **Incision dehiscence**: Typically occurs from failure to obtain a tension-free closure at the time of surgery. May also occur as a result of early and excessive masticatory function.
5. **Septal deviation**: Most cleft orthognathic patients present with some degree of nasal and septal deviation. An inferior septoplasty should be performed when superiorly repositioning the maxilla. Additional rhinoplasty and septoplasty procedures may be required.

Key Points

1. A coordinated treatment plan is established by the surgeon and orthodontist. In cleft-orthognathic surgeries, additional support in surgical planning is provided by other members of the craniofacial team, such as pediatric dentists, speech pathologists, nutritionists, and psychologists.
2. Preoperative considerations unique to cleft patients undergoing orthognathic correction of maxillary hypoplasia and asymmetries include assessment of associated alveolar cleft (unilateral or bilateral, and whether previous and adequate bone grafting was performed or it is unrepaired), assessment of velopharyngeal and speech function, presence of oronasal fistula, psychological evaluation, and required movements to correct the dentofacial deformity (single jaw [Le Fort] vs. double jaw surgery, conventional orthognathic surgery versus maxillary distraction osteogenesis, and the amount of transverse correction required).
3. The majority of cleft-orthognathic patients have an associated alveolar cleft. Ideally, dentoalveolar bone grafting should be completed 5–10 years prior to Le Fort 1 osteotomy, converting a multisegment maxilla into a single-segment unit. In situations where dentoalveolar bone grafting has not been performed or in cases where inadequate bone is present, simultaneous bone grafting combined with orthognathic surgery may be necessary.
4. Repositioning of the maxilla and associated soft tissues may alter the velopharyngeal sphincter. To adequately plan for any potential speech issues after surgery, a speech pathology evaluation and naso-endoscopy (to determine the number of ports) are indicated prior to surgery.
5. The presence of an oronasal fistula requires modification of the standard Le Fort I incision design.
6. Psychological evaluation is a consideration for any young adult undergoing orthognathic surgery; however, children with clefts have a unique situation in which they have undergone multiple surgeries and are often extremely self-conscious about their facial morphology.

7. Surgical imaging is necessary in planning orthognathic surgery. For the cleft-orthognathic patient, a 3D computed tomography (CT) scan is of value to allow the surgeon to familiarize him- or herself with the aberrant bony anatomy of the maxillary, nasal, and palatine bones. Medical models can be made from preoperative CT scans in order to obtain additional information.
8. An angiogram may be of added value to evaluate the vasculature of the palate, oropharynx, and maxilla to evaluate for potential vascular anomalies.
9. The palatal and vestibular tissue surrounding the maxilla in a cleft patient undergoing Le Fort I osteotomy surgery may demonstrate significant scar tissue with minimal elasticity. As such, extreme maxillary movements in the anterior and transverse directions can be particularly challenging, if not impossible. Extreme anterior maxillary movement (>8 mm advancement) may benefit from distraction osteogenesis, and extreme transverse movements (>5 mm) may benefit from a surgically assisted rapid palatal expansion rather than, or in addition to, conventional orthognathic surgery.

References

Phillips, J.H., Nish, I. and Daskalogiannakis, J., 2012. Orthognathic surgery in cleft patents. *Plastic and Reconstructive Surgery*, 129, 535e.

Posnick, J.C., 1997. Maxillary deficiency: unilateral cleft lip and palate. In: *Fundamentals of maxillofacial surgery*. New York: Springer. Ch. 19.

Wolford, L.M., 1992. Effects of orthognathic surgery on nasal for m and function in the cleft patient. *Cleft Palate-Craniofacial Journal*, 29, 546.

PART FIVE

TEMPOROMANDIBULAR JOINT SURGERY

29

Temporomandibular Joint Imaging

Joshua Stone[1] and Christopher J. Haggerty[2]

[1]*Department of Oral and Maxillofacial Surgery, University of Missouri–Kansas City, Kansas City, Missouri, USA*
[2]*Private Practice, Lakewood Oral and Maxillofacial Surgery Specialists, Lees Summit; and Department of Oral and Maxillofacial Surgery, University of Missouri–Kansas City, Kansas City, Missouri, USA*

Indications

1. Evaluation of intra-articular abnormalities (internal derangement)
2. Evaluation of lockjaw
3. Preoperative evaluation of a dysfunctional joint
4. Evaluation of soft tissue changes associated with inflammatory arthritides

Contraindications

1. Implantable metal devices (indwelling pacemakers, intracranial vascular clips, etc.) and foreign body fragments are contraindications for magnetic resonance imaging (MRI)
2. Documented allergy to contrast. Patients with impaired renal function are also contraindicated to receiving intravascular contrast
3. Pregnancy

Relative Contraindications

1. Obesity
2. Claustrophobia
3. Inability to remain motionless

Definitions

Internal derangement: An abnormal relationship involving the articular disc, condyle, and articular eminence.

Magnetic resonance imaging (MRI): A non-ionizing radiation modality utilizing magnetic frequencies and radiofrequencies in image generation. MRI provides cross-sectional multiplanar images that illustrate both soft and osseous tissue abnormalities of the joint, surrounding structures, and dynamic assessment of condylar translation and disc movement (with open and closed views).

T1-weighted MRI images: The anatomy of the temporomandibular joint (TMJ) is clearly defined, and the articular disc is distinctly visible. Fluids are hypointense, whereas fats are hyperintense.

T2-weighted MRI images: Useful for visualizing degenerative periarticular changes and the presence of joint effusions. Fluids are hyperintense in T2-weighted images.

Technitium-99m (T99m) bone scan: T99m is a radioactive compound, which is useful in determining active bone metabolism. The compound uptake depends on osseous blood flow and osteogenesis. Common uses include utilization in determining active condylar growth (i.e., condylar hyperplasia) and bone tumors.

Postgadolinium dynamic enhancement: Contrast agent used to enhance retrodiscal inflammation. Gadolinium can cause nephrogenic systemic fibrosis (i.e., nephrogenic fibrosing dermatopathy) in patients with diminished renal function.

Anatomy

Articular disc: Composed of dense fibrous connective tissue that is nonvascular and non-innervated. The articular disc can be divided into three distinct regions: a thickened anterior and posterior band, and a central intermediate zone. The three distinct regions of the articular disc contribute to the bowtie morphology as seen in sagittal T1-weighted closed-mouth MRI images. The central intermediate zone is the thinnest area, and the area under function between the condylar head and the articular eminence during translation. The posterior band is the thickest area and attaches to the retrodiscal tissues. The normal position of the posterior band in relation to the condyle is the 12 o'clock position in open and closed views. The normal position of the central intermediate zone in relation to the condyle is the 10 o'clock position in the open and closed views.

Retrodiscal tissues: The posterior band of the articular disc is continuous with the highly innervated and highly vascular retrodiscal tissues located within the bilaminar zone. Compression of the retrodiscal tissue is a potential source of TMJ discomfort.

Bilaminar zone: Posteriorly the disc blends with the bilaminar zone, which is composed of the superior and inferior retrodiscal lamina.

Superior retrodiscal lamina: Composed predominately of elastic fibers, which provide the posterior attachment of the articular disc to the tympanic plate and to the external auditory canal perichondrium. Functions to resist extreme translatory disc movements.

Inferior retrodiscal lamina: Composed of dense, longitudinally oriented fibers that attach the articular disc to the posterior condyle. Functions in preventing extreme rotation of the disc with rotational movements of the condyle.

Figure 29.1 shows the articular disc in its normal position.

Atlas of Operative Oral and Maxillofacial Surgery, First Edition. Edited by Christopher J. Haggerty and Robert M. Laughlin
© 2015 John Wiley & Sons, Inc. Published 2015 by John Wiley & Sons, Inc.

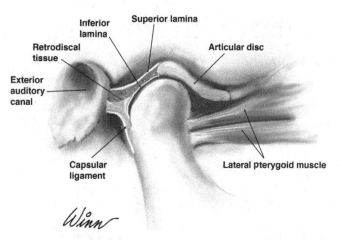

Figure 29.1.   Illustration depicting the normal position of the disc and associated structures on sagittal closed-mouth view.

Five Temporomandibular Joint Ligaments

1. **Medial and lateral collateral (discal) ligament**: Attaches the articular disc to the medial and lateral condylar head (see Figure 29.4 in Case Report 29.1). Separates the joint into superior and inferior compartments. Allows the disc to rotate on the condylar head.
2. **Capsular ligament**: Attaches to the condylar head anteriorly, posteriorly, medially, and laterally to surround the entire joint maintaining the synovial fluid compartment. Originates superiorly from the articular fossa and inserts inferiorly to surround the condylar head. Prevents inferior distracting forces of the condyle.
3. **Temporomandibular ligament**: Originates at the articular tubercle and zygomatic process, and inserts along the lateral pole and lateral aspect of the condyle. Limits inferior distraction and posterior movement of the condyles.
4. **Sphenomandibular ligament**: Originates from the spine of the sphenoid bone and inserts onto the lingula. Provides medial support of the TMJ.
5. **Stylomandibular ligament**: Originates from the styloid process and inserts onto the angle of the mandible. Limits protrusive movements of the TMJ.

Innervation of the TMJ: The auriculotemporal, masseteric, and deep temporal nerves.

Vascularization of the TMJ: Multiple vessels participate in the vascularization of the joint, including the superficial temporal, middle meningeal, internal maxillary, deep auricular, anterior tympanic, and ascending pharyngeal vessels.

Magnetic Resonance Imaging (MRI) Technique

T1- and T2-weighted image with thin slices (1–3 mm) in open- and closed-mouth orientation with axial, coronal, and sagittal reformatting. The technician must ensure that the MRIs are aligned such that the sections will be oriented along the long axis of the condyle and the entire joint space and surrounding structures are captured.

Articular Disc Function and Common Disorders

Normal articular disc function: Normal translation involves maintenance of the central intermediate zone of the disc between the condylar head and the articular eminence during opening and closing. This process is represented on an MRI with the posterior band of the disc located at the 12 o'clock position and the central intermediate zone of the articular disc located at the 10 o'clock position in relation to the condyle on both open and closed views (Figures 29.2, 29.3, and 29.4, Case Report 29.1).

Anterior displaced disc with reduction (ADDWR): Typically presents as a limited opening with or without clicking after excessive function severs the superior retrodiscal lamina. When anteriorly displaced, the classic bowtie appearance of the disc is altered to an elliptical shape. This process is represented on an MRI with the posterior band of the disc located anterior to the condylar head in the closed view, but with a normal disc–condyle relationship in the open view.

Anterior displaced disc with reduction (ADDWOR): Typically presents as the inability to open after excessive function severs the superior retrodiscal lamina. This process is represented on an MRI with the posterior band of the disc located anterior to the condylar head in both open and closed views (Figure 29.5). Adequate open views are frequently difficult to obtain due to limited opening from the mechanical obstruction of the anteriorly displaced disc.

Key Points

1. For patients undergoing MRI evaluation with limited opening due to discomfort, it is important to obtain a vertical opening of at least 20–25 mm in order to ensure adequate translation of the discs for open view evaluation. Failure to obtain adequate opening will impair the ability to evaluate the translation of the disc. Patients are often given a mouth prop or bite block to utilize during imaging to ensure adequate open views and to minimize inadvertent movement.
2. When evaluating a TMJ MRI, the articular disc morphology and the relationship between the articular disc, the mandibular condyle, the articular eminence, and the glenoid fossa are evaluated in both open and closed views.
3. The mandibular condyle is evaluated for irregularities such as erosion, flattening, resorption, sclerosis, osteophytosis, masses, cysts, subchondral marrow edema, and intracapsular fractures. The articular eminence and glenoid fossa are evaluated for morphology and air cells. The joint cavity itself is evaluated for hemarthroses, effusions, masses, and synovitis.
4. Although anterior displacement of the disc is the most common type of displacement, the disc may also be displaced posteriorly, laterally, and/or medially in relation to the condyle.

Case Report 29.1. Normal articular disc position. A 24-year-old female presents with a chief complaint of left-sided facial pain on jaw functioning. The patient has no appreciable joint sounds or dysfunction. On examination, no occlusal discrepancies were identified. The patient demonstrated normal forward and lateral mandibular protrusions and displayed a maximum vertical opening of 25 mm without pain and 40 mm with pain. Bilateral open- and closed-mouth magnetic resonance imaging demonstrated no joint abnormalities, no disc irregularities, and normal translation of the disc on open and closed views. No condyle anomalies or effusions were noted. The patient was diagnosed with myofascial pain and treated with conservative therapy consisting of a monoplane occlusal splint, nonsteroidal anti-inflammatory drugs, and a soft mechanical diet. (See Figures 29.2, 29.3, and 29.4.)

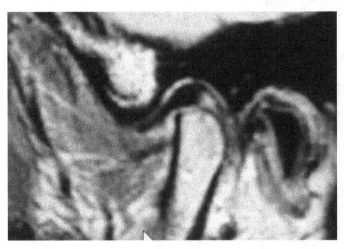

Figure 29.2. T1-weighted sagittal closed-mouth magnetic resonance imaging depicting normal positioning of the biconcave articular disc. The posterior band of the disc is positioned at the 12 o'clock position in relation to the condyle. The central intermediate zone of the disc is positioned at the 10 o'clock position in relation to the condyle.

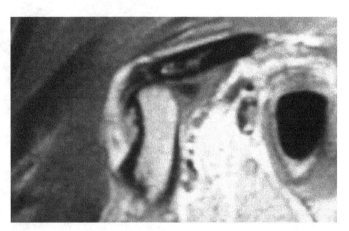

Figure 29.3. T1-weighted sagittal open-mouth magnetic resonance imaging depicting the normal position of the biconcave articular disc.

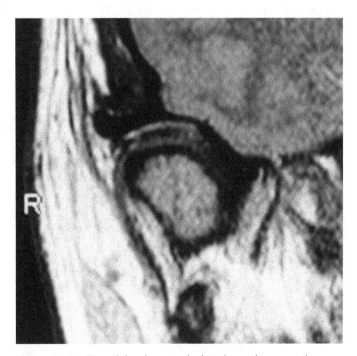

Figure 29.4. T1-weighted coronal closed-mouth magnetic resonance imaging depicting the normal position of the disc over the condylar head and the attachments of the collateral ligaments.

Case Report 29.2. Anteriorly displaced articular disc without reduction (ADDWOR). A 19-year-old male presents with chief complaints of recent left-sided facial pain and limited opening. The patient reports a subluxation of his temporomandibular joint (TMJ) after extreme opening. The subluxation was reduced by an emergency room physician. The patient presents 4 days after reduction with moderate pain located within his left TMJ and limited opening (4 mm). A magnetic resonance imaging (MRI) was obtained, and the T1-weighted sagittal open and closed views demonstrated an anteriorly displaced disc without reduction. The patient was successfully treated with arthrocentesis of the symptomatic joint, a soft mechanical diet, restriction of extreme opening, and a short course of nonsteroidal anti-inflammatory drugs. (See Figure 29.5.)

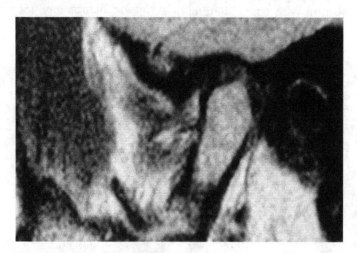

Figure 29.5. T1-weighted sagittal closed-mouth magnetic resonance imaging depicting an anteriorly displaced articular disc. T1-weighted sagittal open-mouth magnetic resonance imaging demonstrated an anteriorly displaced articular disc without reduction.

Case Report 29.3. Temporomandibular joint (TMJ) effusion. A 32-year-old female presents with a chief complaint of right-sided TMJ pain without dysfunction. T1–weighted open and closed images demonstrate no signs of disc displacement, no evidence of condylar anomalies and normal translation of the disc. T2-weighted images demonstrate a hyperintense signal within the right joint space on open and closed views consistent with a joint effusion. The patient was successfully treated with conservative therapy utilizing a soft mechanical diet, nonsteroidal anti-inflammatory drugs, and 3 months of splint usage. (See Figure 29.6.)

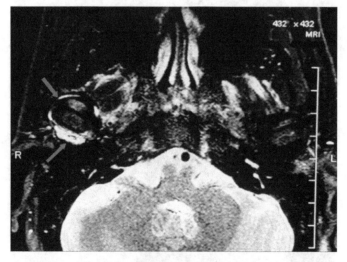

Figure 29.6. T2-weighted axial closed-mouth magnetic resonance imaging depicting an area of high signal intensity within the right joint space representing a large joint effusion. The articular disc has a relatively low signal intensity on T2-weighted images.

Case Report 29.4. Temporomandibular joint (TMJ) mass. A 58-year-old male presents 5 weeks after a blow to the chin with a chief complaint of limited opening (10 mm), right-sided TMJ pain, and malocclusion. The patient did not seek treatment until 5 weeks after the insult. T1- and T2-weighted magnetic resonance imaging was obtained and demonstrated a soft tissue mass within the right joint space and an anteriorly displaced disc without reduction (see Figure 29.7). The patient was treated with open arthroplasty, removal of the mass (granulation tissue), and posterior disc repositioning using a Mitek anchor.

Case Report 29.5. Facial asymetry in growing patient. An 18-year-old patient presents with a chief complaint of increasing facial asymmetry appreciated over the past 12 months. An orthopantomogram demonstrated left condylar hyperplasia. A T99m-scan was attained and noted increased uptake of radiotracer within the left mandibular condyle. The patient was reappointed for a repeat scan in 6 months to determine cessation of his hyperplastic condition. The patient will undergo surgical corection of their skeletal deformity once growth stabilizes. (See Figure 29.8.)

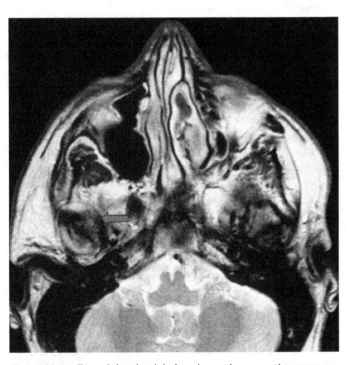

Figure 29.7. T1-weighted axial closed-mouth magnetic resonance imaging depicting an area of hypointense material within the right joint space.

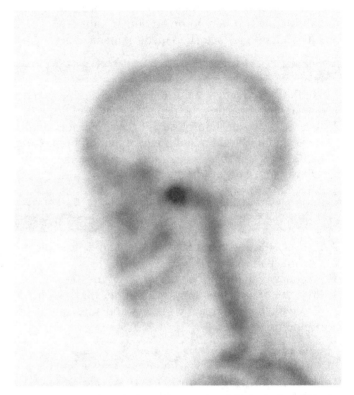

Figure 29.8. T99m scan demonstrating increased uptake within the left condylar head in a patient with active condylar hyperplasia.

References

Brooks, S.L., Brand, J.W., Gibbs, S.J., Hollender, L., Lurie, A.G., Omnell, K.A., Westesson, P.L. and White, S.C., 1997. Imaging of the temporomandibular joint: a position paper of the American Academy of Oral and Maxillofacial Radiology. *Oral Surgery, Oral Medicine, Oral Pathology, Oral Radiology, and Endodontology*, 83(5), 609–18.

Carroll, Q.B., 2011. *Radiography in the digital age: physics, exposure, radiation biology.* Springfield, IL: Charles C. Thomas.

Eastman, G. and Wald, C., 2005. *Getting started in clinical radiology: from image to diagnosis.* New York, NY: TIS.

Kaban, L.B., Cisneros, G.J., Heyman, S. and Treves, S., 1982. Assessment of mandibular growth by skeletal scintigraphy. *Journal of Oral and Maxillofacial Surgery*, 40(1), 18–22.

Koh, K.J., Park, H.N. and Kim, K.A., 2013. Relationship between anterior disc displacement with/without reduction and effusion in temporomandibular disorder patients using magnetic resonance imaging. *Imaging Science in Dentistry*, 43(4), 245–51.

Lewis, E.L., Dolwick, M.F., Abramowicz, S. and Reeder, S.L., 2008. Contemporary imaging of the temporomandibular joint. *Dental Clinics of North America*, 52(4), 875–90, viii.

Okeson, J.P., 2003. *Management of temporomandibular disorders and occlusion.* 5th ed. St. Louis, MO: Mosby.

Shintaku, W.H., Venturin, J.S., Langlais, R.P. and Clark, G.T., 2010. Imaging modalities to access bony tumors and hyperplasic reactions of the temporomandibular joint. *Journal of Oral and Maxillofacial Surgery*, 68(8), 1911–21.

Whyte, A.M., McNamara, D., Rosenberg, I. and Whyte, A.W., 2006. Magnetic resonance imaging in the evaluation of temporomandibular joint disc displacement—a review of 144 cases. *International Journal of Oral and Maxillofacial Surgery*, 35(8), 696–703.

CHAPTER

30

Arthrocentesis of the Temporomandibular Joint

Robert M. Laughlin and James MacDowell
Department of Oral and Maxillofacial Surgery, Naval Medical Center San Diego, San Diego, California, USA

Procedure: Arthrocentesis of the Temporomandibular Joint

A highly successful minimally invasive procedure for the initial treatment of temporomandibular joint (TMJ) pain and dysfunction refractory to medical management.

Indications

1. Medically refractory pain to TMJ muscles, headache, or earache impacting the patient's quality of life
2. Altered jaw mechanics such as closed lock, joint hypomobility, and limited range of motion in maximal incisal opening, excursion, and/or protrusion
3. Alterations of occlusion
4. Joint noises associated with pain

Contraindications

1. Presence of concomitant facial pain of separate etiologies
2. Chronic pain disorders
3. Presence of deformity or pathology of the TMJ
4. Presence of local or systemic conditions that may interfere with normal healing process and subsequent tissue homeostasis

Anatomy

Temporomandibular Joint (TMJ): A compound synovial ginglymoarthrodial joint with rotation of the condyle within the inferior joint space. The TMJ has an overlying highly vascular and innervated fibroelastic capsule, which is thickened on the lateral aspect to form the temporomandibular ligament. The vascular supply to the TMJ is supplied with branches from the superficial temporal and maxillary arteries with an extensive venous plexus within the bilaminar zone.

Articular eminence: A prominent convexity lined with dense, compact connective tissue that is subject to loading during function.

Glenoid fossa: A nonloading, concave structure lined with a thin layer of fibrocartilage separated from the middle cranial fossa by 1–2 mm thickness of temporal bone.

Articular disc: A biconcave avascular fibrocartilage disc that divides the joint space into a 1.2 mL upper compartment and a 0.9 mL lower compartment and allows complex movements of rotation and translation.

Auriculotemporal nerve: Provides sensation to the posterior and lateral capsule.

Masseteric nerve: Provides sensation to the anteriomedial aspect of the joint.

Deep temporal nerve: Provides anterolateral sensation to the joint.

Holmlund–Hellsing line (H-H line): A line extending from the lateral canthus of the eye to a point bisecting the tragus of the ear (Figure 30.1 [all figures cited appear in Case Report 30.1]). The 10-2 point (10 mm anterior and 2 mm inferior to the mid-tragus along the line) correlates with the posterior recess/glenoid fossa. The 20-10 point (20 mm anterior to the mid-tragus point along the line and 10 mm below the line) correlates with the prominence of the articular eminence.

Technique

1. Pre-procedural documentation of maximal incisal opening (MIO), excursive movements, and subjective details of pain and dysfunction are measured and recorded.
2. Bacitracin-soaked cotton is placed within the auditory canal to obtund the canal from blood and fluid accumulation.
3. Landmarks are identified and marked with a skin marker referencing the Holmlund–Hellsing line (H-H line), the 10-2 point, and the 20-10 point (Figure 30.1).
4. Surgical skin prep of the area is performed, with the hair taped superior to the auricle with sterile drape.
5. An auriculotemporal nerve block and local infiltration with a solution of 1% lidocaine with 1:100,000 epinephrine is performed at the marked 10-2 and 20-10 points (Figure 30.2).
6. An 18-gauge needle attached to a 10 mL syringe containing normal saline is inserted in an anterior-superior direction at the 10-2 point into the superior joint space

Atlas of Operative Oral and Maxillofacial Surgery, First Edition. Edited by Christopher J. Haggerty and Robert M. Laughlin.
© 2015 John Wiley & Sons, Inc. Published 2015 by John Wiley & Sons, Inc.

(Figure 30.3). The superior joint space is insufflated with enough normal saline to obtain bouncing-back pressure with the syringe and movement of the jaw.

7. The first syringe is removed, leaving the 18-gauge needle in place to observe for a small amount of fluid backflow.

8. A second 18-gauge needle is placed slightly anterior to the first 18-gauge needle along the same angulation to serve as an exit point for the saline lavage (Figure 30.4).

9. Approximately 100 mL of normal saline lavage should be passed through the superior joint space.

10. At the end of the procedure, 1 mL of betamethasone is injected with 1 mL of 0.5% Marcaine with epinephrine into the superior joint space.

11. The inflow and outflow ports are removed, and pressure is applied over the joint for 5 minutes.

Postoperative Management

1. Ice is applied over the joint for 15–20 minutes of every hour for the first 24 hours.

2. Compression dressings are utilized for the first 24 hours for hemostasis and to minimize swelling.

3. Patients are asked to sleep with 30° head-of-bed elevation for the first 48 hours.

4. A soft mechanical diet is required for the first 72 hours postoperatively.

5. Scheduled nonsteroidal anti-inflammatory drugs and as-needed (pro re nata, or PRN) narcotic analgesics are prescribed.

6. Jaw-opening and range-of-motion exercises are begun the day of the procedure and are encouraged several times per day for the first week.

Complications

1. Iatrogenic scuffing of fibrocartilage covering articular eminence and fossa

2. Injury to temporal vessels or maxillary artery, and/or postsurgical bleeding

3. Neuronal damage (CN V, VII, and VII)

4. Damage to articular disk and/or retrodiskal tissue upon entering the joint space

5. Intra-articular fibrosis and adhesions formed after hemorrhage

6. Ear injury from middle-ear penetration

7. Infection

Case Report

Case Report 30.1. A 17-year-old male presents 5 days after extreme opening with subluxation and self-reduction of his left temporomandibular joint, with a chief complaint of left-sided temporomandibular joint (TMJ) pain, limited opening, and minor malocclusion. On examination, the patient has tenderness to the left TMJ area, a maximum incisal opening of 5 mm, restricted lateral excursive movements, and malocclusion. Based on the patient's history and clinical symptoms, a diagnosis of an anteriorly displaced disc without reduction was made. The patient was successfully treated with left TMJ arthrocentesis, passive physical therapy, a soft mechanical diet, restriction of extreme opening, and a short trial of nonsteroidal anti-inflammatory drugs without recurrence of pain, limited opening, or malocclusion. (See Figures 30.1, 30.2, 30.3, and 30.4.)

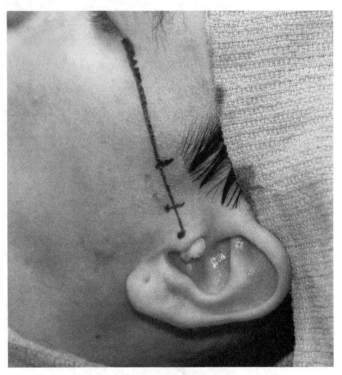

Figure 30.1.   The H-H line and the 10-2 and 20-10 points are marked.

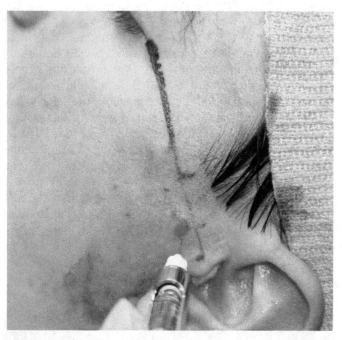

Figure 30.2. Local infiltration and an auriculotemporal nerve block is performed.

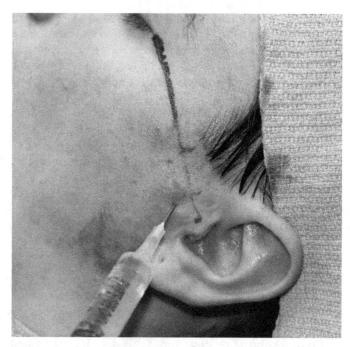

Figure 30.3. An 18-gauge needle attached to a 10 mL syringe is inserted in an anterior-superior direction at the 10-2 point to enter the superior joint space. Entry into the superior joint space is confirmed with superior joint space insufflation and lower jaw movement.

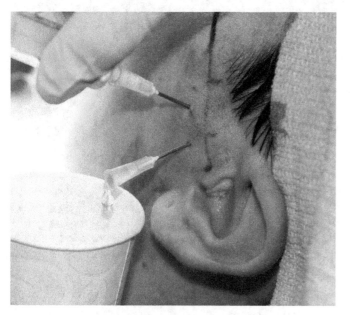

Figure 30.4. A second 18-gauge needle is placed slightly anterior to the first 18-gauge needle and along the same angulation to serve as an exit point for the saline lavage.

References

Carlson, E., 2012. Parameters of care: clinical practice guidelines for oral and maxillofacial surgery—temporomandibular joint surgery (AAOMS ParCare 2012). *Journal of Oral and Maxillofacial Surgery*, 70 (Suppl. 3), e204–31.

Haddle, K., 2001. Arthrocentesis of the TMJ: oral and maxillofacial surgery knowledge update. *TMJ*, 3, 40–50.

Holmlund, A., Hellsing, G. and Wredmark, T., 1986. Arthroscopy of the termporomandibular joint a clinical study. *International Journal of Oral and Maxillofacial Surgery*, 15, 715–21.

Rohen, J.W., Lütjen-Drecoll, E. and Yokochi, C., 2011. *Color atlas of anatomy: a photographic study of the human body*. 7th ed. Philadelphia: Lippincott Williams and Wilkins.

31

Arthroscopic Arthroplasty of the Temporomandibular Joint

Joseph P. McCain[1] and Reem Hamdy Hossameldin[2]

[1]*Private Practice; Baptist Health Systems; and Oral and Maxillofacial Surgery, Herbert Wertheim College of Medicine, Florida International University Miami, Florida, USA; and Nova Southeastern School of Dental Medicine, Fort Lauderdale, Florida, USA*

[2]*Department of Oral and Maxillofacial Surgery, Faculty of Dental Medicine, Cairo University, Cairo, Egypt; and General Surgery Department, Herbert Wertheim College of Medicine, Florida International University, Miami, Florida, USA*

A minimally invasive procedure used to diagnose and/or treat numerous joint pathologies.

Indications

1. Disabling joint conditions refractory to medical management and primary arthroscopy alone that require internal structural modifications of the temporomandibular joint (TMJ)
2. Wilkes stage II, stage III, and/or early stage IV of arthroscopic discopexy

Contraindications

1. Skin infection
2. Possible tumor seeding
3. Medical and other circumstances unique to patients

Anatomy

Temporomandibular joint (TMJ): The TMJ is a diarthrodial joint separated into inferior and superior compartments by the articular disc. The inferior joint space contains approximately 0.9 mL of synovial fluid, whereas the superior joint space contains approximately 1.2 mL of synovial fluid. The inferior joint space is responsible for hinge opening or rotation (ginglymoid), and the superior joint space is responsible for gliding or translation motion (arthrodial), which is the second phase of opening. When the hinge opens, it permits the mandible to open approximately 2 to 3 cm as measured from the edges of the maxillary and mandibular incisor teeth. Translation allows increased opening to a maximum of 4 to 6 cm. The average vertical opening is approximately 45 mm. Anterior translation of the condyle terminates at the anterior peak of the articular eminence.

Articular disk: The articular disk is composed of dense, collagenous connective tissue. The articular disk is biconcave in shape with a length of approximately 22 mm and a width of approximately 16 mm. The disk is firmly attached to the lateral and medial poles of the condyle. The anterior and anterior medial attachments are to the lateral head of the pterygoid muscle. The anterior lateral attachment is to the capsule only. The posterior attachment blends into the retrodiskal tissue, which attaches to the posterior wall of the glenoid fossa. The posterior retrodiskal tissue attachment consists of synovial cells, collagen fibers, nerves, blood vessels, and elastic fibers.

Lateral pterygoid muscle: The most influential muscle involved in TMJ function is the lateral pterygoid muscle due to its attachment to both the disk and the condyle. The lateral pterygoid muscle has an inferior and superior belly. The origin of the inferior belly is the inferior two-thirds of the outer surface of the lateral pterygoid plate, the pyramidal process of the palatine bone, and the maxillary tuberosity. The insertion is into the anterior fovea of the condylar head. The vector of contraction is anterior and medial. The origin of the superior belly is the upper one-third of the lateral pterygoid plate and the infratemporal surface of the greater wing of the sphenoid. The insertion is into the superior aspect of the pterygoid fovea, the articular capsule, the medial aspect of the articular disk, and the condyle. During protrusion and opening, the pterygoid muscle pulls the condyle and disk anteriorly. If the muscle contracts on the right, it causes lateral excursion of the mandible to the left and vice versa.

Glenoid fossa: The mean thickness of the glenoid fossa is 0.9 mm with a range of 0.5 to 1.5 mm. The dura and the temporal lobe are located superior to the glenoid fossa.

Arthroscopic Arthroplasty (Discopexy) Technique

1. The patient is placed supine on the operating room table and nasally intubated. An examination is performed under general anesthesia to evaluate the bilateral joints for joint mobility, condylar translation, and

joint sounds (Figure 31.4 [all figures cited appear in Case Report 31.1]). The patient is prepped, draped, and positioned, allowing for visualization of the entire ear and lateral canthus of the eye. An ear wick impregnated in antibiotic solution or ointment is positioned within the external auditory canal for protection. A Quinn drape is placed (Figure 31.5) to allow for visualization of the ear, TMJ, and lateral canthus of the eye and to provide for a conduit to allow for manipulation of the jaw through the oral cavity without contamination of the extraoral incisions with oral microbes.

2. Standard landmarks are marked and include a line drawn from the lateral canthus of the eye and the tip of the tragus (Holmlund–Hellsing line) (Figure 31.5), the 10–2 point, and the 20–10 point (refer to Chapter 30).

3. The superior joint space is insufflated with 0.5 % Marcaine on a 22-gauge needle. Good plunger rebound confirms adequate insufflation of the space (Figure 31.6). Standard fossa portal entry is obtained with the 2.0 Dyonics operative system. The joint is examined with a 1.9 Dyonics video arthroscope attached to a Stryker camera system.

4. A patent irrigation system is established by placing a 22-gauge needle anterior to the fossa portal (Figure 31.7). Throughout the case, a patent irrigation system is maintained with irrigating fluid consisting of lactated Ringer's and 1:300,000 epinephrine.

5. The superior joint cavity is explored and pertinent diagnostic arthroscopic findings are revealed (Figure 31.8). Operative maneuvers often follow diagnostic arthroscopy.

6. A second cannula is placed at 25 mm anterior to the first, utilizing the vector measuring system (Figure 31.9). For this portal to be most effective in diagnostic and operative arthroscopy, the arthroscope should illuminate the most anterolateral aspect of the anterior recess. Then, swiveling the arthroscope along the intermediate zone and advancing into the anterior recess, identifying the disc synovial crease, the scope is swiveled to the most lateral and anterior aspect of the disc–synovial crease. The second puncture site is placed exactly in the most anterior and lateral corner of the superior joint space to ensure maximum flexibility of the operative cannula. Variations in the second puncture site and technique are dictated by the anterior recess volume and condition of the joint.

7. A 2.0 cannula is inserted into the anterolateral corner of the superior joint space. This second cannula will become the operative cannula, the device channel. The surgeon identifies the disk synovial crease with a straight probe and performs an anterior release (pterygoid myotomy) (Figure 31.10) by splicing the synovial membrane from the most medial component of the disk synovial crease to the vascular hump in the mid-portion of the anterior recess. The synovial

membrane and pterygoid muscle are detached from the disk. The disk is reduced with a straight probe while holding the jaw forward (Figure 31.11).

8. The retrodiscal tissue is contracted utilizing bipolar cautery. Occasionally, a superficial synovectomy (Figure 31.12) is performed, utilizing a stab incision within the posterior lateral gutter of the retrodiscal tissue using a banana blade, and then inserting the cautery into the deep retrodiscal tissues and contracting them.

9. Disk fixation can be accomplished by one of two methods. The first and more traditional method is the suture discopexy. A second method involves rigid fixation with either resorbable or titanium screws.

10. In suture discopexy, the disk is held in reduction, and a 20-gauge needle with a single out poly Dexon suture is inserted through the skin and subcuticular tissues, touching the condyle, into the inferior joint space, and then it angles superiorly to target the superior lateral aspect of the posterior band of the disc (Figure 31.13). The needle is advanced through the posterior band of the disk entering the superior joint space. It is important that the 20-gauge needle is inserted underneath the reduction cannula. A straight meniscus mender is inserted in the pre-auricular crease 5 to 7 mm below the fossa portal into the superior joint space. The snare of the meniscus mender is then inserted through the meniscus mender cannula, and the suture is passed through the 20-gauge needle into the superior joint space to be captured by the snare. Now, both free ends of the suture exit the skin (Figure 31.14). Small skin incisions are made at the exit points of the suture superiorly with a #11 blade. Straight hemostat is used to dissect down the suture tracing anteriorly to the capsule. The dissection is along the course of the facial nerve. Posteriorly, the dissection is carried down halfway to the capsule along the tragal cartilage.

11. A Mayo needle is used to thread the suture from anterior to posterior; both free ends of the suture now exit the skin posteriorly. While the disk is held in reduction, a tight surgeon's knot is tied, plicating the disk to the capsule and to the subcutaneous tissue (Figure 31.15).

12. The joint is evaluated for function arthroscopically and by manual manipulation while the disk is reduced and the sutures are checked for suture tightness (Figure 31.16). After confirmation of no clicking noises and appropriate function or motion of the disk or condyle, the instruments are removed, and steps 15–17 are followed.

13. In rigid screw disk fixation, after the anterior release is accomplished and posterior scarification and disk reduction have been completed, the disk is ready for placement of a fixation screw. The disk is maintained

in reduction, and the condyle is held forward. A third puncture site is placed using the vector measuring system. Ideally, the puncture is approximately 20 mm inferior to the fossa portal. The size of the cannula depends on the size of the screw used. Typically, the authors use a 2.0-mm cannula. The cannula at its distal end has a window so that the screw is visible as it is delivered into the joint and enfacing the disk. The angle of placement of this cannula and screw hole should be from posterior to anterior, superior to inferior, and medial to lateral. This placement avoids angling the drill superiorly toward the glenoid fossa and perforating it. Once the disk is held in reduction and the cannula has been inserted, the target area is the posterior-lateral corner of the disc–condyle assembly. Holding the cannula still, a drill is delivered through the cannula to the disk, and a monocortical screw placed through the condylar head itself. The drill bit is removed, and the screw attached to the screwdriver is delivered through the cannula. The screw is inserted through the disc and into the condyle, screwing it tightly so that the disk is now fastened to the condylar head itself. The window on the cannula enables the surgeon to watch the screw actually being turned into position. Once the screw is rigidly fixated, the cannula is pulled back, and the position of the screw is verified arthroscopically to ensure that it is fully engaged and that its position is ideal. Additionally, one can take a straight probe from the working cannula and wiggle the screw to make sure it is nonmobile and fully engaged.

14. Different types of screws can be applied to the joint. The authors have had success with the Osteomed cannulated screw (Osteomed, TX, USA), an Inion screw (Inion, Tampere, Finland), and a Smart nail (ConMed Linvatec, FL, USA). The ideal situation for rigid disc fixation is an average-sized joint space and a well-formed, nonperforated disc.

15. At the completion of the disk fixation procedure, the joint is lavaged, and one ampule of Healon (hyaluronic acid) is deposited (Figure 31.18) to act as an intra-articular Band-Aid to minimize small microbleeds and also to temporarily replenish the hyaluronic supply of the joint.

16. The external wounds are closed with 5-0 fast-absorbing gut sutures or 6-0 nylon sutures (Figure 31.19). The wound is covered with a thin layer of bacitracin and a light dressing.

17. The patient is positioned face up, and the jaw is manipulated under general anesthesia to confirm a tight motion without eminent subluxation. The TMJ is specifically evaluated for the absence of joint clicks and for smooth translations during functioning. At the completion of the procedure, the occlusion will be shifted to the opposite side as expected.

Postoperative Management

1. Ice packs are placed continuously within the TMJ region.
2. Intravenous antibiotics are utilized during admission. Oral antibiotics are utilized upon discharge for a total antibiotic course of 5 days postoperatively.
3. Corticosteroids are administered postoperatively.
4. Wound care involving cleaning of the incision sites with a mixture of 50% hydrogen peroxide and 50% normal saline is begun on postoperative day 2. A thin layer of bacitracin is applied to all skin incisions after cleaning.
5. A full liquid diet is employed for the first week and then gradually increased.
6. For patients with occlusal appliances, they are instructed to not wear their appliances for the first week after surgery.
7. Patients are instructed to begin physical therapy exercises beginning the day after surgery.

Complications

1. **Facial nerve damage**: Weakness from inadvertent damage or stretching of the temporal and/or zygomatic branches of the facial nerves may occur with arthroscopic entry and manipulation, or from fluid extravasation into the surrounding tissues. Paralysis is typically transient, and most patients recover completely within 4–12 weeks.

2. **Pre-auricular anesthesia and paresthesia**: The auriculotemporal nerve is typically posterior, but in close proximity to, the glenoid fossa puncture site. Damage to the pre-auricular nerve may occur during arthroscopic entry and manipulation, or from fluid extravasation into the surrounding tissues. Postoperative anesthesia around the entry sites is a common occurrence that typically spontaneously resolves within 2–4 weeks.

3. **Iatrogenic scuffing of the fibrocartilage lining**: The cartilage covering the eminence and fossa is prone to iatrogenic damage during instrumentation. Significant scuffing impairs visibility during arthroscopic procedures and may lead to the misdiagnosis of chondromalacia by the inexperienced arthroscopist.

4. **Damage to the middle ear**: The mechanism of entry into the middle ear is through either the bony external auditory canal (EAC) or the soft tissue EAC. Large perforations are identified intraoperatively with leakage of irrigation fluid from the EAC. Attention to detail when inserting the arthroscope and not inserting the arthroscope more than 20 to 25 mm without checking its position are keys to preventing canal perforations. The arthroscope should be inserted anterior and forward to the EAC, not parallel to its external surface. Small tears and perforations of the EAC and

tympanic membrane typically heal without operative intervention and without future sequelae with the use of packings, antibiotics, and corticoid ointment. If the tympanic membrane is perforated and the ossicles appear in the field of view, immediate cessation of the procedure and intraoperative otolaryngologist consultation are warranted.

5. **Inadvertent perforation of the glenoid fossa**: Rare. May occur during inappropriate entrance and instrumentation through the fossa port. Instrumentation toward the tubercle and away from the fossa i recommended to avoid injury to the contents of the cranial fossa. Intraoperative neurosurgical consultation is recommended. Most small cerebrospinal fluid (CSF) leaks will heal spontaneously. If CSF continues to collect within the wound or drain through the incision site, a pressure dressing should be applied and the patient hospitalized with head elevation and antibiotics. Persistence of a leak for more than 48 hours is an indication for consultation with potential lumbar subarachnoid drain placement. A computed tomography scan of the head with bone windows should be obtained to document the site. Surgical repair of the middle fossa dura is rarely necessary.

6. **Excessive hemorrhage within the joint space**: Intracapsular hemorrhage has numerous etiologies to include excessive bleeding upon entering the capsule from tearing of the superficial temporal vessels, excessive bleeding from severely inflamed synovium or retrodiscal tissue upon joint entrance, and bleeding from the pterygoid artery when performing myotomy for anterior release procedures. In arthroscopic surgery, pressure irrigation typically clears the visual field adequately when persistent hemorrhaging occurs. Occasionally, pressure irrigation will not stop the hemorrhaging, leaving behind a joint congested with blood with poor visibility, which prolongs healing, increases postoperative discomfort, and extends recovery time. Several methods are used to control intracapsular bleeding that is refractory to pressure irrigation:

A. Arthroscopic cautery can be applied to the bleeding site. If using laser, apply laser in the synovectomy mode until the tissue blanches. Cautery or laser application is successful in most cases of minor bleeding.

B. Inject small amounts of local anesthetic with vasoconstrictor into the bleeding site. A 3 1/2-inch spinal needle on a 3 mL syringe is passed down the cannula and directly into the involved tissues.

C. Insufflate the joint through the cannula with local anesthetic with vasoconstrictors, bathing all of the joint tissues.

D. Insufflate the joint under pressure using irrigation fluid. Then, tamponade all outflow cannulae for 5 minutes, so the hydrostatic pressure of the irrigation fluid directly tamponades the bleeding site.

E. If bleeding persists after A–D, remove instruments from the joint and apply direct, external tamponading pressure in the pre-auricular area for 5 minutes. For added pressure, seat the condyle into the fossa if the bleeding source is located in the posterior pouch. If it is in the anterior pouch, manipulate the mandible to a protrusive position. After 5 minutes, reinsert the instruments into the original punctures and assess the condition of the joint.

F. Insert a No. 4 catheter balloon through the second portal, inflate the balloon with normal saline, and leave it in the area of bleeding for 5 minutes. Then deflate and reassess.

G. If bleeding persists, approach the joint via open surgery and pack the area. The above steps should be performed in this order (A–G) until the bleeding stops or the procedure is terminated. It is important to examine the contents of the joint space for coagulums deposited in dependent areas and least accessible from the irrigation fluid such as the medial recess. If this is the case, aspiration of joint contents will remove the blood products. However, caution must be observed to not disturb the blood clot over the bleeding site.

7. **Damage to the superficial temporal vessels with or without formation of A-V fistulae**: The superficial temporal vessels (STA and STV) are intimately related to the posterior aspect of the joint capsule. Damage to the STA and STV is initially managed by applying direct controlled pressure. Cases refractory to direct pressure are managed with suture ligation of the offending vessel. Although rare, other investigators have reported the formation of A-V fistulae after injury to the superficial temporal vessels. Typically, patients complain of a constant hissing and whishing sound over the operated TMJ. Superficial temporal A-V fistulae are managed with embolization and fistulectomy.

8. **Instrument failure or loose bodies within the joint**: Instrument failure can be attributed to manufacturing defects, misuse of instruments, and wear of parts within the instrument itself, leading to instrument breakage. Instrument breakage and loose bodies within the joint can be minimized by checking the structural integrity of an instrument before use, using ferromagnetic instruments, having a "golden retriever" available, avoiding excessive force when placing and removing instruments, maintaining visualization of instruments at all times, and keeping movable instruments closed during removal. If breakage of instruments or material

(suture) occurs, the following protocol should be followed:

A. Stop the procedure. Maintain the position of the arthroscope and working cannulae.

B. Keep the instrument in view (arthroscopic visualization).

C. Check inflow bags to make sure there is sufficient irrigation fluid so that the joint is always distended.

D. Record and measure the depth of the instrument with a scored cannula.

E. Have adequate removal instruments available. Extra instruments are a must.

F. Adjust inflow as to ensure optimal visibility.

G. Take a radiograph of the joint if the instrument cannot be found arthroscopically.

H. Consider fluoroscopic assistance to localize the piece if the instrument cannot be found arthroscopically.

I. If using a grabber to remove a fragment, the tips might not fit in a working cannula upon removal. It might therefore be desirable to switch systems to a 3 mm diameter working cannula with a "switch stick" technique and retrieve the broken fragments with instruments or a "golden retriever."

J. If an instrument is broken and cannot be retrieved, the possibility of re-arthroscopy alone or with guided fluoroscopy or open surgery should be contemplated. The attempt should be made in the early postoperative phase (10 days after the first procedure) up to 6 weeks. If this fails, the doctor and the patient must review complications associated with leaving the piece within the joint space. The possibility of future osteoarthrosis or foreign body reaction occurring as a result of leaving the fragment within the joint space must be understood by the patient.

9. **Infection of the puncture sites**: Rare. Minimized with proper sterilization techniques, sterile operating room conditions, prophylactic antibiotics, and a high volume of irrigation used during arthroscopic surgery. Most infections are successfully managed with exploration of the area under local anesthesia, removal of residual suture when found, or breakdown of the suture by the mechanical action of exploring the area and the administration of oral cephalosporin for 7–10 days.

10. **Noninfectious postoperative effusion**: Effusions typically appear as edema of the pre-auricular area, resulting in a higher level of pain upon palpation than that normally encountered postoperatively. Patients are managed with joint rest, a soft diet, application of heat over the affected area, and nonsteroidal anti-inflammatory medication for pain management.

Key Points

1. Ideal patients for discopexy include patients with a class I occlusion, suitable joint space, and an articu-

lar disc that dislocates but does not show remodeling. These conditions are typically found in Wilkes stage II, stage III, and early stage IV joint disease and have an 80% success rate with discopexy. Patients with Wilkes late stage IV and stage V joint disease have a discopexy success rate of only 60%.

2. An efficient anterior release should be established through the disc synovial crease. All muscle fibers are resected from the disc under direct arthroscopic visualization. The cut through the superior belly of the pterygoid muscle is complete when a space between the superior belly of the pterygoid muscle and inferior belly of the pterygoid muscle is encountered and the inferior belly of the pterygoid muscle can be seen to be more purple in color than the superior belly. Care must be taken to avoid cutting to the vascular hump, or significant bleeding will be encountered.

3. During disc reduction, the condyle should be in a closed position, the operative cannula and the scope are within the anterior recess, the anterior release has been completed, and the operative cannula and the scope are then walked back in the lateral sulcus to the posterior pouch. Once these two instruments reach the peak of the articular eminence, the condyle is pulled forward, and then both instruments can drop into the posterior pouch. The disc is reduced by compressing the retrodiscal tissue laterally with a straight probe, while the condyle is in a forward or forward and contralateral position, or occasionally it is necessary to reduce the disc by taking a hook probe and compressing the oblique protuberance.

4. In suture disc fixation, the needle should be advanced through the lasso first, and then the suture is advanced beyond the needle approximately 1 cm. The suture needle is then withdrawn from the lasso, and the lasso is cinched down around the suture material. The disc should be held in reduction while the suture is being passed and retrieved.

5. In order for the knot to be buried in the subcutaneous fatty tissue, a straight hemostat is used to dissect down the suture tracing anteriorly to the capsule through the slit incisions. The dissection is along the course of the facial nerve. Posteriorly, the dissection is carried down halfway to the capsule. The skin is closed primarily with 6–0 nylon interrupted sutures.

6. Caution must be observed when making the myotomy at the most anteromedial corner (anterior release). When the anteromedial synovial drape is incised at the junction with the disk, an artery approximately 1 to 2 mm in diameter usually is found directly underneath this junction. Arthroscopically, it appears as a white tubular structure. If this vessel is incised during the anterior release, copious bleeding will occur.

Case Report 31.1. A 15-year-old female presents with a chief complaint of recurrent locking and pain within her left temporomandibular joint (TMJ) (Figure 31.1). The patient had been refractory to medical management. Plain films showed no advanced arthrosis. Magnetic resonance imaging (MRI) demonstrated a nonreducing disk within the left TMJ (Figures 31.2 and 31.3) and a mild reduction disk within the right joint, which was asymptomatic. The patient was consented for the procedure of arthroscopic discopexy through her mother, as she was a minor. On examination of the paralyzed patient, she was found to have good mobility of both TMJs, with no clicking noted (Figure 31.4).

Pertinent diagnostic arthroscopic findings of the left joint revealed a good joint space with compressed retrodiskal tissue. On function, the retrodiskal tissue was moderately hyperemic and moderately redundant. The medial synovial drape was intact and mildly hyperemic. The pterygoid shadow was purple. The anterior recess demonstrated no significant adhesions, mild to moderate hyperemia, and no chondromalacia. Findings were consistent with a nonreducing disk and a component of synovitis (Figure 31.8). The findings correlated with the MRI depicting a nonreducing disk with a Wilkes early stage IV. After completion of the diagnostic portion of the procedure, a second cannula was placed (Figure 31.9). The disk synovial crease was identified, and an anterior release was performed by splicing the synovial capsule and the pterygoid muscle at their insertion to the disk (Figure 31.10). The patient did not demonstrate a strong muscle attachment to the disk. Conservative muscle resection was performed on the medial aspect of the disk. The scope was directed to the posterior pouch. The disk could now be readily reduced with a probe while the jaw was gently positioned forward (Figure 31.11). The retrodiskal tissue was shortened, and a partial arthrodesis was completed utilizing an Holmium laser on low voltage. A superior synovectomy was also completed at that time of the retrodiskal tissue repositioning (Figure 31.12). The disk was held in reduction, and a suture discopexy was performed (Figures 31.13, 31.14, and 31.15). The disk position was verified arthroscopically and found to be in good position. The joint was functioned with manual manipulation of the lower jaw, and the disc remained in its ideal position and the knot remained tight (Figure 31.16). Additionally, a retrodiskal arthrodesis was completed on the redundant synovium with a low-voltage weld holmium laser (Figure 31.17). One ampule of Healon was deposited (Figure 31.18). The external wounds were closed with 6-0 nylon sutures (Figure 31.19), and the ear was wick removed. The patient was reexamined under anesthesia, and the joint was noted to function ideally with no translation issues and no clicking or popping of the joint. (See Figures 31.1 through 31.19.)

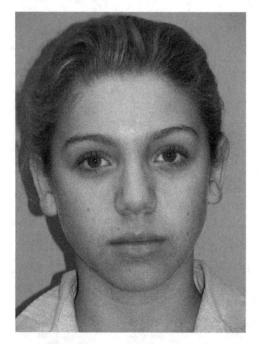

Figure 31.1.   Patient with recurrent left-sided temporomandibular joint locking and pain with no facial asymmetries.

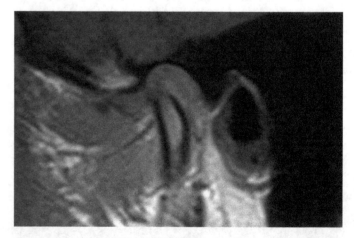

Figure 31.2.   Sagittal T1-weighted open-mouth magnetic resonance imaging demonstrating an anteriorly displaced disk.

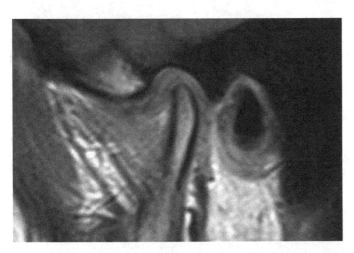

Figure 31.3.   Sagittal T1-weighted closed-mouth magnetic resonance imaging demonstrating a nonreducing anteriorly displaced disk.

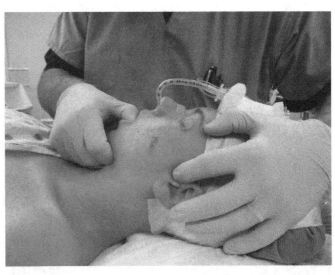

Figure 31.4.   An examination of the joints is performed under general anesthesia.

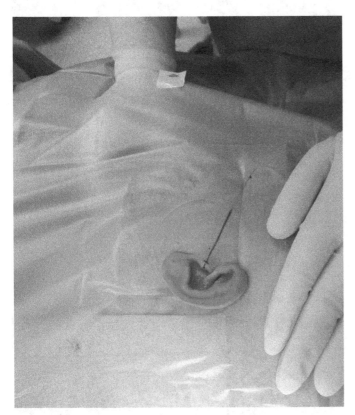

Figure 31.5.   The H and H line is marked, and a Quinn drape is placed to allow instrumentation of the left temporomandibular joint and manipulation of the oral cavity without contamination of the surgical site.

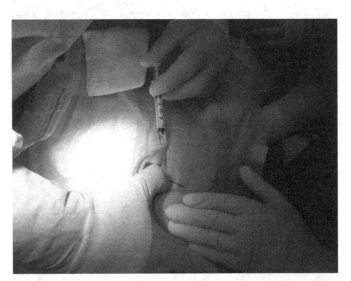

Figure 31.6.   The superior joint space is insufflated with 0.5% Marcaine totaling 5 mL with good plunger rebound.

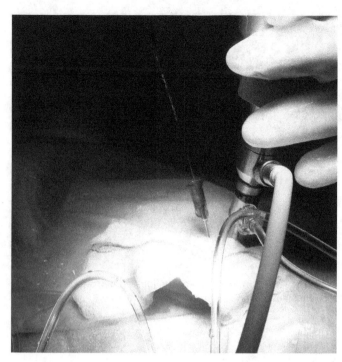

Figure 31.7. A patent irrigation system is established by placing a 22-gauge needle anterior to the fossa portal. The irrigation system is maintained with irrigating fluid consisting of lactated Ringer's and 1:300,000 epinephrine.

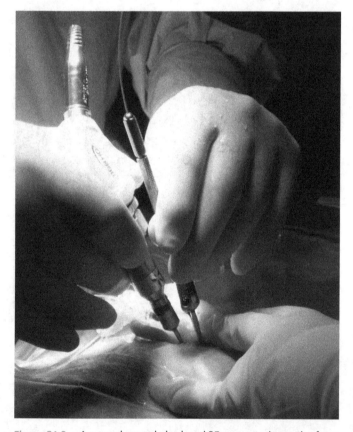

Figure 31.9. A second cannula is placed 25 mm anterior to the fossa portal into the anterolateral corner of the superior joint space with a 2.0 cannula.

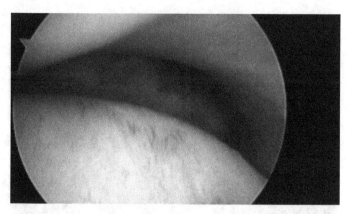

Figure 31.8. Findings consistent with a nonreducing disk and joint synovitis.

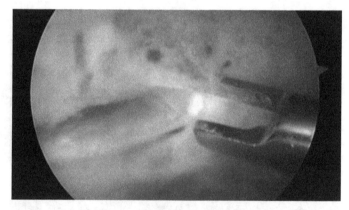

Figure 31.10. The disk synovial crease is identified, and an anterior release is performed by splicing the synovial capsule and the pterygoid muscle at their insertion to the disk.

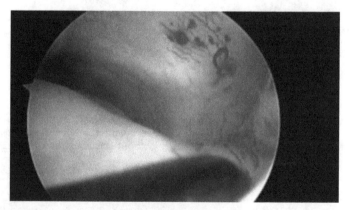

Figure 31.11. Conservative muscle resection is performed on the medial aspect of the disk to allow for reduction. The disk is reduced with a probe while the jaw is positioned forward.

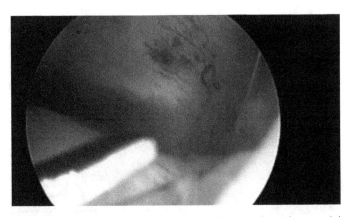

Figure 31.12. The retrodiskal tissue is shortened, and a partial arthrodesis is completed utilizing a holmium laser on low voltage. A superior synovectomy was also performed.

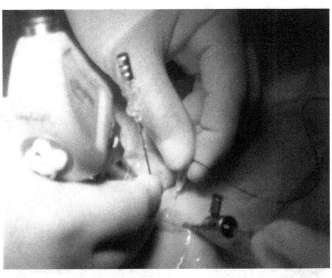

Figure 31.13. Disk fixation is accomplished by holding the disk in place and passing a #1 poly Dexon suture through a 20-gauge needle and through a separate puncture into the joint with a meniscus mender.

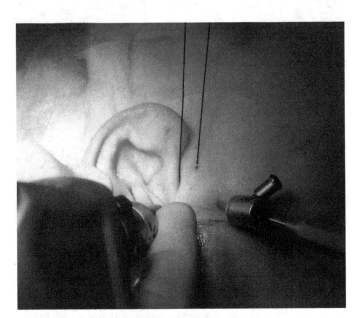

Figure 31.14. Both free ends of the suture exit the skin.

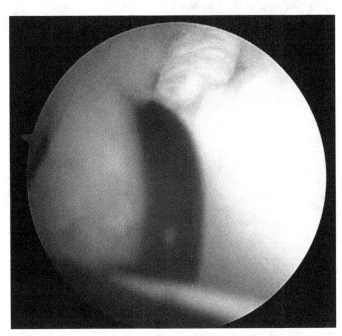

Figure 31.15. While the disk is held in reduction, a tight surgeon's knot is tied, plicating the disk to the capsule and to the subcuticular tissue.

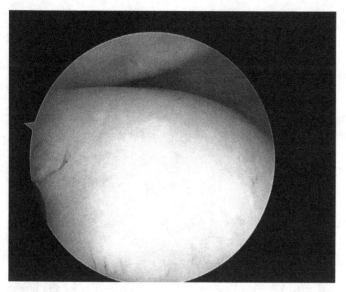

Figure 31.16.   The disk position is verified arthroscopically and found to be ideal. The joint was functioned under arthroscopic visualization, and the disk maintained its position.

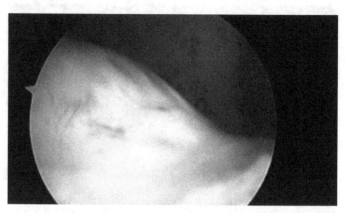

Figure 31.17.   Additionally, a retrodiskal arthrodesis is completed on the redundant synovium with a low-voltage weld holmium laser.

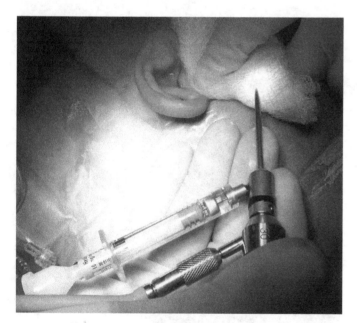

Figure 31.18.   One ampule of Healon is deposited at the completion of the procedure.

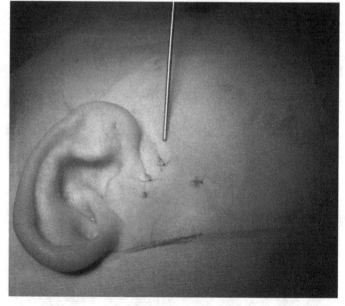

Figure 31.19.   The external ports are closed with 6-0 nylon sutures.

References

McCain, J.P., 1996. *Principles and practice of temporomandibular joint arthroscopy.* St. Louis, MO: Mosby.

McCain, J.P. and Hossameldin, R.H., 2011. Advanced arthroscopy of the temporomandibular joint. *Atlas of the Oral and Maxillofacial Surgery Clinics*, 19 (2), 145–67.

McCain, J.P., Podrasky, A.E. and Zabiegalski, N.A., 1992. Arthroscopic disc repositioning and suturing: a preliminary report. *Journal of Oral and Maxillofacial Surgery*, 50 (6), 568–79.

Perez, R., 2007. Temporomandibular joint arthroscopic arthroplasty with rigid disc fixation—preliminary results in treatment of Wilkes internal joint derangement stages II–V: a 3-year retrospective study. *Journal of Oral and Maxillofacial Surgery*, 65 (9, Suppl.), 38.e3–38.

Tarro, A.W., 1994. A fully visualized arthroscopic disc suturing technique. *Journal of Oral and Maxillofacial Surgery*, 52 (4), 362–9.

32

Alloplastic Reconstruction (TMJ Concepts) of the Temporomandibular Joint and Associated Structures

John N. Kent,[1] Christopher J. Haggerty,[2] Billy Turley,[3] and Robert M. Laughlin[4]

[1]Department of Oral and Maxillofacial Surgery, Louisiana State University Health Sciences Center, New Orleans, Louisiana, USA

[2]Private Practice, Lakewood Oral and Maxillofacial Surgery Specialists, Lees Summit; and Department of Oral and Maxillofacial Surgery, University of Missouri–Kansas City, Kansas City, Missouri, USA

[3]Department of Oral and Maxillofacial Surgery, Navy Medicine Support Command, Jacksonville, North Carolina, USA

[4]Department of Oral and Maxillofacial Surgery, Naval Medical Center San Diego, San Diego, California, USA

A method for reconstructing temporomandibular joints (TMJs) that have become significantly impaired and require alloplastic reconstruction to return form and function.

Indications

1. Ankylosis: An alternative to soft or hard tissue grafting procedures
2. Degenerative joint disease, rheumatoid arthridities, or related arthropathies and autoimmune disorders of the condyle: An alternative to soft or hard tissue grafting procedures
3. Condyle loss from trauma, pathology, or any progressive disease states
4. Failed autogenous joint reconstruction
5. Failed alloplastic joint reconstruction
6. History of multiple joint surgeries
7. Loss of lateral pterygoid function with any of the above
8. Vertical dimension loss of the ramus with occlusal abnormalities
9. Relative indications: Pain, loss of interincisal opening, and/or occlusion disharmony refractory to non-total joint procedures

Contraindications

1. Active or suspected infections in or about the implantation site
2. Proven allergic reactions to any of the prosthetic materials
3. Skeletal immaturity
4. Systemic disease with increased susceptibility to infection
5. Psychiatric disorders
6. Medically compromised individuals: the very elderly, uncontrolled systemic diseases, and drug and/or alcohol addiction

Diagnosis and Surgical Planning

The surgeon must diagnose all preoperative conditions and plan desired outcomes relative to joint pathology, functional goals, desired occlusion, and aesthetics. A one-stage surgical reconstruction using a one-piece or two-piece stereolithic model, or a two-stage surgical procedure (which predominately uses a one-piece stereolithic model), is selected based on the surgeon's preference and desired treatment objectives.

One-Stage Alloplastic Reconstruction Using a One-Piece or a Two-Piece Stereolithic Model

Specific Indications for a One-Piece Stereolithic Model

1. The patient is able to maintain a normal occlusion during the computed tomography (CT) scan. Aesthetics are satisfactory.
2. The surgeon is able to manipulate and maintain a normal occlusion with the use of intermaxillary fixation (IMF) for the CT scan. Aesthetics are satisfactory.
3. The occlusion is ideal or nearly ideal, and it is maintained during the CT scan. Fossa anatomy is easily adjusted with minor corrections at planned surgery. Aesthetics are satisfactory.

To fabricate a one-piece stereolithic model, a manufacturer-specific CT scan is obtained with the jaws in occlusion, utilizing intermaxillary fixation if necessary. The stereolithic model is fabricated in one piece, with the patient's mandibular dentition fused to the maxillary dentition. The custom joints are fabricated based upon the occlusion set during the manufacturer-specific CT scan.

Atlas of Operative Oral and Maxillofacial Surgery, First Edition. Edited by Christopher J. Haggerty and Robert M. Laughlin
© 2015 John Wiley & Sons, Inc. Published 2015 by John Wiley & Sons, Inc.

Specific Indications for a Two-Piece Stereolithic Model

1. A two-piece stereolithic model is preferred when simultaneous mandibular and/or maxillary repositioning is required. A two-piece model is necessary when performing a condylectomy and placing total joints to improve occlusion and aesthetics. In the above instances, the fossa anatomy is normal or near-normal, requiring little alteration, and joint placement improves the occlusion. Simultaneous orthognathic surgery with total joint placement can also be performed in patients with poor occlusion, specific edentulous cases, apertognathia, maxillary or mandibular deformities, and mandibular asymmetries. The surgeon must be comfortable in simultaneously reestablishing the occlusion through orthognathic surgery and performing total joint surgery. When in doubt, it is always best to plan a two-stage surgical reconstruction to reposition the mandible or maxilla through orthognathic surgery first to obtain the desired occlusion. The manufacturer-specific CT scan may then be performed with the patient in normal occlusion, with or without intermaxillary fixation, to obtain a one-piece stereolithic model.

To fabricate a two-piece stereolithic model, a manufacturer-specific CT scan is obtained with the jaws set slightly apart. The stereolithic model is fabricated in two pieces, with the mandible separated from the maxilla. The surgeon establishes the final occlusion during the surgical workup, and the custom joints are fabricated based on the desired final occlusion. The occlusion and desired aesthetics are then corrected at surgery with custom total joint placement and, if required, simultaneous orthognathic surgery.

Note: Many ankylosis patients with acceptable occlusion require only one-stage surgery using a one-piece model as minor alterations of the joint anatomy on the model are easily produced at surgery when placing the prostheses.

Two-Stage Alloplastic Reconstruction

Cases with abnormal joint pathology, mostly extensive bony ankylosis with or without occlusal or aesthetic anomalies, require excision of the ankylosis, shaping of fossa anatomy, and correction of occlusion and facial aesthetics by repositioning the mandible. Intermaxillary fixation is required immediately after the first surgery to obtain the manufacturer-specific, CT scan–generated stereolithic model for a one-piece model. The custom total joint prosthesis is inserted at the second surgical procedure. If orthognathic surgery is planned, it may be performed at either the first or second surgery. If performed at the second surgical procedure, the teeth are separated when obtaining the manufacturer-specific CT scan, and a two-piece stereolithic model will be ordered as described above.

Specific Indications for Two-Stage Alloplastic Reconstruction

1. Fossa or condyle anatomy that requires significant modification or resection
2. Significant bony ankylosis
3. When significant occlusal alterations are necessary with (1) or (2)
4. Resection of large tumors of the temporomandibular region with associated hard tissue defects
5. Removal of failed alloplastic hardware

TMJ Concepts Workup

1. A manufacturer-specific, medical-grade CT scan is ordered to reflect 0.5 to 1.0 mm cuts at zero gantry in an axial plane. The scan must include, at a minimum, 2.5 cm above the glenoid fossa and the complete inferior border of the mandible. The patient is scanned in occlusion (a one-piece model) with or without intermaxillary fixation or with the jaws set apart (a two-piece model), as determined by the surgical plan.
2. DICOM files are sent to the total joint manufacturer on a CD or uploaded directly for the fabrication of a stereolithic model in one or two pieces as prescribed by the surgeon. Stone models, intraoral digital scanner generated data (Figure 32.1), or cone beam CT (CBCT) scanner generated data can be used to remove scan distortion from dental artifacts (i.e., dental restorations, arch bars, and orthodontic brackets), maximize occlusal anatomy, and establish ideal occlusion when a two-piece stereolithic model is used. Utilizing the above modalities will significantly improve the accuracy of the final occlusal result. The dental anatomy data from the laser-scanned stone models, intraoral scanner, or CBCT are registered within the manufacturer's software using surface-based alignment algorithms and are used to replace the maxillary and mandibular teeth (Figures 32.2 and 32.3) within the manufacturer-specific CT scan. Once the dental anatomy is registered

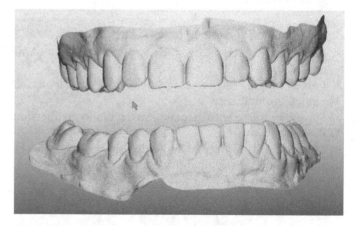

Figure 32.1. Intraoral digital scanner used to capture the surface topography of the dentition. The data is exported to the manufacturer in the form of STL files.

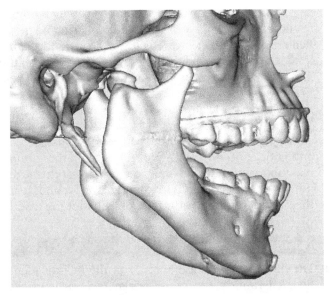

Figure 32.2. Two-piece stereolithic model of a patient with a previously treated medially displaced condyle and symphysis fracture, with resultant temporomandibular joint dysfunction and malocclusion. Stone model dental anatomy has been integrated with manufacturer-specific computed tomography in order to establish dental anatomy free of scan artifacts. Image provided courtesy of TMJ Concepts (Ventura, California).

to the bony anatomy within the manufacturer's software, a hybrid model is generated, and the preferred occlusion can be produced. Either the surgeon can use the improved hybrid pieces in a two-piece model to set the occlusion, or a planned occlusion can be generated using the dental stone models. If dental stone models are used to generate the final occlusion, the stone models are scanned in a prescribed or "ideal" occlusion using one of the methods listed above. The scanned occlusion is registered to the maxilla hybrid component in the CT scan. The hybrid mandible is located to the digitized occlusion. The stereolithic model is then fabricated for subsequent implant design (Figure 32.4).

3. For a one-stage procedure, a one-piece stereolithic model is returned to the surgeon with the teeth in ideal occlusion as placed by the surgeon prior to the manufacturer-specific CT scan, or the ideal occlusion is set by the surgeon on stone models, which are sent to the manufacturer for scanning if the CT was taken with the teeth apart. When the stereolithic model is returned to the surgeon, a condylectomy and coronoidectomy and minor alterations of the fossa are performed by the surgeon on the stereolithic model. The manufacturer will typically place an osteotomy line for the condyle resection and inscribe desired alteration of fossa anatomy or surface of the ramus as a guide for the surgeon.

4. If the surgeon repositions the mandible on the returned stereolithic model, preservation of the coronoid processes may be helpful in maintaining the normal spatial relationships of the mandible to the skull base

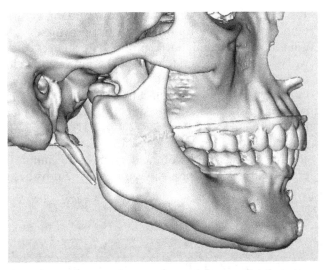

Figure 32.3. Occlusion is determined and transferred to the manufacturer-specific, computed tomography–generated 3D model. Image provided courtesy of TMJ Concepts (Ventura, California).

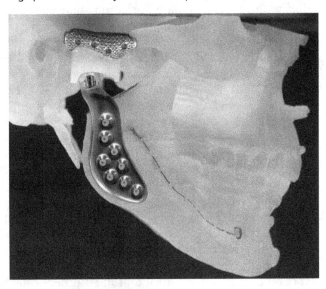

Figure 32.4. Stereolithic model with ideal occlusion established and the right total joint in place after condylectomy with coronoid preservation to allow for orientation of the normal spatial relationships of the mandible to the skull base. Image provided courtesy of TMJ Concepts (Ventura, California).

(Figure 32.4). Once the mandible is secured to the maxilla with hot glue or plates, the coronoids can be removed from the model. Repositioning of the maxilla may also be performed by the surgeon as needed.

5. For two-stage surgical procedures, the condylectomy with fossa shaping and coronoidectomy is completed on the patient. Orthognathic surgery, if necessary, is usually done at this time. A manufacturer-specific CT scan is obtained after resection of the condyle, coronoid, or temporal mass with the patient in occlusion for the fabrication of a one-piece model or not in occlusion for the fabrication of a two-piece model if additional surgery is planned (rarely).

6. The operated model is returned to the manufacturer, who creates a wax-up of the custom prostheses (glenoid fossa and condyle) (Figure 32.22) and sends the wax-up to the surgeon for approval prior to fabrication of the total joints. The surgeon approves or requests modification of the manufacturer's workup. The final custom prosthesis is approved by the surgeon and fabricated (Figures 32.4, 32.7, 32.9, 32.23, and 32.37). Custom-cut guides may be generated for use during condylectomies and coronoidectomies to minimize errors and to allow for a precision fit of the prostheses.

Surgical Technique and Insertion of Custom TMJ Prostheses

Presurgical Preparation

1. Intravenous antibiotics, steroids, and antisialogues are given preoperatively. The patient is positioned supine and nasally intubated. Short-acting paralytics are used during intubation to allow for stimulation and identification of branches of the facial nerve during the procedures. Separate intraoral and facial instrument tray setups are established. Protective draping and/or redraping and prepping are recommended throughout the procedure to avoid cross-contamination between the mouth and face when going back and forth between sterile and nonsterile (oral) environments.

2. A throat pack is placed within the posterior oropharynx. If orthodontic appliances are not in place, mandibular and maxillary Erich arch bars are placed, but intermaxillary fixation is not initiated. The oral cavity is prepped with Betadine paint (Betadine scrub is not recommended for mucous membranes application), and a sterile gauze is placed between the dentition and the internal surface of the lips to prevent the contamination of the extraoral field with saliva.

3. Lacrilube is placed within the orbits. Corneal shields or small occlusive dressings are used to protect the eyes. The use of large, obstructive dressings is contraindicated in order to allow for visualization when testing the temporal branch of the facial nerve. A plastic adhesive drape (i.e., Tegaderm or Opsite) is used to seal the oral cavity to prevent the contamination of the extraoral surgical sites with oral microbes (Figure 32.14). Large occlusive dressings are contraindicated to allow for visualization when testing the buccal and marginal mandibular branches of the facial nerve.

4. The patient's hair is prepped to ensure there is no hair within the surgical field. If the hair is shaved, ensure the underlying skin is not damaged to minimize the risk of infection.

5. The external auditory canals are prepped with Betadine paint, and an antibiotic-impregnated ear wick is placed within the external auditory canals bilaterally. The remainder of the facial skeleton is prepped with Betadine paint from the scalp to the clavicles. The patient is draped to allow for exposure of bilateral pre-auricular and modified retromandibular incisions (even if only anticipating ipsilateral surgery) and the oral cavity. The corner of the mouth and eyes must be exposed within the surgical field to allow for visualization of stimulation of all branches of the facial nerve (Figure 32.14) during the procedure.

6. The prostheses are removed from the manufacturer's sterile wrapping and placed within a broad-spectrum antibiotic concentrated solution (i.e., a mixture of normal saline with Cleocin and Vancomycin) at the beginning of the case. Copious irrigation of the wounds using the same solution is performed throughout the case.

Pre-auricular Approach

1. The natural skin crease anterior to the helix is identified. The anticipated pre-auricular incision is marked with a marking pen from the top of the helix of the ear to the inferior level of the external auditory canal within the natural skin crease (Figure 32.5). A slight antero-superior curved releasing incision may be incorporated into the superior aspect of the incision.

2. A vasoconstrictor (i.e., 1:200,000 epinephrine solution) is injected along the proposed surgical incision within the subcutaneous tissues to assist in hemostasis. A skin incision is initiated along the previously marked line.

3. From the superior aspect of the incision to the zygomatic arch, the incision continues through the underlying subcutaneous tissue to expose the superficial layer of the temporalis fascia (Figure 32.15). A needle-tipped cautery is used to transect through the superficial or outer layer of the temporalis fascia from the root of the zygomatic arch level to the superior aspect of the incision. Once the superficial or outer layer of the temporalis fascia is transected, adipose tissue is recognized between the superficial and deep layers of the temporalis fascia. The deep or inner layer of the temporalis fascia proceeds beneath the zygomatic arch and is not incised. Once the periosteum on the root of the zygomatic arch is incised at the posterior aspect of the fossa, a flap with the outer temporalis fascia and periosteum is elevated and reflected anteriorly. This flap will also include soft tissue over the capsule as described further in this chapter. The superficial temporal vessels are either retracted with the flap or ligated.

4. From the arch to the inferior aspect of the incision-blunt dissection continues approximately 1.5 cm inferior to the level of the arch to expose the TMJ capsule or fibrous connective tissue if the capsule has been operated previously. Exposure of the parotid gland lobule inferiorly should be avoided. During the above-mentioned anterior flap elevation over the root of the zygoma, a periosteal elevator is utilized to slide within a subperiosteal plane over the arch past the articular eminence. Once the articular eminence is reached, the periosteal elevator

Incisions

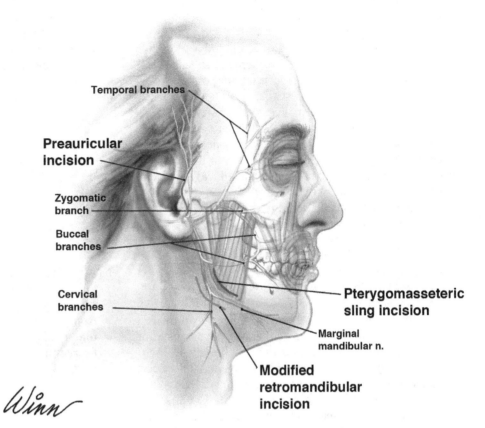

Temporal branches

Preauricular incision

Zygomatic branch

Buccal branches

Cervical branches

Pterygomasseteric sling incision

Marginal mandibular n.

Modified retromandibular incision

Winn

Figure 32.5. Anatomy of the facial nerve and location of the pre-auricular and modified retromandibular approach incisions. The red line depicts the location of the pre-auricular incision. The blue line depicts the location of the modified retromandibular incision. The green line represents the surgical division of the masseter muscle between the marginal mandibular and the buccal branch of the facial nerve to gain access to the lateral ramus.

or a kitner slides inferiorly and anteriorly in a sweeping motion to further expose the lateral capsule of the TMJ.

5. This tissue flap, extending outside the deep layer of the temporalis fascia superiorly and beneath the subperiosteal tissue layer over the arch and over the capsule inferiorly, is elevated and retracted anteriorly just past the articular eminence. Frequent testing of all soft tissues with a nerve stimulator at the level of and below the arch may appreciate the temporal branch of the facial nerve. The nerve must remain within the retracted flap as it passes over the arch (1–3 cm anterior to the postglenoid tubercle), and divides to supply the forehead and the upper eyelid. Posteriorly, care is taken to avoid exposure or damage of the auricular cartilage to minimize chondritis. The postglenoid tubercle is the most posterior aspect of the dissection.

6. A deep incision is made through the soft tissue along the outer edge of the fossa from the postglenoid tubercle across to and slightly past the articular eminence. The incision continues in a large U-shaped fashion surrounding the entire capsule, or, if previously operated, fibrous connective tissue to expose the condyle or fibrous-bony mass. The subperiosteal refection is carried anterior and inferiorly to the level of the condyle neck (Figure 32.16).

Modified Retromandibular Approach

Note: This is the approach that we have predominately used for decades. Standard retromandibular and submandibular techniques are certainly acceptable and occasionally used. This technique provides an aesthetic skin incision and encourages the dissection to pass between the branches of the marginal mandibular and buccal branches of the facial nerve, and continues through the masseter muscle to bone. Selection of this technique provides a more direct access to the ramus and is based on the length of the body portion of the condylar component, anticipated facial nerve involvement, aesthetics, and the surgeon's comfort zone. It gives the surgeon a choice of retracting superiorly or inferiorly the marginal mandibular branch of the facial nerve, usually avoids interaction with the parotid gland, and commonly avoids ligation of the facial vessels.

1. The angle and inferior border of the mandible are palpated and marked with a surgical marking pen. Care should be taken to not stretch the tissue as this can distort the surgical field. A 3 cm slightly curved line is drawn that is not parallel to either the inferior or posterior border of the mandible, is slightly below the angle of the mandible, and is usually parallel to or within a natural skin crease. The line is just below and centered

at the angle of the mandible unless there is anticipation of lowering the angle with the reconstruction.

2. A vasoconstrictor (i.e., 1:200,000 epinephrine solution) is injected subcutaneously along the pre-marked incision line to minimize bleeding.

3. The skin is placed under slight tension, and a #15 blade is used to incise the skin and underlying subcutaneous tissues along the pre-marked incision line to the level of the fascia overlying the platysma. Using a Ray-Tec, gently sweep the overlying subcutaneous tissue superiorly and inferiorly to fully expose the underlying platysma muscle. A #15 blade is used to sharply incise the platysma muscle. Neural testing should be performed deep to the platysma muscle to ensure that the marginal mandibular and buccal branches of the facial nerve are protected (Figure 32.17).

4. After the platysma is incised, the superficial layer of the deep cervical fascia is encountered. At this level, the facial vein and artery may be encountered at the anterior aspect of the dissection at the level of the antigonial notch. Generally, this represents the most anterior aspect of a modified retromandibular dissection, and frequently the facial vessels can be retracted forward, if not ligated. Occasionally, the tail of the parotid gland is encountered and retracted posteriorly and superiorly at the posterior aspect of the dissection. Care must be taken to identify and protect the marginal mandibular and buccal branches of the facial nerve along the superficial layer of the deep cervical fascia. A nerve stimulator set at 2 milliamperes (mA) is used to identify facial nerve branches (Figure 32.17). Once identified, the surgeon must decide whether to proceed inferior or superior to the marginal mandibular nerve. Typically, the procedure extends between the buccal and marginal mandibular nerves (Figure 32.5). In multiply operated patients, the facial nerves are frequently located within scar tissue and/or are encountered outside of normal dissection planes.

5. The pterygomasseteric sling and periosteum are incised over the angle of the mandible close to the inferior border, and a subperiosteal dissection plane is utilized to expose the lateral aspect of the mandibular ramus, the coronoid process, and the sigmoid notch. The posterior border of the mandible is dissected superiorly toward the condylar process and is connected with the pre-auricular dissection. A channel retractor is placed within the sigmoid notch along with toe-in retractors anteriorly and posteriorly to facilitate exposure of the entire ramus (Figure 32.18).

Condylar Resection without Massive Ankylosis

1. Once the pre-auricular and modified retromandibular dissections are completed and connected, the condylar resection is initiated. The previously determined osteotomy line below the condyle is marked via measurements taken from various anatomical landmarks on the model, such as the inferior aspect of the zygomatic arch and angle of the mandible. Alternatively, a custom surgical template can be fabricated prior to the procedure. A reciprocating saw blade is used under copious irrigation to perform the osteotomy, separating the condyle and neck from the ramus of the mandible. A curved Freer or periosteal elevator is placed posteriorly and medially subperiosteally to protect vessels during the osteotomy. A Seldin retractor or curved Freer is used to bring the free condylar segment laterally for removal. On patients with decent lateral and protrusive lateral pterygoid muscle function, the anterior aspect of the condyle with its attached lateral pterygoid muscle can be placed at the top of the middle of the ramus and secured with a single bone screw to preserve such function (Figure 32.6). Generally, the coronoid process is osteotomized and removed at this time. If sufficient opening can be achieved with the coronoid process in place, the surgeon may elect to preserve the coronoid process and the attachment of the temporalis muscle to allow for retraction and elevation of the mandible.

2. After the condylar segment has been removed, the glenoid fossa must be prepped for the fossa component. The remaining soft tissue must be thoroughly debrided from the entire glenoid fossa, zygomatic arch, and articular eminence. If necessary, the glenoid fossa is contoured under copious irrigation to mirror the pre-surgical model from which the prosthesis was fabricated. The zygomatic arch is exposed anteriorly as far as needed to accept the lateral flange of the glenoid fossa component.

Condylar Resection with Massive Ankylosis: Two-Stage Alloplastic Reconstruction

1. A standard preoperative CT scan is obtained to determine the degree of ankylosis and the amount of bone to be removed (Figure 32.10). With severe deformities, a CT angiogram may be helpful (Figure 32.13).

2. Once the condylar mass is identified, a periosteal elevator is used to establish a cleavage plane, if possible, between the area of ankylosis and the natural glenoid fossa (Figure 32.16). A towel clip or large clamp may be placed at the angle of the mandible to facilitate movement of the ankylosis to aid in the identification of the cleavage plane. Once the cleavage plane is identified, a periosteal or Freer elevator is used to separate the mass from the underlying glenoid fossa.

3. For large areas of ankylosis, the mass is typically resected in smaller segments to facilitate the atraumatic removal of pieces through either extraoral incision (Figures 32.18, 32.19, and 32.20). A bur, saw, or piezoelectric device with copious irrigation is used for this process. Care is taken when transecting the lateral portion of the ramus as numerous large vessels are typically found in close proximity to the lateral and medial border of the ramus (Figure 32.13). The segments are removed (Figure 32.20), and the gap is completed by removing any irregularities

from the glenoid fossa to below the neck of the condyle. Any potential areas that may interfere with future prostheses placement or fabrication are removed. The ispilateral coronoid process is also removed.

4. For areas of massive bony ankylosis, a cleavage plane may not be identifiable, and the entire glenoid fossa will need to be recontoured with a round bur. Care is taken to minimize inadvertent middle cranial fossa penetration and exposure of mastoid air cells.

5. Once the condylar mass is resected, the coronoidectomy is completed, and all ascending ramus and glenoid fossa irregularities are removed or recontoured, the incisions are covered and the maximum incisal opening (MIO) of the patient is verified. The MIO of the patient should be 35–40 mm. For unilateral cases where the MIO is less than 35–40 mm, a contralateral coronoidectomy may be necessary. In cases with sufficient resection and mobility of the ramus, but in which a contralateral coronoidectomy does not increase MIO, a contralateral arthroplasty should be considered. In addition, deep fibrous connective-tissue bands medial and anterior to the ramus may be present and require judicious removal. In cases with extensive surgical history and repeated episodes of fibrous-bony ankylosis involving the medial and superior aspects of the ramus, it may be necessary to carefully strip most, if not all, aspects of the medial surface of the ramus and place abdominal fat wherever tissue gaps are present from fibrous connective tissue or bone removal.

6. After completion of the resection and verification of MIO, the oral cavity is covered and reprepped. Spacers should be placed within the site of the gap between the fossa and ascending ramus to prevent dense fibrous connective tissue formation while waiting for stage 2 surgery. Spacers may include homemade acrylic condyles, artificial eyeballs, radial or ulnar forearm and toe prostheses. Occasionally, orthognathic surgery is performed at this surgical stage or during the second surgery when custom total joints are inserted.

7. A manufacturer-specific CT scan is taken postoperatively, with the patient placed into wire intermaxillary fixation to generate a one-piece model (Figure 32.21). If orthognathic or reconstructive procedures are planned at the insertion of the custom TMJ prosthesis, a pediatric bite block is placed to separate the teeth during the scan. A two-piece model is then produced to allow for the correction of the patient's occlusion, as described above in this chapter.

Prostheses Placement: One- or Two-Stage Alloplastic Reconstruction

1. After the condyle is resected and the fossa prepared, the glenoid fossa component is placed. Care is taken to not scratch the plastic bearing surface with sharp instruments during insertion. The glenoid fossa component is seated without soft tissue entrapment in a superior and medial direction using a thin Freer elevator to elevate the flap and slide the fossa prosthesis along the elevator while forcing insertion. A fossa-seating tool provided by the manufacturer is used through the retromandibular or pre-auricular incisions to assist in prosthesis seating. The fossa prosthesis must fit securely within the fossa with no rocking or mobility, and the flange resting along the zygomatic arch should fit snuggly. Failure to seat the fossa component properly may result in failure of the implant or non-ideal articulation of the condylar prosthesis. Any areas that are noted to prevent the fossa prosthesis from seating or that contribute to mobility of the prosthesis are relieved. The fossa component screws are placed using slow speed and copious irrigation to prevent devitalizing the bone. The fossa-seating tool is used to stabilize the implant during fixation.

2. Once the fossa prosthesis is fixated, the patient is placed into intermaxillary fixation with stainless steel wires. In order to minimize the potential contamination of the sterile extraoral incisions with oral microbes, the extraoral incisions are covered prior to entering the oral cavity. Instruments used to place the patient into intermaxillary fixation should not be used for the remainder of the case as they are contaminated with oral microbes. After placing the patient into intermaxillary fixation, the surgeons should replace the oral covering (i.e., Tegaderm or Opsite), re-prep the tissue adjacent to the oral cavity, and change their gowns and gloves before returning to the sterile field.

3. Bony recontouring of the lateral ramus, if conducted on the model, is performed with the patient in intermaxillary fixation. Bone removal should be performed very conservatively with multiple fit tests of the condylar component to ensure proper fit and to minimize unneeded bone removal.

4. The condylar component should be properly aligned with the lateral aspect of the mandible, using the model outlines along the posterior and inferior borders. The articulation is finalized by ensuring that the condylar head is centered within the ultra-high-molecular-weight polyethylene fossa cup in the medial-lateral direction and against the bearing's posterior lip (Figure 32.24). The mandibular component may be held flush against the ramus with the mandibular forceps provided by the manufacture. A Freer elevator is used to check for gapping along the perimeter of the mandibular component, particularly around the superior portion where visualization is limited. Gapping may indicate insufficient condylar resection, inadequate mandibular contouring, or improper fossa component seating.

5. The condylar component is held in position with mandibular forceps, the condylar head position is checked again to ensure its ideal articulation within the fossa, and the condylar prosthesis is fixated using the predetermined size and length screws provided by the manufacturer. The drill

guide provided by the manufacturer should be utilized for each screw placement. Copious irrigation and slow-speed drilling are required to minimize devitalization of the bone. The first two or three screw holes are drilled and screws placed, but not tightened. The remaining screw holes are drilled, and screws are placed sequentially. All screws are then tightened after drilling is completed.

6. The extraoral incisions are covered, and the oral cavity is entered to release intermaxillary fixation and to assess occlusion and function. Using sterile technique, the assistant surgeon directly observes the joint components under function to ensure proper movement without dislocation. While the patient is in occlusion, the condylar heads should continue to be centered in the fossa, bearing in the medial or lateral direction and seated against the fossa bearing's posterior lip.

7. Care must be exercised so as not to cross-contaminate the surgical sites from the oral cavity. Extraoral incisions are copiously irrigated and closed in a layered fashion. A pressure dressing is applied and maintained for 24 hours. Guiding elastics are placed for immediate postoperative comfort and to minimize dislocation of the condyle. Full range of motion testing at the end of the case is performed to observe any tendency for condyle dislocation.

Postoperative Management

1. Pressure dressing for 48–72 hours.
2. Guiding elastics are used for 1–2 weeks postoperatively as necessary, and excessive opening is avoided.
3. Physical therapy should be initiated with jaw-exercising devices (i.e., Therabite, Atos Medical, West Allis, WI, USA) at 7–10 days. Nighttime elastics are used up to 3–6 weeks postoperatively.
4. A full liquid diet is employed for 2–3 weeks postoperatively, and then the patient is advanced to a soft chew diet.
5. Orthodontic brackets or arch bars are retained for a minimum of 6 weeks to allow the use of training elastics.
6. Patients are followed weekly for 4–6 weeks to monitor function and occlusal, and to observe for remote postoperative complications.
7. Nonresorbable sutures are removed at 7–10 weeks postoperatively.
8. Sunscreen is placed along the incision lines to prevent potential hyperpigmentation.
9. If occlusal adjustments are necessary, it is best to wait until mandibular opening is maximum, smooth, and demonstrates repetitive articulation. Occlusal adjustments are not recommended until 6–8 weeks postoperatively.

Complications

Early

- Continued or increased pain levels
- Worsening of present or previous TMJ symptoms
- Any issue related to multiply operated patients
- Infection
- Intermittent myofascial spams on the affected side
- Temporary or permanent injury to cranial nerve VII
- Temporary or permanent numbness of skin overlying the incisions
- Otologic issues, including tinnitus, infections, external canal damage, equilibrium imbalances, and hearing loss (temporary or permanent)
- Formation of scar tissue (adhesions)
- Malocclusion
- Allergic or foreign body reaction
- Objectionable scarring of the incisions
- Perforation through the glenoid fossa into the cranial base
- Noncompliance with physical therapy
- Postsurgical neuroma
- Frey's neuralgia
- Failure to maintain initial postsurgical opening

Late

- Excessive fibrous connective tissue or heterotopic bone leading to ankylosis
- Material wear or fracture
- Unrecognized design flaw or treatment planning
- Infection, local or systemic etiology
- Otologic complications
- Any issue related to multiply operated patients
- Need for revision surgery

Key Points

1. For patients with craniofacial syndromes, large ankylosis masses, or those who have undergone multiple previous approaches to the TMJ, a CT angiogram (Figure 32.13) may be beneficial to determine the exact location of major vessels prior to surgery.
2. Virtual Surgical Planning (Figure 32.11), with or without the fabrication of custom cut guides, will give the operator a better understanding of the patient's hard tissue anatomy and the extent of tissue that requires excision prior to fabrication of custom TMJ implants.
3. For multiply operated patients, facial nerves and blood vessels are frequently located in atypical locations and/or within scar tissue. The surgeon should always adhere to strict surgical principles during dissection to prevent neural or vascular injuries.
4. The prostheses and the seating tool are removed from the manufacturer's sterile wrapping and placed within a broad-spectrum antibiotic concentrated solution (i.e., a mixture of normal saline and Vancomycin and Cleocin) at the beginning of the case. During repeated try-ins, the prostheses are stored within the antibiotic solution to impregnate the prostheses with antibiotics to minimize the opportunity for postoperative infections.

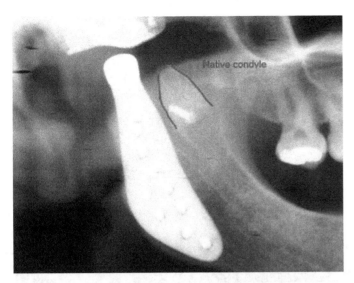

Figure 32.6.   When possible, the anterior aspect of the condyle can be secured to the superior mid-ramus to preserve the function of the lateral pterygoid muscle.

5. Perforation or severance of the external auditory canal is managed with reapproximation of the cartilage with 4-0 Vicryl sutures, placement of an ear wick impregnated with ciprodex or ciprofloxacin drops and postoperative otolaryngology consultation.

6. It is very important to follow a subperiosteal tissue plane during dissection along the zygomatic arch and to stay between the inner and outer layers of the temporal fascia to minimize damage to the facial nerve.

7. For ankylosed joints, a cleavage plane is often identified between the ankylotic mass and the glenoid fossa (Figure 32.16). A Freer elevator may be used to elevate within this plane. Care is taken to minimize excessive pressure along the base of the skull to prevent fractures/perforations of the skull base, ear canal and/or mastoid air cells.

8. The gap arthroplasty/mandibular resection must be adequate for placement of the prosthesis. Typically this involves creating a 15–20 mm space between the glenoid fossa and the ascending ramus.

9. Resurfacing of the mandible and fossa should be carefully completed to ensure that the prosthesis does not rock and fits passively. All fibrous and granulation tissue and irregular bone should be completely removed from the glenoid fossa, particularly the hard to visualize medial aspect of the joint cavity.

10. For one and two stage reconstructions, always adhere to the manufactures CT scan protocol.

11. Use the fossa-seating tool only to prevent fossa prosthesis damage when testing its fit.

12. Secure the fossa component and the mandibular component with the indicated screws from the manufacturer (Figures 32.4, 32.7, 32.9, 32.23, and 32.37).

13. One and two-piece models may be fabricated dependent on the patient's occlusion. One-piece models are ideal for patients with a stable occlusion before or after condylectomy. Two-piece models are best suited for patient's requiring correction of severe preoperative deformity or malocclusion by repositioning the mandible through total joint placement with or without simultaneous maxillary surgery.

14. As a general rule, case involving condylar degeneration and small ankylosis are best suited for one stage reconstruction. Cases involving facial reconstruction surgery, combined orthognathic surgery and large bony ankylosis may be better suited for two stage reconstruction.

15. Examples of atypical cases involving total temporomandibular joints and adjacent anatomical reconstruction include hemimandiblectomies (Figure 32.7), glenoid fossa/temporal bone reconstruction (Figures 32.8 and 32.9) and combined orthognathic surgery (Figures 32.27 through 32.42).

16. In patients with reasonably good lateral pterygoid and temporalis function, the preservation of their muscular attachments to the condyle and coronoid process will allow for increased post-operative mandibular range of motion, specifically lateral excursive and protrusive movements. If sufficient mandibular opening can be achieved after condylotomy, the coronoid process may be left to allow for function of the temporal muscle (mandible elevation and retraction). If the condyle can be resected with preservation of the lateral pterygoid attachments, the condyle may be rigidly fixated to the superior aspect of the mid-ramus (Figure 32.6) to preserve the function of the lateral pterygoid muscle (protrusive and lateral excursive movements).

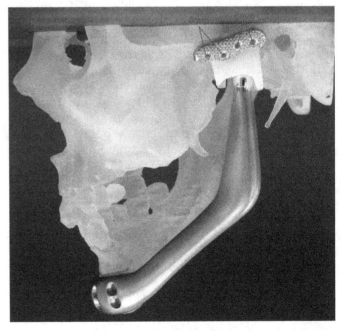

Figure 32.7.   One-piece stereolithic model depicting reconstruction of the left mandible with a custom total temporomandibular joint prostheses following hemi-mandiblectomy for ameloblastoma.

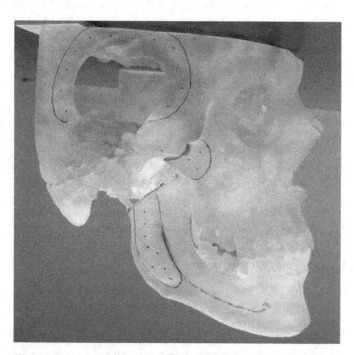

Figure 32.8. One-piece stereolithic model depicting pathological loss of the glenoid fossa, a significant portion of the squamous portion of the temporal bone, the zygomatic arch and the condylar head. Image provided courtesy of TMJ Concepts (Ventura, California).

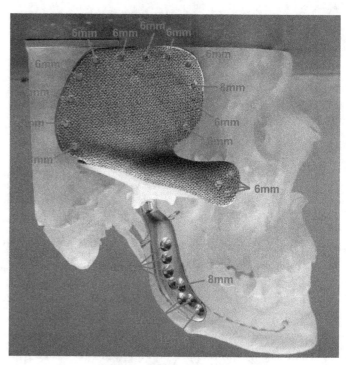

Figure 32.9. One-piece stereolithic model depicting complex reconstruction of the glenoid fossa, temporal bone, zygomatic arch, and condyle. Image provided courtesy of TMJ Concepts (Ventura, California).

Case Reports

Case Report 32.1. A 24-year-old male presents 4 years after closed reduction of bilaterally displaced condyle fractures at an outlying facility with a chief complaint of limited opening, inability to adequately nourish himself and weight loss. Review of the initial CT scan from the incident demonstrated bilateral medially displaced condyles and a moderately displaced symphysis fracture. No other facial fractures were identified. The patient was definitively treated with 6 weeks of intermaxillary fixation. The patient was lost to follow-up and progressively developed a limited range of motion, condylar dysfunction, and progressive weight loss. Physical examination demonstrated a MIO of 5 mm with a lack of lateral excursive movements. A CT scan was obtained that demonstrated bilateral bony ankylosis of the TMJs (Figure 32.10). Due to the degree of ankylosis, the decision was made to perform a two-stage reconstruction. Virtual Surgical Planning (Medical Modeling Inc., Golden, CO, USA) allowed for 3D visualization of the bilateral ankylosed TMJs and enabled virtual treatment planning to determine the exact osteotomy location and design (Figure 32.11). A CT angiogram was obtained that demonstrated extreme proximity of the internal maxillary artery to the medial aspect of the ramus bilaterally. The Stryker Navigation System (Stryker, Kalamazoo, MI, USA) was used to allow for exact osteotomy placement and to avoid damage to anatomical structures (the internal maxillary artery and the inferior alveolar nerve) (Figures 32.12 and 32.13). Electrodes were positioned that allowed for the identification of exact bony reference points identified by the Navigation System throughout the procedure (Figure 32.12). After completion of the bilateral ankylosis resection, a protomed CT scan was obtained with the patient in intermaxillary fixation the day after surgery (Figure 32.21). A one-piece TMJ Concepts (Ventura, CA, USA) stereolithic model was fabricated, and bilateral total joints were waxed-up, approved, manufactured, and inserted (Figures 32.22, 32.23, 32.24, 32.25, and 32.26). The patient's maximum vertical opening immediately status post bilateral total joint insertion was 40 mm. The patient has maintained a maximum vertical opening of 44 mm postoperatively. (See also Figures 32.13 through 32.20.)

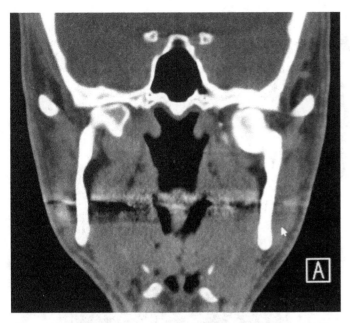

Figure 32.10. Coronal computed tomography scan demonstrating bilateral temporomandibular joint ankylosis from previous medially displaced condyle fractures.

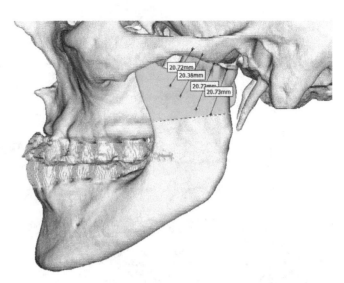

Figure 32.11. Virtual Surgical Planning (VSP) permits the identification of anatomical markers and allows for determination of osteotomy location and design. Measurements are taken from known, uninvolved structures such as the zygomatic arch. Custom cut guides may be fabricated based on VSP treatment sessions.

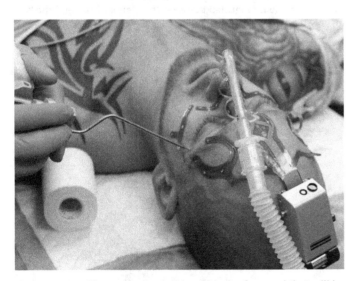

Figure 32.12. Electrodes are positioned and referenced that will be detected with the Stryker Navigation System's software. The Navigation System enables exact osteotomy planning and execution.

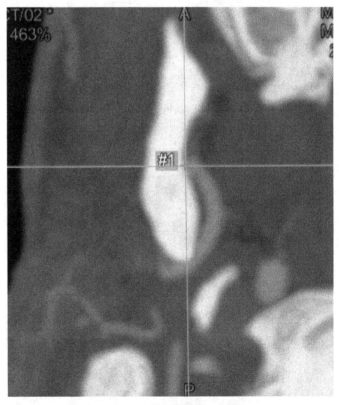

Figure 32.13. The computed tomography (CT) scan and CT angiogram are integrated into the Stryker Navigation System, and a cut plane is determined superior to the internal maxillary artery.

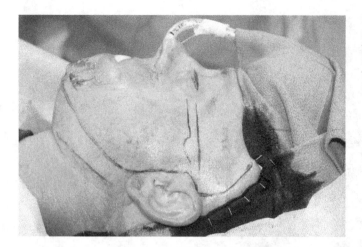

Figure 32.14. The patient is prepped and draped, a sterile, antibiotic-impregnated ear wick is placed within the bilateral external auditory canals, and the oral cavity is covered with a plastic adhesive drape to prevent the contamination of the extraoral surgical sites with oral microbes.

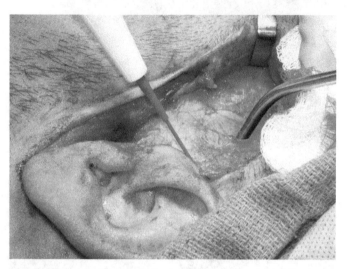

Figure 32.15. The pre-auricular incision is initiated, and the superficial layer of the temporalis fascia is exposed above the zygomatic arch.

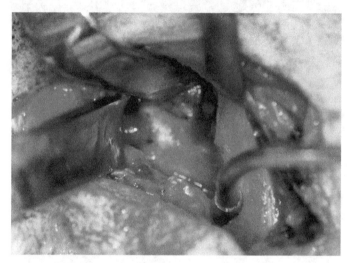

Figure 32.16. The zygomatic arch is exposed anterior to the eminence, the head of the condyle and ankylosed mass is exposed, and a cleavage plane is identified between the glenoid fossa and the condyle and ankylosed mass.

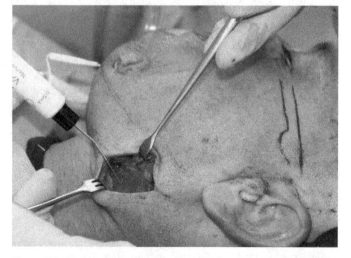

Figure 32.17. A nerve stimulator set at 2 mA is used to test for branches of the facial nerve during both the modified retromandibular and the pre-auricular approaches.

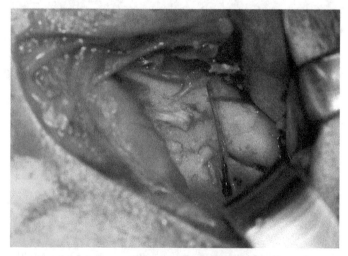

Figure 32.18. A Sonopet Ultrasonic Aspirator (Stryker, Kalamazoo, MI, USA) is used to section the ankylosed mass into small segments to facilitate the atraumatic removal of the bone from the modified retromandibular incision.

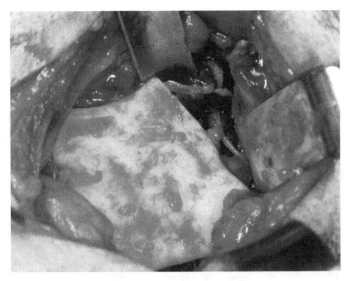

Figure 32.19. The upper ramus resection is completed and includes the medially displaced condyle, the coronoid process and the ankylosed mass. All bony irregularities that could interfere with custom joint fabrication and seating are removed from the ramus and glenoid fossa.

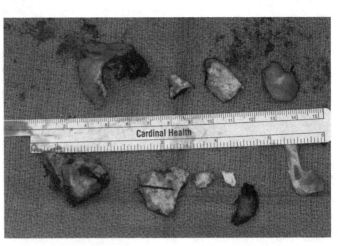

Figure 32.20. Resected ankylosed bone from the bilateral upper ramus resections, condylectomies, and coronoidectomies.

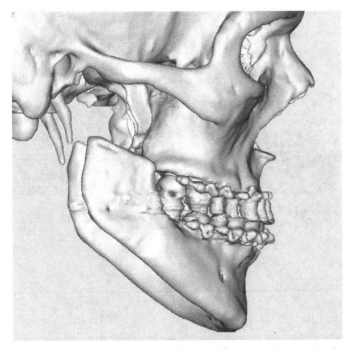

Figure 32.21. Postoperative sagittal 3D scan depicting bilateral temporomandibular joint resections. The patient is placed within intermaxillary fixation during this scan in order to establish the postoperative occlusion and to create a one-piece stereolithic model.

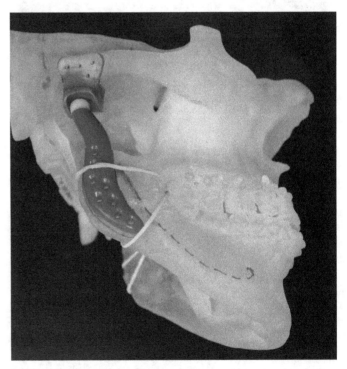

Figure 32.22. Wax-up of temporomandibular joint custom prostheses on a one-piece stereolithic model.

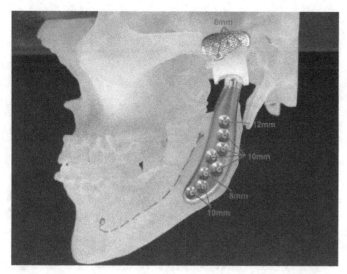

Figure 32.23.   Manufacturer image depicting precise placement of the prostheses on the stereolithic model. Fixation screw length and placement are predetermined based on the patient's anatomy and the extent of the upper ramus resections.

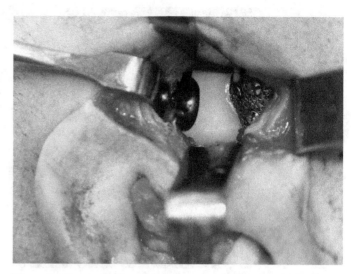

Figure 32.24.   At the second stage surgery, the glenoid fossa and ramus prostheses are fixated in position, with the artificial condyle seated within the ultra-high-molecular-weight polyethylene fossa cup.

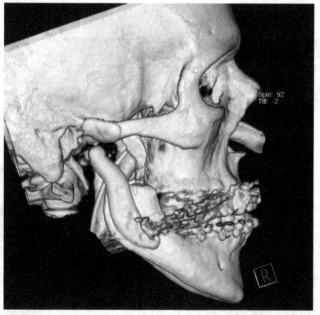

Figure 32.25.   Immediate postoperative 3D reconstruction depicting ideal placement of the prostheses.

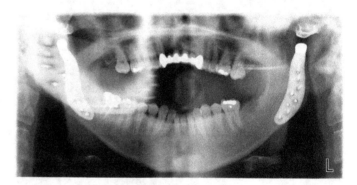

Figure 32.26.   Two-year postoperative orthopantomogram demonstrating a maximum incisal opening of 4 cm.

Case Report 32.2. A 26-year-old patient with a history of progressive right TMJ degenerative disease over a 3-year period presents with a 10 mm loss of right condylar height (Figure 32.27), malocclusion consisting of premature contact of the right posterior teeth, an anterior open bite, and a maxilla tilted downward on the left (Figure 32.28). After biopsies, the patient was diagnosed with severe osteoarthritis of her right mandibular condyle. No anomalies were identified within the left TMJ. Orthodontic appliances were placed prior to surgery (Figure 32.29). A manufacturer-specific CT scan was taken, and a one-piece stereolithic model was fabricated. Due to limited occlusal contact within the one-piece stereolithic model, the mandible was easily separated from the maxilla and the case was worked up as a two-piece model. A right condylectomy and coronoidectomy were performed on the stereolithic model, and the right ramus was lowered to reestablish lost condyle height. The mandible was glued to the maxilla with a splint in position to allow for superior elevation of the left maxilla at surgery (Figure 32.30; see also Figure 32.31). The maxilla was leveled with a one-piece Le Fort I osteotomy, and the right ascending ramus height was reconstructed with a custom TMJ Concepts prostheses (Figure 32.32; see also Figure 32.33).

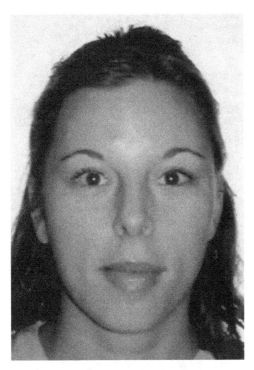

Figure 32.27. A 26-year-old female with decreased height to her right mandibular condyle with resulting maxillary canting and dentofacial asymmetry.

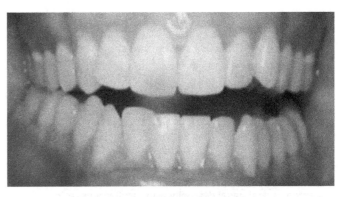

Figure 32.28. Preoperative malocclusion depicting severe dysgnathia, apertognathia, and a canted maxilla.

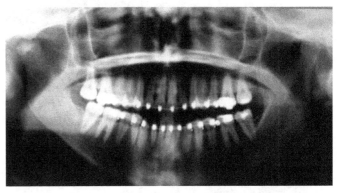

Figure 32.29. Preoperative orthopantomogram demonstrating a degenerative process of the right condyle, dysgnathia, and a maxillary yaw deformity.

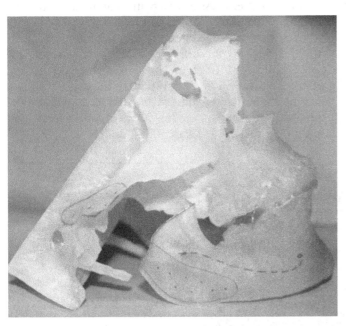

Figure 32.30. One-piece stereolithic model after right condylectomy, coronoidectomy, and restoration of ramus height. Hot glue is used to reposition the mandible to the maxilla prior to the fabrication of the right-sided total joint.

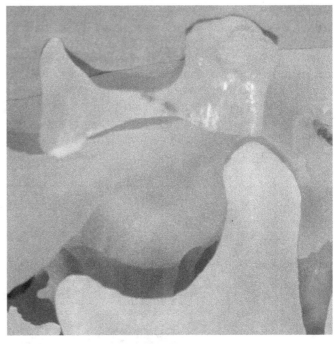

Figure 32.31. Note loss of condyle height when the resected right condyle is positioned next to the normal left condyle.

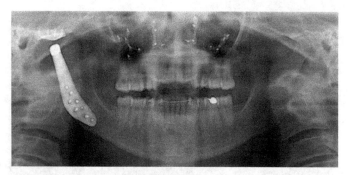

Figure 32.32. 8-year postoperative orthopantomogram demonstrating correction of dentofacial deformity with simultaneous Le Fort I osteotomy leveling of the maxilla and the placement of a right TMJ Concept total joint.

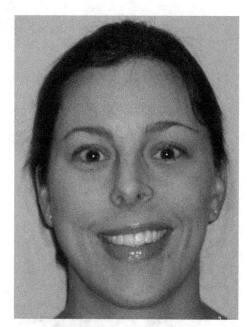

Figure 32.33. 8-year postoperative appearance illustrating restoration of occlusion and facial balance.

Case Report 32.3. An 11-year-old female presented with a chief complaint of left mandibular deviation with restricted opening and significant facial asymmetry after resection of a desmoplastic fibroma involving the left glenoid fossa, condyle, and ramus of the mandible at an age of 3. Reconstruction with a costochondral graft was attempted at the age of 8 (Figure 32.34). The costochondral graft reconstruction resulted in graft resorption and ankylosis, contributing to the patient's severe mandibular asymmetry, retrognathism, and dysgnathia. At age 11, the patient was referred to the senior author's facility for definitive surgical treatment. The patient's treatment plan was delayed 2 years until skeletal maturity was achieved as measured by serial lateral cephalograms and wrist films. Once skeletal maturity was reached, orthodontic therapy was initiated to upright the dentition, but not to correct the malocclusion or cant of the jaws. At age 15, at the completion of ortho-

dontics, the occlusion was leveled, and a 10 mm transverse malocclusion discrepancy was established (Figure 32.35). This allowed full surgical correction of the patient's dentofacial deformity through a combined Le Fort I, one-piece osteotomy and a right bilateral sagittal split ramus osteotomy (BSSO) with degloving of the left body of the mandible to permit mandibular advancement and rotation of the mandible to the right. Due to this extreme transverse surgical movement, associated with degloving of the left body of the mandible, the patient was kept in fixation for 12 weeks to prevent the lateral shift of the mandible to the pathology side. Six months later, a left-sided custom TMJ Concepts total joint (Figures 32.36, 32.37, and 32.38) and an 8 mm anterior sliding osteotomy of the symphysis was performed. The patient has no functional anomalies and has a maximum vertical opening of 4 cm at 10 years of follow-up (Figures 32.39, 32.40, 32.41, and 32.42).

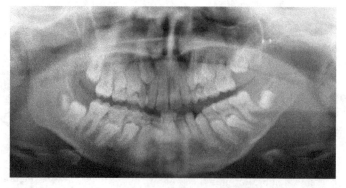

Figure 32.34. Radiograph of the patient at age 8 following removal of desmoplastic fibroma and failed rib graft.

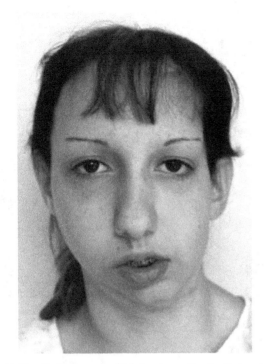

Figure 32.35.   Patient at age 15 following orthodontic treatment in preparation for orthognathic surgery and total joint reconstruction.

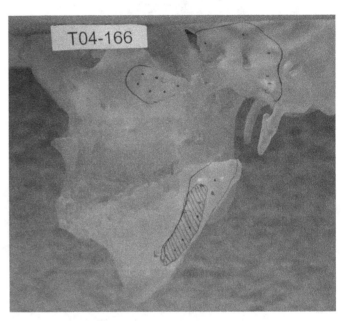

Figure 32.36.   One-piece stereolithic model fabricated with the patient in intermaxillary fixation after bilateral sagittal split ramus osteotomy and Le Fort I osteotomy surgery to correct mandibular asymmetry, retrognathism, and canted jaws.

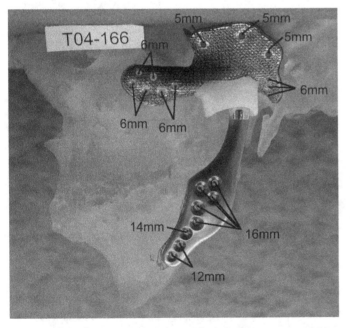

Figure 32.37.   One-piece custom prostheses depicting reconstruction of the left zygomatic arch, glenoid fossa, and mandibular condyle.

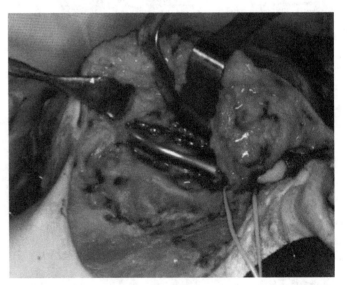

Figure 32.38.   The temporomandibular total joint prostheses are placed and secured to the defect site with fixation screws through a cranial facial approach. Vessel loops indicate the location of the upper trunk of the facial nerve.

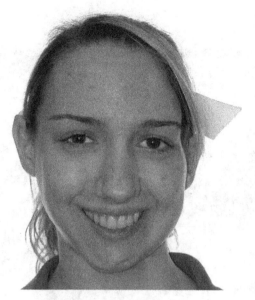

Figure 32.39.   Postoperative appearance of the patient demonstrating restoration of facial symmetry.

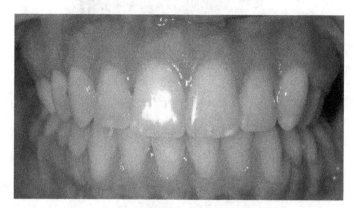

Figure 32.40.   8-year postoperative occlusion.

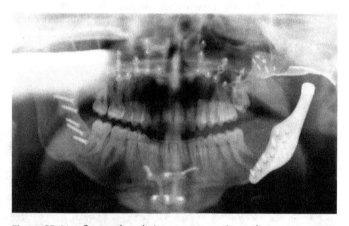

Figure 32.41.   8-year closed-view postoperative orthopantomogram depicting ideal articulation of the condylar prosthesis within the glenoid fossa polyethylene cup.

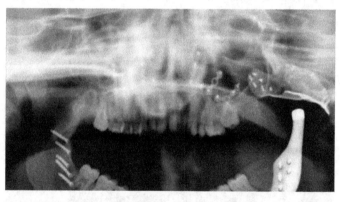

Figure 32.42.   8-year open-view postoperative orthopantomogram depicting appropriate function of the prostheses and a maximum vertical opening of greater than 4 cm.

References

Mercuri, L.G., 2000. The TMJ concepts patient fitted total temporomandibular joint reconstruction prosthesis. In: W.C. Donlon, ed. *Oral and Maxillofacial Surgery Clinics of North America*, 12 (1), 73–91.

Mercuri, L.G., 2011. Patient-fitted ("custom") alloplastic temporomandibular joint replacement technique. In: G. Ness, ed. *Atlas of the Oral & Maxillofacial Surgery Clinics of North America*. Vol. 19. Philadelphia: Elsevier Saunders, 233–242.

Mercuri, L.G. 2012a. Alloplastic TMJ replacement: rationale for custom devices. *International Journal of Oral and Maxillofacial Surgery*, 41, 1033–1040.

Mercuri, L.G., 2012b. Avoiding and managing temporomandibular joint total joint replacement surgical site infections. *Journal of Oral and Maxillofacial Surgery*, 70, 2280–2289.

Mercuri, L.G., 2014. Temporomandibular joint replacement periprosthetic joint infections: a review of early diagnostic testing options. *International Journal of Oral and Maxillofacial Surgery*, 43, 1236–1242.

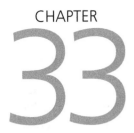

CHAPTER

33

Autogenous Reconstruction of the Temporomandibular Joint

John N. Kent[1] and Christopher J. Haggerty[2]

[1]*Department of Oral and Maxillofacial Surgery, Louisiana State University Health Sciences Center, New Orleans, Louisiana, USA*

[2]*Private Practice, Lakewood Oral and Maxillofacial Surgery Specialists, Lees Summit; and Department of Oral and Maxillofacial Surgery, University of Missouri–Kansas City, Kansas City, Missouri, USA*

A means of reconstructing acquired and congenital temporomandibular joint (TMJ) abnormalities.

Indications

1. Reconstruction of defects resulting from acquired joint abnormalities (primary fibrous and bony ankylosis, infection, osteoarthritis, idiopathic condylar resorption, rheumatic diseases, neoplasms, and posttraumatic deformities)
2. Reconstruction of defects resulting from congenital joint abnormalities caused by malformations of the structures of the first and second branchial arches (hemi-facial microsomia, Goldenhar syndrome [oculo-auriculo-vertebral syndrome], otomandibular dysostosis, and lateral facial dysplasia)
3. Failure of components of alloplastic joint prosthesis, if scar bed is not excessive
4. When reconstruction with an alloplastic prosthesis is cost-prohibitive
5. Severe occlusal discrepancies involving the TMJ and associated structures that are not amendable to conventional orthognathic surgery

Contraindications

1. Children without the complete eruption of the primary dentition
2. Multiple operated joints
3. Active infection
4. Psychiatric disorders
5. Medically compromised individuals: the very elderly, those with uncontrolled systemic diseases (chronic obstructive pulmonary disease, unstable cardiovascular issues, and poorly controlled diabetes), and those with drug and/or alcohol addiction
6. Patients unable or unwilling to perform recommended postoperative physical therapy and cooperate with rehabilitation protocols

Autogenous TMJ Replacement Procedure: Costochondral Graft

1. Intravenous antibiotics, steroids, and antisialogues are given preoperatively. The patient is positioned supine on the operating room table and nasally intubated. Short-acting paralytics are used in order to test for branches of the facial nerve during the procedure. Separate intraoral and facial–chest instrument tray set-ups are created. Protective draping and/or redraping and prepping are always recommended throughout the procedure to avoid cross-contamination between the mouth and face–chest when going back and forth between sterile and nonsterile (oral) environments.
2. A throat pack is placed within the posterior oropharynx. If orthodontic appliances are not in place, mandibular and maxillary Erich arch bars are placed, but maxillomandibular fixation (MMF) is not initiated.
3. The patient is prepped in a sterile fashion. The oral cavity is prepped with Betadine paint (Betadine scrub is not recommended for mucous membranes application), and a sterile gauze is placed between the dentition and the internal surface of the lips to prevent the contamination of the extraoral field with saliva. The external auditory canals are prepped with Betadine paint, and an antibiotic impregnated ear wick is placed within the external auditory canals bilaterally. The remainder of the facial skeleton is prepped with Betadine paint from the scalp to the clavicles. The patient is draped to allow for exposure of bilateral pre-auricular and retromandibular incisions (even if only anticipating ipsilateral surgery) and the oral cavity.
4. The head is turned 45° to the contralateral side. The affected joint is approached via a combined pre-auricular and modified-retromandibular approach (refer to Chapter 32). A nerve stimulator is used to test for branches of the facial nerve.
5. A gap arthroplasty is performed from the glenoid fossa to the sigmoid notch. Diseased or deformed bone, scar tissue, and/or the involved condyle is removed, leaving

a gap of approximately 15–20 mm from the ascending ramus osteotomy to the glenoid fossa. An ipsilateral coronoidectomy is performed. On occasion, if the patient has appreciable lateral pterygoid muscle function, the anterior aspect of the mandibular condyle with lateral pterygoid muscle attachment can be placed beneath the sigmoid notch area with a bone screw to preserve a portion of the lateral pterygoid function.

6. The glenoid fossa is smoothed or reshaped (Figure 33.6 [all figures cited in this list appear in Case Report 33.1]), and, if present, the native disc is preserved.

7. After completion of the gap arthroplasty, the oral cavity is entered and mandibular movement is assessed to confirm unrestricted function. If mandibular movement is less than 35 mm, the gap arthroplasty site is inspected for interferences. Areas of scar tissue are removed from the ascending ramus, lateral and medial surfaces, and inferior border of the mandible. If interferences are identified on the contralateral side, a contralateral coronoidectomy should be performed. If contralateral interferences are present after coronoidectomy, contralateral open arthroplasty should be considered.

8. After obtaining and confirming adequate mandibular movement, the patient is placed into MMF, the oral gauze located between the dentition and the internal surfaces of the lips is replaced, the patient is reprepped and draped extraorally with betadine paint, and the surgeon's gloves are changed to prevent contamination of the extraoral surgical sites with oral microbes.

9. The autogenous graft is harvested after the gap arthroplasty is completed and all interferences are addressed (Figure 33.7).

10. For costochondral grafts (CCGs), the cartilage head is reshaped to mimic a condylar head and to seat ideally within the glenoid fossa (Figure 33.8). Five to ten millimeters of cartilage are preserved at the rib–cartilage junction. The CCG should fit passively along the lateral surface of the ascending ramus while the CCG's cartilaginous cap is seated within the glenoid fossa (Figure 33.10).

11. In order to maximize CCG contact with the lateral ascending ramus, autogenous interpositional grafting may need to be performed between the CCG and the lateral ascending ramus as the rib may be slightly curved as it opposes the flat ramus surface. It is prudent to harvest 1–2 cm of rib beyond the intended graft length. Sources of potential autogenous bone include the distal aspect of the rib harvested and/or adjacent ribs.

12. The CCG is secured to the lateral ascending ramus with rigid fixation in the form of plate fixation using 3–4 screws (Figure 33.9).

13. After fixation of the CCG, the face is draped out, and the oral cavity is entered. MMF is removed, and mandibular movement and occlusion are confirmed prior to closing the extraoral incisions in a layered fashion. Drains are typically not necessary. The patient is placed into light guiding elastics, and a pressure dressing is applied to the facial skeleton.

Postoperative Management

1. Antibiotics are given immediately preoperatively and for 2 weeks postoperatively.

2. The patient is functioned immediately after surgery with nonforceful, passive jaw exercises.

3. For the first 10–12 weeks, patients are allowed to function with a soft mechanical (nonchew) diet and guiding elastics during the day. At night, patients are placed into MMF via heavy elastics.

4. Arch bars or orthodontic appliances are removed at 3 months provided occlusion is satisfactory and the interincisal opening is reaching a 30 mm range. Aggressive physiotherapy is continued for 3–12 months in order to maintain a maximum opening of 30–35 mm and to minimize recurrent ankylosis.

Complications

1. **Donor site morbidity**: Refer to Chapter 57.

2. **Reankylosis**: Minimized with complete removal of the ankylotic mass and appropriate physiotherapy.

3. **CCG overgrowth and undergrowth**: Minimized by leaving 10 mm or less of a cartilaginous cap at the rib–cartilage junction and with postpubertal CCGs.

4. **Facial nerve damage or paralysis**: Minimized with appropriate incision placement, meticulous dissection, and the use of a nerve stimulator.

5. **Fracture at the costal cartilage–rib interface**: Can be minimized by leaving 10 mm or less of cartilage at the rib–cartilage junction and avoiding early, excessive loading of the CCG.

6. **Fracture or splintering of the rib**: Minimized by using plate fixation instead of lag or positional screw fixation.

7. **Hardware failure or graft mobility**: Minimized with the use of screw and plate rigid fixation of the graft to the lateral ascending ramus. A minimum of three screws should be utilized to fixate the CCG to the ascending ramus.

8. **Infection**: Minimized with strict attention to sterile technique and wound closure in a layered fashion. Gowns and gloves should be changed when alternating from the oral cavity to extraoral incisions in order to minimize contamination of the extraoral sites with oral microbes. Separate instruments and instrument tables should be established for oral and extraoral instruments in order to avoid cross-contamination.

9. **Malocclusion**: Minimized with the use of a prefabricated occlusal splint, rigid fixation of the graft material, and the use of heavy elastic MMF at night for 3 months postoperatively.

10. **Graft resorption**: Rare. When graft resorption occurs, it is typically seen in children and young adults.

1. TMJ reconstruction not only aids in correcting functional disorders (restricted mouth opening, malocclusion, and malnutrition), but also can improve cosmetic disabilities and dentofacial deformities.

2. Autogenous sources for TMJ reconstruction include CCG, metatarsal, fibula, distraction osteogenesis, and the posterior border of the ascending ramus (sliding osteotomy).

3. Advantages of CCG include a low complication rate, the ability to shape the cartilage to the anatomy of the glenoid fossa, the capacity for remodeling into an adaptive mandibular condyle, and possessing an adaptive growth center for growing patients. CCG should not be used in areas of recurrent ankylosis or active infection.

4. The CCG is the graft of choice for growing pediatric patients.

5. Prior to any surgical intervention, a thorough CT evaluation should be performed to evaluate both the involved and uninvolved joint to identify areas of potential abnormalities and/or restrictions to movement.

6. For patients with moderate to severe dysgnathia, a prefabricated occlusal splint should be used in order to establish ideal intraoperative and postoperative occlusion.

7. When performing gap arthroplasty on ankylosed joints, the ankylosed mass is typically removed en bloc. For larger ankylosed masses (Figure 33.1; see also Figure 33.2), the mass is sectioned and removed in smaller segments (Figure 33.3). When removing ankylosed masses, a line of separation or cleavage plane is frequently present between the ankylosed mass and the glenoid fossa. If present, a periosteal elevator can be placed within this plane to identify the caudal aspect of the glenoid fossa and to allow for the dissection of the ankylotic mass from the glenoid fossa. The removal of the ankylotic mass from the medial aspect of the glenoid fossa is imperative to allow for maximal function and to minimize the risk of recurrent ankylosis.

8. In ankylosis cases resulting from condyle trauma, the fractured condyles are completely removed during excision of the fibrous or bony ankylotic mass.

9. When securing the CCG to the lateral ascending ramus, positional and lag screws may propagate a fracture within the CCG and distract the costal cartilage cap from the glenoid fossa. Plate fixation will minimize the risk of fracture of the CCG by acting as a washer and distributing the forces of compression along the lateral surface of the CCG.

10. When possible, the native disc should be preserved and maintained. Temporalis muscle fascia flaps, temporoparietal galea flaps, and dermis grafts can also be used to line the glenoid fossa. Well-contoured cartilage caps that articulate ideally within the glenoid fossa often require no lining.

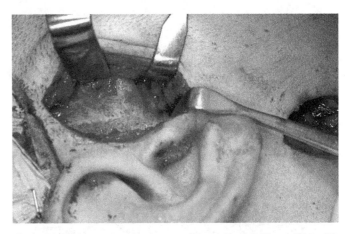

Figure 33.2. Intraoperative image of the patient in Figure 33.1 with complete bony ankylosis of the right temporomandibular joint space.

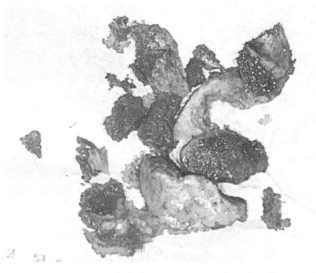

Figure 33.3. Larger ankylotic masses are sectioned and removed in smaller pieces.

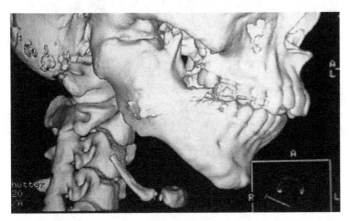

Figure 33.1. 3D reconstruction demonstrating a complete right-sided temporomandibular joint bony ankylosis.

Case Report

Case Report 33.1. A 42-year-old patient presents with a chief complaint of pain, malocclusion, an anterior open bite, decreased vertical ramus height (bilateral degenerative condyles), and a medical history significant for rheumatoid disease. (See Figures 33.4 through 33.13.)

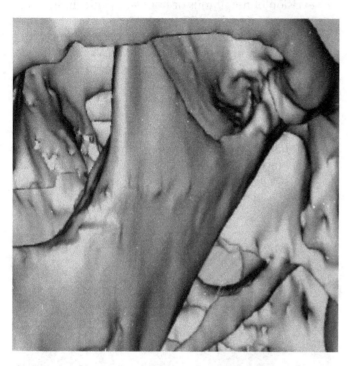

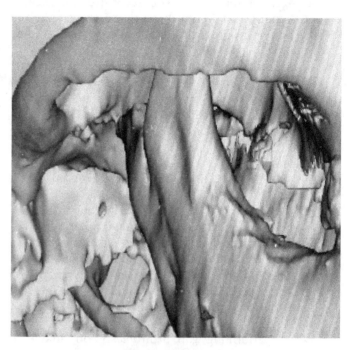

Figure 33.4.   3D reconstruction views demonstrating bilateral condylar degeneration secondary to rheumatoid disease.

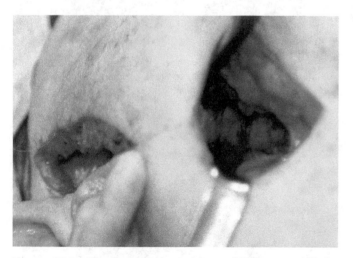

Figure 33.5.   The preauricular and modified-retromandibular approaches allow access to the mandibular condyle, coronoid process and ascending ramus.

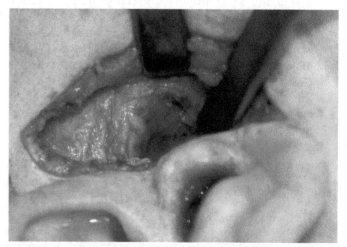

Figure 33.6.   The degenerative condyle and coronoid process have been excised, establishing a 15–20 mm gap between the ascending ramus and the glenoid fossa. The glenoid fossa has been reshaped and all interferences have been removed.

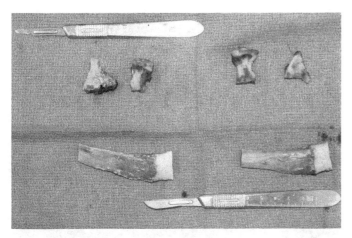

Figure 33.7.   Bilateral degenerative condyles and coronoid processes. Ribs 5 and 6 prior to reshaping.

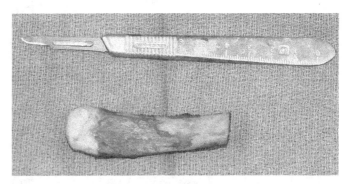

Figure 33.8.   The costal cartilage is reshaped to function as a condyle and to articulate ideally within the glenoid fossa.

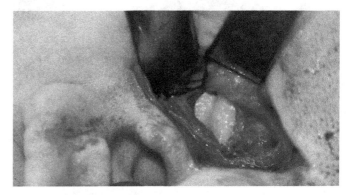

Figure 33.10.   The cartilaginous cap of the costochondral graft articulates ideally within the glenoid fossa.

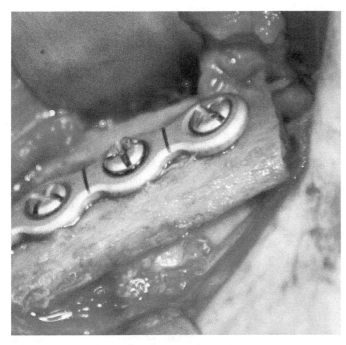

Figure 33.9.   The costochondral graft (CCG) is secured to the lateral surface of the ascending ramus with plate fixation. The titanium plate acts as a washer and distributes the compression forces along the lateral surface of the CCG.

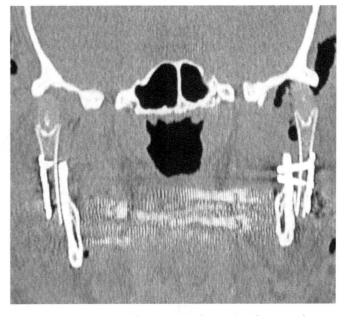

Figure 33.11.   Postoperative computed tomography scan demonstrating costochondral grafts secured to the lateral aspect of the ascending ramus with articulation within the glenoid fossa.

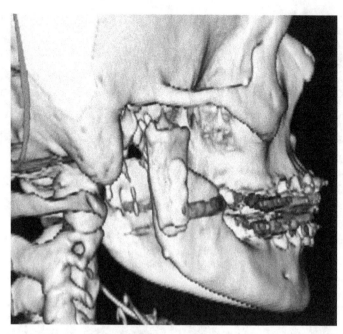

Figure 33.12. Postoperative 3D reconstruction demonstrating placement of the right costochondral graft.

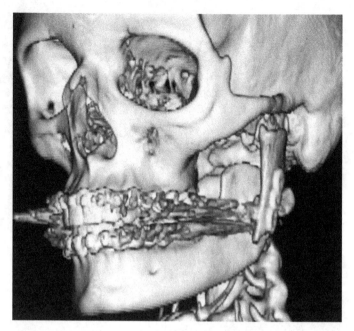

Figure 33.13. Postoperative 3D reconstruction demonstrating placement of the left costochondral graft.

References

El-Sayed, K.M., 2008. Temporomandibular joint reconstruction with costochondral graft using modified approach. *International Journal of Oral and Maxillofacial Surgery*, 37, 897–902.

Kaban, L.B., Bouchard, C. and Troulis, M.J., 2009. A protocol for management of temporomandibular joint ankylosis in children. *Journal of Oral and Maxillofacial Surgery*, 67, 1966–78.

Khadka, A. and Hu, J., 2012. Autogenous grafts for condylar reconstruction in treatment of TMJ ankylosis: current concepts and considerations for the future. *International Journal of Oral and Maxillofacial Surgery*, 41, 94–102.

Medra, A.M., 2005. Follow up of mandibular costochondral grafts after release of ankylosis of the temporomandibular joints. *British Journal of Oral and Maxillofacial Surgery*, 43, 118–22.

Saeed, N.R. and Kent, J.N., 2003. A retrospective study of the costochondral graft in TMJ reconstruction. *Journal of Oral and Maxillofacial Surgery*, 32, 606–9.

Sahoo, N.K., Tomar, K., Kumar, A. and Roy, I.D., 2012. Selecting reconstruction option for TMJ ankylosis: a surgeon's dilemma. *Journal of Craniofacial Surgery*, 23, 1796–801.

Vega, L.C., Gonzalez-Garcia, R. and Louis, P.J., 2013. Reconstruction of acquired temporomandibular joint defects. *Oral and Maxillofacial Surgery Clinics of North America*, 25, 251–69.

34

Eminectomy

Joseph P. McCain[1] and Reem Hamdy Hossameldin[2]

[1]*Private Practice; Baptist Health Systems; and Oral and Maxillofacial Surgery, Herbert Wertheim College of Medicine, Florida International University Miami, Florida, USA; and Nova Southeastern School of Dental Medicine, Fort Lauderdale, Florida USA*

[2]*Department of Oral and Maxillofacial Surgery, Faculty of Dental Medicine, Cairo University, Cairo, Egypt; and General Surgery Department, Herbert Wertheim College of Medicine, Florida International University, Miami, Florida, USA*

A procedure performed to correct chronic dislocation or closed lock of the mandible with surgical reduction of the articular eminence.

Indications

1. Habitual chronic dislocation of the mandible, where all conservative and minimally invasive methods are either unsuccessful or contraindicated
2. Treatment of closed lock of the temporomandibular joint (TMJ) (modified eminectomy)

Contraindications

1. Chronic mandibular dislocation cases involving a shallow articular eminence
2. Radiological evidence of a pneumatized eminence (increased risk of infection as a result of communication between the joint space and the mastoid air cells)
3. Radiographic evidence of a vascularized eminence (intracranial hemorrhage)

Anatomy

Superficial temporal vessels: Emerge from the superior aspect of the parotid gland and accompany the auriculotemporal nerve (Figure 34.1). The superficial temporal artery (STA) arises from the parotid gland as a bifurcation of the external carotid artery (ECA). The STA is a common source of bleeding during approaches to the TMJ. The superficial temporal vein lies superficial and usually posterior to the artery.

Transverse facial vessels: Branch off of the superficial temporal vessels and course inferior and relatively parallel to the zygomatic arch (Figure 34.1).

Auriculotemporal nerve: Courses from the medial aspect of the posterior neck of the condyle and turns superiorly, coursing superficial to the zygomatic root of the temporal bone (Figure 34.1). Just anterior to the auricle, the nerve divides into its terminal branches within the skin of the temporal area. The auriculotemporal nerve accompanies, and is posterior to, the STA. Pre-auricular exposure of the TMJ area almost always invariably injures this nerve. Damage is minimized by incision and dissection in close apposition to the cartilaginous portion of the external auditory meatus. Temporal extension of the skin incision should be located posteriorly so that the main distribution of the nerve is dissected and retracted forward within the flap. Patients rarely complain about sensory disturbances that result from damage to the auriculotemporal nerve.

Pre-auricular Dissection Layers

Temporoparietal fascia (superficial temporal fascia): The temporoparietal fascia, which is the most superficial fascia layer beneath the subcutaneous fat, is the lateral extension of the galea and is continuous with the superficial musculoaponeurotic layer (SMAS). The blood vessels of the scalp, such as the superficial temporal vessels, run along its superficial aspect closely related to the subcutaneous fat. Motor nerves, such as the temporal branch of the facial nerve, run on the deep surface of the temporoparietal fascia.

Subgaleal fascia: The subgaleal fascia within the temporoparietal region is well developed and can be dissected as a discrete fascial layer if desired, but it is usually used only as a cleavage plane in the standard pre-auricular approach.

Temporalis fascia (deep temporal fascia): The dense, white fascia overlying the temporalis muscle. This thick fascia arises from the superior temporal line and fuses with the pericranium. The temporalis muscle arises from the deep surface of the temporal fascia and the whole of the temporal fossa. Inferiorly, the temporal fascia splints into a superficial and a deep layer above the zygomatic arch. A small quantity of fat between the two layers is referred to as the superficial temporal fat pad. A large vein frequently runs just deep to the superficial layer of temporalis fascia.

Atlas of Operative Oral and Maxillofacial Surgery, First Edition. Edited by Christopher J. Haggerty and Robert M. Laughlin
© 2015 John Wiley & Sons, Inc. Published 2015 by John Wiley & Sons, Inc.

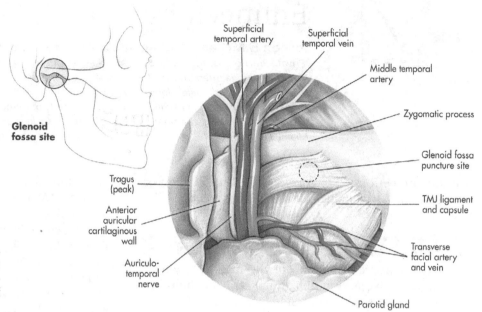

Glenoid fossa site

Superficial temporal artery

Superficial temporal vein

Middle temporal artery

Zygomatic process

Glenoid fossa puncture site

TMJ ligament and capsule

Transverse facial artery and vein

Parotid gland

Auriculo-temporal nerve

Anterior auricular cartilaginous wall

Tragus (peak)

Figure 34.1. Image depicting the orientation of the superficial temporal artery and vein, auriculotemporal nerve, and transverse facial artery and vein at the root of the zygoma.

Technique

1. The patient is placed supine on the operating room table and nasally intubated.
2. The patient is prepped and draped, allowing for visualization of the entire ear and lateral canthus of the eye. The pre-auricular hair is shaved, and the remainder of the patient's hair is positioned under a surgical head cap. An ear wick soaked in antibiotic solution is placed within the external auditory canal.
3. No local anesthetic or vasoconstrictors are injected.
4. The pre-auricular incision is marked along an actual skin crease, contouring the incision around the tragal cartilage (Figure 34.5 [all figures cited in this list appear in Case Report 34.1]). The incision originates at the top of the ear and extends just inferior to the tragal cartilage. The incision does not extend to the pinna. The incision initially transverses skin and subcutaneous tissue only (Figure 34.6). Small bleeding points are cauterized with needlepoint cautery at the coagulation mode of 20.
5. The dissection can be divided into thirds. The upper third is performed first. A curved hemostat is used to dissect bluntly through the horizontal auricular muscles down to the glistening white temporalis fascia (Figure 34.7). The neurovascular bundle is kept forward. Occasionally, a horizontal vessel is encountered arising from the superficial temporal artery or vein that crosses the dissection site (transverse facial vessels) and requires cauterized or suture ligation. Once the glistening white temporalis fascia is identified, a Messer retractor is placed to confirm that position and to reflect the flap anteriorly.

6. The second part of the dissection is within the lower third of the incision. The tragal cartilage is skeletonized (Figure 34.8) to its apex with a curved hemostat. A small tag of tissue may be retained (4 to 6 mm) along the tragal cartilage to provide a point to place subcutaneous sutures during closure. With the upper and the lower aspects of the dissection completed, two points of depth are established: one within the superior third of the dissection at the level of the temporalis fascia, and a second at the inferior third of the dissection at the level of the tragal cartilage apex that goes to the capsule.
7. The third part of the dissection connects the middle third of the incision to the superior and inferior thirds of the dissection (Figure 34.9). Sharp dissection proceeds through the horizontal auricular muscles to expose and connect the temporalis fascia with the superior dissection and the tragal tip with the inferior dissection.
8. A periosteal elevator is utilized in a sweeping motion to flap forward the tissue within the layer superficial to the temporalis fascia (Figure 34.10). A sharp incision from the apex of the tragal cartilage to the superior aspect of the incision is made. Methylene blue mark can be used to mark the incision site (Figure 34.12). The Messer retractor is used to pull the flap superior to allow for a release of the temporalis fascia so that the skin incision does not need to be extended for additional exposure. The incision extends from the tip of the tragal cartilage, superiorly through the temporalis fascia and temporalis muscle, and down to bone (Figure 34.13). The temporalis muscle is transected with the cautery mode at 20 to 30. The parotid

gland can be swept inferiorly with a Messer retractor if encountered.

9. A periosteal elevator is used to dissect within the subperiosteal plane from the root of the zygoma anteriorly to expose the articular eminence (Figures 34.14 and 34.15). The periosteal elevator is used in an inferior sweeping motion to expose the capsule of the TMJ.

10. The capsule of the TMJ is incised with a #15 blade from the posterior glenoid process onto the maximum concavity of the fossa located at the back slope of the articular eminence. A periosteal elevator is used to dissect free the superior joint space from the articular eminence, trying to preserve articular cartilage (Figure 34.16). In articular eminectomy, it is not necessary to enter the inferior joint space.

11. After disarticulation of the superior joint space and isolation of the articular eminence (Figure 34.17), a 101 bur is utilized to score the anticipated osteotomy at the level of the zygomatic process of the temporal bone (Figure 34.18). The osteotomy of the articular eminence is completed with a sharp straight osteotome angled inferiorly 10° (Figure 34.19). Failure to angle the chisel slightly inferiorly will increase the risk of inadvertent damage or penetration of the skull base.

12. It is important to resect the articular tubercle so that laterally the eminence and medially the tubercle are preserved. If the articular tubercle is not resected, there is a high incidence of future dislocation.

13. Once the bulk of the eminence is resected, a reciprocating bone rasp is used to further flatten and smooth the remaining portion of the articular eminence. Care is taken to maintain a 10° inferior angulation and to flatten the difficult-to-visualize medial aspect of the eminence.

14. Copious irrigation is used to debride any bony remnants within the surgical field. The site is inspected for hemostasis, and any areas of concern are managed prior to closing or proceeding to the contralateral side. In cases involving bilateral eminectomy, the same procedure is performed on the contralateral side.

15. The patient is functioned to verify no areas of entrapment or dislocation and to ensure smooth translations of the condyles.

16. The pre-auricular incision is closed in a layered fashion (Figure 34.20) with closure of the deeper fascial layers, subcuticular tissues, and skin. Bacitracin ointment is applied to skin incisions, and the wound is dressed.

Postoperative Management

1. Following eminectomy, ice packs are applied to the surgical area for 24 hours postoperatively.

2. Dressings on surgical wounds are to be removed after 24 hours. Incisions are cleaned with a mixture of half normal saline and half hydrogen peroxide. A thin layer of bacitracin ointment is applied to all skin incisions to minimize the risk of infection.

3. Intravenous antibiotics are employed for inpatients. Oral antibiotics are prescribed for 7 days after discharge. Cephalosporin is typically selected unless the patient is allergic to penicillin. Clindamycin is used for penicillin-allergic patients.

4. One or two doses of postoperative corticosteroids are administered for anti-inflammatory purposes.

5. Prescription analgesics are prescribed for pain management.

6. Patients are placed on a clear to full liquid diet, which advances to a soft mechanical diet once the patient is capable.

7. Patients are instructed in Stage I exercises for the first 2 weeks, followed by Stage II full-range-of-motion exercises afterward.

8. Skin sutures are removed routinely after 6 days.

Complications

Early Complications

1. **Hemorrhage**: Minimized with a meticulous dissection and reduction technique. Controlled via direct compression, the use of hemostatic packs and materials, cauterization, and/or ligation of any visible bleeding vessels.

2. **Infection**: Minimized by maintaining a sterile environment. Infections are initially managed with antibiotic administration, local irrigation, and close follow-up. For cases refractory to conservative measures, surgical intervention and debridement are warranted.

3. **Facial nerve palsy**: Typically transient and results from tissue traction during surgery or subsequent postoperative edema and swelling of the surgical site. No intervention is required as the condition typically resolves within 6–9 months.

Late Complications

1. **Wound dehiscence**: May be attributed to infection, poorly placed sutures, and poor tissue handling and management resulting in diminished blood supply of the dissected tissues. Conservative management is required using antibiotics and local debridement for secondary-intention wound healing.

2. **Recurrence of mandibular dislocation**: Commonly from insufficient articular eminence reduction and/or unremoved articular tubercle. Treatment involves reoperation.

Key Points

1. The key to a successful eminectomy procedure is proper patient selection. Ideal candidates possess steep articular eminences and have a history of chronic mandibular dislocation.
2. Preoperative computed tomography scans are necessary to determine the anatomy of the surgical site and to rule out pneumatization of the articular eminence. Knowledge of the dimensions of the articular eminence prior to the eminectomy procedure will minimize the risk of infratemporal fossa or middle cranial fossa penetration.
3. Postoperative rehabilitation is crucial to obtaining and maintaining a full range of motion after eminectomy procedures.
4. With the success of arthroscopic procedures, arthroscopic eminoplasty can be performed in select cases according to Segami's method. With the patient under general anesthesia, diagnostic arthroscopy by means of the infero-lateral approach can be undertaken to visualize the shape of the eminence. The articular eminence is then reduced and smoothed using an electric shaver with a triangulation technique.

Case Report

Case report 34.1. A 73-year-old female presents with a chief complaint of a longstanding history of dislocation of her mandible (Figures 34.2 and 34.3). Two minimally invasive endoscopic posterior scarification therapies including autologous blood injections were attempted with no success. Due to the chronic history of dislocation and failed conservative therapies, the decision was made for bilateral open eminectomies. The patient was taken to the operating room, intubated, and prepped and draped in a sterile fashion. The patient's jaw was manipulated anteriorly in a protrusive fashion. 0.5% Marcaine was used to insufflate the superior joint capsule and a trocar was placed into the superior joint space. The scope was entered and manipulated into the posterior space. The medial synovial drape, the medial pterygoid shadow, all retrodiscal tissue and the joint function were evaluated. The patient demonstrated appropriate function and no evidence of joint irregularities or pathology (Figure 34.4). After arthroscopic evaluation of the bilateral temporomandibular joints, bilateral open eminectomies were performed. (See also Figures 34.5 through 34.21.)

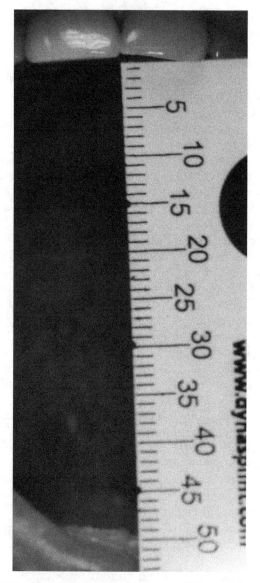

Figure 34.2.   Chronic dislocation of the mandible as evidenced by a maximum vertical opening of over 5 cm.

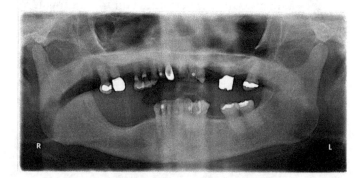

Figure 34.3.   Orthopantomogram demonstrating steep bilateral articular eminences and dislocations.

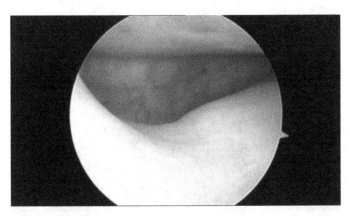

Figure 34.4. Arthroscopic evaluation of the left temporomandibular joint demonstrating a normal-appearing joint with appropriate position and function of the disc. The joint space is free of chondromalcia, synovitis, and adhesions.

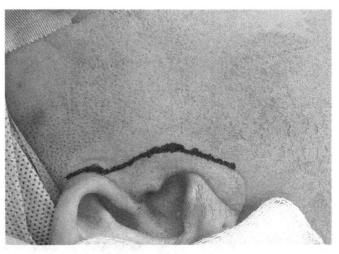

Figure 34.5. A standard pre-auricular incision is marked within a well-developed pre-auricular skin crease.

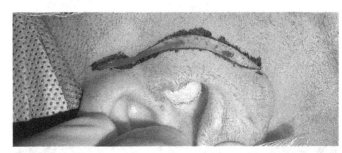

Figure 34.6. A #15 blade is used to transect skin and subcutaneous tissues.

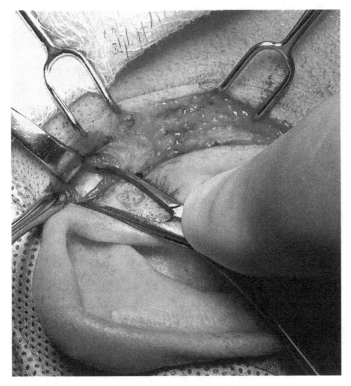

Figure 34.7. Blunt dissection through the horizontal auricular muscles to expose the glistening white temporalis fascia.

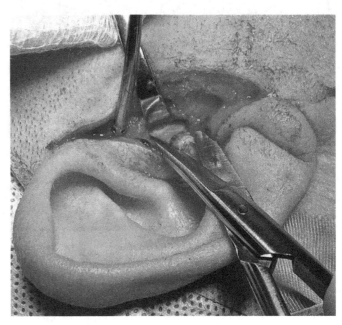

Figure 34.8. Sharp dissection over the tragal cartilage in close proximity to the perichondrium to expose the tip of the tragal cartilage.

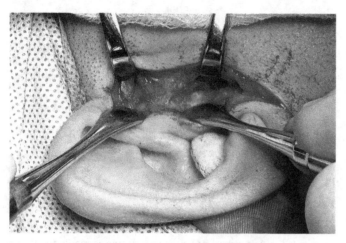

Figure 34.9.   The pre-auricular soft tissue is transected down to the temporalis fascia.

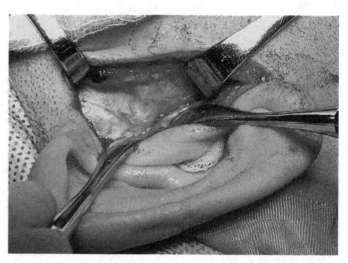

Figure 34.10.   A periosteal elevator is utilized in a sweeping motion to flap forward the tissue within the layer superficial to the temporalis fascia. The parotid is bluntly swept inferiorly with a periosteal elevator and retracted with a Messer retractor.

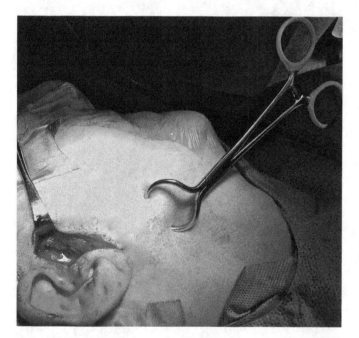

Figure 34.11.   A towel clamp was placed at the angle of the mandible, and the condyle was palpated.

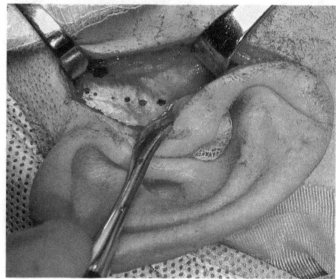

Figure 34.12.   Methylene can be used to mark an incision line from the superior aspect of the incision inferiorly to the apex of the tragal cartilage.

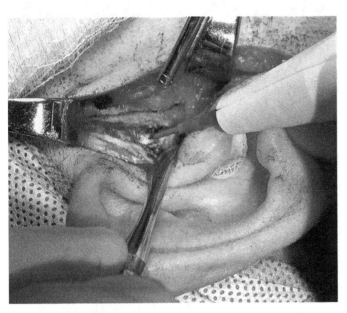

Figure 34.13. A releasing incision is made with the cautery from the posterior glenoid process to the tip of the incision; through the temporalis fascia, temporalis muscle, and periosteum; down to the bone.

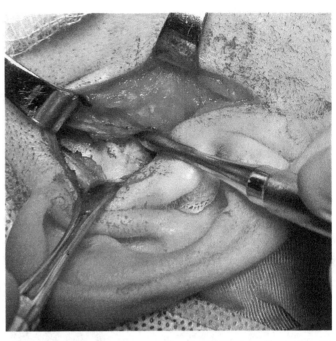

Figure 34.14. The flap is swept subperiosteally along the zygomatic process of the temporal bone anterior to the articular eminence.

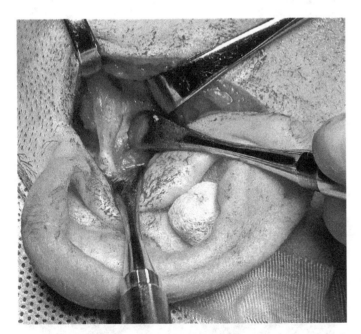

Figure 34.15. A periosteal elevator is used to dissect in a subperiosteal plane from the root of the zygoma anteriorly to expose the articular eminence.

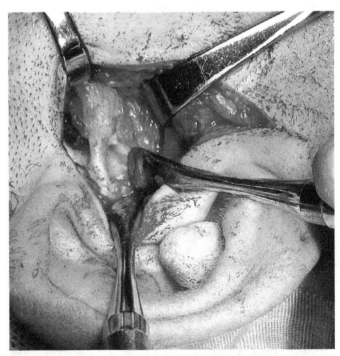

Figure 34.16. Once ample visualization of the eminence is achieved, a periosteal elevator is used to carefully dissect the superior joint space free from the eminence.

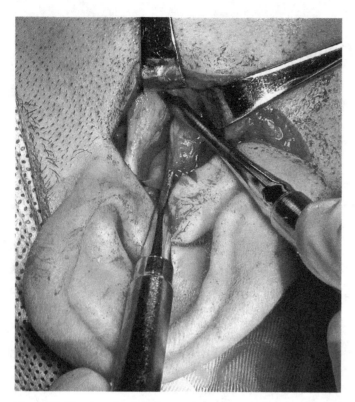

Figure 34.17.   A periosteal elevator is used to protect the disk and condyle from further instrumentation.

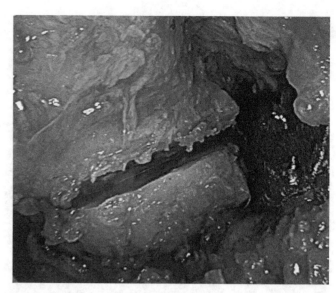

Figure 34.18.   A 101 bur was used to identify and score the osteotomy site, which is planed in a 10° plane perpendicular to the superior most concavity of the glenoid fossa.

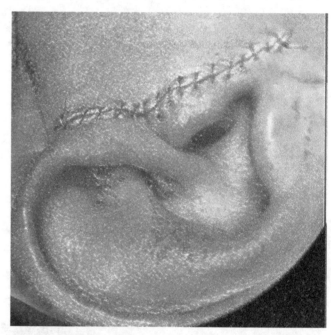

Figure 34.20.   Layered closure of the pre-auricular incision.

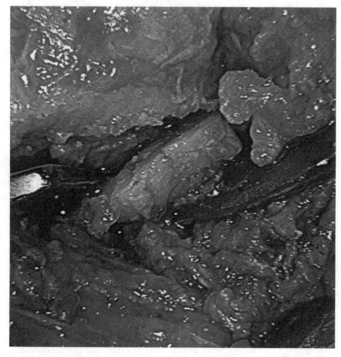

Figure 34.19.   The medial osteotomy is completed with a sharp straight chisel, and the eminence is fractured laterally and inferiorly. Irregular edges are re-contoured using a reciprocal rasp or bone files.

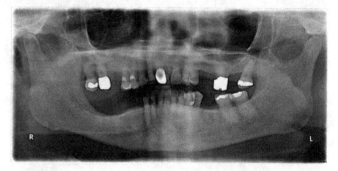

Figure 34.21.   Postoperative orthopantomogram demonstrating bilateral eminectomies.

References

Ellis, E. and Zide, M.F., 2005. *Surgical approaches to the facial skeleton.* 2nd ed. Philadelphia: Lippincott Williams & Wilkins.

Hall, M.B., Randall, W.B. and Sclar, A.G., 1984. Anatomy of the TMJ articular eminence before and after surgical reduction. *Journal of Craniomandibular Practice*, 2, 135–40.

Kulikowski, B.M., Schow, S.R. and Kraut, R.A., 1982. Surgical management of a pneumatized articular eminence of the temporal bone. *Journal of Oral and Maxillofacial Surgery*, 40, 311.

Sato, J., Segami, N., Nishimura, M., Suzuki, T., Kaneyama, K. and Fujimura, K., 2003. Clinical evaluation of arthroscopic eminoplasty for habitual dislocation of the temporomandibular joint: comparative study with conventional open eminectomy. *Oral Surgery, Oral Medicine, Oral Pathology, Oral Radiology, and Endodontology*, 95 (4), 390–95.

Segami, N., Kaneyama, K., Tsurusako, S. and Suzuki, T., 1999. Arthroscopic eminoplasty for habitual dislocation of the temporomandibular joint: preliminary study. *Journal o Craniomaxillofacial Surgery*, 27, 390–97.

Tremble, G.E., 1934. Pneumatization of the temporal bone. *Archives of Otolaryngology*, 19, 172.

Undt, U., 2011. Temporomandibular joint eminectomy for recurrent dislocation. *Atlas of the Oral and Maxillofacial Surgery Clinics*, 19 (2), 189–206.

Williamson, R.A., McNamara, D. and McAuliffe, W., 2000. True eminectomy for internal derangement of the temporomandibular joint. *British Journal of Oral and Maxillofacial Surgery*, 38 (5), 554–60.

PART SIX

FACIAL COSMETIC SURGERY

CHAPTER

35 Botulinum Toxin Type A (Botox)

Antoine J. Panossian[1] and Christopher J. Haggerty[2]

[1]Panossian Oral and Maxillofacial Surgery, Massapequa, New York, USA
[2]Private Practice, Lakewood Oral and Maxillofacial Surgery Specialists, Lees Summit; and Department of Oral
and Maxillofacial Surgery, University of Missouri–Kansas City, Kansas City, Missouri, USA

The injection of a neuromodulator for the temporary paralysis of specific muscles for the aesthetic management of facial rhytids resulting from repeated muscle animation.

Facial Aesthetic Indications

1. Glabellar rhytids
2. Horizontal forehead rhytids
3. Crow's feet
4. Bunny lines
5. Nasal flaring
6. Perioral lip lines
7. Mouth frown
8. Platysmal banding
9. Peau d'orange chin
10. Blepharospasm

Contraindications

1. Hypersensitivity to ingredients (albumin, sodium chloride, and botulinum toxin type A [Botox]) (Allergan, Irvine, California, USA)
2. Infection at the proposed injection site
3. Pregnancy or lactation
4. Patients with neuromuscular disorders or diseases (Eaton–Lambert, myasthenia gravis, and motor neuron disease)
5. Medications that interfere with neuromuscular transmission (aminoglycosides, penicillamine, quinine, calcium channel blockers, neuromuscular blocking agents, anticholinesterases, magnesium sulfate, and quinidine)
6. Unrealistic expectations (patients who would be better treated with surgical intervention or patients with psychological disorders)

Anatomy

Frontalis muscle: Originates from the galea aponeurotica and inserts within the dermis at the level of the eyebrow, procerus, corrugator, and orbicularis oculi muscles. Elevates the eyebrow and produces horizontal forehead rhytids.

Corrugator supercilii muscle: Originates from the medial supraorbital ridge and inserts at the caudal aspect of the frontalis muscle, the medial aspect of the orbicularis oculi, and the skin in the region of the mid-brow. Contraction produces vertical glabellar rhytids (#11) and/or a dimpled radix depression.

Procerus muscle: Originates at the periosteum of the nasal bone and inserts into the mid-forehead dermis. Contraction produces transverse rhytids over the nasal bridge (bunny lines).

Orbicularis oculi: Originates from the frontal process of the maxilla, the nasal portion of the frontal bone, and the medial palpebral ligament, and inserts laterally around the orbit and at the lateral palpebral raphe. The lateral orbicularis oculi are responsible for lateral canthal rhytids (crow's feet).

Technique

1. The patient is placed in an upright position, and the injection sites are cleansed with alcohol pads. EMLA cream can be applied to the areas of injection. Local anesthesia is typically not utilized.
2. The patient is asked to contract their facial muscles in the areas to be treated. Facial animation will allow the practitioner to delineate the extent, size, and strength of the muscles to be treated. Figure 35.1 illustrates the muscles used in facial animation.
3. Injection sites can be marked (see Figures 35.4 and 35.5 in Case Report 35.1) with a sterile marking pen for less experienced practitioners. More experienced practitioners will modify injections to suit individual patient needs and anatomic variation for best results.
4. A total of 25–35 units of Botox for women and 35–45 units in men is injected to treat horizontal forehead rhytids and glabellar rhytids. These units are patient dependent and can vary greatly with gender and anatomic variation.
5. Injections are a minimum of 1–1.5 cm above the supraorbital rim to avoid unwanted eyelid ptosis, and even higher lateral to the midpupillary line in women to maintain a high lateral brow.
6. Lateral canthal rhytids are evaluated with the patient smiling and squinting. Six to ten units are injected on each side. Injections are placed a minimum of 1–1.5 cm lateral to the lateral orbital rim and above the zygomatic arch (Figure 35.4, Case Report 35.1).

Atlas of Operative Oral and Maxillofacial Surgery, First Edition. Edited by Christopher J. Haggerty and Robert M. Laughlin
© 2015 John Wiley & Sons, Inc. Published 2015 by John Wiley & Sons, Inc.

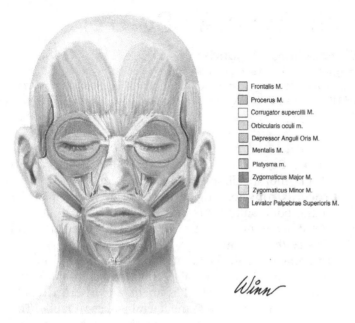

Frontalis M.
Procerus M.
Corrugator supercilli M.
Orbicularis oculi m.
Depressor Anguli Oris M.
Mentalis M.
Platysma m.
Zygomaticus Major M.
Zygomaticus Minor M.
Levator Palpebrae Superioris M.

Winn

Figure 35.1. Illustration depicting the muscles of facial animation.

7. Bunny lines are treated with 2–4 units on each side injected into the transverse nasalis muscle. Injecting four units into the alar part of the nasalis muscle on each side will decrease nasal flaring.
8. Perioral lip lines are treated with two units injected in each quadrant at the vermillion border.
9. Mouth frown is caused by lack of balance between the depressor anguli oris (DAO) and zygomaticus muscles. To allow the commissures to return to a more horizontal position, two units are injected into the DAO on each side. Two units can also be injected into the mentalis muscle, which contributes to the unpleasant appearance.
10. Peau d'orange chin is treated with two 5-unit injections into the mentalis muscle.
11. Platysmal bands are treated with 15 units/3 injection sites per band, not to exceed 45 units per session.

Postoperative Management

1. Immediately after the application of Botox, the patient is kept seated, and ice is applied to the treated areas for 10–15 minutes.
2. For 4–6 hours after treatment, the patient is instructed to remain upright and to avoid strenuous activity.
3. The patient is encouraged to animate their facial muscles for 2–4 hours after treatment.
4. The patient is asked to not rub or manipulate the injection sites as this may redistribute the Botox into undesirable locations.

5. The patient is asked to lightly remove their makeup later that evening with a single alcohol pad and to not reapply makeup or wash their face until the next day.

Complications

Early Complications

1. **Injection site pain**: Can be minimized by applying ice or EMLA cream to the proposed injection site, not injecting into a contracting muscle, and injecting superficial to the periosteum.
2. **Injection site ecchymosis**: Caused by injecting into a blood vessel (commonly, the supratrochlear vessels) or injecting deep in the region of the lateral orbicularis oculi.
3. **Injection site edema**: Can be minimized by applying ice after the procedure and by appropriate injection technique.
4. Headaches
5. Transient flu-like symptoms

Late Complications

1. **Facial asymmetry**: Caused by asymmetrical injection technique, aberrant muscle patterns, or preexisting facial asymmetry.
2. **Brow ptosis (frozen face)**: Caused by overtreating the frontalis muscle. Conservative treatment of the frontalis muscle lateral to the midpupillary line will allow for lateral brow animation, a more natural appearance, and a minor lateral eyebrow lift.
3. **Eyelid ptosis**: Caused by injections in close proximity to the superior orbital rim, resulting in paralysis of the levator palpebrae superioris. Injections should be kept 1–1.5 cm from the orbital rim. Treatment consists of apraclonidine 0.5% drops in the affected eye to stimulate a contraction of Müller's muscle to allow an additional 1–3 mm of upper eyelid elevation.
4. **Diplopia**: Caused by injections in close proximity to the lateral orbital rim with resultant paralysis of the lateral rectus muscle. Injections should be kept 1–1.5 cm lateral to the lateral orbital rim.
5. **Spock eyebrow**: Excessive elevation of the lateral brow caused by undertreatment of the lateral frontalis. Treated with a touchup dose of Botox placed lateral to the midpupillary line in the area of the lateral suprabrow.
6. **Oral muscular incompetence or asymmetry**: Caused by injections in close proximity to the zygomaticus major. Injection should be kept above the zygomatic arch.

Key Points

1. A Botox 100-unit vial is reconstituted with 0.9% preservative-free sterile saline. Depending on the amount of Botox to be injected per patient, the authors either reconstitute a Botox 100-unit vial with 2 mL of 0.9% preservative-free sterile saline (two 1.0 mL syringes with 5 units/0.1 mL) or 3 mL of 0.9% preservative-free sterile saline (three 1.0 mL syringes with 3.3 units/0.1 mL). The reconstituted Botox is drawn into 1.0 mL Luer-Lok syringes with a 25-gauge needle. A 32-gauge half-inch needle tip is then used for the injections.

2. Botox should be used within 24 hours after reconstitution.

3. Reloxin (Dysport) is an alternative to Botox.

4. Facial cosmetic patients typically receive between 25 and 100 units of Botox at 3–6-month intervals. Men typically require more units of Botox than women due to their increased muscle mass and larger brows.

5. Facial animation will allow the practitioner to inject directly into the mass of the muscle.

6. Patient discomfort can be minimized by not injecting into a contracting muscle and by injecting superficial to the periosteum. Injections into the crow's feet should be more superficial to decrease potential pain and bruising.

7. Botox can diffuse 1–1.5 cm from the injection site. It is important to remain a distance of at least 1–1.5 cm from the supraorbital and lateral orbital rim in order to minimize eyelid ptosis.

8. Higher doses of Botox delivered in smaller volumes will keep the effects more localized and allow for the more precise placement of the toxin with less diffusion. The injection of a lower concentration of Botox delivered in larger volumes contributes to a wider diffusion, a shorter duration, and an increased number of complications associated with the diffusion pattern.

9. The clinical effects of Botox typically appear 1–4 days after injection, peak at 1–4 weeks, and decline after 3–4 months. The duration of action is highly variable.

10. Touch-up injections with 5–20 units of Botox are common and are performed 2–4 weeks after the initial treatment.

Case Report

Case Report 35.1. A 26-year-old female with a chief complaint of deep facial rhytids. (See Figures 35.2 through 35.9.)

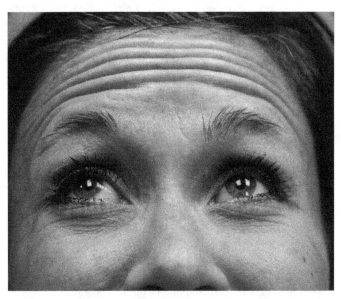

Figure 35.2.   Contraction of the frontalis muscle produces deep horizontal rhytids as the brow is elevated.

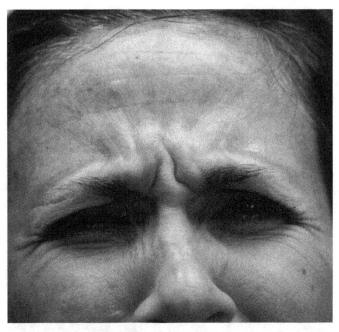

Figure 35.3.   Contraction of the corrugator supercilii muscle produces vertical glabellar rhytids (#11) and a dimpled radix depression.

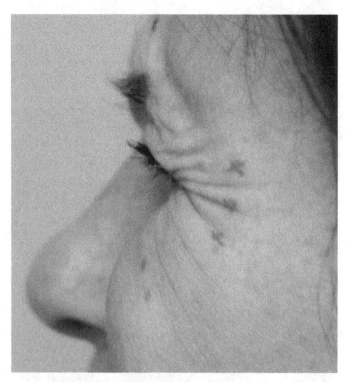

Figure 35.4.   Smiling and squinting produces lateral canthal rhytids (crow's feet). The red X's mark the locations for the injections to paralyze the lateral orbicularis oculi muscle. The injection should be superficial, at least 1–1.5 cm lateral to the lateral orbital rim, and above the zygomatic arch.

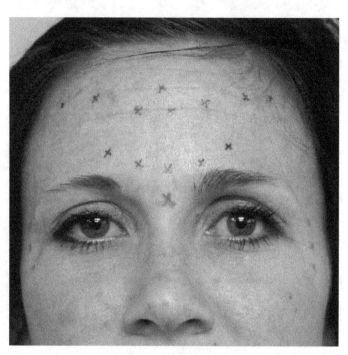

Figure 35.5.   Botox markings. The blue markings represent the sites for injection of the frontalis muscle. The black markings represent the sites for injection of the corrugator supercilii muscle. The red markings within the midline represent the sites for injection of the procerus muscle, and the lateral red markings represent the sites for injection of the lateral orbicularis oculi muscle.

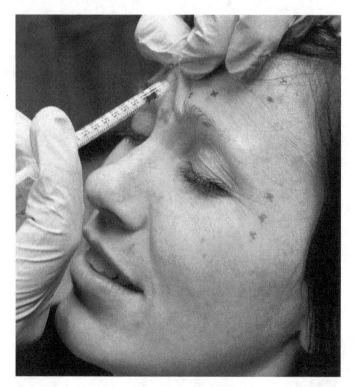

Figure 35.6.   Injections should be made within the mass of the targeted muscle.

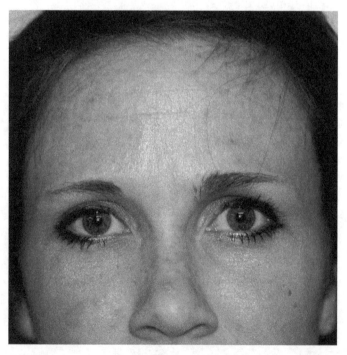

Figure 35.7.   Patient at repose 6 weeks after injection of frontalis, corrugator supercilii, procerus, and lateral orbicularis oculi muscles.

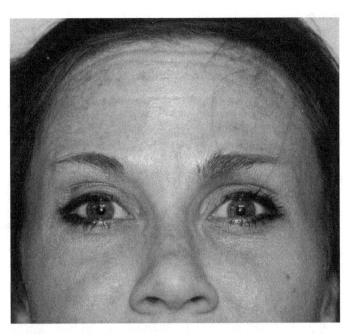

Figure 35.8. Patient at animation 6 weeks after Botox treatment.

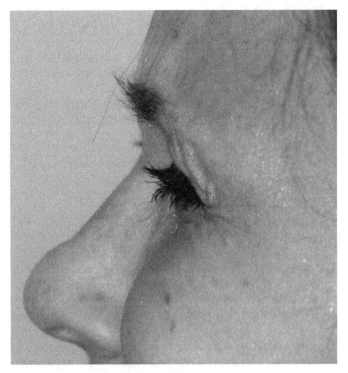

Figure 35.9. Patient squinting 6 weeks after Botox treatment of lateral canthal rhytids (crow's feet).

References

Carruthers, A. and Carruthers, J., 2008. Practical botulinum toxin anatomy. In: *Botulinum toxin*. 2nd ed. Philadelphia: Saunders; pp. 31–42.

Carruthers, J. and Carruthers, A., 2006. The use of botulinum toxin type A in the upper face. *Facial and Plastic Surgery Clinics of North America*, 14, 253–60.

Finn, J.C. and Cox, S.E., 2008. Practical botulinum toxin anatomy. In: *Botulinum toxin*. 2nd ed. Philadelphia: Saunders; pp. 19–29.

Matarasso, A. and Shafer, D., 2009. Botox cosmetic. In: *Minimally invasive facial rejuvenation*. Philadelphia: Saunders; pp. 1–20.

Nettar, K. and Maas C. Facial filler and neurotoxin complications. *Facial and Plastic Surgery*, 28, 288–93.

Niamtu, J., 2009. Complications in fillers and botox. *Oral and Maxillofacial Surgery Clinics of North America*, 21, 13–21.

36

Soft Tissue Augmentation

Antoine J. Panossian[1] and Christopher J. Haggerty[2]

[1]*Panossian Oral and Maxillofacial Surgery, Massapequa, New York, USA*
[2] *Private Practice, Lakewood Oral and Maxillofacial Surgery Specialists, Lees Summit; and Department of Oral and Maxillofacial Surgery, University of Missouri–Kansas City, Kansas City, Missouri, USA*

Injection of autogenous, synthetic biodegradable and permanent soft tissue fillers for facial aesthetic augmentation and rejuvenation.

Autogenous fat: A semipermanent filler for all forms of facial soft tissue augmentation, in particular for patients undergoing liposculpting procedures and with previous hypersensitivity to injectable fillers

Temporary synthetic fillers: Juvederm (Allergan, Irvine, California, USA) (hyaluronic scaid {HA}), Perlane (Medicis Aesthetics Inc, Scottsdale, Arizona, USA) (HA), and Restylane (Medicis Aesthetics Inc, Scottsdale, Arizona, USA) (HA)

Semipermanent synthetic fillers: Radiesse (Merz Aesthetics Inc, Franksville, Wisconsin, USA) (calcium hydroxylapatite [CaHa]) and Sculptra (Valeant Pharmaceuticals Inc, Laval, Quebec, Canada) (ploy-L-lactic acid [PLLA])

Permanent fillers: ArteFill (Suneva Medical Inc, Santa Barbara, California, USA) (polymethyl methacrylate microspheres [PMMA]), which is currently the only US Food and Drug Administration–approved permanent injectable filler for facial soft tissue augmentation

Facial Aesthetic Indications

1. Lip augmentation
2. Effacement of nasolabial folds
3. Perioral rhytids and marionette lines
4. Cheek enhancement
5. Defining lower jaw
6. Elevation of lateral brow
7. Glabellar lines
8. Horizontal forehead lines
9. Temporal fossa wasting
10. Asymmetrical facial features
11. Scars
12. HIV lipoatrophy

Contraindications

1. Hypersensitivity to injectable material and ingredients
2. Infection at the proposed injection site

Anatomy

Epidermis: Layers, from superficial to deep, are the stratum corneum, stratum granulosum, stratum spinosum, and stratum basale.

Dermis: Layers, from superficial to deep, are the papillary dermis and reticular dermis.

Hypodermis: Contents include fat, connective tissue, neural tissue, and blood vessels.

Injection Technique

1. Patients are advised to avoid anticoagulant substances or medications prior to facial soft tissue augmentation procedures.
2. For lip augmentation, local anesthesia in the form of mental and infraorbital nerve blocks are employed. Care must be taken to minimize local anesthetic distortion of the anatomy of the site to be injected. For areas not amendable to local anesthesia, topical anesthetic (EMLA) cream can be applied 10–30 minutes prior to the procedure.
3. Makeup is removed, and injection sites are prepped with an alcohol pad.
4. Patients are positioned seated and upright.
5. Depth of injection (dermis, mid-dermis, and hypodermis) is dependent on the type of filler used. In general, nonpermanent fillers are injected more superficially, whereas semipermanent and permanent fillers are injected deeper.
6. Injection of filler is slow, deliberate, and in a retrograde fashion with aspiration. The filler is injected with the needle bevel facing superiorly.
7. The noninjecting hand is used to feel and mold the filler as it is injected into the appropriate tissue plane.
8. Patients are allowed to visualize and make recommendations during the procedure. The surgeon always has the final determination of the amount of filler used.

Atlas of Operative Oral and Maxillofacial Surgery, First Edition. Edited by Christopher J. Haggerty and Robert M. Laughlin
© 2015 John Wiley & Sons, Inc. Published 2015 by John Wiley & Sons, Inc.

Postoperative Management

1. Cold compresses are immediately applied to the injected areas.
2. Strenuous activities are avoided for 8–10 hours immediately post injection.
3. Makeup can be applied 4–6 hours post injection.
4. Vigorous massage of the injected areas is avoided.

Complications

Early Complications (0–7 Days)

1. **Injection site–related sequelae and hypersensitivity reactions**: Redness, pruritis, pain, edema, and ecchymosis at the injection sites. Typically resolves spontaneously after 3–7 days.
2. **Overcorrection**: Overcorrection can be minimized by injecting slowly and allowing the patient to provide feedback during the process. HA overcorrection can be decreased to some extent with massaging the filler into adjacent tissues. HA can be degraded with the use of hyaluronidase.
3. **Infection**: Infections are rare. Infections can be minimized by cleaning the injection sites with alcohol or a similar prep. Abscesses, cellulitis, and skin infections are treated with oral antibiotics and, if necessary, surgical drainage.
4. **Vascular compromise and necrosis**: Occurs with the intravascular injection of a filler, direct needle injury to a vessel, or external compression of a vessel by surrounding filler. Acute symptoms include severe pain, blanching, duskiness, and ecchymosis immediately post injection. Treatment includes immediately massaging the area, applying heat, a course of aspirin therapy, and nitroglycerine paste applied to the affected area. Hyaluronidase may also be used if the patient was injected with HA; however, it is recommended to first perform prick testing for immediate hypersensitivity. Vascular compromise and necrosis can be minimized by injecting slowly and with minimal pressure, aspirating prior to injection, injecting small volumes per pass, and using small-caliber needles. High-risk areas for vascular compromise and necrosis include the glabella, nose, and nasolabial folds.

Late Complications (Greater than 7 Days)

1. **Subcutaneous nodular formation, lumps, and beading**: Occurs from the injection of filler too superficially, injection of too much filler, and poor injection technique. Treatment for HA is time or hyaluronidase. Treatment for semipermanent and permanent fillers is intralesional steroids.
2. **Granulomatous reaction**: All fillers can potentially cause granuloma formation. CaHa is frequently linked to the formation of granulomas. Treatment involves intralesional steroids.
3. **Filler migration**: Minimized by avoiding strenuous activity and vigorous massage immediately after filler placement.

Key Points

1. Pre- and postoperative photographs are always taken in order to demonstrate to the patient their change in facial appearance.
2. Fillers can be utilized to lessen facial rhytids; however, they should be utilized as an adjunct to Botox and surgery, which treat the underlying dynamic muscle contractions and excessive skin laxity.
3. It is the author's recommendation to utilize synthetic biodegradable products (HA) for first-time patients. This will allow patients to evaluate outcomes and develop realistic expectations. It may also avoid complications of unsatisfied patients with permanent fillers.
4. Filler selection is extremely important as different fillers are more ideal for certain areas of the facial skeleton and vary in viscosity, length of degradation, and injection depth. The manufacturer's recommendations should be followed with respect to filler site, depth, and frequency.
5. Certain fillers are more prone to complications than others (nodules and granulomas with PLLA and CaHa). Hyaluronic acids, when injected properly, have the advantage of temporary augmentation and few side effects.
6. It is generally better to err on the side of injecting too deep versus too superficial. Superficial injections may overcorrect or overcontour defects, lead to surface irregularities, and cause the epidermis to become transparent (HA), which may lead to bluish spots (known as th Tyndall effect).
7. It is better to undercorrect an area and have the patient return in 2–4 weeks for a minor touchup than to overcorrect the area. This is especially true with permanent fillers.

Case Report

Case Report 36.1. A 29-year-old female presents with a chief complaint of lack of definition and volume to her upper and lower lips, upper lip asymmetry, and deep nasolabial folds. The patient will be treated with Juvederm Ultra Plus to redefine the upper lip vermillion border, to correct her minor upper lip asymmetry, to add philtrum definition, and to add volume to the body of the upper and lower lips. Volume will also be restored to the nasolabial folds. (See Figures 36.1 through 36.7.)

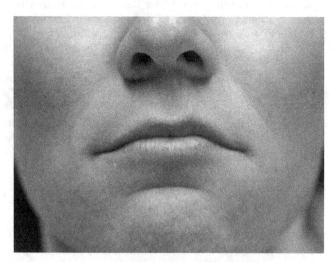

Figure 36.1. Pre-injection photograph demonstrating thin upper and lower lips, upper lip asymmetry, and deepened nasolabial folds.

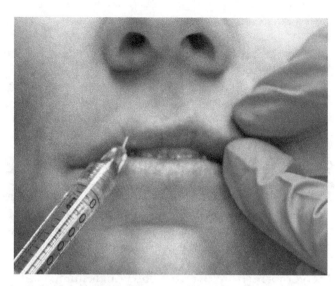

Figure 36.2. Volume is added to the bilateral philtrum columns.

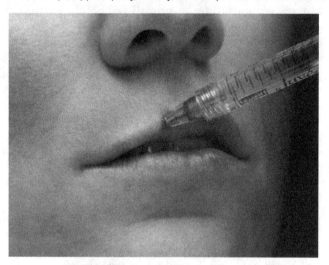

Figure 36.3. The vermillion border of the upper lip is injected in a retrograde fashion to add definition and volume.

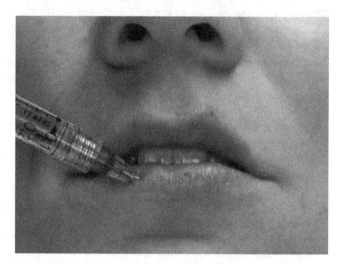

Figure 36.4. Additional volume is added to the body of the upper and lower lips.

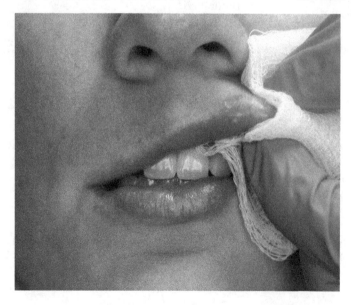

Figure 36.5. Gauze is utilized to smooth the Juvederm Ultra Plus and to minimize filler beading.

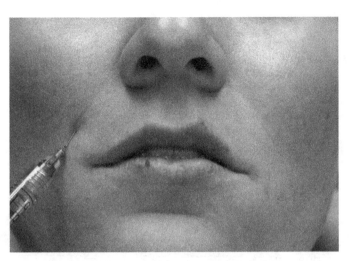

Figure 36.6.   Volume is added to the nasolabial folds. Injections should be kept medial to the nasolabial folds and within the dermis. Superficial injections may result in unaesthetic beading of the soft tissue filler.

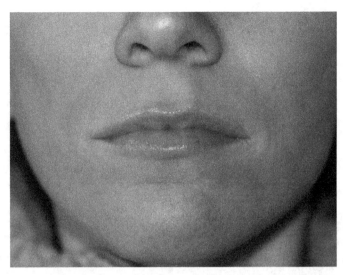

Figure 36.7.   Two-week postoperative result. Note the added definition to the vermillion border and philtrum, added volume to the lower lip and nasolabial folds, and correction of minor upper lip asymmetry.

References

Daines, S.M. and Williams, E.F., 2013. Complications associated with injectable soft-tissue fillers: a 5-year retrospective review. *JAMA Facial Plastic Surgery*, 15, 226–31.

Narins, R.S., Michales, J. and Cohen, J.L., 2012. Hylans and soft tissue augmentation. In: J. Carruthers and A. Carruthers, eds. *Soft tissue augmentation*. 3rd ed. Amsterdam: Elsevier.

Ozturk, C.N., Tung, R., Parker, L., Piliang, M.P. and Zins, J.E., 2013. Complications following injection of soft-tissue fillers. *Aesthetic Surgery Journal*, 33, 862–77.

Wilson, Y.L. and Ellis, D.A., 2011. Permanent soft tissue fillers. *Facial Plastic Surgery*, 27, 540–46.

CHAPTER 37

Chemical Peels

Jon D. Perenack[1] and Brian W. Kelley[2]

[1]*Department of Oral and Maxillofacial Surgery, Louisiana State University Health Sciences Center, New Orleans, Louisiana, USA*

[2]*Private Practice, Carolinas Center for Oral and Maxillofacial Surgery, Charlotte, North Carolina, USA*

The use of a chemical exfoliant to injure specific tissue layers to lessen fine facial rhytids, decrease dispigmentation and actinic changes, and rejuvenate damaged areas in a minimally invasive manner.

Indications

1. Photo dyspigmentation
2. Superficial rhytids
3. Melasma
4. Acne vulgaris
5. Ephelides

Contraindications

1. Active cutaneous infection (i.e., herpes)
2. Ice-pick or deep atrophic acne scars
3. Allergy to agent
4. Extreme sunburn
5. Open wounds (open acne wounds will propagate peel depth)
6. Unrealistic patient expectations
7. Patient is unable or unwilling to perform postoperative management
8. Caution with patients using skin sensitizers (e.g., Retin-A, Retinol, and Accutane)

Anatomy

Epidermis: Layers from superficial to deep: stratum corneum, stratum granulosum, stratum spinosum, and stratum basale

Dermis: Layers from superficial to deep: papillary dermis and reticular dermis

Pretreatment Protocol for Chemical Peel Patients

1. Commercially prepared skin systems that contain tretinoin 0.05–0.1% and 4% hydroquinone, such as Obagi Nu-Derm (Skin Specialists PC, Omaha, NE, USA), are available and are recommended for 4–6 weeks prior to the application of a peel in order to allow for a more uniform depth of peel and to minimize complications associated with melasma and postinflammatory pigmentation.
2. Valacyclovir (Valtrex) is recommended beginning the day prior to the peel and for 7–14 days post peel.

Procedure: Medium-Depth Chemical Peel

1. All patient consents are reviewed and signed, and all patient questions are answered. All patient makeup is removed, and the maxillofacial skeleton is prepped with alcohol from the hairline to a point several inches below the inferior border of the mandible.
2. For medium-depth and deep peels, intravenous sedation is performed.
3. The patient is positioned supine on the surgical table. The skin is degreased with acetone, and standard nerve blocks are performed with long-acting a local anesthetic within the areas of the anticipated peel.
4. A pre-peel is performed with Jessner's solution to include the forehead, the periorbital region (the upper lids and thin tissue below the lower lid lash lines are avoided), the nasal bridge, the perioral region, and the lower face to the inferior border of the mandible (Figure 37.2). After the Jessner's solution has dried and a thin layer of frosting has occurred, 25–35% trichloracetic acid (TCA) is applied to the above-mentioned regions with 4 × 4 gauze (Figure 37.3).
5. When using TCA solution, it is important to wait several minutes after the application of the solution in order to allow for frosting of the tissue to assess the depth of the peel. The peel is typically carried into the hairline in order to minimize any demarcations of the peel. Areas such as the central forehead, glabellar region, and peri-oral region contain thicker tissue and are resilient to peels. Additional solution may be applied to these areas. The use of a cotton-tipped applicator may be used to rub the solution into areas such as deep peri-oral and glabellar rhytids. The upper eyelids are avoided in medium to deep peels, and the ciliary margin is the upper extent of the lower lids' involvement. The solution is feathered as the inferior border of the mandible is reached in order to prevent a line of demarcation to the thinner and more vulnerable cervical tissue. Additional layers of TCA may be applied until the desired amount of frosting is observed (Figure 37.4) and the desired depth of penetration is reached.
6. Once the desired depth of the peel has been reached, a facial moisturizing cream is applied to the facial skeleton. In the immediate recovery period, the use of cool

Atlas of Operative Oral and Maxillofacial Surgery, First Edition. Edited by Christopher J. Haggerty and Robert M. Laughlin

© 2015 John Wiley & Sons, Inc. Published 2015 by John Wiley & Sons, Inc.

compresses and/or a fan will aid in minimizing immediate postoperative discomfort.

Postoperative Management

1. **Moisturizing cream**: The patient is required to keep the peeled area moisturized at all times during the postpeel period. Moisturizing creams prevent drying and crusting of the peeling areas, and they provide patient comfort while the skin re-epithelializes. Depending on the depth of the peel, moisturizing creams may be combined with topical antibiotics.
2. **Analgesics**: Prescribed based on the depth of the peel and adjunct procedures performed at the time of the peel.
3. **Valacyclovir**: Continued 7–14 days post peel.
4. **Wound care**: Should be initiated on postpeel day 2. Involves lightly washing the peeled area with mild soap in a blotting fashion several times a day and then reapplying the moisturizing cream. Avoid scrubbing, itching, picking, or pulling at sloughing skin as this may cause scar and keloid formation. Pre-peel skin care systems are typically restarted 2 weeks after the chemical peel.
5. **Sunblock**: Direct sun exposure is avoided, and SPF 30 or above is necessary to minimize the stimulation of melanocytes and further postinflammatory hyperpigmentation (PIH).

Complications

Early Complications

1. **Discomfort, edema, and tissue erythema**: Common to all peels; corresponds to the depth of the peel.
2. **Hyperpigmentation**: Frequently occurs within the recovery period, especially with early sun exposure. Hyperpigmentation is typically transient and responds to tretinoin and 4% hydroquinone.
3. **Prolonged flaking after a peel**: Requires generous moisturizer application and avoidance of restarting topical retinoids.
4. **Milia formation**: Treated by sterilely unroofing the lesion.
5. **Wound infection (bacterial or fungal)**: Symptoms include increasing deep erythema, pruritis, and discomfort around the third to fifth days after the peel. Early suspicion of an infection should be managed with cultures and sensitivities, systemic antibiotics, and acetic acid solution rinses. Fungal infections are managed with topical and systemic antifungal agents.
6. **Herpes labialis**: Suspected if the classic vesicular eruption appears. Antiviral therapy dosage is changed from a preventative to a treatment dosage.

Late Complications

1. **Persistent erythema (greater than 2–3 months)**: May be caused by early sun exposure; however, persistent erythema may be an early indicator of scarring and future keloid formation.
2. **Scarring and keloid formation**: If an eschar forms post peel that does not shed for greater than 14 days, one can expect some degree of scarring, keloid formation, and pigmentary disturbances. Thickening consistent with keloid formation may be treated upon recognition with monthly intralesional injections of triamcinolone acetomide (10 mg/ml) and/or 5-fluorouracil (off-label use). Selective treatment with CO_2 or an erbium-doped yttrium aluminum garnet (Er:YAG) laser can be helpful in releasing and smoothing scars.
3. **Depigmentation**: Areas of depigmentation are typically observed for 3 to 6 months for return of pigmentation. After 6 months, it can be assumed that a permanent depigmentation has occurred.

Key Points

1. As a general rule, the deeper the depth of the peel, the greater the possible improvements, and the greater the potential complications.
2. Superficial peel depth varies (0.02–0.06 mm) depending on the chemical exfoliant used and the number of applications. Superficial peels injure the epidermis without extending into the dermis. Indications for superficial-depth peels include superficial dispigmentation, solar lentigines, and/or minimal photo damage.
3. Medium-depth peels span from the superficial papillary dermis to the upper reticular dermis (0.45 mm). Indications for medium-depth peels include moderate rhytids, melasma, pigmentary dyschromia, actinic keratosis, depressed scars, and ephelides.
4. Deep chemical peels have a goal depth of the midreticular dermis (0.6 mm). They are the most aggressive type of chemical exfoliant, are associated with the highest potential for complications, and are indicated for moderate to deep rhytids and depressed scars.
5. Jessner's solution (14 g each of resorcinol, salicylic acid, and lactic acid [85%] mixed in 95% ethanol to make a quantity of 100 mL) may be used to perform superficial peels or as a pre-peel for medium and deep chemical peels. The use of acetone and Jessner's solution prior to the application of a stronger chemical exfoliant will remove the oily, keratinized superficial layer of the skin and allow the second, more aggressive chemical agent a more uniform depth of penetration and a better final result.
6. Peel depth may be assessed based upon the type of frosting achieved after the application of the peeling solution. A thin, transparent frost with a pinkish background indicates that the peel has reached the papillary dermis. A solid, thick frost indicates that the peel has reached the upper reticular dermis. A thick, white-gray frost indicates that the peel has reached the midreticular dermis and that subsequent application of solution should be avoided.

Case Report 37.1. Medium-depth peel. A 42-year-old female presents with a chief complaint of "inconsistent skin tone and fine wrinkles." The patient admits to excessive sun exposure through her second and third decades of life as well as a 15-pack/year history of smoking. Physical exam demonstrates a Glogau II Fitzpatrick II skin type, ephilides, pigmentary dyschromia, depressed acne scars, and moderate rhytids (Figure 37.1). The patient was placed on a 6-week pre-peel skin regimen of Obagi Nu-Derm followed by a medium-depth skin-resurfacing procedure utilizing Jessner's solution and 30% trichloracetic acid. (See also Figures 37.2, 37.3, 37.4, 37.5, and 37.6.)

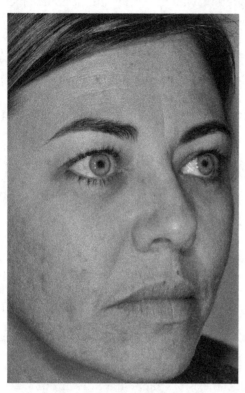

Figure 37.1. Pre-peel patient demonstrating a Glogau II Fitzpatrick II skin type.

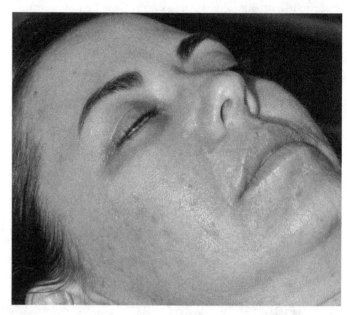

Figure 37.2. After application of acetone and Jessner's solution. Note light frosting to the face.

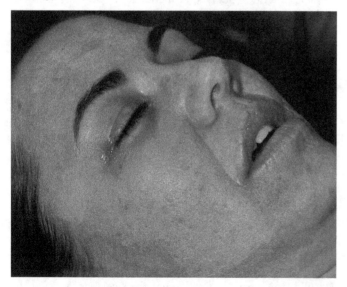

Figure 37.3. After first application of 30% trichloracetic acid. Note a thin transparent frost indicating that the papillary dermis has been reached. Also note the avoidance of the thin tissue of the periorbital and cervical regions.

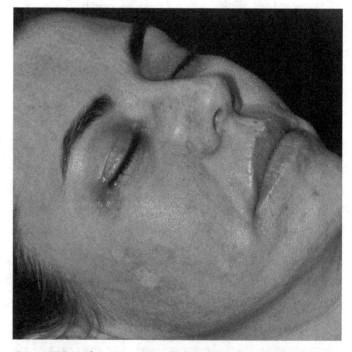

Figure 37.4. After second application of 30% trichloracetic acid. Note a solid, thicker frost indicating that the upper reticular dermis has been reached. This layer indicated the stopping point for the medium-depth peel.

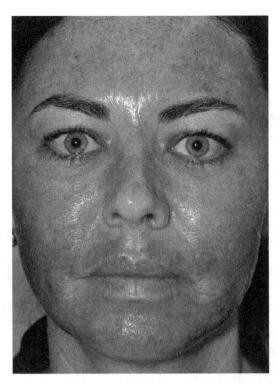

Figure 37.5.   Postpeel day 3. Patient demonstrates tissue erythema, edema, and evidence of early peeling.

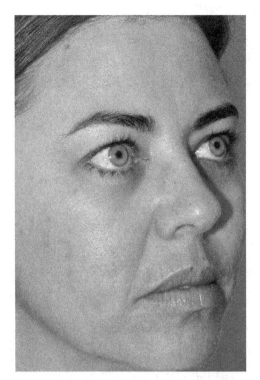

Figure 37.6.   Two months post peel with dramatic improvements to facial rhytids, acne scars, and pigmentary disturbances.

References

Avrum M.R., Tsao, S., Tannous, Z. and Avram, M., 2007. *Color atlas of cosmetic dermatology.* New York: McGraw-Hill; pp. 38–40.

Bensiman, R.H., 2009. Chemical peels. In: F.R. Nahai and F. Nahai, eds. *Minimally invasive facial rejuvenation.* Amsterdam: Elsevier.

Coleman, W.P., 3rd. 2001. Dermal peels. *Dermatologic Clinics,* 19(3), 405–11.

Coleman, W.P. and Lawrence, N., 1998. *Skin resurfacing.* Baltimore: Williams & Wilkins; 10–84.

Saags, H., 1989. *Civilization before Greece and Rome.* New Haven, CT: Yale University Press.

Wolff, K., Goldsmith, L.A., Katz, S.I., Gilchrest, B.A., Paller, A.S. and Leffell, D.J., 2008. *Fitzpatrick's dermatology in general medicine.* 7th ed. New York: McGraw-Hill; pp. 2369–70.

Facial CO_2 Laser Resurfacing

Matthew Robert Hlavacek

Private Practice, Kansas City Surgical Arts, Liberty, Missouri and Truman Medical Center and St. Luke's Hospital, Department of Surgery and Oral and Maxillofacial Surgery, Kansas City, Missouri, USA

Laser ablation of the mid-dermis and above to remove senescent changes.

Indications

1. Facial rhytidosis
2. Coarse skin texture
3. Mild skin laxity
4. Minor dyspigmentation
5. Acne scarring or facial scars
6. Dermatopathologic entities (rhinophyma, xanthelasma, or actinic keratosis)

Contraindications

1. Patients with poorly controlled comorbidities
2. Anticoagulated patients
3. Patients with collagen or vascular diseases
4. Isotretinoin use within the last 6 months
5. History of facial radiation
6. Dysmorphic patients with unrealistic expectations
7. Patients with malignant facial skin pathology
8. Caution in patients with preexisting eczema, rosacea, or atopic dermatitis
9. Caution in patients with a history of hypertrophic scarring or keloids
10. Caution in patients with darker Fitzpatrick skin types
11. Caution in patients with previous facial-lifting procedures (primarily lower blepharoplasty)

Anatomy

The epidermis is the most superficial layer of the skin and contains continuously regenerating squamous epithelial cells from its basal layer. It is limited at its deepest extent by the basement membrane. The epidermis also contains varying numbers of melanocytes, Langerhans cells, and Merkle cells depending on the location in the body. This layer produces the color and texture of the skin; however, it is devoid of collagen. Deep to the epidermis is the dermis, which is divided into the more superficial papillary layer and the deeper reticular layer. The main function of the dermis is to provide support both structurally and metabolically for the epidermis. The papillary layer is a minor part of the dermis that abuts the basement membrane and contains a concentrated vascular supply. The reticular layer forms the majority of the dermis and contains collagen and elastin fibers produced by fibroblasts, the main cell of the dermis.

Technique

1. Pretreatment conditioning with retinoic acid and hydroquinone is performed 4 weeks prior to the procedure.
2. Preoperative antiviral medication is initiated 24–48 hours preoperatively and for 2 weeks postoperatively. Single-dose intravenous preoperative antibiotics are administered prior to the procedure.
3. Ensure fire precautions are in place.
4. Intravenous conscious sedation or endotracheal general anesthesia may be employed depending on if adjunctive invasive procedures will be performed.
5. An equal mixture of 2% lidocaine with epinephrine and 0.5% marcaine without epinephrine is utilized to block the supratrochlear, infratrochlear, infraorbital, mental, and transverse facial-cervical plexus nerves.
6. Laser-resistant corneal shields with lacrilube are placed.
7. A laser setting is selected that is appropriate for the laser system and the patient Fitzpatrick skin type using a random pattern or fractionated setting.
8. Ensure that the face is dry. The face is lasered in subunits, protecting the follicles of the hairline and the brow with a tongue blade (Figure 38.2 [all figures cites appear in Case Report 38.1]). Start with the forehead, and laser caudally to the inferior border of the mandible in subunits. Care is taken to not overlap laser passes.
9. Withdraw the laser off of the skin, defocus, and angle at 45° to blend the laser over the inferior border of the mandible (Figure 38.3). Feathering of the thin cervical tissue may be performed with lighter laser settings.
10. A second pass is made with or without debridement, depending on the surgeon's preference. (Figure 38.4). Problem areas may require additional passes with the laser. Make consideration to reduce the energy around the eyes and increase the energy around the mouth and deeper acne scars.

Atlas of Operative Oral and Maxillofacial Surgery, First Edition. Edited by Christopher J. Haggerty and Robert M. Laughlin.
© 2015 John Wiley & Sons, Inc. Published 2015 by John Wiley & Sons, Inc.

11. At the completion of the laser treatment, the face is covered with a thin layer of emollient (aquaphore) (Eucerin, Montreal, Quebec, Canada) (Figure 38.5).

12. The corneal shields are removed and the eyes are irrigated with balanced salt solution (BSS).

Postoperative Management

1. Elevate head and use ice packs cautiously (facial numbness) for the first 2–3 days.

2. Antibiotics are recommended for one week postoperatively, and antiviral medications are recommended for 2 weeks postoperatively.

3. Patients are instructed to gently wash their face with hands and fingers (no towels or washcloths) with very mild soap (Dove, Unilever US, Inc, Englewood Cliffs, New Jersey, USA) followed by the application of a thin layer of emollient 3-4 times a day.

4. Patients are encouraged to not pick at their face to avoid prematurely removing involved skin.

5. The use of a diluted vinegar mist and a fan will provide comfort to a hot and itchy peeling face.

6. Mineral-based makeup can be used to cover erythema 1–2 weeks post ablation.

7. Retinoids and bleaching agents may be restarted after one month if tolerated.

8. Sun exposure is avoided.

Complications

Early Complications

1. **Pruritis**: Common and usually associated with re-epithelialization. Treat with a cool packs to the face and antihistamines, consider steroid ointment in severe cases. If pruritis continues after 3–4 days postoperatively, consider a superficial skin infection.

2. **Acne**: If there is reoccurrence within the first 2 weeks, consider a different emollient. Consider topical or systemic antibiotic (benzaclin) if severe after re-epithelialization.

3. **Bacterial infection**: Weeping crusting lesions with pain and pruritis. Attempt to culture and initially treat for *Staphylococcus aureus*.

4. **Viral infection**: Distinct pattern of markedly painful erythematous ulcerative lesions. Increase the currently utilized antiviral to the maximum dose, or switch to another antiviral.

5. **Fungal infection**: Pruritis with white patches. Diagnosis with KOH prep. Begin systemic antifungal therapy.

6. **Contact dermatitis**: Diffuse intense facial erythema and pruritis. Identify and discontinue the offending agent.

Late Complications

1. **Prolonged erythema**: Consider other causes, including incipient scar formation, infection, and dermatitis.

Typically related to the depth of ablation. Treated with reassurance and topical steroids if severe. Also consider pulse dye laser.

2. **Scarring**: Marked by inappropriately tender erythema, especially in prone patients. Initially treat with topical steroids, silicone sheeting, and massage. Consider steroid and/or 5-fluorouracil injections for severe cases.

3. **Hyperpigmentation (3–4 weeks)**: Typically seen in darker skin types and those unable to avoid ultraviolet (UV) exposure post laser treatment. Most cases resolve without treatment. Bleaching agents and avoiding UV exposure will hasten resolution. Consider nonablative laser treatments in refractive cases.

4. **Hypopigmentation (6–12 months)**: Typically presents as a delayed phenomenon that occurs 6–12 months after laser treatment. Frequently results from overaggressive resurfacing or resurfacing in subunits that heal adjacent to photodamaged skin (pseudo-hypopigmentation). Pigmentation frequently resolves with time. Refractory cases are managed with retreatment of the entire face to blend areas or with makeup to camouflage.

5. **Milia (3–4 weeks)**: Microcyst formation with re-epithelialization of follicles. Treatment involves sterilely unroofing and removing the microcysts with a large bore needle and manual expression.

Key Points

1. Appropriate patient selection and utilization of the laser energy will avoid most complications. For example, use caution when treating patients with a "thinner" dermis (to avoid scarring and prolonged erythema) and with darker skin types (to avoid dyspigmentation and scarring).

2. Patients with lighter Fitzpatrick skin types have a lower incidence of postoperative hyperpigmentation and a higher incidence of prolonged postoperative erythema.

3. Laser ablation will not treat marked skin laxity. Deep facial rhytids and moderate to severe skin laxity are best treated with surgical intervention.

4. Attempt to laser the full facial unit when possible to avoid lines of demarcation.

5. Care is taken to minimize overlapping laser passes. Overlapping passes result in excessive thermal damage, deep wounds, and scarring.

6. Areas that typically require additional laser passes include the thicker tissues of the forehead, glabellar, nasolabial, and perioral regions.

7. When treating perioral rhytids, care is taken to not cross the vermillion border. Overtreatment of this area will lead to blunting, scarring, and thickening of the vermillion border.

Case Report

Case report 38.1. A 54-year-old Caucasian female with a Fitzpatrick II Glogau II skin profile presents with a chief complaint of desiring to look younger and refreshed. Simultaneous full-face laser resurfacing, endoscopic brow lift, upper and lower lid blepharoplasties, and facial fat grafting procedures were performed with general endotracheal intubation. (See Figures 38.1 through 38.5.)

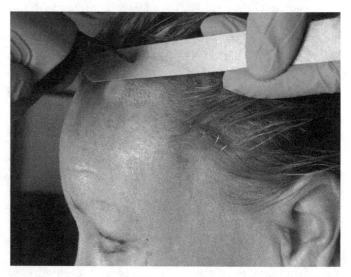

Figure 38.2.   The hair follicles are protected with a tongue blade, the patterns are not markedly overlapped, and the face is carefully lasered in subunits.

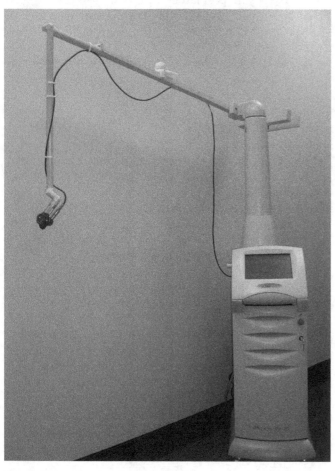

Figure 38.1.   The laser unit utilized at the author's facility, the Lumenis Ultrapulse Total FX system (San Jose, California, USA), which enables random pattern fractionated laser resurfacing.

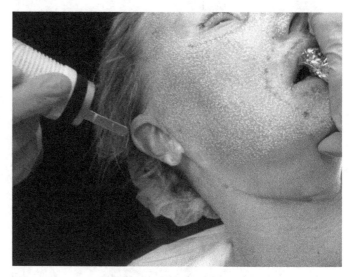

Figure 38.3.   The hand piece is defocused and angled at the inferior border of the mandible to blend this area into the thinner cervical tissue.

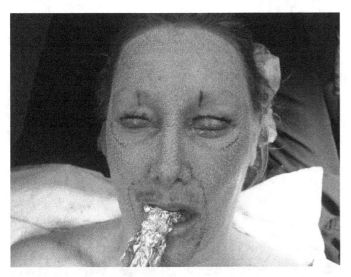

Figure 38.4.   Note the char pattern on the skin; the second pass is made without debridement.

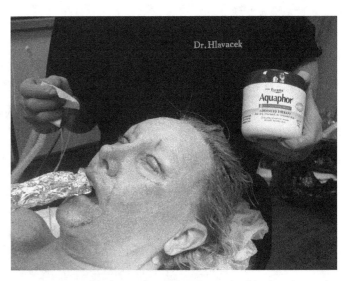

Figure 38.5.   A thin layer of emollient (aquaphor) is placed over the resurfaced areas after laser treatment is completed.

References

Beeson, W.H. and Rachel, J., 2002. Valacyclovir prophylaxis for herpes simplex viral infection recurrence following laser skin resurfacing. *Dermatologic Surgery*, 28, 331–36.

Bernstein, I.J., Kauvar, A.B., Grossman, M.C. and Geronemus, R.G., 1997. The short and long term side effects of carbon dioxide laser resurfacing. *Dermatologic Surgery*, 23, 519–25.

Burkitt, H.G., 1993. Skin. In: H.G. Burkitt, B. Young and J.W. Heath, eds. *Wheater's functional histology*. 3rd ed. Edinburgh: Churchill Livingston; pp. 152–69.

Fulton, J.E., Rahimi, A.D., Mansoor, S., Helton, P. and Shitabata, P., 2004. The treatment of hypopigmentation after skin resurfacing. *Dermatologic Surgery*, 30, 95–101.

Hevia, O., Nemeth, A.J. and Taylor, J.R., 1991. Tretinoin accelerates healing after trichloroacetic acid chemical peel. *Archives of Dermatology*, 127, 678–82.

Manuskiatti, W., Fitzpatrick, R.E. and Goldman, M.P., 1999. Prophylactic antibiotics in patients undergoing laser resurfacing of the skin. *Journal of the American Academy of Dermatology*, 40, 77–84.

Niamtu, J., 2008. To debride or not to debride: that is the question. *Dermatologic Surgery*, 34, 1200–11.

Zachary, C.B., Rokhsar, C.K. and Fitzpatrick, R.E., 2008. Laser skin resurfacing. In: D. Goldberg, ed. *Lasers and lights*. Vol. 2. Philadelphia: Saunders.

Brow Lift

Jon D. Perenack and Earl Peter Park
Department of Oral and Maxillofacial Surgery, Louisiana State University Health Sciences Center, New Orleans, Louisiana, USA

Procedures aimed toward addressing brow ptosis and forehead and glabellar rhytids. Approaches include endoscopic, trichophytic (subgaleal and subcutaneous), and coronal. Although all techniques address brow ptosis, treatment planning is often guided by cosmetic diagnoses, surgeon preference, and supplemental procedures such as bony orbital recontouring, muscle resection, hairline repositioning, and concomitant upper blepharoplasty.

General Indications

1. Brow ptosis
2. Brow asymmetry
3. Deep rhytids and furrows traversing the forehead, glabella, and/or nasal radix
4. Appearance of heavy or redundant forehead or temporal skin
5. Pseudo-blepharoptosis and/or visual field restriction

General Contraindications

1. Lagopthalmos
2. Previous or current dry-eye symptoms
3. Unrealistic patient expectations

Anatomy

Supraorbital nerve: Exits the superior orbit parallel to the medial limbus. The nerve forms branches, which innervate the frontoparietal skin (deep branch) and upper eyelid (superficial branch).

Supratrochlear nerve: Exits the superomedial orbit and is located 9.0 mm (+/− 3 mm) medial to the supraorbital nerve. Innervates the skin of the lower forehead (midline glabella), the medial upper eyelid, and a portion of the conjunctiva.

Sentinel vein: Located approximately 10 mm lateral to the zygomaticofrontal suture. Serves as a warning for the proximity of the temporal branch of the facial nerve.

Temporal branch of the facial nerve: As the temporal branch courses superior to the zygomatic arch, it is located within or along the undersurface of the temporoparietal fascia. The temporal branch provides motor innervation to the brow musculature and the superior portion of the orbicularis oculi muscle. The anticipated course of the temporal branch can be approximated by drawing a line from a point 5 mm anterior to the tragus to a point 15 mm lateral to the lateral taper of the ipsilateral brow.

Conjoint (*conjoin*) tendon: The fusion of the galea, superficial and deep temporal fascia and periosteum (pericranium) within the anterior temporal region.

Preoperative Markings

1. Patients are marked preoperatively while sitting upright.
2. The brow lift is simulated with manual manipulation of the brows prior to placing the patient supine, and the desired vectors of pull are marked.
3. Important markings include the incision sites, the skin to be resected, and the anticipated location of nerves (supraorbital, supratrochlear, and temporal nerve).
4. Standard preoperative photographs are taken and placed in the operatory within the surgeon's field of view for reference during the procedure.

Endoscopic (Closed) Brow Lift

Indications

1. Circumvent the placement of more visible scars associated with open techniques (trichophytic and coronal)
2. Patient preference for a less invasive procedure
3. Patient with short to normal upper facial third (less than 6 cm from brow to hairline)

Note that the endoscopic brow lift procedure may raise the hairline.

Contraindications

1. Excessive hairline recession
2. Excessively curved forehead inhibiting the passing of endoscopic instruments to the periorbita

Technique

1. Preoperative markings are made with the patient sitting upright (Figure 39.1 [all figures cited in this section appear in Case Report 39.1]).
2. Intravenous sedation or oral endotracheal intubation is employed. A single dose of intravenous antibiotics is recommended prior to the start of the procedure.

Atlas of Operative Oral and Maxillofacial Surgery, First Edition. Edited by Christopher J. Haggerty and Robert M. Laughlin
© 2015 John Wiley & Sons, Inc. Published 2015 by John Wiley & Sons, Inc.

3. The patient is positioned supine (Figure 39.2) with the endoscope monitor within view of the surgeon and surgical assistant, typically at the foot of the operating table.

4. Tumescent solution is injected within the anticipated tissue planes to be elevated. Local anesthetic is injected supraperiosteally along the supraorbital and lateral orbital rims. Nerve blocks of the auriculotemporal and zygomaticotemporal nerves is recommended with intravenous sedation.

5. Five incisions (ports) are placed and hidden posterior to the patient's hairline: a single vertical 2 cm midline incision (Figure 39.3), two 1.5 cm vertical paramedian (parasagittal) incisions (Figure 39.4) located superior to the proposed highest point of the brow arch (lateral limbus of the eye), and two beveled 2–3 cm horizontal incisions (Figure 39.9) located within the temporal hair-bearing region 1–2 cm lateral to the temporal crest and 2–3 cm posterior to the hairline. The midline and paramedian incisions are made through all layers of the scalp to the cranium, and the temporal incisions are carried to the superficial layer of the deep temporal fascia.

6. Blind dissection (without the endoscope) is performed with a curved periosteal elevator to develop a full-thickness subperiosteal flap using the midline and paramedian ports (Figure 39.5). Blindly, a curved endoscopic elevator is utilized to dissect within a subperiosteal tissue plane posteriorly to the coronal suture (vertex of the skull), anteriorly to a point 2 cm cephalic to the supraorbital rims, and laterally along the lateral orbit rims below the lateral canthus approaching the infraorbital rim. Care is taken to fully release the arcus marginalis from the orbital margins (Figure 39.6).

7. A 30° endoscope with a protected sheath is inserted through the midline port (Figure 39.7). Endoscopic instruments are inserted through the paramedian ports, and dissection proceeds caudally toward the supraorbital rim, glabella, and lateral orbital rims. The endoscope is used to visualize the central compartment and to allow instrumentation to dissect the remaining central periosteum and to expose the brow (galeal) fat pad. The supraorbital nerves are often visualized (Figure 39.8) through the overlying tissue, and the periosteum is subsequently released around the nerve bundles. Below the brow fat pad, a horizontal release of the periosteum is typically carried out with a scoring instrument. The periosteal release is enlarged until the defect is at least 1 cm. This allows passive mobilization of the forehead and minimizes relapse. Care is taken not to tear the supraorbital neurovascular bundles as they are often denuded at this point.

8. With periosteum exposure and scoring completed, resection or ablation of the corrugators and procerus muscles may be carried out if desired. The authors typically recommend scoring with the electrocautery as an alternative to muscle resection to minimize postoperative soft tissue defects and an unnatural brow appearance.

9. Laterally, utilizing the temporal ports (Figure 39.9), a curved elevator is used to blindly dissect (Figure 39.10) within a tissue plane created between the temporoparietal fascia (superficial temporal fascia) and the temporalis fascia (deep temporal fascia) overlying the temporalis muscle. The entire superficial temporal space is released anteriorly and posteriorly to allow passive posterior movement of the scalp. Inferiorly, the dissection comes to a "soft" stop approximately 1 cm above the zygomatic arch where the temporoparietal fascia fuses with the temporalis fascia. Aggressive dissection below this point raises significant risk of injuring the facial nerve as it crosses the arch. The sentinel (medial zygomatic temporal) vein is located 1 cm lateral to the zygomaticofrontal suture and should also be avoided.

10. The lateral subgaleal and the central subperiosteal dissection planes are connected by dividing the conjoint tendon (Figure 39.11) at the superior temporal line. A sharp dissector is placed through the temporal port and is driven through the conjoint tendon into the frontal pocket slightly above the supraorbital rim. The conjoint tendon is then opened posteriorly with a sweeping motion until there is a complete connection between the two pockets.

11. Fixation is accomplished at the temporal ports first and then at the paramedian ports. A 0-0 Nurolon (Ethicon US, LLC, Somerville, New Jersey, USA) suture is utilized to grasp the temporoparietal fascia on the medial aspect of the incision (Figure 39.12). The suture is superiorly and posteriorly ligated to the temporalis fascia (Figure 39.13). The vector follows the line formed from the ala to lateral canthus (Figure 39.1). Occasionally, a second suture is required to secure the flap. This suture placement is performed bilaterally to a symmetrical endpoint. (*Note:* If the corrugators were aggressively released earlier, this step has the risk of excessively widening the interbrow distance.) Fixation is accomplished at the paramedian incisions with the placement of resorbable 3.5 mm Endotine (Microaire Aesthetics, Charlottesville, Virginia, USA) devices. Skin hooks are utilized to retract the paramedian incision laterally. The Endotine drill is used to engage the cranium to the depth of the Endotine drill bit along the anticipated vertical vector (typically, the lateral limbus of the eye) of the brow lift. The osteotomy (Figure 39.14) site is irrigated to remove any residual bone shavings. The Endotine insertion tool is used to secure the Endotine into the predrilled Endotine osteotomy. The Endotine is fully seated when it is flush with the cranium. Endotines

are placed bilaterally at each of the two paramedian incisions. The forehead scalp is elevated and positioned onto the Endotine devices. This maneuver sets the height and arch of the brows. Care is taken not to over- or underelevate the brow. If resistance to elevation is noted, additional periosteal release along the lateral supraorbital rims may be required. We recommend leaving the forehead scalp secured to the anchors for at least 10 minutes, and then reassess for any soft tissue creep and resulting laxity. If necessary, the lax scalp is then gently lifted off of the Endotine devices, re-elevated to the proper height with tension, and then resuspended.

12. Scalp incisions are closed with either skin staples or sutures, and bacitracin is applied. Drains are usually not necessary. Light pressure dressing may be placed depending on the preference of the surgeon.

Key Points

1. Advantages of the endoscopic brow-lifting technique include a minimally invasive approach, rapid recovery time, decreased alopecia, decreased bleeding, decreased tissue edema, decreased scalp anesthesia and paresthesia, and minimal scarring compared to open techniques.
2. Endoscopic brow lifts may elevate the hairline, particularly in patients with thick, redundant forehead skin, and should be used cautiously in patients with excessive vertical brow height.
3. Failure to maintain a subperiosteal tissue plane while performing the central dissection will result in poor hemostasis of the surgical field and will make further endoscopic visualization difficult.

Case Report

Case Report 39.1. Endoscopic brow lift. A 37-year-old female presents with a chief complaint of brow ptosis, forehead rhytids, and an "angry" appearance. Physical examination reveals brow asymmetry and brow ptosis. Chronic corrugator activation is noted. Forehead height is normal to slightly short. (See Figures 39.1 through 39.14.)

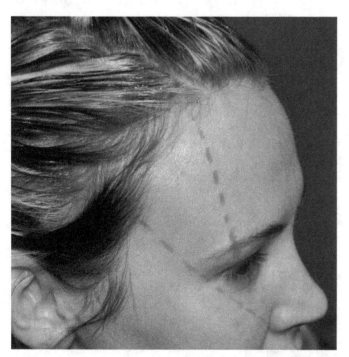

Figure 39.1. Preoperative markings are made with the patient in the upright position. The pink lines represent the anticipated vectors of pull.

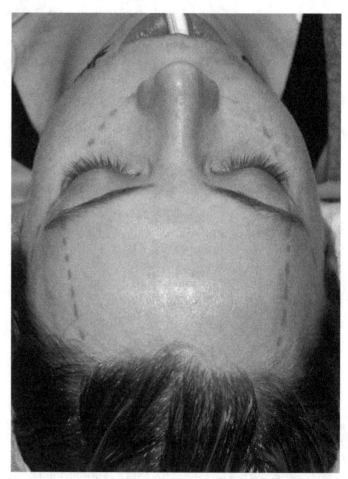

Figure 39.2. The patient is orally intubated, and the anticipated vectors of pull and the sites of the incisions are marked.

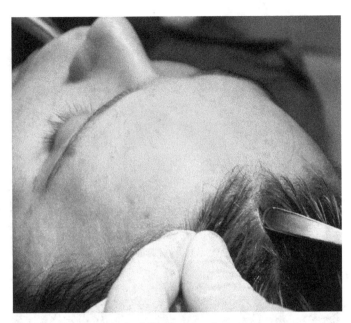

Figure 39.3. A vertical midline incision is created posterior to the hairline.

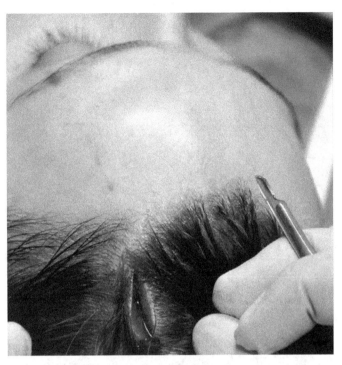

Figure 39.4. Two vertical paramedian incisions are created posterior to the hairline and along the anticipated vector of pull to elevate the apex of the brow.

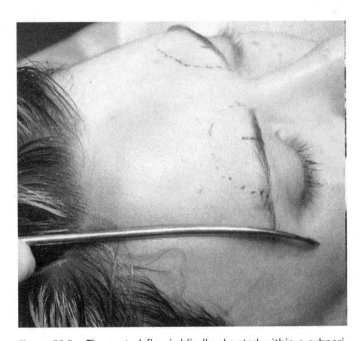

Figure 39.5. The central flap is blindly elevated within a subperiosteal tissue plane. The supraorbital markings demonstrate the inferior extent of the blind dissection.

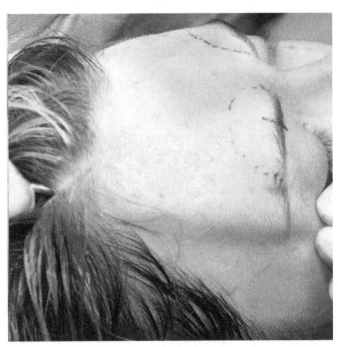

Figure 39.6. The arcus marginalis must be freed in order to sufficiently mobilize the tissue flap.

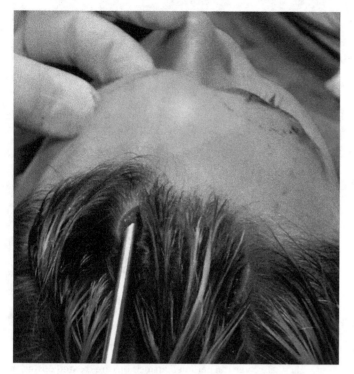

Figure 39.7. A 30° endoscope is inserted through the midline port and allows for dissection of the central flap under visualization.

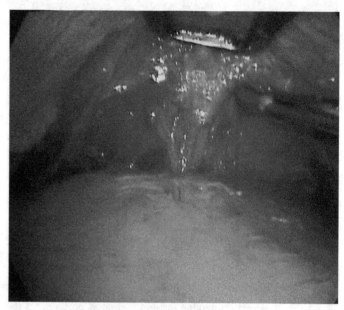

Figure 39.8. The endoscope allows for visualization of the peri-osteal release and the supraorbital nerve.

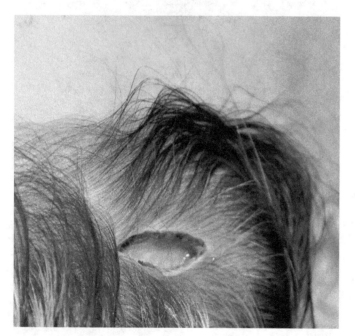

Figure 39.9. The temporal incision is carried down to the glistening white temporalis fascia (deep temporal fascia).

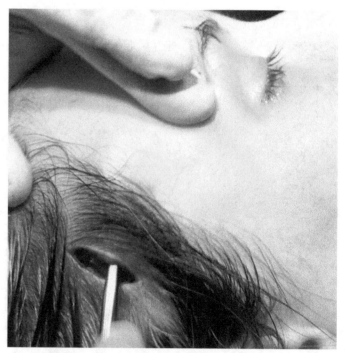

Figure 39.10. Blind dissection within the temporal space in a tissue plane between the temporoparietal fascia and the temporalis fascia to protect the temporal branch of the facial nerve.

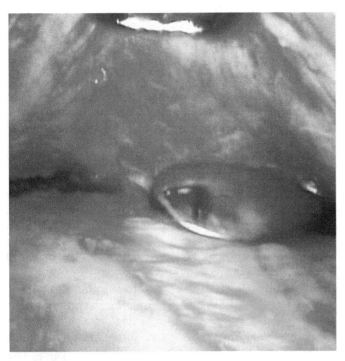

Figure 39.11.   The temporal dissection and conjoint tendon release as seen by endoscopic visualization.

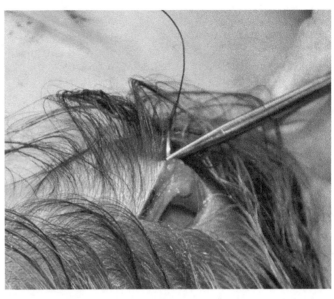

Figure 39.12.   0-0 nonresorbable sutures are used to secure the temporoparietal fascia. The suture is pulled posteriorly and superiorly to resuspend the brow.

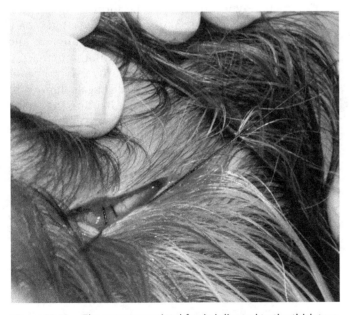

Figure 39.13.   The temporoparietal fascia is ligated to the thick temporalis fascia.

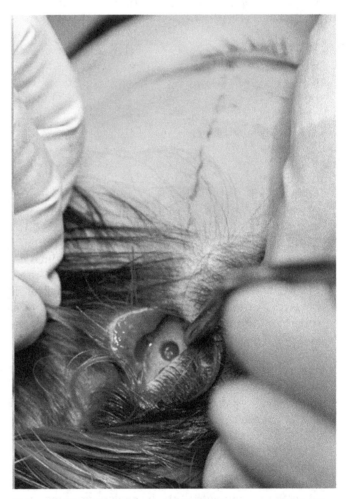

Figure 39.14.   Osteotomy created within the paramedian incision for the insertion of an Endotine. The Endotine placement corresponds with the superior vector of pull (the lateral limbus of the eye).

Trichophytic Brow Lift

Indication

1. Excessively high hairline and tall forehead with supplemental desire to lower the hairline

Contraindications

1. Progressive recession of hairline in female patients, which may expose the transverse trichophytic surgical scar
2. Male patients
3. Simultaneous medium-depth skin resurfacing

Technique (Subgaleal Brow Lift)

1. Preoperative markings are made with the patient sitting upright. The amount of tissue (scalp) to be excised should be determined prior to the initiation of the procedure.
2. Intravenous sedation or oral endotracheal intubation is employed. A single dose of intravenous antibiotics is recommended prior to the start of the procedure.
3. The patient is positioned supine, and tumescent solution is injected within the subgaleal tissue planes to be elevated. Local anesthetic is injected supraperiosteally along the supraorbital and lateral orbital rims. Nerve blocks of the auriculotemporal and zygomaticotemporal nerves is recommended with intravenous sedation.
4. Three to four millimeters of the thin hair located at the anterior hairline is trimmed with scissors (Figure 39.16 [all figures cited in this section appear in Case Report 39.2]), and the lateral extension of the proposed incision is shaved for 5 cm as it enters the temporal region.
5. A wavy trichophytic incision is initiated 4–5 mm posterior to the anterior hairline and is continued to the depth of the galea. The trichophytic aspect of the incision extends to the middle of the lateral hairline curvature. The trichophytic incision is beveled in three distinct regions. The anterior aspect of the incision is beveled to transect the hair follicles, and the lateral aspect of the incision is beveled to parallel (not transect) the hair follicles.
6. The frontal and temporal flaps are elevated within the subgaleal plane (Figure 39.17). Frontal dissection is carried to the level of the supraorbital rim. The supraorbital neurovascular bundle is identified and preserved. The temporal flap is elevated just superficial to the temporalis fascia in order to preserve the temporal branch of the facial nerve as it courses within the overlying temporoparietal fascia. If brow elevation with flap manipulation is easily achieved, the frontal dissection is complete. If the brow does not move passively to the extent desired, dissection is continued within a subperiosteal plane around the supraorbital

ridge, inferior to the nasal radix, and inferiorly along the lateral orbital rim. Flap elevation posterior to the hairline is typically not required. Once the entire forehead flap is mobilized, the glabellar musculature may be addressed.

7. The subgaleal forehead flap is retracted superiorly, allowing the flap to be drawn upward from the lateral brow over the undissected scalp. The amount of tissue to be excised is determined by the position of the brows and the vertical height of the forehead after the superior elevation of the forehead flap (Figure 39.18). Vertical-guide cuts (Figure 39.19) may be made within the forehead flap as it overlaps the undissected scalp to aid in determining the amount of tissue to be excised. A 1–2 cm wedge of tissue is removed with a #15 blade (Figure 39.20). A slight overcorrection may be necessary.
8. A #15 blade is used to create a reverse beveling of the recipient skin site to incorporate a trichophytic hair-sparing flap margin. Fibrin sealant is applied under the forehead flap to facilitate fixation and to minimize hematoma formation. Alternatively, or in cases with moderate muscle oozing, a closed suction drain may be placed.
9. The galea is closed with interrupted 3-0 Vicryl sutures, the subcutaneous tissue is closed with 4-0 Monocryl sutures, and the skin edges are reapproximated with a running 6-0 plain gut suture (Figure 39.21). Incisions within the temporal hair-bearing areas are closed with staples.

Key Points

1. The trichophytic lift may be performed in either a subcutaneous or a subgaleal tissue plane. Both share a frontal hairline incision that extends laterally and inferiorly into the temporal hairline. Both approaches allow for the correction of forehead rhytids, brow ptosis, and brow asymmetries, but the subgaleal brow lift approach allows for lowering of the hairline and shortening of the vertical forehead.
2. With the trichophytic incision, the bevel has three separate parts or segments. In the anterior segment of the incision, the beveling transects the follicles and allows for hair growth through the incision to hide the scar. Thus, the bevel is at an angle that transects the shaft of the hair follicle while maintaining the base of the hair follicle. The lateral segment of the incision is located within the hair-bearing areas, similar to the coronal incision. In the lateral segment of the incision, the incision is parallel to the hair follicles in order to not transect the hair follicles.
3. The trichophytic incision may become visible with time as the anterior hairline recedes.

Case Report

Case Report 39.2. Trichophytic brow lift. A 35-year-old female presents with a chief complaint of a high hairline and brow asymmetry. Physical examination reveals an elongated upper facial third and mild brow ptosis with slight asymmetry. (See Figures 39.15 through 39.22.)

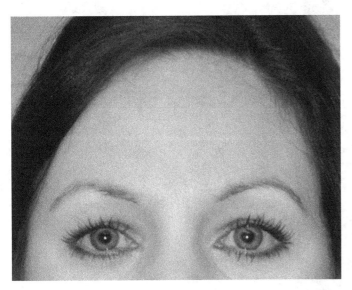

Figure 39.15.   The patient demonstrates mild brow asymmetry and a tall forehead.

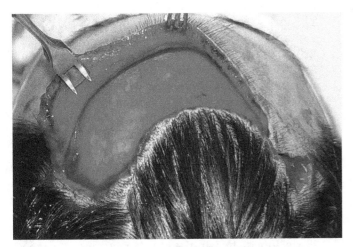

Figure 39.17.   The subgaleal frontal flap is elevated with minimal temporal elevation down to the level of the brow (galeal) fat pad.

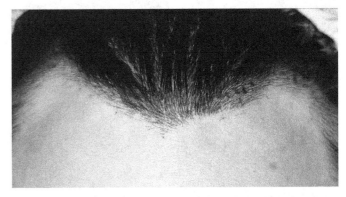

Figure 39.16.   Planned trichophytic incision. The hair inferior to the incision is trimmed, and the incision is tattooed with methylene blue.

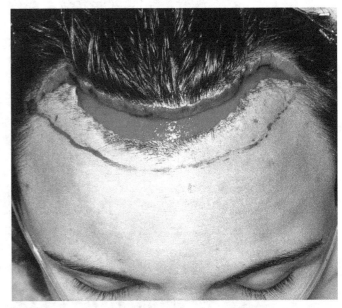

Figure 39.18.   A 2.0 cm section of tissue is outlined for excision.

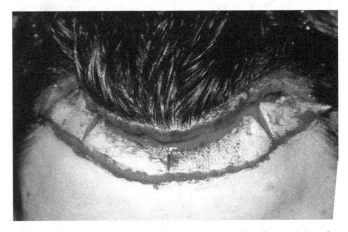

Figure 39.19.   Vertical cuts guides are used to aid in determining the amount of tissue to be excised.

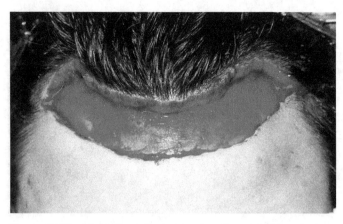

Figure 39.20.   Tissue is excised, exposing the underlying pericranium–subgalea.

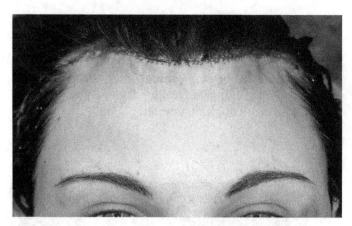

Figure 39.21.   Flap placement and closure.

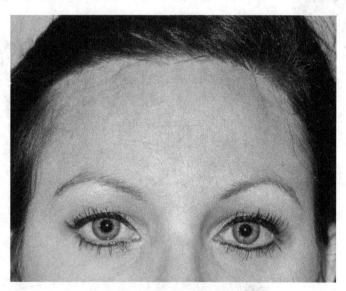

Figure 39.22.   Patient at 1-year follow-up after trichophytic subgaleal brow lift. Note shortening of the vertical length of the forehead, the well-concealed scar, and the retained brow elevation.

Coronal Brow Lift

Indications

1. Excessive supraorbital bone protrusion requiring recontouring
2. Subcutaneous fat loss accentuating supraorbital bony protrusion

Contraindications

1. Progressive recession of the hairline in female patients
2. Male patients

Technique

1. Preoperative markings are made with the patient sitting upright.
2. Intravenous sedation or oral endotracheal intubation is employed. A single dose of intravenous antibiotics is recommended prior to the start of the procedure.
3. The patient is positioned supine, and tumescent solution is injected within the anticipated tissue planes to be elevated. Local anesthetic is injected supraperiosteally along the supraorbital and lateral orbital rims. Nerve blocks of the auriculotemporal and zygomaticotemporal nerves is recommended with intravenous sedation.
4. The hair is parted with hair clips to expose a horizontal segment of scalp 5–6 cm posterior to the hairline (Figure 39.24 [all figures cited in this section appear in Case Report 39.3]). An undulated, beveled incision is created parallel to the hair follicles (Figure 39.25) from temporal tuft to temporal tuft. Centrally, the incision is carried through the galea, and a subgaleal dissection proceeds to a point several centimeters above the supraorbital rim. A subperiosteal dissection is then initiated and continues to expose the supraorbital rims, the radix of the nose, and the lateral orbital rims (Figure 39.26). The supraorbital neurovascular bundles are identified and preserved (Figure 39.27).
5. Depending on the depth of bony removal planned, the dissection is carried subperiosteally into the

orbits with care not to detach the lateral canthal tendons. Supraorbital neurovascular bundles within their foramina may need to be released with a small osteotome and mobilized into the scalp flap.

6. The temporal flap is elevated just superficial to the temporalis fascia in order to protect the temporal branch of the facial nerve. The lateral subgaleal and the central subperiosteal dissection planes are connected by dividing the conjoint tendon at the superior temporal lines bilaterally.

7. Subperiosteal dissection allows for exposure of the osseous orbital structures, thus allowing the recontouring of the supraorbital and lateral orbital rim prominences. Preoperatively, a determination should be made as to the three-dimensional osseous changes desired. Depth (guide) cuts (Figure 39.28) are placed within the bone to be reduced with a crosscut fissure burr to map out the extent of reduction. The reduction is carried out with a 4 mm egg bur (Figures 39.28 and 39.29) with copious irrigation. Periodic redraping of the coronal flap over the upper brow is necessary to observe progress and symmetry.

8. After bony recontouring is completed, the periosteum is released below the brow (galeal) fat pads to allow for flap advancement. Glabellar musculature may be addressed at this time.

9. Towel clamps are used to retract the tissue flap superiorly, allowing the scalp to be drawn upward from the lateral brow. If necessary, paramedian bone tunnels or Endotine devices may be used to further suspend the central component of the flap and to stabilize the arch of the brows. The temporal portion of the flap is secured with heavy, nonresorbable sutures passed from the temporoparietal fascia to the temporalis fascia in a superolateral vector.

10. A #10 blade is used to trim the excessive flap tissue. Fibrin sealant is applied under the forehead flap to facilitate fixation and to minimize hematoma formation. Alternatively, or in cases with moderate muscle oozing, a closed suction drain may be placed. The galea is closed with interrupted 3-0 Vicryl sutures, and the scalp is secured with staples.

Key Points

1. For women, recontouring of the supraorbital region allows for feminizing of the nasofrontal angle and brow prominences.

2. Care should be taken when recontouring the supraorbital rim to avoid penetration into the frontal sinus. Preoperative computed tomography scans will allow the surgeon to map out frontal sinus anatomy and minimize inadvertent perforation.

Case Report

Case Report 39.3. Coronal brow lift. A 40-year-old female presents with a chief complaint of deep-set eyes, deep wrinkles, and a "tired" appearance. Physical examination reveals normal upper facial third height, vertical glabellar rhytids, prominent superolateral bony orbital rims, and mild brow ptosis with slight asymmetry. (See Figures 39.23 through 39.32.)

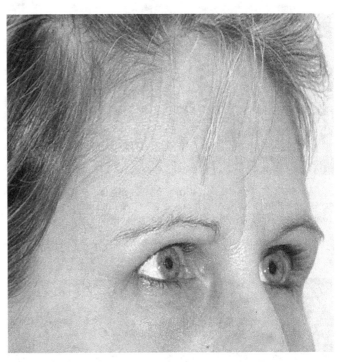

Figure 39.23. The patient demonstrates brow ptosis, vertical glabellar rhytids, and prominent superolateral bony orbital rims.

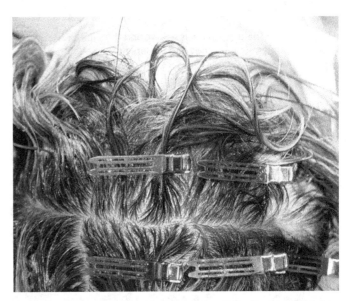

Figure 39.24. The site of the proposed scalp incision is defined by parting the hair with clips. The shaving of sections of hair is often not warranted.

343

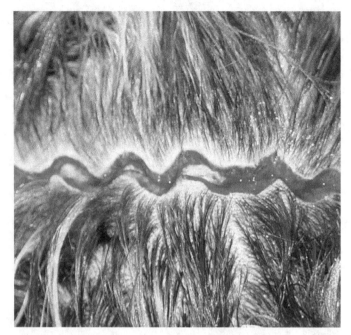

Figure 39.25. An undulated incision is initiated 5–6 cm posterior to the hairline. The wavy appearance of the incision will aid in flap reapproximation and will camouflage the scar.

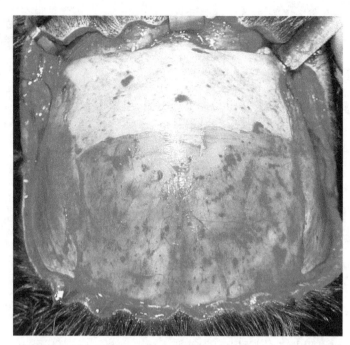

Figure 39.26. Frontal and temporal flaps are elevated and connected, and the orbital rims are exposed in a subperiosteal tissue plane.

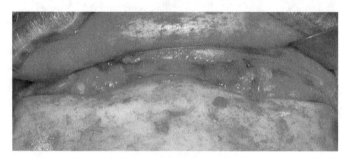

Figure 39.27. The periosteum is scored, and the supraorbital neurovascular bundles are identified and preserved.

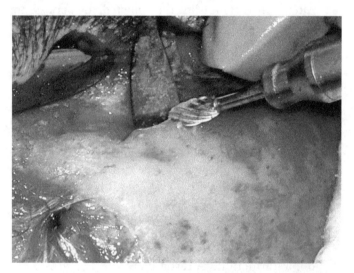

Figure 39.28. After the depth of bone to be reduced is marked with depth cuts with a fissured bur, an egg or round bur is used to recontour the bony prominences of the supraorbital rims.

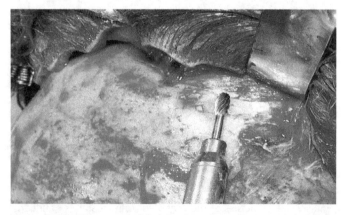

Figure 39.29. The supraorbital rims have been recontoured without penetrating the frontal sinus.

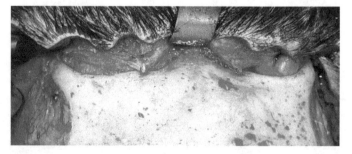

Figure 39.30. Bony recontouring is completed.

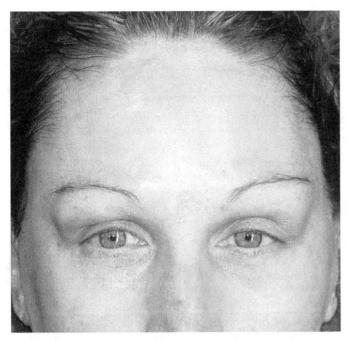

Figure 39.31. Patient appearance immediately postoperatively.

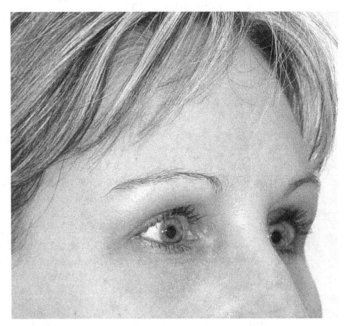

Figure 39.32. Patient appearance at one year postoperatively.

Postoperative Management for Brow Lift Procedures

1. A thin layer of bacitracin is placed over all skin incisions, and a light pressure dressing is placed at the time of surgery.
2. Antibiotics and analgesics are prescribed postoperatively.
3. The patient is asked to sleep with their head of the bed elevated for the first week postsurgery.
4. On postoperative day 2, the pressure dressing is removed, and all incisions are cleaned with a 50–50 mixture of hydrogen peroxide and sterile water to minimize incision site crusting.
5. Patients are allowed to gently shampoo their hair on postoperative day 3.
6. Patients are advised to avoid hot curlers, straightening irons, excessive blow drying, and caustic hair chemicals as surgical anesthesia may lead to self-inflicted tissue damage.
7. Staples are removed 7 to 10 days postoperatively.
8. Patients are asked to minimize strenuous activities for 3 weeks postoperatively.

Complications

Early Complications

Hematoma: Unrecognized hematoma formation may lead to flap necrosis. Once a hematoma is recognized, immediate evacuation and flap repositioning are performed.

Supraorbital or supratrochlear paresthesia–hypothesia: Typically resolves with conservative management and tincture of time. For persistent cases, consider short-course steroid treatment or low-dose amitriptyline.

Muscle weakness: Weakness of the brow elevators due to injury of the temporal branch of the facial nerve. Typically resolving within 3–4 months. To mask resolving or permanent brow paralysis, adjunctive botulinum toxin can be used to weaken the contralateral frontalis to create symmetry.

Late Complications

Lagophthalmos: Typically from overelevating the brow. Minor lagophthalmos typically resolves with time and with inferior massage of the eyelids. Severe cases often result from simultaneous brow lifting and upper blepharoplasty procedures performed by an inexperienced surgeon. Severe cases require resuspension of the brow lift if noticed early. Late lagophthalmos is treated with upper-lid skin grafts, muscle resuspension procedures, botulinum toxin, and gold weight application.

Unnatural appearance (operated look): Aggressive resection of the corrugator and procerus may lead to a widened interbrow distance and movement abnormalities. Complete or partial removal of muscle may lead to a soft tissue deficit once edema resolves. Movement abnormalities may be masked with botulinum toxin therapy. Soft tissue topography deficits may be camouflaged with injectable soft tissue fillers.

Incisional scarring: Thickened scars are amenable to dermabrasion or laser resurfacing at 6–8 weeks. Keloids are treated with serial Kenalog injections.

Alopecia: May be temporary or permanent along areas of incision tension or fixation. Hair follicles typically display hair regrowth within 4–5 months. However, hair loss can be permanent with overzealous cautery and ischemia of the hair follicles. Follicular unit hair grafting or scar excision with scalp advancement may camouflage troubled areas.

Key Points

1. Brow-lifting surgery is often not just about brow elevation. Flattening of forehead skin, lowering of the hairline, and bony recontouring are frequently primary and/or secondary goals. Open approaches allow for direct access and more aggressive muscle resection (frontalis, procerus, and corrugator). The trichophytic approach allows the surgeon the opportunity to shorten a tall forehead. The coronal approach allows the surgeon the best access to perform osseous recontouring.

2. Novice surgeons should be cautious of combining brow-lifting procedures with upper eyelid blepharoplasty due to the risk of lagophthalmos. Lagophthalmos can be minimized by performing the procedures in two stages with the elevation of the brow first, followed by upper blepharoplasty after 3 months.

3. Tumescent solution (25 mL 1% lidocaine + 1 mL 1:1000 epinephrine in a 500 mL bag of normal saline) is diffusely injected with a 22 g spinal needle into all tissue planes that are expected to be elevated during the surgery. Tumescent anesthesia facilitates hydrodissection of the desired tissue planes and aids in hemostasis. A 7–10-minute delay after tumescent infiltration allows sufficient time for the ideal vasoconstrictive (hemostatic) properties of the tumescent solution.

4. The vectors of pull should coincide with the final placement of the brow (Figure 39.1). The ideal placement of the highest point (apex) of the brow typically coincides with a vertical line drawn from the lateral limbus of the eye. The lateral margin of the brow ideally terminates along an oblique line connecting the lateral canthus and the lateral nasal ala.

5. Failure to achieve desired flap elevation and/or long-term results is frequently a result of failure to fully release the arcus marginalis from the orbital rims.

6. If excessive skin has been excised with an open lifting procedure, a posterior subgaleal dissection can often facilitate closure while minimizing lagophthalmos.

7. Methods of fixation along the paramedian vector may include resorbable Endotines, bone tunnels, percutaneous screws, and cranial plates. Bone fixation is never placed within the midline in order to prevent inadvertent damage to the superior sagittal sinus.

8. Some surgeons prefer to place botulinum toxin 10–14 days prior to brow lifting procedures. Eighteen to twenty-four units of botulinum toxin deposited within the brow depressors will weaken the inferior pull of the depressors and promote maintenance of the new position of the brow during the immediate postoperative period.

References

Cilento, B.W. and Johnson, C.M., 2009. The case for open forehead rejuvenation: a review of 1004 procedures. *Archives of Facial and Plastic Surgery*, 11 (1), 13–17.

Cuzalina, A.L. and Holmes, J.D., 2005. A simple and reliable landmark for identification of the supraorbital nerve in surgery of the forehead: an in vivo anatomical study. *Journal of Oral and Maxillofacial Surgery*, 63 (1), 25–7.

Javidnia, H. and Sykes, J., 2013. Endoscopic brow lifts: have they replaced coronal lifts? *Facial Plastic Surgery Clinics of North America*, 21 (2), 191–9.

Johnson, C.M. and Alsarraf, R., 2002. *The aging face: a systematic approach*. Philadelphia: Saunders.

Puig, C.M. and LaFerriere, K.A., 2002. A retrospective comparison of open and endoscopic brow-lifts. *Archives of Facial and Plastic Surgery*, 4 (4), 221–5.

Terella, A.M. and Wang, T.D., 2013. Technical considerations in endoscopic brow lift. *Clinics in Plastic Surgery*, 40, 105–15.

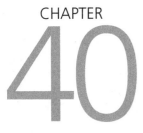

CHAPTER

40 Rhytidectomy

Jennifer Elizabeth Woerner and Ghali E. Ghali

Department of Oral and Maxillofacial Surgery, Louisiana State University Health Sciences Center, Shreveport, Louisiana, USA

A procedure used to correct changes of the lower face and neck caused by the gravitational forces of physiologic aging.

Indications

1. Moderate to severe cervicofacial skin laxity
2. Jowling
3. Platysmal banding

Contraindications

1. Poorly controlled medical conditions
2. Patients seeking surgery due to psychological motivation or with unrealistic expectations
3. Uncontrolled mental illness or body dysmorphic disorder
4. Cigarette smoking, alcoholism, and illicit drug use are relative contraindications

Anatomy

Great auricular nerve: With the head turned 45°, the greater auricular nerve can be identified as it crosses the sternocleidomastoid (SCM) muscle 6.5 cm below the bony external auditory meatus (Erb's point). The greater auricular nerve provides sensation to a portion of the cheek and earlobe. Along with the external jugular vein, this nerve remains deep to the superficial musculoaponeurotic system (SMAS). The greater auricular nerve is the most commonly injured nerve during a facelift procedure.

Superficial musculoaponeurotic system (SMAS): Fibromuscular layer between the subcutaneous tissue and the parotid-masseteric fascia. The facial nerve runs deep to this layer. The SMAS transfers the forces of the muscles of facial expression to the overlying skin through septal connections. It is continuous with the frontalis and galea superiorly and the platysma inferiorly.

McGregor's patch: The area overlying the malar eminence of ligamentous attachments between the periosteum and the dermis. Dissection in this region is difficult, and bleeding may be encountered due to its high vascularity.

Mesotemporalis: Contains the superficial temporal artery and the frontal branch of the facial nerve. It marks the transition from the sub-SMAS dissection to the subcutaneous dissection.

Superficial (supra-SMAS) Rhytidectomy Technique

1. Proposed incision lines and anticipated areas of undermining are marked while the patient is seated in an upright position prior to anesthesia (Figures 40.3 and 40.4 [all figures cited in this chapter appear in Case Report 40.1]).
2. The procedure may be performed with intravenous sedation or with laryngeal mask airway (LMA) or oral endotracheal general anesthesia.
3. After induction of anesthesia, the patient is placed supine on the operating room table; the hair, face, and neck are treated with surgical prep; and the patient is draped in a sterile fashion.
4. Local anesthetic is administered along the proposed incision lines with 2% lidocaine solution with 1:100,000 epinephrine.
5. A #11 blade is used to create bilateral temporal (Figure 40.5), infralobular (Figure 40.6) and mastoid (Figure 40.7) trochar incisions and a single, midline submental (Figure 40.8) trochar incision. Tumescent solution (a mixture of 20 mL of 2% lidocaine with 1:100,000 epinephrine solution with 180 mL of normal saline, creating a solution of 0.2% lidocaine with a 1:1,000,000 epinephrine concentration) is used to hydrodissect through the trocar sites within the supra-SMAS plane 1 cm beyond the planned area of dissection. 75 mL of tumescent solution should be placed on each side, and 50 mL should be deposited within the submental region. The tumescent solution should be allowed at least 10 minutes to take effect before further dissection is carried out. The contralateral side should not be infiltrated until just prior to closure of the first side.
6. Blunt cannula dissection is performed through the trocar sites without suction to bluntly dissect the cervicofacial supra-SMAS rhytidectomy flap. A 5 mm incision is made just posterior to the submental crease for open liposuction. Open liposuction is performed within the supraplatysmal plane with a 3 mm blunt cannula facing the platysma (Figure 40.9). The liposuction is performed inferiorly to the superior aspect of the thyroid cartilage and laterally to the anterior border of the SCMs. Care is taken to leave a uniform layer of fat against the skin to prevent developing an

Atlas of Operative Oral and Maxillofacial Surgery, First Edition. Edited by Christopher J. Haggerty and Robert M. Laughlin
© 2015 John Wiley & Sons, Inc. Published 2015 by John Wiley & Sons, Inc.

unnatural atrophic appearance of the neck (cobra deformity).

7. If a neck lift is indicated, a 2 cm long transverse incision (Figure 40.10) is placed within the submental skin 1-2 mm posterior to the dominant (submental) crease. Do not place this incision within the dominant crease, or upon healing it may create a "double-chinned" deformity.

8. The cervical dissection is initiated within the subcutaneous plane. The medial borders of the platysma muscle are identified and released along their deep surface to the level of the thyroid cartilage to allow for sufficient mobilization (Figure 40.11).

9. The medial borders of the platysma muscle are plicated using a 2-0 slowly resorbing suture from the level of the thyroid cartilage as far superiorly as possible. Partial myotomy of the inferior aspect of the muscles may be needed for adequate mobilization and relief of tension at the anterior surface of the neck. A diamond-shaped portion of the midline platysma muscle may be removed and reapproximated with 3-0 Mersilene sutures.

10. The rhytidectomy incision is initiated along the conchal bowl cartilage on the posterior surface of the ear. The incision rises superiorly onto the back of the conchal bowl (Figure 40.12) approximately 3 mm until reaching the level of the postauricular sulcus. The incision courses posteroinferiorly approximately 4 to 5 cm into the scalp of the retromastoid region.

11. In the pre-auricular region, the incision follows the natural curvature of the inferior ear lobule and is curved inferiorly 2 mm below the junction of the lobule with the cheek. The incision courses superiorly just above the base of the incisura intertragica, following the margin of the tragus and staying anterior to the curve of the crus helicis (Figure 40.13). The temporal incisions are placed at least 2 cm posterior to and parallel to the hairline (Figure 40.14).

12. Considerations for incision design in male patients:

    a. Modification of incision design in the temporal area must be considered in those with thinning hair, temporal recession, or significant male pattern baldness.

    b. When assessing the pre-auricular region, the incision should extend in a linear fashion, following a natural skin crease adjacent, parallel, and anterior to the sideburn in order to leave the non-hair-bearing area anterior to the ear intact.

    c. Place the posterior extension of the incision along the postauricular hairline. This will prevent a step deformity or posterior displacement of the hairline.

13. Flap elevation begins by undermining 1 cm along the entire length of the rhytidectomy incision (Figure 40.15) using blunt-tipped scissors (face-lift scissors) in a push-cutting motion (Figure 40.16). The appropriate level of dissection is within the subdermal plane, leaving approximately 4 mm of subcutaneous fat on the underside of the flap. Rees T-clamps are placed along the flap edges for countertraction. In the temporal region, the dissection is carried through the temporoparietal fascia (subgaleal) down to the loose areolar tissue overlying the deep temporal fascia. Dissection within this plane creates a thicker flap, preserving hair follicles and therefore preventing alopecia. The dissection is continued across the cheek within the subcutaneous plane. This transition from the sub-SMAS to the subcutaneous plane marks the mesotemporalis. The dissection is carried superiorly to the level of the lateral canthus and within 1 cm of the oral commissure. When a neck lift is also planned, the dissection is carried inferiorly to the level of the thyroid cartilage bilaterally. Below the earlobe, it is important to stay within the subcutaneous plane in order to protect the great auricular nerve and external jugular vein.

14. Hemostasis is obtained with the use of bipolar cautery (Figure 40.17). Avoid excessive use of cautery to minimize the potential for damage to the facial nerve and necrosis of the skin flap.

15. Once the rhytidectomy flap is fully elevated, SMAS plication is performed (Figure 40.18). The SMAS is plicated in a bidirectional fashion, independent of the skin flap. SMAS plication is initiated by placing two key sutures utilizing a 2-0 slowly resorbing suture on a tapered needle. The first suture extends from the fascia overlying the angle of the mandible to the fascia immediately inferior to the tragus. The second suture extends from the fascia lateral to the oral commissure to the fascia immediately superior to the tragus. Additional sutures can be placed if additional stabilization or vectors of pull are required. All knots should be buried.

16. Once SMAS plication is completed, excessive skin is trimmed from the posterior aspect of the rhytidectomy incision. The patient's head is placed within a neutral position, and the rhytidectomy flap is redraped (Figure 40.19) in a posterior-superior direction. Key suspension sutures or staples (anchor points) are placed (Figure 40.20). The root of the helix is the first anchor point; once this anchor point is secured, excessive temporal hair tuft skin is removed above this anchor point. The second anchor point is at the level of the tragus. Care is taken to not remove excessive skin anterior to the tragus. Excessive skin removal will prevent obtaining a tension-free closure and may result in the development of a wide, visible scar that will pull the tragus anteriorly. Anchor point 3 is the most posterior and superior aspect of the flap within the postauricular area. The long axis of the earlobe should be inset 10–15° posterior to the long axis of the ear proper (Figure 40.21).

17. After securing the anchor points, excessive skin is trimmed with a blade or sharp scissor. Closure begins in the hair-bearing areas with subdermal 3-0 resorbable sutures and staples to approximate the scalp. The postauricular region is closed with a 4-0 plain gut suture, without the need for deep sutures. The pre-auricular region is closed with subdermal 4-0 resorbable sutures, and the skin edges are reapproximated with 6-0 or 7-0 nylon running sutures. If a neck lift was performed, the submental incision is closed following both sides of the facelift. The subdermal layer is closed with 4-0 resorbable sutures, and the skin is closed with 6-0 nylon sutures.

18. Drains are rarely needed. Prior to extubation, the face and hair are gently cleansed with antiseptic soap, triple antibiotic ointment is applied to all incisions, and fluff pads are placed within the submental, pre-auricular, and postauricular regions. The entire face is gently wrapped with an elastic bandage, while placing the ears in the appropriate position underneath the dressing. Avoid excessive tightness of the bandage to prevent ischemia of the flaps.

Postoperative Management

1. Ice is applied for the first 72 hours.
2. Patients are asked to sleep with head-of-bed elevation for the first several days.
3. Patients are seen at postoperative day 1. The patients are evaluated for hematoma formation and flap discoloration, all wounds are cleaned, and a layer of antibiotic ointment is reapplied.
4. Patients are allowed to wash their hair on postoperative day 3.
5. Patients wear their facial pressure dressing for 3–4 days and then at night only for one week.

Complications

Early Complications

1. **Hematoma formation**: Typically occurs early within the postoperative period. An expanding hematoma is considered an emergency and should be evacuated immediately with control of bleeding to prevent compression of the dermal plexus and necrosis of the skin flap. Small hematomas may be treated by needle aspiration and compression.
2. **Seroma formation**: Can be treated with needle aspiration; frequently requires several treatments until complete resolution.
3. **Facial nerve injury**: The marginal mandibular branch is the most commonly injured facial nerve during supra-SMAS rhytidectomy. The frontal branch may also be injured if the dissection is carried over the zygomatic arch. Most facial nerve injuries are temporary, with return of facial animation within 3 to 6 months.
4. **Great auricular nerve injury**: The subcutaneous layer is very thin within the region of the mastoid, and the dermis is in close contact with the sternocleidomastoid muscles. Because of this, it is possible to damage the greater auricular nerve as it courses over the sternocleidomastoid muscle, causing numbness of the skin overlying the earlobe, the postauricular region, and the mastoid process.

Late Complications

1. **Flap necrosis or wound dehiscence**: Necrosis of the skin or breakdown of the incisions typically results from aggressive cauterization of the underside of the flap, hematoma formation, developing a thin flap that does not preserve the subdermal plexus, excessive tension on the wounds during closure, and applying a postoperative bandage that is too tight. Smokers are at increased risk for poor wound healing and flap necrosis.
2. **Hypertrophic scarring**: Treated with later re-excision and closure, steroid injections, and/or CO_2 laser resurfacing.

Key Points

1. Proper patient selection and treatment planning are imperative. It is not enough to only evaluate a patient's facial features; overall health and psychological stability must also be determined. Documenting the patient's preoperative condition with photos; discussing the procedure in detail with the patient, including what to expect within the postoperative period; and obtaining a detailed informed consent are necessary prior to any procedure.
2. Patients with severe actinic damage or elastosis do not achieve the same results as patients with only signs of physiologic aging alone.
3. Patients who are smokers must be informed that nicotine use increases the risk of poor wound healing and skin slough. A more conservative undermining may be warranted. Smokers should be counseled on smoking cessation for at least 2 weeks, and preferably 1 month, prior to surgery.
4. Platysma plication procedures, with or without myotomy, are aimed at lessening platysma banding, elevating the neck, and redefining the cervicomental angle.
5. In SMAS plication, the SMAS is folded upon itself and sutured into position. In SMAS imbrication, the SMAS is incised or excised so that the distal portion is repositioned to overlap the proximal tissue and then secured with sutures.

Case Report 40.1. A 59-year-old female presents with complaints of "sagging skin around her face, jowls, neck, and eyelids." Clinical examination demonstrated jowling, redundancy and sagging of facial skin, poor cervicomental angle, and the accumulation of submental fat (Figures 40.1 and 40.2). The patient also exhibits blepharptosis and dermatochalasis. The patient will be treated with a superficial plane (supra-SMAS) rhytidectomy and cervical (neck) lift with SMAS and platysmal plication with simultaneous upper lid blepharoplasty. (See Figures 40.1 through 40.23.)

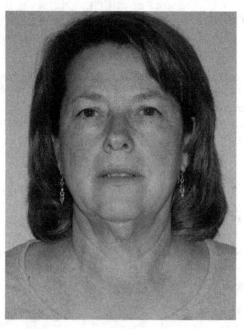

Figure 40.1.   Frontal preoperative photograph demonstrating jowling, moderate cervical skin laxity, and midface changes associated with aging.

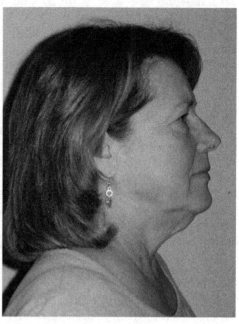

Figure 40.2.   Lateral preoperative photograph demonstrating an obtuse cervicomental angle, submental fat accumulation, jowling, and redundant and sagging skin.

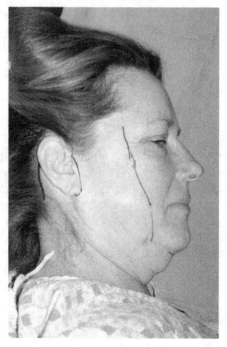

Figure 40.3.   Preoperative marking are made with the patient in an upright position and include the sites of the proposed skin incisions and the extent of the supra-SMAS dissection.

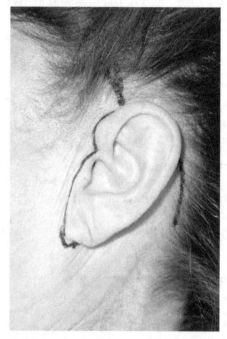

Figure 40.4.   Proposed pre- and postauricular incisions with temporal extension are marked.

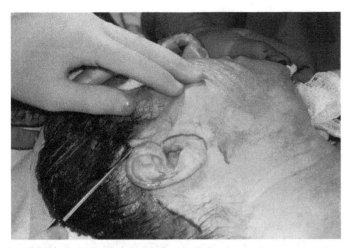

Figure 40.5. The temporal trocar site.

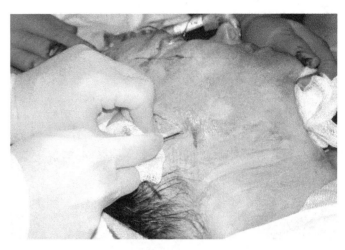

Figure 40.6. The infralobular trocar site.

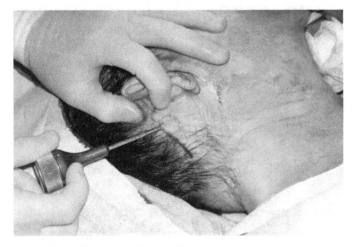

Figure 40.7. The mastoid trocar site.

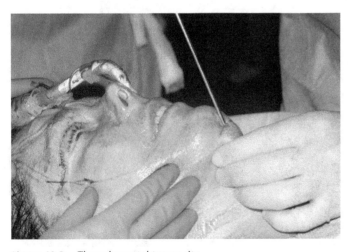

Figure 40.8. The submental trocar site.

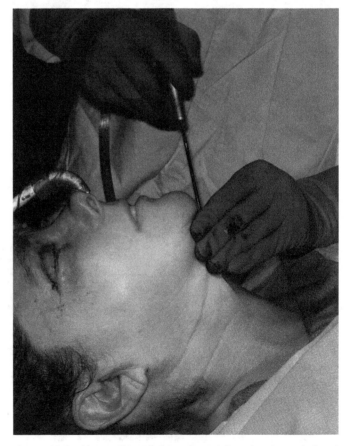

Figure 40.9. Liposuction of the submental region is carried out within a supraplatysmal plane with the opening on the cannula facing away from the skin (towards the platysma muscle).

351

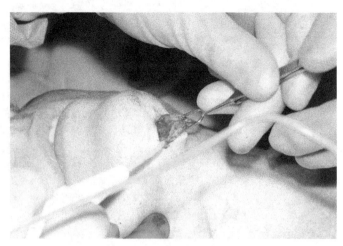

Figure 40.10.   A 2 cm incision is placed just posterior to the submental fold.

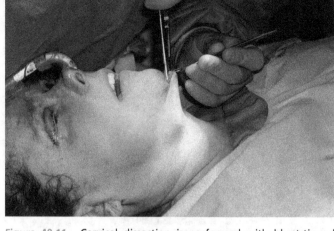

Figure 40.11.   Cervical dissection is performed with blunt-tipped scissors within the subcutaneous plane. The platysma muscles are identified along their medial border and dissected along their deep surfaces to the level of the thyroid cartilage.

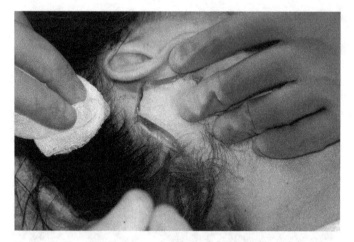

Figure 40.12.   The rhytidectomy incision is directed posteriorly along the back of the conchal bowl until reaching the postauricular sulcus. The incision is then directed posterior-inferiorly approximately 4 to 5 cm into the retromastoid region along the hairline.

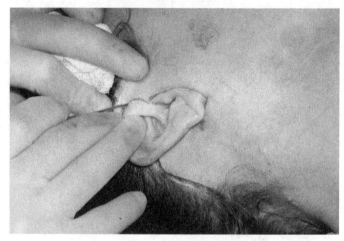

Figure 40.13.   In the pre-auricular region, the incision is made just above the base of the incisura intertragica, following the margin of the tragus and staying anterior to the curve of the crus helicis.

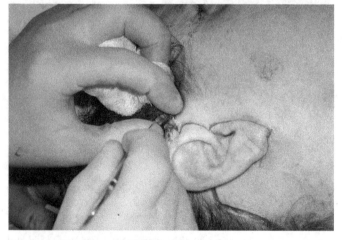

Figure 40.14.   The temporal incision is placed at least 2 cm posterior to and parallel to the hairline.

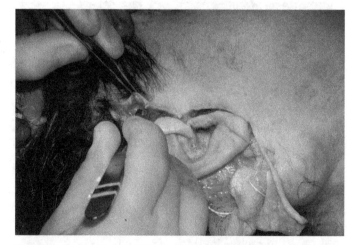

Figure 40.15.   The facial flap is developed by undermining 1 cm along the entire length of the incision. Approximately 4 mm of subcutaneous fat is preserved along the undersurface of the facial flap.

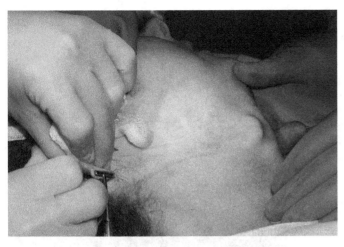

Figure 40.16.   Blunt-tip scissors (facelift scissors) are used in a push-cutting motion within the subdermal plane. This is aided by counter-traction with Rees T-clamps.

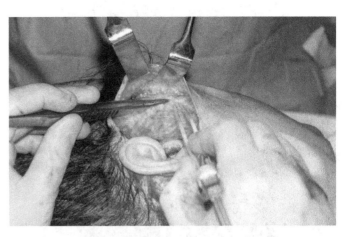

Figure 40.17.   Once flap development is complete, hemostasis is achieved with bipolar electrocautery.

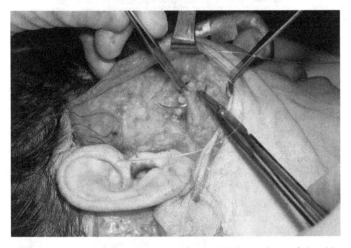

Figure 40.18.   SMAS plication is performed independent of the skin flap.

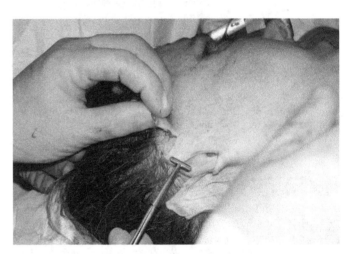

Figure 40.19.   The skin is redraped in a posterior-superior direction.

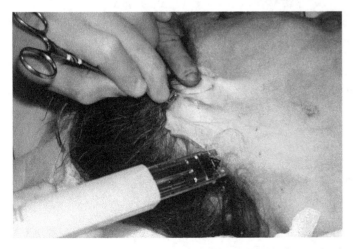

Figure 40.20.   Key suspension sutures or staples (anchor points) are placed prior to trimming excessive skin from the rhytidectomy flap.

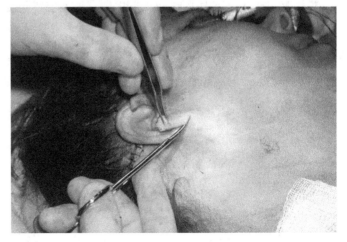

Figure 40.21.   The long axis of the earlobe is inset 10–15° posterior to the long axis of the ear proper, and the excess skin is trimmed with sharp scissors.

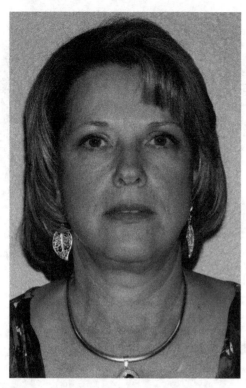

Figure 40.22. Frontal view of the patient 3 months post surgery with correction of redundant and sagging skin and redefining of the mid- and lower face anatomy.

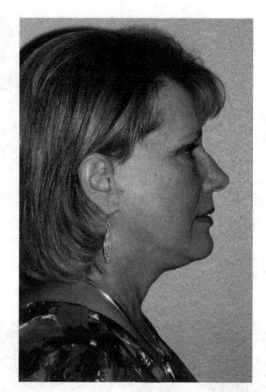

Figure 40.23. Lateral postoperative view demonstrating a less obtuse cervicomental angle, more defined lower third of the face, and correction of jowling, submental fat accumulation, and skin laxity or redundancy.

References

Baker, D.C. and Conley, J., 1979. Avoiding facial nerve injuries in rhytidectomy: anatomical variation and pitfalls. *Plastic and Reconstructive Surgery*, 64, 781–95.

Baker, T.J. and Gordon, H.L., 1969. Rhytidectomy in males. *Plastic and Reconstructive Surgery*, 44, 219–22.

Ghali, G.E. and Banker, A.R., 2012. Rhytidectomy. In: M. Miloro, G.E. Ghali, P. Larsen and P. Waite, eds. *Peterson's oral and maxillofacial surgery*. 3rd ed. Shelton, CT: People's Medical Publishing House; Ch. 67.

Ghali, G.E. and Smith, B.R., 1998. A case for superficial rhytidectomy. *Journal of Oral and Maxillofacial Surgery*, 56, 349–51.

McKinney, P. and Gottlieb, J., 1985. The relationship of the great auricular nerve to the superficial musculoaponeurotic system. *Annals of Plastic Surgery*, 14, 310–4.

Webster, R., Smith, R. and Hall, B., 1984. Facelift—better results with safer surgery of the head and neck. In: P. Ward and W. Berman, eds. *Plastic and reconstructive surgery of the head and neck*. St. Louis, MO: CV Mosby; pp. 321–3.

41

Upper and Lower Lid Blepharoplasty and Tear Trough Implants

Dustin M. Heringer[1] and L. Angelo Cuzalina[2]
[1]*Department of Ophthalmology, University of Arizona, Tucson, Arizona, USA*
[2]*Cosmetic Surgery Fellowship Director, American Academy of Cosmetic Surgery, Tulsa, Oklahoma, USA*

Upper Lid Blepharoplasty Procedure

The excision of excess upper lid skin and/or fat for cosmetic or functional improvement.

Indications

1. Dermatochalasis
2. Psuedoherniation or prolapsing of central and medial orbital fat that is cosmetically troublesome to the patient
3. Upper lid ptosis
4. Asymmetries
5. Vision blocked by excess upper lid skin (lateral hooding). In order to qualify for a functional procedure, loss of the visual field must be documented with visual field testing and photographs

Contraindications

1. **Blepharoptosis**: Blepharoptosis will not be corrected with blepharoplasty alone and requires identification prior to surgery. Blepharoptosis and lid malposition should be addressed prior to, or concurrently, with blepharoplasty to minimize postoperative complications.
2. **Eyebrow ptosis**: Eyebrow ptosis is frequently the patient's chief complaint, and should be recognized and treated with a brow lift instead of upper blepharoplasty.
3. **Active thyroid disease**: Patient's with active thyroid eye disease should avoid cosmetic upper and lower lid blepharoplasty until their disease has been stable for 12 months.
4. **Refractive eye surgery**: upper and lower lid blepharoplasty should be avoided in patients who have undergone lamellar refractive surgery within the previous 6 months or surface ablative refractive surgery within the previous 3 months.
5. **Severe dry eye syndrome (relative contraindication)**: An upper lid blepharoplasty may exacerbate the condition, especially if postoperative lagophthalmos is present. It is important to obtain a detailed ophthalmic history with attention to eye drop and ointment usage. Basal tear secretion testing (Schirmer testing) can be helpful, but the results of this test are sometimes unpredictable.
6. **Lack of orbicularis oculi strength and/or absent Bell's phenomenon (relative contraindications)**: Both increase the incidence of postoperative corneal trauma.

Anatomy and Definitions: Upper Lid

Dermatochalasis: Excessive or redundant skin of the upper and lower eyelid. Often associated with excessive skin laxity as well.

Blepharoptosis: Ptosis of the upper eyelid resulting in a low-lying upper eyelid margin.

Lagophthalmos: The inability to completely close the eyelids.

Bell's phenomenon: The ability of the eyeball to move superiorly with eyelid closure. A protective reflex that aids in preventing corneal trauma, especially if postoperative lagophthalmos is present.

Marginal reflex distance (MRD): A means of identifying the position of the upper and lower lids in reference to the eye by measuring the distance of the upper and lower lid margin from the pupillary light reflex.

Margin reflex distance-1 (MRD1): The distance from the center of the pupillary light reflex and the upper eyelid margin with the eye in primary gaze. The normal range for MRD1 distance is 4–5 mm. An MRD1 of less than 4 mm may indicate blepharoptosis. An MRD1 of greater than 5 mm may indicate proptosis from hyperthyroidism.

Margin reflex distance-2 (MRD2): The distance from the center of the pupillary light reflex and the lower eyelid margin with the eye in primary gaze. The normal range for MRD2 distance is 5 mm. An MRD2 of greater than 5 mm may indicate lower lid retraction.

Layers of the upper eyelid superior to the tarsal plate (9–10 mm high centrally), from external to internal (Figure 41.1):

1. Skin
2. Orbicularis oculi
3. Orbital septum
4. Preaponeurotic fat
5. Levator palpebrae superioris
6. Müller's muscle
7. Conjunctiva.

Atlas of Operative Oral and Maxillofacial Surgery, First Edition. Edited by Christopher J. Haggerty and Robert M. Laughlin
© 2015 John Wiley & Sons, Inc. Published 2015 by John Wiley & Sons, Inc.

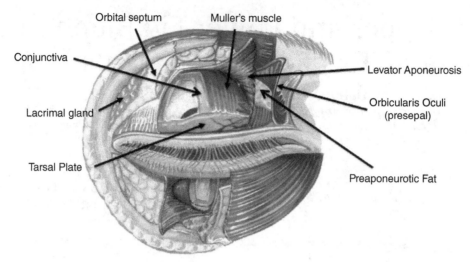

Figure 41.1.   Anatomy of the upper eyelid. Image by Randy Sappo.

Orbicularis oculi muscles: Innervated by the frontal (temporal) and zygomatic branches of the facial nerve located on the underside of the muscle. Functions to close the eyelid.

Orbital septum: A tough fibrous layer that lies anterior to the preaponeurotic fat and posterior to the orbicularis muscle. The orbital septum extends from the orbital rim to the tarsal plate and separates the eyelid from the orbit.

Preaponeurotic fat: Consists of fat pads that lie anterior to the levator aponeurosis and posterior to the orbital septum. The upper lid contains only two fat pads: a central and a medial fat pad. The central fat pad is more yellow in appearance, whereas the medial fat pad is whiter in appearance. There is no lateral fat pad. The lacrimal gland lies in the preaponeurotic space laterally and appears whitish-gray, glandular, and irregular.

Levator palpebrae superioris muscle: Innervated by the oculomotor nerve and is the primary muscle responsible for opening the eyelid. Fibrous extensions from the levator palpebrae superioris muscle pass through the orbicularis muscle to insert on the skin and help create the upper lid crease.

Müller's muscle: Innervated by sympathetic nerves and functions to involuntarily open the eyelid. Müller's muscle is located between the conjunctiva posteriorly and the levator muscle anteriorly. Originates on the inferior aspect of the levator palpebrae muscle and inserts onto the superior border of the tarsal plate.

Conjunctiva: A mucous membrane that lines the posterior surface of the eyelid (palpebral) and anterior eyeball (bulbar). The conjunctiva is composed of nonkeratinized squamous epithelium that contains goblet cells that protect and lubricate the eye.

Upper Blepharoplasty Preoperative Assessment and Markings

1. Prior to any upper and lower blepharoplasty procedure, a thorough history and physical should be performed that assesses and documents visual acuity, facial nerve function, asymmetries, dryness of the eyes, lagophthalmos, orbicularis oculi strength, and Bell's phenomenon. Preoperative photographs should be taken and should include frontal, three-quarter, and lateral views (Figures 41.2 through 41.7).

2. Preoperative markings are performed with the patient in a seated and upright position. The patient's natural upper lid skin crease is marked. The upper lid skin crease is typically 7–8 mm superior to the lid margin in males (Figure 41.8) and 8–10 mm superior to the lid margin in females. A pinch test is performed to define the upper extent of the excision. A pinch test is conducted by gently pinching the excess skin superior to the marked eyelid crease with blunt pickups until there is slight eversion of the upper lid eyelashes without lagophthalmos. The upper mark for the blepharoplasty incision is designed to maintain 10–15 mm of skin between the inferior brow hairs and the upper mark to prevent overresection. Therefore, the total amount of skin remaining from the lid margin to the inferior brow hairs is at least 20 mm. When marking laterally, make sure to extend the skin incision upward into one of the crow's feet starting at the lateral canthus to prevent the incision from extending too low.

Upper Lid Blepharoplasty Procedure

1. The procedure may be performed with local anesthesia alone, intravenous sedation, laryngeal mask airway (LMA), or endotracheal anesthesia.

2. After induction of anesthesia, the patient is placed supine, and 1 to 1.5 mL of local anesthetic containing epinephrine is injected just below the skin within the areas of excision in both upper lids with a 30-gauge needle.

3. The patient is prepped and draped in a sterile fashion.

4. The incision is initiated along the preoperative markings with a #15 blade, CO_2 laser, or needlepoint cautery. If using a CO_2 laser, make sure to place metallic eye shields prior to making an incision. The depth of the incision extends through the orbicularis muscle to the septum. You will observe a color change from pink to white when the septum is reached.

5. Remove the excess skin and orbicularis muscle with needlepoint cautery or scissors within the tissue plane just anterior to the septum (Figure 41.9).

6. If prolapsing pre-aponeurotic fat removal is required, needlepoint cautery is utilized to open the septum and to expose the central and medial fat pads. The medial fat pad is easily differentiated from the central fat pad due to its whiter appearance than the central fat pad. In the preaponeurotic space laterally, the lacrimal gland may prolapse and create fullness or a contour irregularity. A 6-0 polyglycolic acid suture (Vicryl) can be used to suspend and reposition the prolapsing gland to the medial aspect of the superolateral orbital rim periosteum.

7. If performing the procedure under local anesthesia alone, local anesthesia is injected into each fat pad prior to removal to minimize patient discomfort.

8. The herniated fat is gently teased out with a hemostat or forceps and excised with needlepoint cautery using the coagulation mode (Figure 41.10). Attempt to remove equal amounts of fat from each side for symmetry, unless an asymmetry was identified preoperatively.

9. If lower lid laxity or malposition is present, a canthopexy procedure can be performed through the upper lid incision to resuspend the lateral canthal tendon. Scissors are used to dissect down to the lateral canthal tendon posterior to the skin and orbicularis oculi muscle. Using forceps, the tendon is identified, and a 6-0 polyglycolic acid suture (Vicryl) is passed first through the tendon and then through the medial aspect of the superolateral orbital rim periosteum. The suture is tightened until the canthus has a pleasing appearance. The lateral canthus usually has a slight superior angle in females and is level with the medial canthus in males.

10. Skin closure is performed with a running 6-0 polypropylene (Prolene) or fast-absorbing gut suture. If the patient exhibits a poorly defined lid crease, fixation of the inferior skin edge to the levator aponeurosis at the superior aspect of the tarsal plate with a 6-0 polyglycolic acid suture (Vicryl) will help define the fold. One suture should be placed centrally with additional sutures placed at the medial and lateral limbus.

Complications

1. **Asymmetry**: Minimized with a thorough preoperative examination with eyelid measurements to identify preexisting conditions (i.e., blepharoptosis) and asymmetries, meticulous preoperative markings, and surgeon experience.

2. **Blepharoptosis**: Typically occurs secondary to postoperative edema and resolves within 2–4 weeks after surgery. Occasionally, prolonged edema can lead to attenuation of the levator palpebrae superioris muscle, resulting in a persistent blepharoptosis. Excessive tension during the surgical removal of upper eyelid skin can result in a dehiscence of the levator palpebrae superioris, causing ptosis. Blepharoptosis that persists for greater than 6 months after surgery usually requires surgery for correction.

3. **Lagophthalmos**: Frequently the result of the removal of excessive upper eyelid tissue. A good rule of thumb is to leave 20 mm of skin between the eyelid margin and the inferior brow hairs. In addition, incorporating the septum into the closure can cause adhesions and prevent adequate closure. Untreated or unrecognized lagophthalmos will lead to corneal exposure and dry eye. Mild cases of lagophthalmos are managed with lubricants and massage until the condition resolves. Severe cases are managed with skin grafting to the upper lids.

4. **Hematoma**: Typically result from bleeding of the orbicularis oculi muscle postoperatively. Small hematomas are observed and resolve without sequelae. Larger hematomas require evacuation to prevent fibrosis and scarring of the eyelid. Expanding hematomas require immediate surgical exploration with evacuation and control of the source of bleeding.

5. **Retrobulbar hematoma**: Minimized with appropriate use of cautery and wound hemostasis prior to the termination of the procedure. Posterior bleeding may result in a compartment syndrome, which places pressure on the blood supply to the retina and, if unrecognized or untreated, can lead to permanent vision loss. Signs and symptoms include severe ocular pain, proptosis, massive edema, limited or absent extraocular movement, elevated intraocular pressure, vision loss, and an unreactive pupil. Retrobulbar hematomas are a medical emergency and require immediate action to prevent permanent loss of vision. Initial treatment involves opening the surgical incision and attempting to visualize and evacuate the forming hematoma. If the evacuation of the hematoma though the incision site fails, a lateral canthotomy with cantholysis of the upper and lower limbs of the lateral canthal tendon is performed to increase the volume of the orbit. In rare cases, decompression of the bony orbit may be accomplished by pushing a hemostat through the medial wall and orbital floor. After decompression, an ophthalmology consult

is warranted to monitor vision and for serial intraocular pressure checks.

6. **Infection**: Rare due to the rich blood supply to the eyelids. Signs and symptoms of an eyelid infection include increased erythema, edema, pain, and purulent discharge from the surgical site. Infections are treated with the administration of broad-spectrum oral antibiotics. If an abscess is present, drainage of the abscess with culture and sensitivities is indicated.

7. **Corneal abrasion**: Present as pain and increased light sensitivity in the affected eye after surgery. Diagnosis may be made via symptoms alone or in conjunction with fluorescein drops and a cobalt blue light to visualize the abrasion and to confirm the diagnosis. Treatment consists of ophthalmic antibiotic ointment to the affected eye 4–6 times per day until symptoms resolve. Corneal abrasions typically heal in 24 to 48 hours depending on the size of the abrasion.

Key Points

1. Excessive fat pad removal is avoided to prevent creating an "A-frame" deformity or hollow appearance to the upper lid. Only fat that prolapses anterior to the septum with light pressure to the globe should be excised.

2. Always remove herniating fat with coagulation in order to cauterize small vessels traveling through the fat and to minimize postoperative bleeding and hematoma formation.

3. Avoid removing excess skin. The surgeon should leave approximately 20 mm of skin between the eyelid margin and lower brow hairs to avoid postoperative lagophthalmos.

4. Always evaluate the patient to see if he or she has brow ptosis and would benefit from a brow lift instead of, or in addition to, an upper lid blepharoplasty. Always perform the brow lift first to ensure the upper eyelid skin is not over-resected. Performing upper lid blepharoplasty in a patient with brow ptosis will further lower the position of the brow.

References

Gentile, R., 2005. Upper lid blepharoplasty. *Facial and Plastic Surgery Clinics of North America*, 13, 511–24.

Lelli, G.J. and Lisman, R.D., 2010. Blepharoplasty complications. *Plastic and Reconstructive Surgery*, 125, 1007–17.

Nerad, J., 2001. Clinical anatomy. In: J.Nerad, *Oculoplastic surgery: the requisites in ophthalmology*. St Louis, MO: Mosby; pp. 25–69.

Parikh, S. and Most, S., 2010. Rejuvenation of the upper eyelid. *Facial and Plastic Surgery Clinics of North America*, 18, 427–33.

Victoria, A.C., Chuck, R.S., Rosenberg, J. and Schwarcz, R.M., 2011. Timing of eyelid surgery in the setting of refractive surgery: preoperative and postoperative considerations. *Current Opinion in Ophthalmology*, 22, 226–32.

Case Reports

Case Report 41.1. A 50-year-old female presents with a chief complaint of always looking tired and that her upper lid skin was rubbing her eyelashes. On exam, the patient has significant upper lid dermatochalasis and lateral hooding. The patient has a secondary complaint of a large asymmetric nose with a dorsal hump. The patient was treated with upper lid blepharoplasty and open rhinoplasty. (See Figures 41.2 through 41.7.)

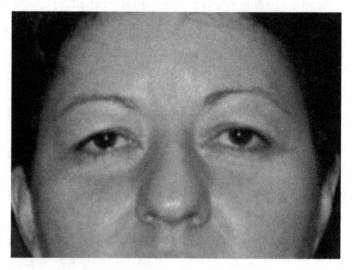

Figure 41.2. Frontal preoperative view depicting a tired and aged look to the eyes.

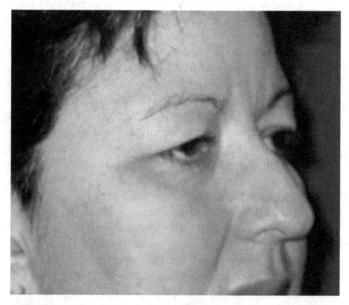

Figure 41.3. Three-quarters preoperative view depicting upper lid dermatochalasis, nasal asymmetry, and a dorsal nasal hump deformity.

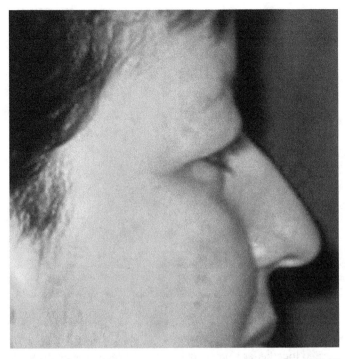

Figure 41.4.   Lateral preoperative view depicting lateral hooding of the upper, lateral quadrant of the upper lid.

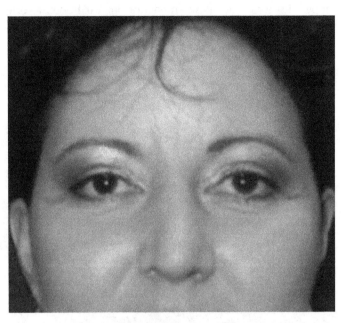

Figure 41.5.   Frontal postoperative view depicting a more youthful appearance of the eyes after correction of dermatochalasis with upper lid blepharoplasty.

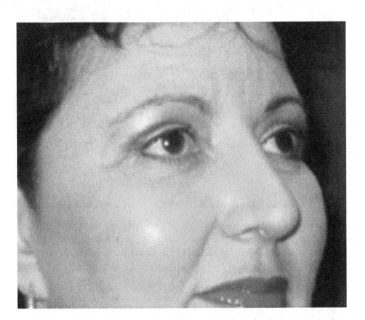

Figure 41.6.   Three-quarters postoperative view depicting correction of dermatochalasis, nasal asymmetries, and dorsal hump reduction.

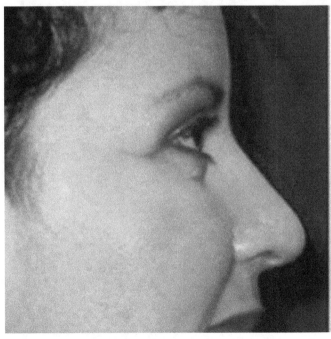

Figure 41.7.   Lateral postoperative view depicting correction of lateral hooding.

Case Report 41.2. A 52-year-old male presents with a chief complaint of tired-looking eyes. On exam, the patient has upper lid dermatochalasis, moderate lateral hooding, and prolapsing upper and lower fat pads. The patient was treated with upper and lower lid blepharoplasty with prolapsed fat pad reduction. (See Figures 41.8, 41.9, and 41.0.)

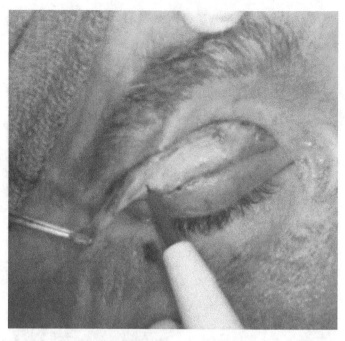

Figure 41.9. The skin and orbicularis muscle of the upper lid are excised together as a unit with needlepoint cautery. Note the white septum beneath the orbicularis muscle.

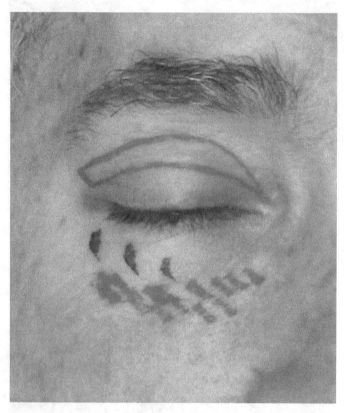

Figure 41.8. Preoperative markings for upper lid blepharoplasty are shown in red.

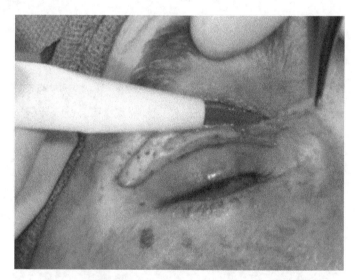

Figure 41.10. The medial fat pad is gently teased out from its capsule with forceps, and the prolapsing fat is removed with cautery to coagulate small perforating vessels within the fat pad. After fat removal is completed, the skin incision will be closed with a running suture.

Lower Lid Blepharoplasty Procedure

The excision of excess lower lid skin and/or prolapsing fat, often in combination with lid-tightening procedures, for cosmetic improvement. This procedure is often performed in conjunction with fat grafting, fat repositioning, or the placement of soft tissue filler or cheek implants to optimize results.

Indications

1. Dermatochalasis
2. Herniated or prolapsing fat that is cosmetically troublesome to the patient
3. Lower lid laxity
4. Asymmetries

Contraindications

1. A negative vector between the cornea and the inferior orbital rim is a relative contraindication because its correction requires additional procedures to minimize postoperative lid malposition
2. Malpositioned lower eyelids (ectropion, entropion, and lower lid retraction) are relative contraindications as they require additional procedures to correct the underlying pathology causing the malposition
3. Contraindications 3–6 of upper lid blepharoplasties

Anatomy and Definitions: Lower Lid

Ectropion: A condition where the lower lid is everted (turned outward) away from the globe, leaving the inner eyelid surface and cornea exposed and prone to irritation. Symptoms include excessive dryness, eyelid crusting, chronic epiphora, conjunctivitis, keratitis, pain, and ultimately a breakdown of the cornea.

Entropion: A condition where the lower lid is inverted (turned inward), allowing the inturned lashes to rub and damage the cornea. Symptoms include a feeling that something (i.e., foreign body) is within the eye, pain, chronic epiphora, sensitivity to wind, photophobia, eyelid crusting, and ultimately scarring of the cornea.

Malar edema: Fluid that collects over the malar eminence, inferior to the inferior orbital rim.

Malar mounds: Chronic soft tissue swellings or bulges located within the region of the malar eminence between the inferior orbital rim and the cheek. Differs from malar edema in that the bulges contain an excess of soft tissue, rather than edema.

Festoons: Cascading hammocks of lax skin and orbicularis muscle that hang between the medial and lateral canthi. Festoons may or may not contain herniated lower lid fat.

Layers of the lower eyelid inferior to the tarsal plate (4–6 mm high) from external to internal (Figure 41.11):

1. Skin
2. Orbicularis oculi
3. Orbital septum
4. Postseptal fat
5. Lower lid retractors
6. Conjunctiva.

Retroseptal lower lid fat pads: Consists of three fat pads (lateral, central, and medial) located posterior to the orbital septum and anterior to the lower lid retractors. Just as in the upper lid, the medial fat pad of the lower lid has a more whitish appearance than the more lateral fat pads. The inferior oblique muscle courses between the medial and central fat pads and should be protected during lower lid blepharoplasty.

Lower lid retractors: Includes the capsulopalpebral fascia and inferior tarsal muscle. The capsulopalpebral fascia is a band of fibrous tissue that originates

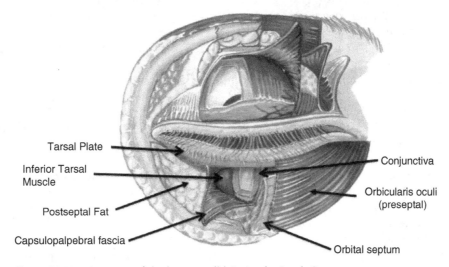

Figure 41.11. Anatomy of the lower eyelid. Image by Randy Sappo.

Labels: Tarsal Plate · Inferior Tarsal Muscle · Postseptal Fat · Capsulopalpebral fascia · Conjunctiva · Orbicularis oculi (preseptal) · Orbital septum

from the inferior rectus muscle, and as it travels anteriorly, it splits to surround the inferior oblique muscle and then ultimately inserts on the inferior border of the lower lid tarsal plate. The inferior tarsal muscle travels from Lockwood's ligament to the inferior border of the tarsal plate and is located posterior to the capsulopalpebral fascia and anterior to the conjunctiva.

Lateral canthal tendon: Attaches the eyelid to the lateral orbital rim. The pretarsal and preseptal orbicularis oculi muscles taper as they extend laterally to form the upper and lower limbs of the lateral canthal tendon. These limbs then join to form the lateral canthal tendon that inserts on Whitnall's tubercle. The lateral canthal tendon is normally 2–3 mm higher than the medial canthal tendon.

Transconjunctival Lower Lid Blepharoplasty Procedure

1. The procedure may be performed with local anesthesia alone, intravenous sedation, LMA, or endotracheal anesthesia.
2. After induction of anesthesia, the patient is positioned supine or with a slight reverse Trendelenburg position.
3. Topical anesthetic (i.e., tetracaine) is placed into each eye. 1.5 to 2 mL of local anesthetic containing epinephrine is injected into the palpebral conjunctiva and anteriorly within the eyelid.
4. Corneal shields are placed bilaterally, and the patient is prepped and draped in a sterile fashion.
5. The lower lid is everted with a Desmarres retractor, and needlepoint cautery is utilized to initiate an incision through the conjunctiva and lower lid retractors approximately 6–8 mm below the inferior border of the tarsal plate (Figure 41.16).
6. A hemostat or forceps are used to gently tease fat from the medial, central, and lateral fat pads (Figure 41.17). The herniated fat is removed with coagulation to cauterize small vessels within the fat pads. When removing fat, care is taken to ensure symmetry between sides and to avoid injury to the inferior oblique muscle located between the medial and central fat pads (Figure 41.18).
7. No closure of the conjunctiva is required.
8. Fractionated CO_2 laser resurfacing to the lower lids may be performed to tighten minor to moderate skin laxity and to improve fine lines and wrinkles (Figure 41.21). Two to three passes are conducted using the settings recommended by the manufacturer of the laser. If a fractionated CO_2 laser is unavailable, a 20–35% trichloroacetic acid (TCA) peel may be used.
9. Fat grafting to the tear trough and cheek is performed to smooth and improve the contours of the lid–cheek junction (Figures 41.19 and 41.20). Fat is typically harvested from the abdomen and placed within 1 mL or 10 mL Luer lock syringes with 0.9 mm × 5 cm blunt-tipped fat-grafting microcannulae. The fat is injected into the tear trough areas and cheeks using a microdroplet technique just anterior to the periosteum to a pleasing cosmetic endpoint. Typically, 5–10 mL of fat are placed within the tear trough areas and cheeks bilaterally.

Transcutaneous Lower Lid Blepharoplasty Procedure

1. A subciliary mark is placed 2 to 3 mm inferior to the lower lid eyelashes (Figure 41.22). The mark originates lateral to the puncta and extends toward the lateral canthus. The mark terminates 6 mm lateral to the lower lid within a natural rhytid.
2. Steps 1–4 of the transconjunctival lower lid blepharoplasty procedure.
3. A #15 blade, a CO_2 laser, or needlepoint cautery is used to initiate an incision along the subciliary mark.
4. A skin flap is developed, and the dissection proceeds inferiorly for 6–8 mm, preserving a rim of pretarsal orbicularis oculi muscle. This cuff of muscle will provide tone to the lower lid, minimizing lower lid retraction and ectropion postoperatively.
5. The dissection then extends through the muscle, and the orbital septum is identified (Figure 41.23). Dissection proceeds to the inferior orbital rim in a dissection plane just anterior (superficial) to the orbital septum.
6. If horizontal laxity is noted prior to surgery, a lateral canthopexy must be performed to support the lower lid (Figure 41.24). This is accomplished by passing a 5-0 polyglycolic acid suture (Vicryl) through the periosteum of the medial aspect of the lateral orbital rim and then through the lateral edge of the tarsal plate, and tightening the suture to the appropriate tension. It is helpful to perform this procedure before removing fat because additional fat will prolapse after the lower lid is tightened.
7. The orbital septum is opened with scissors or needlepoint cautery, and the medial, central, and lateral fat pads are identified.
8. If performing the procedure under local anesthesia alone, local anesthesia is injected into each fat pad prior to removal to minimize patient discomfort.
9. A hemostat or forceps are used to gently tease out fat from the medial, central, and lateral fat pads. The herniated fat is removed with coagulation to cauterize small vessels within the fat pads. When removing fat, care is taken to ensure symmetry between sides and to avoid injury to the inferior oblique muscle located between the medial and central fat pads.
10. In select cases, the surgeon will choose to redrape the fat over the inferior orbital rim to correct a tear

trough deformity. This is accomplished by dissecting inferior to the orbital rim in a preperiosteal plane with a Colorado needle to create a pocket within the area of the tear trough for 1.5 to 2 cm. Care must be taken to avoid injuring the infraorbital nerves. The fat from the medial and central fat pads can be teased out of their capsules, redraped over the inferior orbital rim, and sewn to the periosteum with 6-0 polyglycolic acid sutures (Vicryl) in a horizontal mattress fashion. The fat from the lateral fat pad is almost always excised and typically not redraped.

11. The lower lid skin is redraped in a tension-free manner, and the excess skin is excised at the lower lid margin.

12. If additional lateral support is required or if excessive skin was excised, an orbicularis sling can be performed. A 5-0 polyglycolic acid suture (Vicryl) is passed through the anterior aspect of the lateral orbital rim and then through the orbicularis muscle in the lateral aspect of the skin flap. The suture is tied in a manner that supports the flap in a more superior location. Frequently, the skin is dissected off of the underlying orbicularis muscle laterally for a short distance to assist in redraping.

13. The skin is closed with a running 6-0 plain gut suture.

Key Points

1. It is important to identify lower lid horizontal laxity and tone prior to lower lid blepharoplasty surgery. Lower lid horizontal laxity and tone can be assessed with the eyelid distraction test and eyelid snap test. The distraction test is performed by pulling the lower lid away from the eyeball and should measure less than 6 mm. The snap test is performed by pulling the lower lid inferiorly toward the inferior orbital rim and releasing it. The lower lid should snap back to its normal position without a blink. If the distraction test is greater than 7 mm or the lower lid fails the snap test, a canthopexy with or without an orbicularis sling procedure is required. These procedures will correct the laxity and support the lower lid to minimize the risk of lower lid retraction and ectropion. If the patient has significant lower lid laxity, a horizontal lid-shortening procedure with lateral canthoplasty may be required.

2. Avoid creating a hollowed look to the lower lid by resisting the urge to remove excessive fat. Only remove fat that herniates anterior to the orbital septum with light pressure on the globes. The lateral fat pad is more difficult to identify, and underresection often occurs with inexperienced surgeons. Underresection of the lateral fat pad will result in a contour deformity of the lateral lid and usually requires revision surgery.

3. With any blepharoplasty procedure (upper and lower), always err on the side of conservative skin excision to avoid lid retraction and lagophthalmos.

4. For patients with a deep nasojugal fold (i.e., tear trough), combine lower lid blepharoplasty procedures with fat grafting, soft tissue fillers, repositioning of the orbital fat, or tear trough implants to enhance the aesthetics of the volume-deficient regions.

5. Many patients have a negative vector to the lower face and are at much higher risk of lower lid retraction after a traditional transcutaneous lower lid blepharoplasty. Typically, the cornea lies parallel or slightly posterior to the orbital rim. In patients with a negative vector, the cornea is anterior to the inferior orbital rim. These individuals are at a higher risk for lower lid retraction after traditional transcutaneous lower lid blepharoplasty and need additional support to minimize this complication. Extra support can be provided by a canthopexy or canthoplasty in mild cases, or with a cheek lift and/or a cheek implant in more severe cases. A transconjunctival lower lid blepharoplasty reduces the risks associated with patients with a negative vector because the middle lamellae are not violated and no skin is removed.

6. The correction of lower lid malar mounds and festoons can be a challenging endeavor. Procedures typically involve combinations of skin–muscle flaps, direct excision, and midface lifts in combination with previously described techniques in this chapter.

Complications

Lower lid retraction and/or ectropion: Often results in lagophthalmos and inadequate protection of the cornea with resultant dry-eye symptoms. Minimized with conservative skin excision and repair of horizontal lid laxity during lower lid blepharoplasty. The incidence of lid retraction is much higher with a transcutaneous approach versus a transconjunctival approach. If lid retraction develops postoperatively, the patient is managed with aggressive lid massage and injections of a 50–50 mixture of 5 fluorouracil and triamcinolone (0.2–0.4 mL). Injecting a hyaluronic acid filler into the lower lid may help splint the lid up and prevent severe scar retraction. If conservative therapies fail, spacer grafts (i.e., ear cartilage or hard palate grafts) or skin grafts are indicated to repair lid retraction.

Chemosis: Occurs more commonly with lower lid blepharoplasty than upper lid blepharoplasty, and can cause persistent aggravation and discomfort in the postoperative period. Treatment consists of combinations of artificial tears, ophthalmic lubricating ointments, topical steroid drops (i.e., fluorometholone or prednisolone acetate), and/or an eye patch. For severe cases and/or cases that do not resolve after 7 days, a temporary tarsorrhaphy or conjunctivotomy should be performed.

Diplopia: Typically results from injury to the inferior oblique muscle or inferior rectus muscle. Intramuscular hemorrhage or edema may also cause transient extraocular muscle dysfunction, leading to diplopia. Diplopia should be followed closely, and a referral to an ophthalmologist is warranted for cases that do not resolve within 6–8 weeks. Patients with persistent diplopia (greater than 8 weeks) may require surgical exploration of the extraocular muscle and possible strabismus surgery.

Postoperative Management: Upper and Lower Lid Blepharoplasties

1. Cold compresses are applied to the lids for the first 48 to 72 hours after surgery.
2. Topical ophthalmic antibiotic ointment is applied to the incision four times a day for 5 days.
3. Have the patient monitor vision, and if any visual changes, proptosis, or increased pain occurs, the patient should contact the surgeon immediately.
4. Systemic antibiotics are typically not required.
5. Head-of-bed elevation is used for the first 24 hours to decrease postoperative edema.
6. Restricted physical activity with no heavy lifting (greater than 15 lbs.) the first week after surgery.
7. Avoid aspirin and nonsteroidal anti-inflammatory drugs in the immediate postoperative period.
8. Nonabsorbable sutures are removed at 7 days postoperatively.

References

Grant, J.R. and LaFerriere, K.A., 2010. Periocular rejuvenation: lower eyelid blepharoplasty with fat repositioning and the suborbicularis oculi fat. *Facial and Plastic Surgery Clinics of North America*, 18, 399–499.

Kpodzo, D.S., Nahai, F. and McCord, C.D., 2014. Malar mounds and festoons: review of the current management. *Aesthetic Surgery Journal*, 43, 235–48.

Lee, A.S. and Thomas, J.R., 2005. Lower lid blepharoplasty and canthal surgery. *Facial and Plastic Surgery Clinics of North America*, 13, 541–51.

Lelli, G.J. and Lisman, R.D., 2010. Blepharoplasty complications. *Plastic and Reconstructive Surgery*, 125, 1007–17.

Nassif, P.S., 2005. Lower blepharoplasty: transconjunctival fat repositioning. *Facial and Plastic Surgery Clinics of North America*, 13, 553–9.

Nerad, J., 2001. Clinical anatomy. In: J.Nerad, ed. *Oculoplastic surgery: the requisites in ophthalmology*. St Louis, MO: Mosby; pp. 25–69.

Pak, J. and Putterman, A.M., 2005. Revisional eyelid surgery: treatment of severe postblepharoplasty lower eyelid retraction. *Facial and Plastic Surgery Clinics of North America*, 13, 561–9.

Case Reports

Case Report 41.3. A 65-year-old male presents with a chief complaint of a decreased peripheral field of vision, bags under his eyes, and feeling as though his eyes make him appear old and tired. On exam, the patient has significant upper and lower lid dermatochalasis, steatoblepharon, horizontal lower lid laxity, and moderate festoons (Figures 41.12 and 41.13). The patient underwent simultaneous upper lid blepharoplasty and transconjunctival lower lid blepharoplasty with lateral canthopexies. (See also Figure 41.14 and 41.15.)

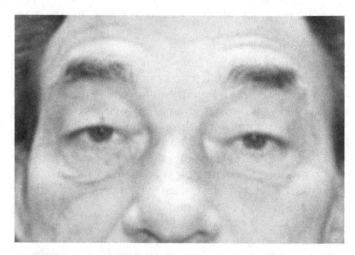

Figure 41.12. Frontal preoperative view depicting dermatochalasis, lid laxity, and lower lid festoons.

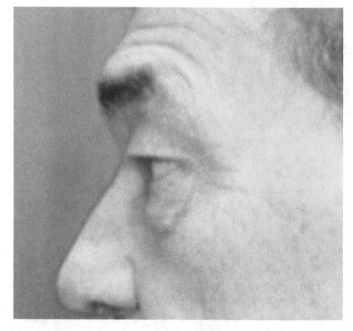

Figure 41.13. Lateral preoperative view depicting dermatochalasis, lateral hooding, and festoons.

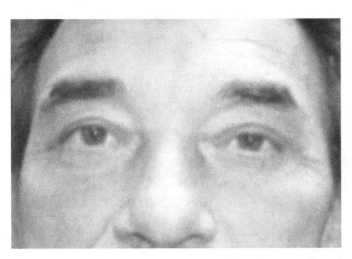

Figure 41.14. Frontal postoperative view depicting correction of dermatochalasis, lid laxity, and lower lid festoons.

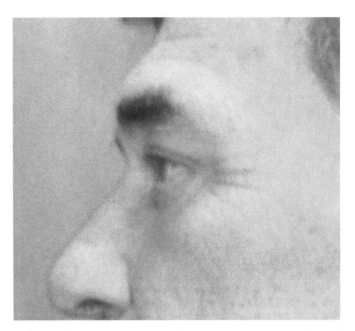

Figure 41.15. Lateral postoperative view depicting correction of lateral hooding, lower lid laxity, and festoons.

Case Report 41.4. A 48-year-old man presents with a chief complaint of always looking tired and having bags under his eyes. On exam, the patient has significant upper and lower lid dermatochalasis, bilateral horizontal lower lid laxity, and moderate loss of volume to the tear trough areas. The patient underwent upper lid blepharoplasty, transconjunctival lower lid blepharoplasty with removal of prolapsed lower lid fat and lateral canthopexies, fractionated CO_2 laser resurfacing of the lower lid skin, and autogenous fat grafting to the tear trough areas. (See Figures 41.16 through 41.21.)

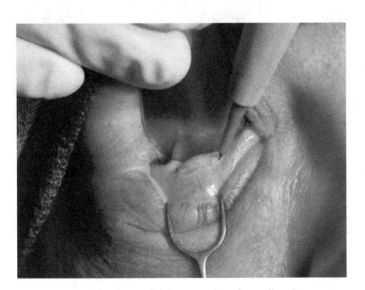

Figure 41.16. The lower lid is everted and needlepoint cautery is used to make an incision through the conjunctiva and lower lid retractors.

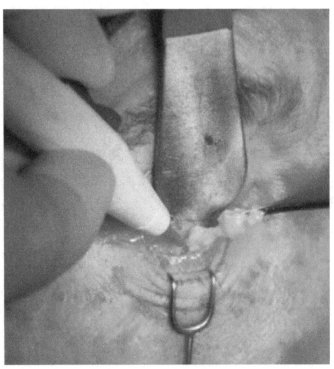

Figure 41.17. The medial, central, and lateral fat pads are identified. The fat pads are gently teased out of their surrounding capsules, and the prolapsing fat is removed with needlepoint cautery on coagulation mode.

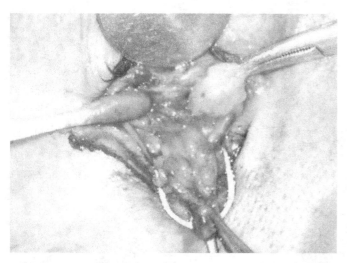

Figure 41.18.   The inferior oblique muscle is visualized during the lower lid blepharoplasty coursing between the medial and central fat pads. Care must be taken to avoid injuring this muscle during lower fat pad removal.

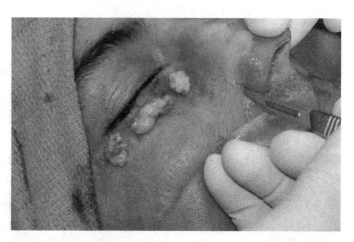

Figure 41.19.   Herniated fat is removed from the medial, central, and lateral fat pads. A small stab incision is made with an #11 blade in preparation for abdominal fat grafting to the tear trough area and cheek.

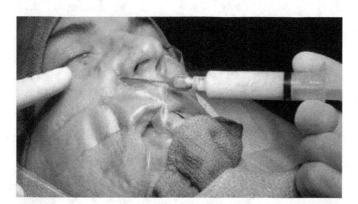

Figure 41.20.   Autogenous purified fat harvested from the abdomen is grafted to the areas of volume deficiency within the tear trough and cheek with a fat-grafting microcannula. This technique works well for patients with mild to moderate tear trough deformities.

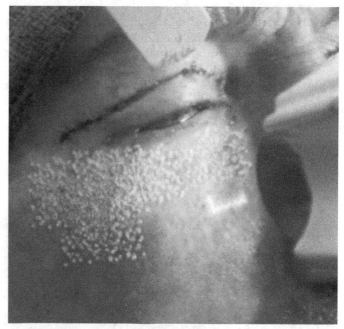

Figure 41.21.   Fractionated CO_2 laser resurfacing after a transconjunctival lower lid blepharoplasty is used to resurface and tighten the lower lid skin. Note the use of metal eye shields when using laser therapy.

Case Report 41.5. A 54-year-old female with a chief complaint of bags under her eyes and lower lid asymmetry. On exam, the patient has lower lid orbital fat herniation, mild asymmetry, and lower lid horizontal laxity. The patient underwent transcutaneous lower lid blepharoplasty with lateral canthopexy. (See Figures 41.22, 41.23, and 41.24.)

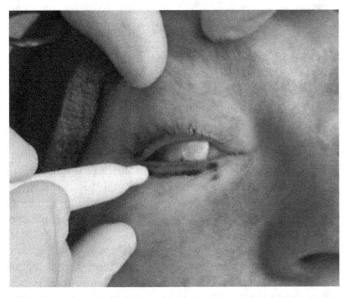

Figure 41.22. A subciliary mark is made 2 to 3 mm inferior to the lower lid eyelashes in preparation for the transcutaneous lower lid blepharoplasty. Laterally, the mark is extended into a rhytid within the area of the crow's feet.

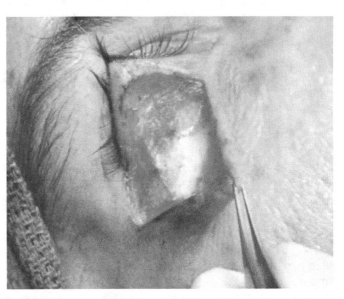

Figure 41.23. The dissection is initially preorbicularis for 6–8 mm and then changes to a preseptal dissection inferiorly. This change can be appreciated by the color change from pink to white. The yellow postseptal fat can also be seen behind the white septum centrally.

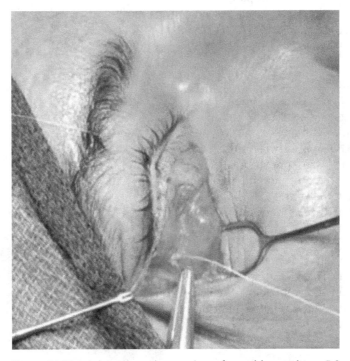

Figure 41.24. A lateral canthopexy is performed by passing a 5-0 polyglycolic acid (Vicryl) suture through the periosteum along the medial aspect of the lateral orbital rim and through the lateral aspect of the tarsal plate.

Tear Trough Implants

The placement of a silicone implant to correct a deep nasojugal fold or tear trough deformity.

Indications

1. A tear trough deformity (e.g., a deep nasojugal fold)
2. A negative vector that is caused by maxillary or zygomatic bone deficiency

Contraindications

1. Silicone sensitivity or allergy
2. Deep-set eyes or a patient with maxillary or zygomatic bone excess. In these patients, the implant will worsen the appearance of the patient's already deep-set eyes

Anatomy

The nasojugal fold is the medial fold that demarcates the lid–cheek junction and is also known as the tear trough. The malar fold is the lateral fold that demarcates the lid–cheek junction. These folds become more pronounced with aging as the malar fat pads descend, facial volume is lost, and septal laxity allows the orbital fat to prolapse anteriorly. These factors contribute to the contour changes of the lower lid with aging, resulting in a double convexity deformity.

Tissue layers in the lid–cheek junction from superficial to deep:

1. Skin
2. Subcutaneous tissue (location of malar fat pad)
3. Orbital portion of the orbicularis oculi (part of the superficial musculoaponeurotic system [SMAS])
4. Suborbicularis oculi fat (SOOF; invested by SMAS)
5. Periosteum.

Malar fat pad: Lies within the subcutaneous tissue plane. A triangular fat pad that gives fullness to the midface and is invested by the SMAS. The malar fat pad lies anterior to the orbicularis oculi muscle.

Suborbicularis oculi fat (SOOF): A fatty layer that rests anterior to the inferior orbital rim in a preperioteal plane. The SOOF is thickest lateral to the infraorbital foramen and envelops the zygomaticus major and minor muscles.

Arcus marginalis: The anatomical name for the location where the orbital septum, periorbita, and periosteum meet at the orbital rim.

Infraorbital nerve: A branch off of the maxillary division of the trigeminal nerve. The nerve exits its foramen within the maxillary bone 6–9 mm below the inferior orbital rim in a straight line extending inferiorly from the medial limbus in primary gaze. After exiting the foramen, the infraorbital nerve provides sensation for the lower eyelid, cheek, and upper lip.

Zygomaticofacial nerve: A branch off of the maxillary division of the trigeminal nerve. The nerve exits its foramen within the zygomatic bone and provides sensation to the malar region of the cheek. The zygomaticofacial nerve is often encountered during subperiosteal dissection for larger malar, submalar, or combined implants.

Transcutaneous Approach to the Placement of a Tear Trough Implant

1. Steps 1–5 of the transcutaneous lower lid blepharoplasty procedure.
2. The dissection is continued 4–6 mm inferior to the orbital rim within the SOOF, preserving a cuff of periosteum and the arcus marginalis.
3. A #15 blade or needlepoint cautery is used to incise the periosteum and a Freer elevator is used to create a subperiosteal pocket within the tear trough area.
4. The infraorbital nerve is identified, and a subperiosteal dissection is performed for 360° around the nerve.
5. The subperiosteal pocket is enlarged until the pocket is large enough to accomodate the tear trough implant.
6. The implant is soaked in Betadine solution prior to placement.
7. Using a #11 blade, a keyhole is created within the implant to accommodate the infraorbital nerve to prevent compression of the nerve (Figure 41.25).
8. The implant is positioned in its proper position within its subperiosteal pocket with the keyhole surrounding the infraorbital nerve.
9. Three 4-0 polyglycolic acid (Vicryl) sutures are used to secure the implant to the cuff of preserved periosteum to prevent migration or rotation of the implant. Alternatively, the implant can be secured with two or three 2 mm × 5 mm titanium screws (Figure 41.26). The secured implant should rest just below the inferior orbital rim to prevent a palpable or visual contour irregularity (Figure 41.27).
10. With the implant secured, additional procedures may be performed (i.e., a lateral canthopexy) if needed.
11. Perform the identical procedure on the opposite side, and then compare for symmetry.
12. The skin is closed with a running 6-0 fast-absorbing plain gut suture.

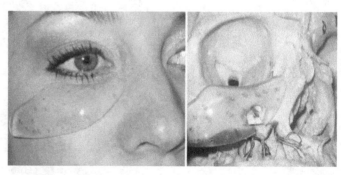

Figure 41.25. The location for the placement of a tear trough implant is shown. The silicone implant is trimmed during surgery to provide adequate space for the infraorbital nerve.

Transconjunctival Approach to Placement of a Tear Trough Implant

1. Steps 1–4 of the transconjunctival lower lid blepharoplasty procedure.
2. The lower lid is everted with a Desmarres retractor, and needlepoint cautery is utilized to initiate an incision through the conjunctiva and lower lid retractors approximately 2–3 mm below the inferior border of the tarsal plate from the lateral canthus to the puncta.
3. Inferior dissection proceeds within a plane between the orbicularis muscle and the orbital septum to the inferior orbital rim. This plane preserves the orbital septum and prevents orbital fat prolapse into the plane of dissection.
4. The dissection continues for 4–6 mm inferior to the orbital rim within the SOOF, preserving a cuff of periosteum and the arcus marginalis.
5. The periosteum is incised, and a subperiosteal pocket is created within the tear trough region.
6. Steps 4–11 of the transcutaneous approach to the placement of a tear trough implant are performed.
7. The conjunctiva is closed with a running 6-0 fast-absorbing plain gut suture.

Intraoral Approach to Placement of a Tear Trough Implant

1. The procedure may be performed with local anesthesia alone, intravenous sedation, LMA, or oral endotracheal anesthesia.
2. 2–4 mL of local anesthetic containing epinephrine is injected within the maxillary vestibule, the suborbital area just above the periosteum, and to block the infraorbital nerves bilaterally.
3. The patient is prepped and draped, and the oral cavity is prepped with Chlorohexidine Gluconate 0.12% oral rinse.
4. A 2–3 cm horizontal full-thickness mucoperiosteal incision is created above the canine, leaving a cuff of mucosa. A periosteal elevator is used to dissect within a subperiosteal tissue plane to expose the maxilla, infraorbital nerve, and inferior orbital rim. A pocket is made within the tear trough area large enough to encompass the desired implant.
5. Steps 4–11 of the transcutaneous approach to the placement of a tear trough implant are performed.
6. The intraoral incisions are closed with deep interrupted 3-0 polyglycolic acid sutures (Vicryl), and the mucosa is reapproximated with a continuous 3-0 chromic suture.

Complications

Infection: Typically presents as a subperiosteal abscess. Treatment incudes drainage of the abscess, culture and sensitivities of purulence, and removal of the implant. Broad-spectrum antibiotics are initiated until culture and sensitivity results return.

Migration or rotation of the implant: Results in contour changes to the implant site. Minimized with securing the implant with 2–3 screws or deep sutures. Treatment involves revision surgery to reposition and resecure the implant.

Asymmetry: Frequently the result of a poorly positioned implant. Treatment involves revision surgery to reposition the implant, reshape the implant, or place a differently shaped implant.

Paresthesia: Due to stretching of the infraorbital nerve during implant placement or dissection. Most cases are transient and resolve over time.

Key Points

1. The implant should be secured with screws or sutures to prevent postoperative migration.
2. An alternative to implant placement in patients with mild to moderate tear trough deformities is autogenous fat grafting. Advantages of autogenous fat grafting include a technically simpler procedure and minimal morbidity. Disadvantages of autogenous fat grafting include the variability in fat survival from patient to patient and the occasional need for a second fat-grafting session or the addition of further filler.
3. In patients with a significant negative vector, the authors' preferred method for treatment is with a malar or a combined malar-submalar implant in combination with fat grafting. A tear trough implant alone often does not provide sufficient volume within the entire cheek to adequately correct the deficiency.

References

Flowers, R.S., 2006. Correcting suborbital malar hypoplasia and related boney deficiencies. *Aesthetic Surgery Journal*, 26, 341–55.

McCord, C.D. Jr. and Codner, M.A., 2008. Classical surgical eyelid anatomy. In: C.D.McCord Jr. and M.A.Codner, eds. *Eyelid and periorbital surgery*. St Louis, MO: Quality Medical Publishing; pp. 23–7.

Terino, E.O. and Edwards, M.C., 2008. Alloplastic contouring for suborbital, maxillary, zygomatic deficiencies. *Facial and Plastic Surgery Clinics of North America*, 16, 33–67.

Case Report 41.6. A 55-year-old male presents with a chief complaint of aged eyes, specifically excessive skin to his upper lids and a loss of volume to the areas under his eyes. On exam, the patient demonstrated dermatochalasis, lateral hooding, and bilateral volume deficiency to the tear trough areas and along the inferior orbital rims. The patient underwent simultaneous upper lid blepharoplasty and the placement of large tear trough implants bilaterally. (See Figures 41.26 and 41.27.)

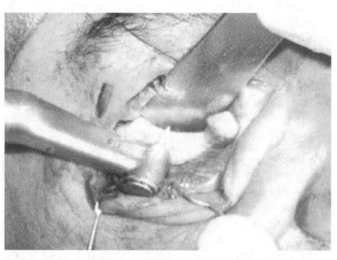

Figure 41.26. The tear trough area is accessed via a subciliary transcutaneous lower lid blepharoplasty approach. After reaching the orbital rim, a subperiosteal pocket is created in preparation for the tear trough implant. A hand piece is used to create osteotomies for fixation of the implant.

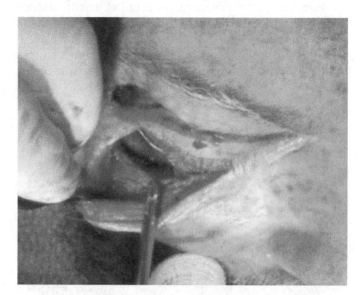

Figure 41.27. The tear trough implant is secured within the subperiosteal pocket with at least two screws to prevent rotation and/or migration of the implant. After fixation, the implant should rest just below the inferior orbital rim to prevent a palpable or visual contour irregularity.

Rhinoplasty

Jon D. Perenack and Shahrouz Zarrabi
Department of Oral and Maxillofacial Surgery, Louisiana State University Health Sciences Center, New Orleans, Louisiana, USA

Procedures aimed at improving the form and/or function of the nose and associated structures.

Indications

Correction of Functional Nasal Deformities

1. **Septal deformity**: deviated nasal septum, bone spurs, and internal and external nasal valve deformities
2. **Intranasal abnormalities**: turbinate hypertrophy, septal perforations, synechiae, and intranasal pathology

Correction of Aesthetic Deformities as a Result of Congenital and Acquired (Trauma) Deformities

1. **Upper nose deformities**: high or low dorsal hump, lateral dorsal hump, elongated nose, thin or broad nasal dorsum, and nasal deviations
2. **Lower nose deformities**: poorly defined nasal tip, nasal tip deviation, over- or underprojection of the nasal tip, large or asymmetrical nostrils, and excessive columella show
3. **Posttraumatic deformities**: crooked nose and saddle nose deformities
4. **Revision rhinoplasty**: undesired cosmetic result from prior rhinoplasty

Contraindications

1. Uncontrolled systemic illness
2. Large septal perforations
3. Unstable nasal support structures secondary to trauma
4. Multiply operated rhinoplasty patient with a scarred or avascular skin–soft tissue envelope (S-STE)
5. Heavy smoker
6. Psychological disorders, such as body dysmorphic disorder, depression, and personality disorders

Anatomy

Membranous septum: The portion of the septum located between the cartilaginous septum and the columella.

Nasal septum: The nasal septum is a combined bony and cartilaginous structure that separates the nasal vault into two halves, provides support to the nasal tip, and stabilizes the upper and lower lateral cartilages (LLC). The anterior aspect of the nasal septum is cartilaginous, and the posterior and cephalic aspect of the nasal septum is osseous. The cartilaginous septum is quadrangular in shape and is fused to the paired upper lateral cartilages (ULC) dorsally and to the anterior nasal spine and maxillary crest anteriorly and inferiorly. The osseous septum is composed of the bones of the vomer and the perpendicular plate of the ethmoid. The vomer bone articulates with the posterior maxillary crest. The perpendicular plate of the ethmoid articulates with the nasal bones, frontal bone, and cribriform plate.

Septal Procedures

Caudal septoplasty: Procedures performed to address the deviated cartilaginous portion of the nasal septum to improve obstructive nasal breathing, correct cosmetic deformities or deviations, and/or harvest a section of cartilage for adjunctive grafting procedures. A large quantity of cartilage may be harvested from the central cartilaginous septum (quadrangular resection). It is paramount to leave at least a 10 mm dorsal and caudal cartilaginous strut (Figure 42.1) for support of the nasal complex. During revision rhinoplasty, if the septum has been previously harvested, alternative sites for cartilage harvesting include the conchal bowl of the ear and the costochondral cartilage obtained from the sixth and seventh ribs.

Septal repositioning: Repositioning of a deviated cartilaginous septum within the midline of the nasal cavity. The cartilaginous septum may be repositioned with or without cartilage resection. A mucoperiochondrial dissection is initiated along the inferior aspect of the cartilaginous septum to mobilize the septum from the anterior nasal spine and maxillary crest. The cartilaginous septum is mobilized and positioned along the midline of the nasal cavity. More commonly, a "swinging-door" technique is utilized to resect a conservative inferior strip of cartilage to allow repositioning along the midline of the nasal vault. A nonresorbable suture is frequently placed

---

Atlas of Operative Oral and Maxillofacial Surgery, First Edition. Edited by Christopher J. Haggerty and Robert M. Laughlin

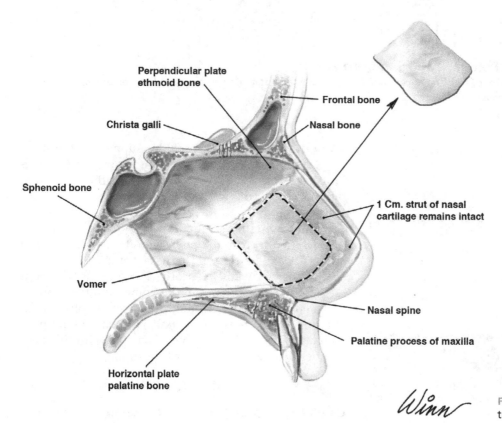

Winn

Figure 42.1. Anatomy of the nasal septum and quadrangular cartilage harvest.

through the anterior and inferior portion of the cartilaginous nasal septum and secured to the anterior nasal spine or the periosteum overlying the anterior nasal floor or maxillary crest (Wright suture).

Cartilage scoring: Cartilage scoring is performed to facilitate septal cartilage straightening. Scoring is done perpendicular to the orientation of the deviation and is frequently required on both sides of the involved cartilage to soften and reform deviated cartilage.

Spreader grafting: A section of cartilage, typically harvested from the nasal septum, is positioned bilaterally between the superior articulation of the cartilaginous septum and the ULC (see Figures 42.31, 42.32, and 42.33 in Case Report 42.2). Spreader grafts are utilized to open the internal nasal valve (increase nasal airflow), to reconstruct or widen a narrow middle nasal vault, to increase nasal length in patients with a short nose, and to reconstruct hump deformities during revision rhinoplasty.

Turbinate Anatomy and Procedures

Turbinates: The three paired nasal turbinates (superior, middle, and inferior) are positioned along the lateral nasal wall via thin turbinate bones. Their function is to humidify and warm inspired air. The inferior turbinate is a common cause of obstructive nasal breathing.

Total inferior turbinectomy: Involves the out-fracture of the turbinate bone and the resection of the entire inferior turbinate along its lateral attachment to the lateral nasal wall. This procedure is infrequently performed due to its alteration of nasal physiology, which leads to postoperative epistaxis, crusting, atrophic rhinitis, and dryness.

Partial anterior turbinectomy: Involves the removal of the anterior one-third to one-half of the affected inferior turbinate. Minimizes the risks associated with total inferior turbinectomy.

Submucous resection: Involves removal of the inferior turbinate bone while preserving the overlying mucosa. By maintaining the overlying mucosal flaps, the normal mucosal functions are preserved and complications (crusting, atrophic rhinitis, and dryness) are minimized.

Other methods of turbinate treatment include electrocautery, radiofrequency and laser reduction, cryosurgery, and out-fracture without reduction or removal.

Nasal Valves: Anatomy and Procedures

Internal nasal valve: The junction of the nasal septum and the caudal margin of the ULC (normally, 10–15°). The internal nasal valve comprises the narrowest portion of the nasal airway and is commonly associated with obstructive nasal breathing. Narrowing of the internal nasal valve is corrected with spreader grafts to increase the internal valve angle and to stent the airway open.

External nasal valve: Located caudal to the internal nasal valve and bounded laterally by the ala and medially by the septum and columella. The external nasal valve is essentially the vestibule that serves as the entrance to the nose. A collapsed external nasal valve frequently presents as a collapse of the alar rim during inspiration. Collapsed external nasal valves are treated by correcting any underlying septum deviations and with alar rim grafts to open the angle of the external nasal valve.

Nasal Skin–Soft Tissue Envelope (S-STE)

Thick S-STE: Thick and sebaceous tissues are more adapt to concealing deformities and hiding minor irregularities and asymmetries. However, it is more difficult to obtain well-defined cosmetic results with thicker nasal tissues.

Thin S-STE: Underlying definition of the nasal skeleton is readily visible. Allows for well-defined nasal tip anatomy. Readily shows nasal irregularities, imperfections, and asymmetries.

Nasal Skeleton

Nasion: The intersection of the nasal bone and the frontal bone. Represents the deepest aspect of the nasofrontal angle. A deep nasion can be augmented with alloplastic (expanded polytetrafluoroethylene) and/or autogenous (morselized septal cartilage, costochondral cartilage, and temporal fascia) grafts to increase the nasofrontal angle.

Nasal bones: The paired nasal bones form the bony roof of the nose and articulate with each other medially, with the maxilla laterally, the frontal bone superiorly, the ULC inferiorly, and the perpendicular plates of the ethmoid posteriorly.

Upper lateral cartilages: Attach to the midline septum and form the cartilaginous midvault. The cephalic portion of the ULC is attached and overlapped by the paired nasal bones.

Lower lateral cartilages (or alar cartilages): The C-shaped and paired LLC are each composed of a medial, middle, and lateral crura. Supported inferiorly by the caudal aspect of the septum and the pyriform aperture. The LLC determine the majority of the nasal tip shape, size, and projection.

Scroll region: The junction where the LLC overlap the ULC.

Keystone area: The junction of the ULC, the nasal bones, and the septum.

Initial Nasal Examination

1. Discussion regarding the patient's chief complaints regarding nasal function and aesthetics.
2. Preoperative photographs are taken that will allow the surgeon to manipulate the images in their preferred computer software package (to be used as a visual aid for evaluation with the patient) and will allow for an intraoperative reference during the rhinoplasty surgery.
3. Aesthetic evaluation of the entire face and nasal anatomy to include the nasal tip, dorsum, nasal base, alar rims, columella, nasal bones, radix, and S-STE, as well as overall symmetry during both animation and repose.
4. Intranasal examination with a nasal speculum to view the nasal septum to identify areas of deviation, mucosal condition, septal perforations, synechiae, and intranasal masses. Particularly important in patients with functional complaints, with previous nasal surgery, and requiring septal harvest and grafting. The inferior turbinates are also evaluated for hypertrophy contributing to obstructive nasal breathing.
5. Either a treatment plan may be created at the initial visit and reviewed with the patient, or it may be developed and reviewed with the patient at a subsequent visit prior to surgery. The treatment plan should address both functional and aesthetic patient concerns and allow for an open discussion with the patient and surgeon regarding treatment.

Septal Access: Killian and Transfixion Incisions

Killian Incision

Indications

1. Provides access to harvest a quadrangular graft specimen
2. Provides access to the midseptum (quadrangular septum), vomer, and ethmoid
3. Minimal disturbance of adjacent structures

Contraindications

1. Poor access to caudal and dorsal septal deformities

Technique: Killian Approach Septoplasty

1. Anesthesia options include intravenous sedation, laryngeal mask airway (LMA) or oral endotracheal general anesthesia. A single dose of intravenous antibiotics is administered prior to the start of the procedure.
2. The patient is positioned supine, and a countable throat pack is placed within the posterior oropharynx. The external and internal nose are prepped with Hebiclense solution and draped so that the forehead, chin, and ears are visible.
3. The nasal cavities are packed with oxymetazoline-soaked half-inch ribbon gauze. One percent lidocaine

with 1:100,000 epinephrine is injected into the septum with a 27- or 30-gauge needle. The septum is injected bilaterally within a subperichondrial (anterior cartilaginous septum) and subperiosteal (posterior osseous septum) plane. An appropriate injection technique allows the hydrodissection of the tissue from the underlying septum and blanching of the overlying tissues. The pyriform aperture, nasal floor, and inferior turbinates (if inferior turbinectomy is to be performed) are also injected. Blocks are performed at the supratrochlear and infraorbital neurovascular bundle locations.

4. For access to the cartilaginous septum, a Kilian incision is placed 3–5 mm posterior to and parallel to the caudal border of the cartilaginous septum (Figure 42.2, Case Report 42.1). The Killian incision may be placed on either side of the septum, depending on the surgeon's hand preference and/or the nature and location of the septal deformity. A #15 blade is utilized to transverse the mucoperichondrium without penetrating the underlying cartilaginous septum. The discoid end of a Cottle elevator is used to dissect within a subperichondrial (cartilaginous septum) and a subperiosteal (bony septum) tissue plane just beyond the area of deviation and/or the site of cartilage harvest. A #15 blade is used to incise through the cartilaginous septum 5–7 mm posterior and parallel to the Killian incision, thus preserving at least a 10 mm caudal strut. Subperichondral dissection is performed on the opposite side of the septum with the Cottle elevator. Care is taken to not perforate the opposing side's mucoperichondrium. With the mucoperichondrial tissue flaps protected, a Ballenger swivel knife is used to resect the deviated cartilage or the cartilage to be harvested, preserving at least a 10 mm strut of dorsal septum. The resected cartilage is delivered with Debakey pickups (Figure 42.3, Case Report 42.1). The harvested cartilage is placed within moist gauze if it will be used as a grafting material for adjunctive procedures.

5. The site is irrigated, and the Killian incision is closed with a 6-0 plain gut suture on a P3 needle. Quilting sutures are placed within the area of the cartilage defect to eliminate the dead space (minimizing hematoma formation) with a 4-0 plain gut suture on a Keith needle.

Key Points: Killian Access

1. Although traditionally placed 3–5 mm posterior and parallel to the caudal edge of the cartilaginous septum, the exact location of the Killian incision may vary depending on the location of the septal deformity. A Killian incision can be used to address vomer and ethmoid deviations and bone spurs with the Killian incision placed just anterior to the site of bony abnormality, with or without extension of the incision onto the floor of the nose for increased access.

Case Report 42.1. Obstructed nasal breathing (deviated cartilaginous nasal septum). A 46-year-old patient presents with a chief complaint of right-sided nasal obstruction not relieved with medical management. Nasal speculum examination demonstrated significant deviation of the cartilaginous septum and hypertrophy of the right inferior turbinate. Treatment included resection of the deviated septal cartilage via Killian incision and submucous resection of the right inferior turbinate. (See Figures 42.2 and 42.3.)

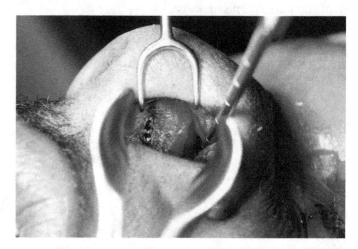

Figure 42.2.   A Killian incision placed 5 mm posterior and parallel to the caudal margin (blue surgical marking) of the cartilaginous septum.

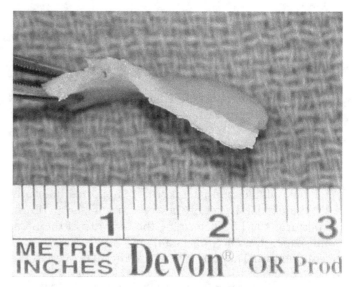

Figure 42.3.   Resected deviated cartilage. A 10 mm dorsal and caudal strut of the cartilaginous septum was preserved.

Transfixion Incisions

Indications

1. Provides access to the anterior caudal septum to correct caudal septal deviations and to harvest graft material
2. Provides access to the anterior nasal spine and floor of the nose
3. Need for tip deprojection

Contraindications

1. When less invasive procedure are indicated (i.e., a Killian incision)

Technique: Three Variations

1. **Full transfixion incision**: An incision is made completely through the membranous septum, beginning superiorly from the caudal-dorsal septal angle and terminating inferiorly through the footplate attachments. Subperichondrial dissection allows for cartilage graft harvest and correction of septal deformities. Provides tip deprojection and access to the anterior nasal spine.
2. **Hemitransfixion incision**: An incision is made through only one side of the membranous septum. A #15 blade sharply accesses the caudal septum without complete disruption of footplate attachments. Subperichondrial dissection allows for cartilage graft harvest and correction of septal deformities.
3. **Partial transfixion incision**: An incision is made completely through the membranous septum above the footplate attachments. Subperichondrial dissection allows for cartilage graft harvest and correction of septal deformities.

Key Points: Transfixion Access

1. Transfixion incisions allow for excellent access to the caudal septum.
2. Incisions are placed as close as possible to the caudal margin of the septum in order to minimize disruption of the membranous septum.

Open Approach Rhinoplasty

Indications

1. Anticipated complex shaping or grafting rhinoplasty, particularly to the nasal tip
2. Severely deviated or twisted nose deformity
3. Complex revision rhinoplasty
4. Surgeon preference, or novice surgeon

Contraindications

1. When minimal changes are required (i.e., isolated dorsal hump) that may be accomplished by limited dissection (endonasal approach) or with injectable fillers

Technique

1. A preoperative treatment plan is reviewed with the patient, and surgical markings are placed.
2. Anesthesia options include intravenous sedation, LMA or oral endotracheal general anesthesia. A single dose of intravenous antibiotics is administered prior to the start of the procedure.
3. The patient is positioned supine, and a countable throat pack is placed within the posterior oropharynx. The external and internal nose is prepped with Hebiclense solution and draped so that the forehead, chin, and ears are visible.
4. The nasal cavities are packed with oxymetazoline-soaked ½-inch ribbon gauze. 1% lidocaine with 1:100,000 epinephrine is injected into the septum with a 27- or 30-gauge needle. The septum is injected bilaterally within a subperichondrial (anterior cartilaginous septum) and subperiosteal (posterior osseous septum) plane. An appropriate injection technique allows the hydrodissection of the tissue from the underlying septum and blanching of the overlying tissues. The pyriform aperture, nasal floor, and inferior turbinates (if an inferior turbinectomy is to be performed) are injected. The marginal incision sites, nasal tip, nasal dorsum, lateral nasal walls, and columella are injected. With any nasal procedure, the minimal amount of local anesthetic required for hemostasis is used to limit tissue distortion (typically, 7–8 mL total). A 10–15-minute delay after the administration of local anesthesia should be observed in order to allow for the ideal vasoconstrictive properties of the local anesthetic and to allow post injection tissue distortion to resolve.
5. A stair-stepped, Chevron, or "W" transcolumellar incision is marked (Figure 42.15 [all figures cited in this list appear in Case Report 42.2]) just cephalad to the medial crural footplates, (typically the narrowest part of the columella) and incised with an #11 blade (Figure 42.16). The incision is carried out in a sawing motion and perpendicular to the skin. The columellar artery is frequently encountered superficial to the medial crura and should be managed with conservative bipolar cautery.
6. Marginal incisions are created with a #15 blade. A finger is placed on the outer surface of the LLC, and a two-pronged skin hook is used to evert the nostril. This maneuver will show the demarcation of the caudal aspect of the LLC. The marginal incision is created along this caudal aspect of the lateral crura with care to not transect the underlying cartilage. The marginal incision extends medially along the caudal margin of the middle and medial crura, and joins the transcolumellar incision (Figure 42.17).
7. Angled converse or iris scissors are used to dissect across the columella from the medial marginal incisions, and the columellar flap is freed with a #11 blade (Figure 42.18).
8. Angled converse or iris scissors are used to elevate the S-STE within the relatively avascular tissue plane superficial to the domes (Figure 42.19) until

the paired LLC can be delivered with an 8 mm double hook (Figure 42.20).

9. Dissection is carried from the LLC cephalically to the ULC. The ULC are exposed within the same relatively avascular plane until the nasal bones are reached. A subperiosteal dissection is performed over the nasal bones with a Cottle or #9 periosteal elevator (Figure 42.21) to reveal the upper vault. Residual fibrous attachments are swept off of the ULC with a Joseph knife (Figure 42.22) or #9 periosteal elevator. An Aufricht retractor is placed to retract the S-STE and to allow direct visualization of the entire nasal skeleton.

10. Open septoplasty is performed to harvest cartilage for additional grafting procedures and to resect, score, and reposition the septal cartilage.

11. Modifications to the nasal tip and dorsum are performed as planned. Surgeon preference dictates the order, but throughout, the S-STE is redraped after adjustments to visualize changes until the planned result is obtained.

12. Nasal tip modifications frequently involve the placement of columellar struts (Figure 42.24), cephalic trim (Figure 42.25), intradomal sutures, interdomal sutures (Figure 42.26), and nasal tip grafting (42.27).

13. Dorsal modifications may include dorsal hump reduction (Figures 42.28, 42.29, and 42.30), augmentation, and/or correction of deviations. Cartilaginous dorsal reductions are performed with either a #10 or a #15 blade. Bony dorsal reductions are performed with a sharp monobeveled osteotome. Open roof deformities may occur after large dorsal reductions and are managed with spreader grafts (Figures 42.31, 42.32, and 42.33) and nasal osteotomies.

14. Osteotomies are performed as needed (Figures 42.5 and 42.34). Lateral osteotomies are typically used to correct nasal bone deviations or asymmetries and to close open roof deformities. A #15 blade is used to create a stab incision for lateral osteotomies at the pyriform aperture just superior to the inferior turbinate. A #9 periosteal elevator develops a subperiosteal path for the osteotomes. The lateral osteotomies are created using a guarded osteotome so that the direction of the osteotome can be palpated through the skin at all times and to minimize tissue damage. Occasionally, a transcutaneous osteotomy using a 2 mm straight osteotome is necessary to mobilize the fractured nasal bones.

15. Alar modifications are performed as planned. Alar rim grafts (Figures 42.35 and 42.36) may be placed to correct for collapse of the external nasal valve during inspiration and to provide support to the lateral nasal sidewall. Cartilage struts are placed within pockets developed superficial, lateral, and superior to the LLC.

16. The columellar incision is closed with interrupted 6-0 plain gut sutures.

17. Intranasal incisions are closed with 5-0 plain gut sutures, and a 4-0 plain gut suture on a Keith needle is used to perform a septal quilting stitch.

18. Lidocaine blocks are given at the sites of the supratrochlear and infraorbital neurovascular bundle locations.

19. Mastisol is applied to the external nose, and ¼-inch steri-strips are applied to the external nose to create compression of the dissected spaces. A thermoplastic Aquaplast splint (Aquaplast Corp., Wyckoff, NJ, USA) is trimmed with heavy scissors and heated within a hot-water bath to allow shaping of the material. The splint should provide coverage from the supratip region to the glabella and laterally to the nasojugal groove. Properly trimmed and positioned, the splint applies compression to close dead space, limits edema, supports the position of osteotomized nasal bones, and serves as a reminder to the patient to not sleep on their stomach during the healing period. If the nasal bones appear to medialize more than desired, intranasal silastic splints (Doyle splints) are placed within each nasal cavity and secured to each other with a 2-0 nylon transseptal (membranous septum) suture. Antibiotic ointment and a moustache dressing are applied. The nose is rarely packed.

20. The throat pack is removed, the patient's posterior oropharynx is suctioned, and the patient is extubated and recovered per standard protocol.

Key Points: Open Rhinoplasty

1. The open approach allows the surgeon to perform complex procedures to the nasal skeleton in a relatively undistorted fashion. Complex grafting and corrective techniques may be accomplished under direct vision. Disadvantages include the columellar incision scar and increased nasal tip edema.

2. A stair-stepped, Chevron, or "W" columellar incision aids in camouflaging the incision scar. Care is taken when performing the transcolumellar incision to not transect the underlying medial crura.

3. During nasal skeletonization, it is important to stay just superficial to the LLC and ULC to maximize the S-STE thickness in order to minimize damage to the S-STE, maintain blood flow, and minimize scar tissue formation, edema, and intraoperative and postoperative bleeding.

Closed (Endonasal) Rhinoplasty

Indications

1. Surgeon preference
2. Primary rhinoplasty or minor revision rhinoplasty
3. Need for limiting skin incisions (keloid formers)

Contraindications (Relative)

1. Complex rhinoplasty requiring numerous grafting procedures
2. Complex revision rhinoplasty
3. Complex posttraumatic rhinoplasty with severe deviation or twisted component
4. Novice surgeon unfamiliar with endonasal technique

Technique: Closed (Endonasal) Rhinoplasty

1. Steps 1–4 of the open rhinoplasty technique.
2. The septum is accessed first and addressed as needed. If necessary, a septal cartilage graft is harvested for structural and shaping grafts as planned preoperatively.
3. Attention is turned to the closed rhinoplasty incisions. Access is through a transcartilaginous incision between the LLC and the ULC (scroll area) (Figure 42.4). The tip is manually displaced caudally until the ULC–LLC junction (scroll area) is visualized within the nasal vestibule. A #15 blade is used to incise nasal mucosa and to transverse the scroll area parallel to the lateral aspect of the ULC. Dissection is carried onto the nasal dorsum with blunt (Cottle elevator) and sharp (iris scissors) dissection. Care is taken to dissect just superficial to the cartilage to minimize bleeding, maintain a uniform S-STE thickness, and minimize tissue trauma and edema.
4. The same access is performed on the opposing side, and the tissue planes are joined.
5. Once the bony dorsum is reached, a subperiosteal dissection with a Cottle or #9 periosteal elevator creates a pocket over the upper bony vault.
6. A Joseph knife is used to sweep any remaining soft tissue attachments from the lateral ULC. Lateral dissection is necessary to allow passive redraping of S-STE after hump resection.

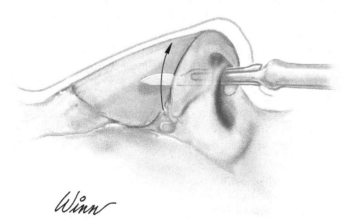

Figure 42.4. Endonasal rhinoplasty incision transecting the scroll area.

7. Dorsal height modifications are carried out with a combination of #10 and #15 blades, chisels, and/or rasps.
8. Medial, intermediate, and lateral osteotomies are performed as needed. Medial and intermediate osteotomies are carried out with a straight 2 mm osteotome through the transcartilaginous incision. Lateral osteotomies are carried out through a vestibular approach as described previously within this chapter.
9. Attention is next turned to the nasal tip. To expose the LLC, a #15 blade is used to create bilateral marginal incisions along the LLC caudal margins. The incisions extend along the entire caudal aspect of the LLC from the lateral crura to the medial crura. Using iris or converse scissors, dissection continues superficial to the LLC and domes until the previous transcartilaginous dorsal dissection is connected.
10. The LLC may be delivered through one nostril or the other to carry out the planned shaping, grafting, and suturing maneuvers.
11. Alar rim modifications and grafting are performed if required.
12. Incisions are closed with a 5-0 plain gut suture. A quilt stitch utilizing a 4-0 gut suture on a Keith needle is performed if nasal cartilage was reshaped or resected.
13. Steps 18–20 of the open rhinoplasty technique.

Key Points: Closed (Endonasal) Rhinoplasty

1. Advantages of endonasal rhinoplasty include no external scar, minimal postoperative edema, decreased operating time, and quicker patient recovery. Nasal tip edema after open rhinoplasty may take up to 9–12 months to completely resolve, thus delaying the final appearance of the surgery.
2. Disadvantages of endonasal rhinoplasty include difficulty in performing complex grafting and tip work, prohibits direct visualization of anatomy, and typically requires a more experienced surgeon. Many modifications are done blindly or require significant tissue distortion to view the changes directly. For this reason, complex procedures and grafting should be attempted only by experienced surgeons who are familiar with the endonasal approach.

Correction of Specific Nasal Deformities

Upper Bony Vault and Middle Cartilaginous Vault

Excessive width: Small reductions may be corrected with reductive lateral osseous rasping and cartilage scoring. Large reductions require nasal osteotomies to medialize nasal bones (Figure 42.5).
Narrow width: Frequently seen after previous aggressive rhinoplasty. Treatment typically involves nasal osteotomies and spreader graft placement. Medial and

lateral osteotomies are performed to lateralize the nasal bones from the bony septum. The cartilaginous septum is dissected from the ULC, and spreader grafts are inserted to maintain the new position. Consider camouflage onlay grafts or injectable filler for small defects.

High dorsum: Small dorsal reductions may be rasped (bony) and sharply planed (cartilage) lower. Larger dorsal reductions require en bloc resection of cartilage and bone (Figures 42.28, 42.29, and 42.30, Case Report 42.2). The cartilage is first incised at the proposed height along each ULC. Intranasal mucosa at the height of the vault is elevated and rolled 2–4 mm inferiorly into the nasal cavity. The cartilaginous septum is incised at the new height until the bony septum is encountered. The nasal mucosa is elevated from the underside of the bony vault. A monobevel chisel is used to reduce the bony dorsum to slightly higher than the desired final position. Sharp bony edges are smoothed with a push rasp and finished with a diamond rasp. A gap will frequently exist between the septum and the ULC–nasal bones on each side (open roof deformity). Depending on the presence of pre-existing nasal obstruction and the planned cosmesis, the gap is typically filled with septal cartilage spreader grafts (Figures 42.31, 42.32, and 42.33, Case Report 42.2), and lateral osteotomies (Figure 42.34, Case Report 42.2) are performed to complete the closure. Any planned correction of a deviated septum must be completed prior to the closure of the open roof deformity. The spreader grafts will also act as batton grafts in reinforcing the straightened septum.

Low dorsum: Typically corrected with dorsal onlay grafting to augment the dorsal height. Augmentation materials include morselized septal cartilage, deep temporal fascia, carved autologous rib, and alloplastic materials. A variant of the low dorsum is the saddle nose deformity. Correction involves large dorsal onlay grafts, frequently silicone implants placed via endonasal access.

Deviated and/or twisted dorsum: Typically results from fractures of the nasal bones, the septum, the ULC, and/or the ULC insertion on the underside of the nasal bones. Corrected with lateral, intermediate, and medial osteotomies (Figure 42.5). High septal deformities may require osteotomies of the bony septum. Small defects and asymmetries may be corrected with camouflage onlay grafts or injectable fillers. Septal scoring with batton and spreader grafts may be indicated depending on the specific type of deformity.

Nasal Tip

Overprojected nasal tip: Separating the caudal septum from the LLC footplates by performing a full transfixation incision alone will deproject the nasal tip 1–2 mm.

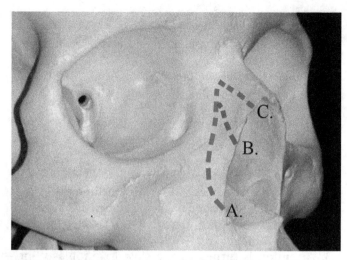

Figure 42.5. Sites of (A) lateral, (B) intermediate, and (C) medial nasal osteotomies.

Significant overprojection may be treated with a combination of a full transfixion incision, cephalic trim and crura division, resection, and reconstitution.

Underprojected nasal tip: Minor cases are treated with a columellar strut graft. Significant cases are treated with combinations of columellar strut grafting, shield grafting, and Goldman tip procedures.

Ptotic or derotated nasal tip: Treatment includes cephalic trim, resection of the caudal-dorsal septal angle with the dome rotated toward the septum, and augmentation of the anterior nasal spine for a deficient, acute nasolabial angle. Most techniques that project the tip also cause cephalad tip rotation, particularly if the medial crura are lengthened (columellar strut, shield graft, cap graft, and suturing techniques).

Overrotated nasal tip: Often seen secondary to previous aggressive rhinoplasty. Treated with camouflage grafts to increase the infratip lobule (shield graft, and mastoid fascia graft to infratip). When seen concomitantly with alar rim retraction, alar rim cartilage graft or composite ear graft to the alar vestibule should be considered.

Broad, bulbous, or boxy nasal tip: A wide intermediate crura is frequently responsible for broad- or boxy-tip deformities. This condition may be corrected with a combination of intermediate crura resection, cephalic trim, interdomal sutures, intradomal sutures, structural cartilage grafts (columellar strut, shield, and cap graft), and selective defatting of the S-STE in patients with thick sebaceous skin.

Alar Base and Nostrils

Asymmetric nostrils: Frequently due to caudal septal deviation from the maxillary crest. The caudal septum is straightened with concave surface scoring and reinforced with batton grafting. The cartilaginous septum is secured to the midline maxillary crest periosteum with 4-0 poly-l-lactic suture (Wright suture).

Wide alar base: Consider an alar cinch suture with a 2-0 Nurolon suture. The periosteum must be released around the nasal aperture to facilitate medialization of the ala. Consider alar base resection (Weir incisions) for excessively wide nostrils.

Postoperative Management

1. The Aquaplast splint and nasal tape are maintained for 7–10 days.
2. Incisions receive topical antibiotic ointment for 2 days, and then moist occlusive petroleum ointment for 5 days.
3. Plain gut sutures are trimmed flush at 7 days.
4. Arnica gel is applied to any areas of ecchymosis after 3 days.
5. Patient are typically seen at postoperative weeks 1, 2, 4, 12, and 24. Patients are reminded that the final result of their rhinoplasty may not be apparent until 9–12 months after surgery due to resolving nasal edema, especially with open rhinoplasty procedures.

Early Complications

Hemorrhage: Bleeding in the immediate postoperative period is typically from improper usage of local anesthetic, inadvertent mucosal trauma, and bleeding from the vascular turbinate incision after inferior turbinectomy. Bleeding may be minimized with appropriate local anesthetic injection technique, meticulous flap dissection, placing oxymetazoline-impregnated sponges into the nasal passages for 5–10 minutes after inferior turbinectomy, and administering additional local anesthetic containing a vasoconstrictor at the end of the procedure if hemostasis is not ideal.

Infection: Rare. Rhinoplasties are generally considered contaminated procedures. Infections are managed with antibiotics, wound debridement, hematoma evacuation, and the removal of infected materials (nasal packing, and alloplastic and autogenous grafts).

Septal hematoma: An unrecognized septal hematoma may lead to infection, ischemia, and necrosis of the septal cartilage and decreased tip support, resulting in a saddle nose deformity. Septal hematoma prevention includes meticulous dissection of the mucoperichondrium flaps, hemostasis upon termination of the procedure, the placement of quilting (horizontal mattress) sutures, and early recognition. Treatment involves early evacuation, elimination of the dead space (nasal packing, drain placement, and horizontal mattress or quilting sutures), and antibiotic coverage.

Cerebral spinal fluid (CSF) rhinorrhea: Rare complication. Symptoms include headaches, a clear nasal discharge, and a salty or metallic postnasal drip. Causes include mucoperichondrium tunneling too far posterior and superior with a Cottle elevator and extending beyond the ethmoid roof and fracturing the cribriform plate with excessive force during osteotomy or resection of an osseous septal deviation or bone spur. Initial treatment involves prophylactic coverage of meningitis with antibiotics. Persistent CSF rhinorrhea is treated with lumbar drain placement and/or layered repair.

Late Complications

Septal perforations: Occurs with septal cartilage resection and bilateral mucosal tears in corresponding segments of the septum. Symptoms include nasal crusting, obstruction, dryness, epistaxis, pain, and whistling during nasal inspiration. Large perforations may compromise the structural integrity of the nose and may lead to cosmetic changes, including saddle nose deformity. Septal perforations are minimized with meticulous mucoperichondrium flap dissection, repair of intraoperative tears immediately, and close follow-up with excellent nasal hygiene. Delayed repair is often accomplished with bilateral bipedicled mucosal flap advancements.

Synechiae: Typically occurs with opposing damaged mucosal surfaces, but may also occur with infection and nasal trauma. Often occurs at the site of inferior turbinectomy, due to the denuded turbinate site contacting the nasal septal mucosa. Patients with posterior synechiae are frequently asymptomatic. Patients with symptomatic synechiae typically present with obstructive nasal breathing and/or a Starling defect. Prevention of synechiae involves meticulous flap dissection, avoidance of inadvertent and accidental mucosal damage, utilizing nasal splints or nasal packings for 1–2 weeks post surgery, and septal sutures.

Overresection: These complications are often the most devastating and difficult to correct. Revision surgery is almost always warranted, and plans should be made to harvest structural cartilage grafts from the ear or rib as necessary.

1. **Ptotic nasal tip (overrotated tip and deprojected tip)**: Often, the result of aggressive cephalic trimming, an overresected caudal septum, scar tissue formation, and/or a weakened, unsupported medial crura. Treated with columellar strut grafting and/or nasal tip grafting.
2. **Alar rim retraction**: Due to aggressive cephalic trim. Consider an alar rim strut graft for small retractions. Larger retractions may require composite skin–cartilage grafts from the anterior conchal bowl to the nasal vestibule.
3. **Uni-tip deformity**: Frequently associated with overzealous narrowing and grafting of the nasal tip

coupled with aggressive cephalic trimming, leading to collapse of ala. Treatment typically consists of alar strut grafts or composite grafts.

4. **Keel deformity**: Due to closure of an open roof with inadequately sized or absent spreader grafts. The dorsum cross-section comes to a point instead of a rounded or square dome. Corrected with nasal osteotomies and generous spreader graft placement.

5. **Internal and external nasal valve collapse**: A frequent cause of revision rhinoplasty. Treatment is based on the site of valve collapse.

6. **Saddle nose deformity**: Results from undiagnosed septal hematoma with resulting cartilage necrosis, overresection of the dorsal hump (uncorrected open roof deformity), and failure to preserve sufficient septal cartilage (10 mm dorsal and caudal struts). Corrected with a combination of spreader grafting, onlay grafting, and nasal osteotomies.

Underresection: These complications are the result of an incomplete treatment plan or suboptimal execution. They are generally easier to correct than overresection complications.

1. **Pollybeak deformity**: Presents as a thick and humped nasal dorsum accompanied with underrotation of the nasal tip, resembling a parrot's beak. Frequently due to underresection of the caudal dorsal septum during correction of a dorsal hump and a loss of tip support. Treatment includes revision rhinoplasty with adequate hump reduction and the placement of columellar and nasal tip grafts.

2. **Residual dorsal lumps or bumps**: Most noticeable on profile. Typically corrected with reoperation. Small irregularities may be amenable to injectable filler to augment deficiencies.

3. **Residual or new deviation or twisted deformity**: Patients with traumatic nasal deformities should always be cautioned preoperatively that complete symmetry is rarely achieved. If gross asymmetry remains after surgery, consider revision rhinoplasty or injectable fillers or grafts to camouflage deficient areas.

Key Points

1. When performing aesthetic rhinoplasty, the surgeon should always be cognizant of racial and cultural anatomical norms and desires.
2. The patient's cosmetic and functional goals must be discussed and understood. The unrealistic patient should be educated about likely surgical outcomes.
3. Imaging provides a tool to facilitate the surgeon–patient conversation. Imaging also provides a framework for the surgeon to develop an anatomically based rhinoplasty technique treatment plan (Figures 42.13 and 42.14, Case Report 42.2). Various computer software programs offer imaging analysis of digital photographs that allows the surgeon to measure and evaluate facial angles, facial proportions, and symmetry and to make visual modifications to preoperative photos that simulate results that are felt to be achievable (Figures 42.10 and 42.11, Case Report 42.2). The pre- and postoperative imaging allows the surgeon the ability to virtually plan treatment procedures and outcomes (Figure 42.12, Case Report 42.2). The pre- and postoperative imaging is reviewed with the patient to ensure that the patient agrees with the treatment plan and has realistic expectations of surgery. It should be stressed that the imaging is not a guarantee of the final result. Typically, a final treatment plan or outcome is reached between the surgeon and the patient. Alternatively, it may become apparent that the patient has unrealistic goals, and the decision to not proceed with surgery may be determined.
4. The surgical approach should be chosen to maximize the opportunity to achieve the desired results while minimizing the destructive nature of the rhinoplasty dissection. The surgeon should choose the technique that is the most familiar and predictable.
5. A Cottle test is performed by applying lateral traction to the cheek and lateral nostril and assessing nasal airflow. A positive Cottle test occurs when lateral cheek–lateral nostril traction improves nasal breathing. The positive Cottle test suggests collapse of the nasal valves in general. A more specific test to differentiate between collapse of the internal versus the external nasal valve involves placing a cotton-tip applicator into the nostril and selectively elevating the LLC and ULC on the affected side. Improved breathing with elevation of the LLC coincides with a collapse of the external nasal valve, whereas improved breathing with elevation of the ULC coincides with a collapse of the internal nasal valve.
6. Medical management (topical steroids, antihistamines, anticholinergics, and sympathomimetics) is recommended prior to any nasal obstructive surgery procedure in order to assess the true need for surgery. For cases refractory to medical management, surgical intervention is warranted.
7. For patients with nasal obstruction, a complete workup to include a radiographic evaluation with computed tomography (CT) scanning, speculum examination, evaluation of the internal and external nasal valve, and a trial of medical management is required prior to surgical intervention. CT scanning is not only beneficial to evaluate turbinate

hypertrophy and septal deviation, but also crucial for identifying nontraditional causes of obstruction such as neoplasms, congenital disorders (choanal stenosis), and foreign bodies. Speculum examination should be performed to evaluate for conditions such as turbinate hypertrophy, septal deviation, synechiae, papilloma formation, tissue inflammation, and septal perforations. Identification of preoperative nasal septal perforations in the previously unoperated patient may be a sign of cocaine abuse.

8. Consideration should be given to the thickness of the skin–soft tissue envelope. Appropriate dorsal hump reduction and tip-refining techniques are directly affected by this often underappreciated aspect of the nose.

9. Care should be taken when elevating a mucopericondrial flap over areas of septal deviation and bone spurs in order to minimize tears.

10. When harvesting septal cartilage, the largest feasible caudal and dorsal strut should be preserved (minimum of 10 mm) in order to provide support for the nose.

11. When performing a cephalic trim, at least 7 mm of LLC width must be preserved to ensure adequate support and to avoid nasal tip and columella deformities.

12. In general, it is better to err on the side of undertreatment and underresection as complications are easier to correct. Overtreatment typically requires complex grafting techniques and distant graft harvest.

Case Report 42.2. A 42-year-old female presents with a chief complaint that she has an "old-looking" nose and would like the tip "elevated and narrowed." She reports mild nasal obstruction on the left while working out. Her past medical history is unremarkable. Her physical examination reveals Fitzpatrick sun reactive type II, Glogau wrinkle score III, and moderately thick, sebaceous skin. The upper vault is mildly wide with a slight depression of the left nasal bone. The middle vault is similarly wide with depression of the left lateral wall. A moderate dorsal hump is present that is equally bony and cartilaginous. The nasal tip is wide, bulbous, and slightly ptotic. The alar base is an appropriate width. A profile exam of the nasal tip shows a retracted columella with a 90° nasolabial angle. The tip is slightly overprojected. An intranasal exam reveals a deviated septum within the midbody to the dorsum. Turbinates are normal in size and appearance. A functional examination reveals no obstruction with normal breathing and left middle vault collapse–obstruction with dynamic breathing. A Cottle test was positive on the left.

Standard preoperative photographs were taken and consisted of an anterior-posterior view (Figures 42.6 and 42.13), a three-quarter view (Figure 42.7), lateral views (Figure 42.8 and 42.14), and a worm's-eye view (Figure 42.9). All preoperative and postoperative photographs are taken in the same manner and with the Frankfurt plane (auriculo-orbital plane) parallel to the floor. (See also Figures 42.15 through 42.39.)

Treatment Plan

1. Full transfixion incision for septal access: quadrangular resection of septum with preservation of dorsal-caudal struts, release of footplate–septum attachment, and tip set back 1.5 mm with reattachment of footplates to septum.
2. Open approach rhinoplasty.
3. Nasal tip modifications: columellar strut, cephalic trim, interdomal sutures, and shield graft.
4. Dorsum modifications: resection of dorsal hump (cartilage and bone), correction of deviated septum with scoring, and batton and spreader graft placement.
5. Lateral nasal osteotomies

Postoperative photographs are taken at 1 year (Figures 42.40, 42.41, and 42.42) and 7 years (Figures 42.43, 42.44, and 42.45). The patient has undergone facial volumizing with fillers and fat grafting and a necklift. Subtle refining changes are noticeable within the nose between the 1- and 7-year follow-up.

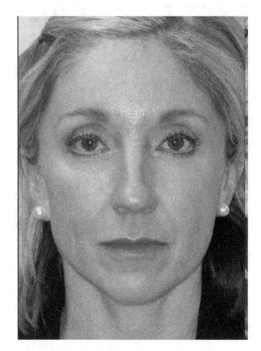

Figure 42.6.   Preoperative anterior-posterior view.

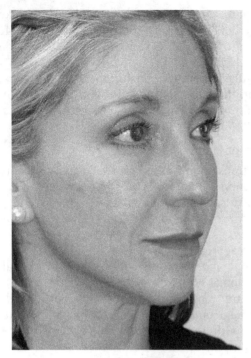

Figure 42.7.   Preoperative three-quarters view.

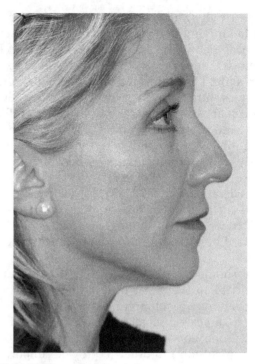

Figure 42.8.   Preoperative lateral view.

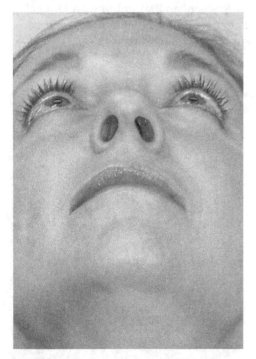

Figure 42.9.   Preoperative worm's-eye view.

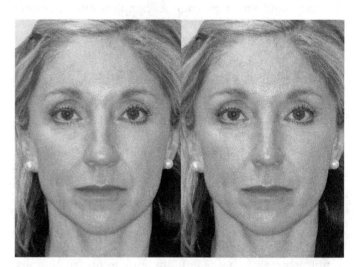

Figure 42.10.   Software generated before and after anterior-posterior views depicting correction of the excessively wide nasal vault, nasal vault deviations and asymmetries, and the bulbous nasal tip.

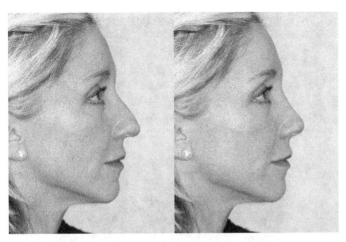

Figure 42.11. Software generated before and after lateral views depicting correction of the high nasal dorsum, ptotic nasal tip, and excessive columella show.

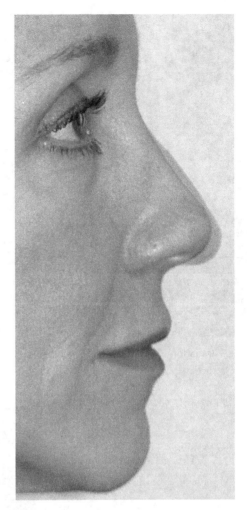

Figure 42.12. Software-generated lateral view depicting before and after results within the same image.

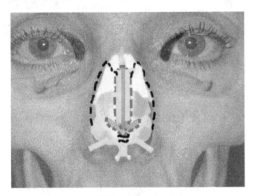

Frontal

█ Reduction   █ Graft

Figure 42.13. Schematic treatment plan, anterior-posterior view.

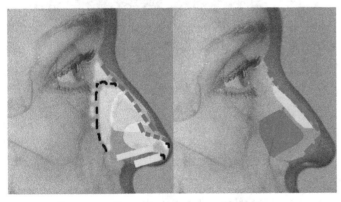

Lateral   Septum

Figure 42.14. Schematic treatment plan, lateral view.

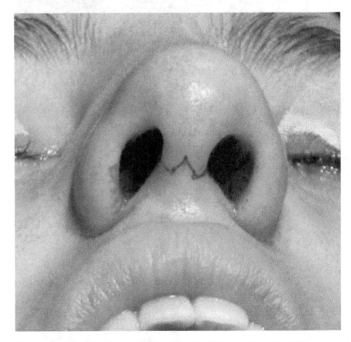

Figure 42.15. Marking of W-shaped transcolumellar incision.

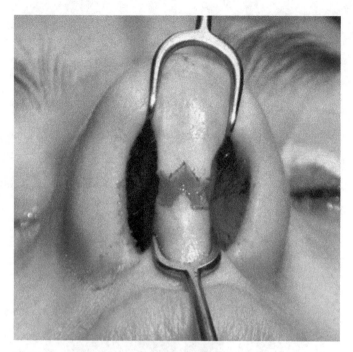

Figure 42.16.   Initiation of transcolumellar incision.

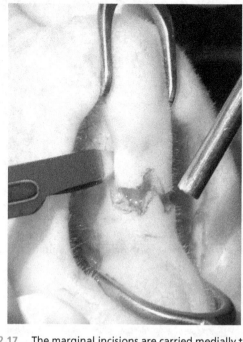

Figure 42.17.   The marginal incisions are carried medially to join the transcolumellar incision.

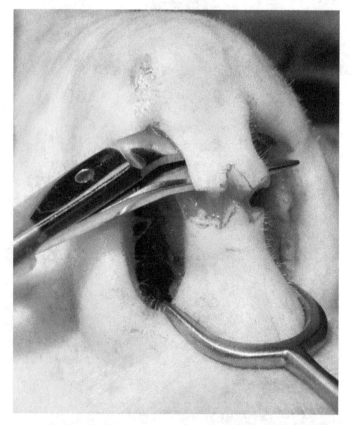

Figure 42.18.   Angled scissors are used to dissect superficial to the medial crura to connect the bilateral marginal incisions with the columellar incision.

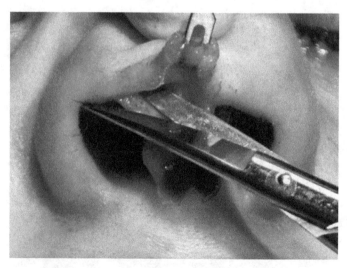

Figure 42.19.   Marginal incision is completed along the caudal aspect of the lower lateral cartilages, and iris scissors are used to dissect the overlying skin–soft tissue envelope.

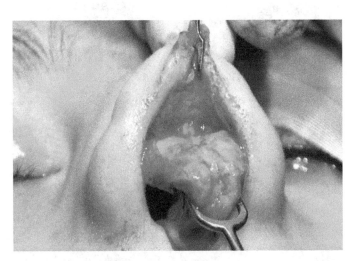

Figure 42.20.   The lower lateral cartilages are freed from the skin–soft tissue envelope and fully exposed.

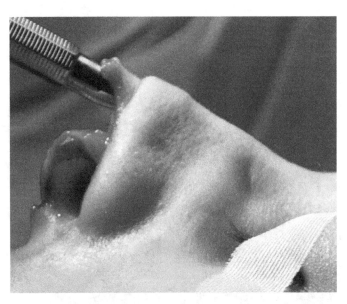

Figure 42.21.   A #9 periosteal elevator is used to expose the upper lateral cartilages and the nasal bones.

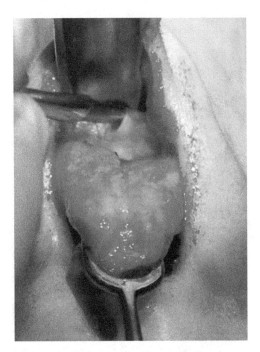

Figure 42.22.   An Aufricht nasal retractor is placed to expose the upper vault, and a Joseph knife is used in a sweeping motion to remove residual fibrous attachments from the lateral aspect of the upper lateral cartilages.

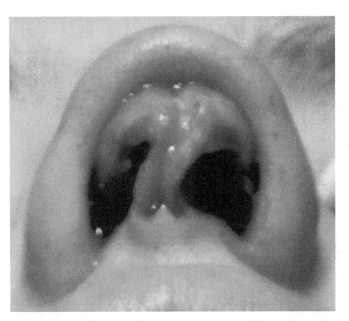

Figure 42.23.   Open view reveals septal deviation, a bulbous nasal tip, and deviation of the nasal tip.

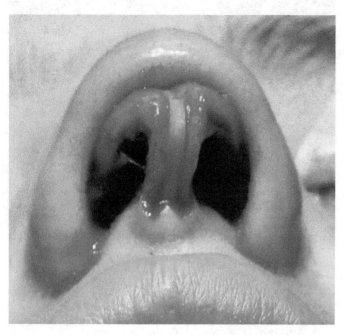

Figure 42.24. After correction of the deviated nasal septum, a 2×12×1 mm columellar strut is placed within a pocket formed between the medial crura to further correct the deviated nasal tip and to provide tip projection.

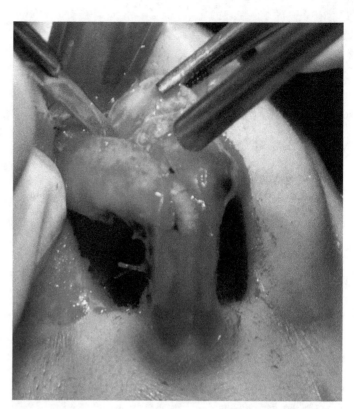

Figure 42.25. The columellar strut is secured with interrupted prolene sutures, and a cephalic trim is performed with a #15 blade.

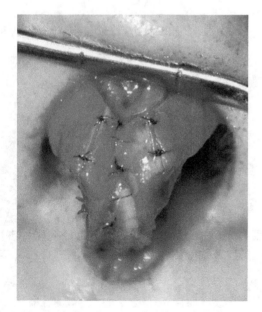

Figure 42.26. Cephalic trim completed, and interdomal sutures placed.

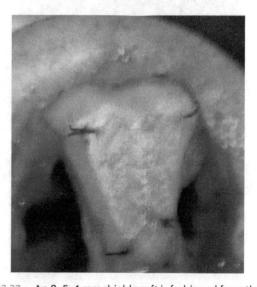

Figure 42.27. An 8×5×1 mm shield graft is fashioned from the quadrangular septal harvest, the edges are beveled to minimize visibility, and the graft is fixated to the infratip region with 6-0 nylon sutures. Shield grafts provide definition and added support to the nasal tip.

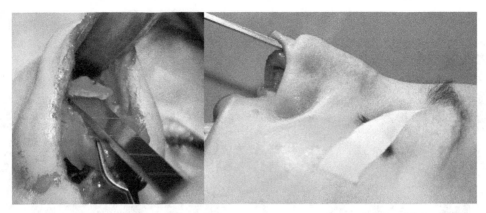

Figure 42.28.   A #15 blade and a sharp monobevel chisel are used to resect the dorsal hump.

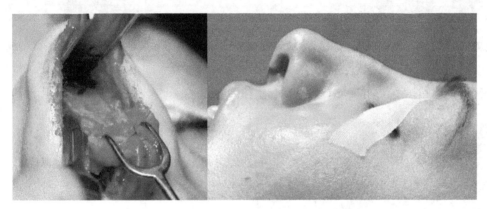

Figure 42.29.   An Aufricht nasal retractor is inserted to directly visualize the dorsal reduction. The skin–soft tissue envelope was redraped to evaluate the dorsum after hump reduction.

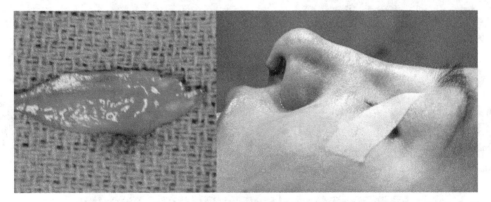

Figure 42.30.   The resected portion of the cartilaginous-bony dorsal hump. A push rasp was used to further reduce the dorsum and to remove any irregularities. The skin–soft tissue envelope is redraped to assess hump reduction and symmetry.

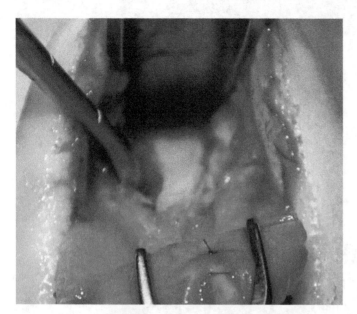

Figure 42.31. The development of pockets between the nasal septum and the upper lateral cartilages for the placement of spreader grafts.

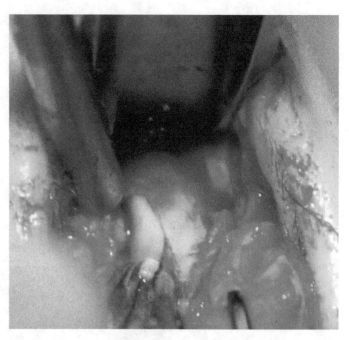

Figure 42.32. Spreader grafts were fashioned from the inferior straight segment of the quadrangular septal cartilage and placed within pockets adjacent to the septum.

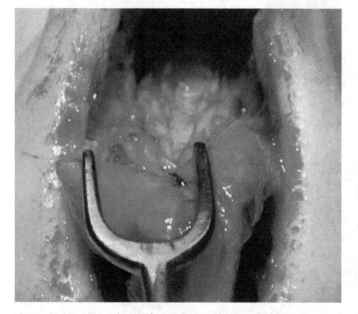

Figure 42.33. Spreader grafts in place and secured with interrupted 5-0 gut sutures.

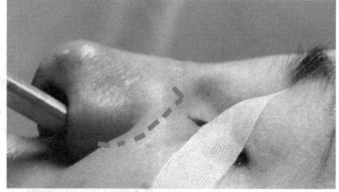

Figure 42.34. Path of lateral nasal osteotomies. The lateral osteotomies will straighten and narrow the nasal dorsum.

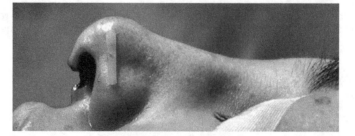

Figure 42.35. Cartilage harvested and shaped for use as alar rim grafts. The alar rim grafts will aid in minimizing alar retraction and will function to stent the external nasal valve open.

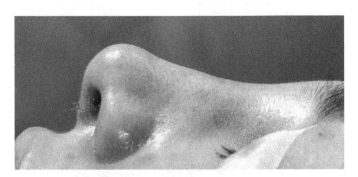

Figure 42.36.   Bilateral alar rim grafts in place.

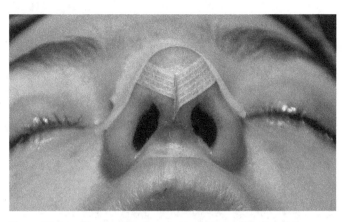

Figure 42.37.   Closure of columellar incision and taping of the nose.

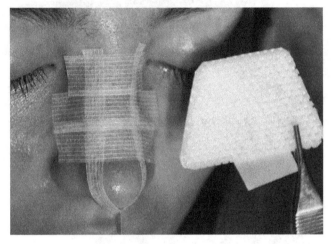

Figure 42.38.   Aquaplast splint is trimmed with heavy scissors.

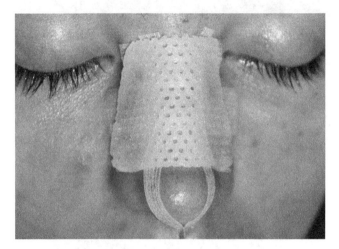

Figure 42.39.   Nasal taping and Aquaplast splint in place.

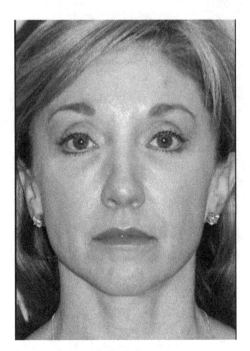

Figure 42.40.   1 year postoperative.

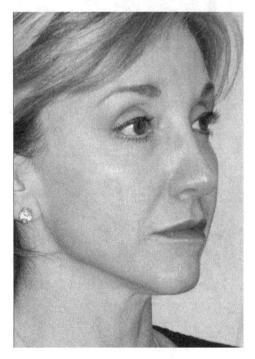

Figure 42.41.   1 year postoperative.

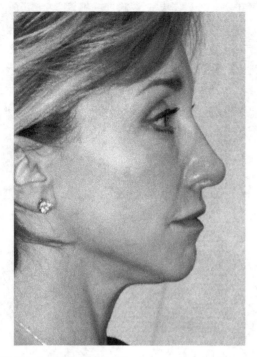

Figure 42.42.   1 year postoperative.

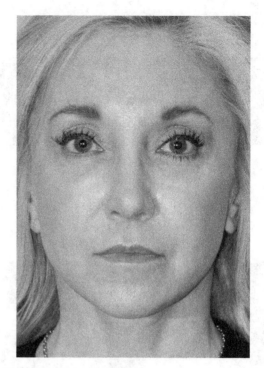

Figure 42.43.   7 years postoperative.

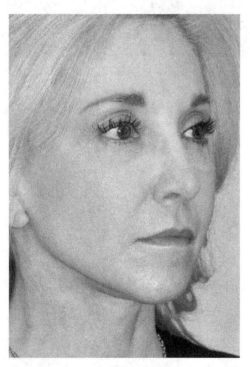

Figure 42.44.   7 years postoperative.

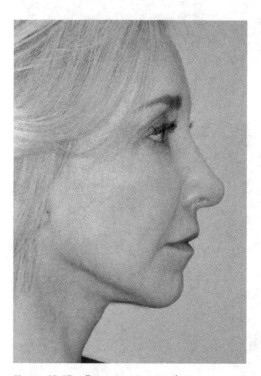

Figure 42.45.   7 years postoperative.

References

Aston, S.J. and Martin, J., 2009. Primary closed rhinoplasty. In: S.J.Aston, D.S.Steinbach and J.L.Walden, eds. *Aesthetic plastic surgery*. Philadelphia: Saunders/Elsevier; pp. 437–72.

Bloom, J.D., Kaplan, S.E., Bleier, B.S. and Goldstein, S.A., 2009. Septoplasty complications: avoidance and management. *Otolaryngologic Clinics of North America*, 42 (3), 463–81.

Ghali, G.E. and Harris, C.M., 2007. Cosmetic surgery considerations in the female patient. *Oral and Maxillofacial Surgery Clinics of North America*, 19, 235–44.

Griffin, J.E. and Caloss, R., 2004. Nasal deformities. *Atlas of Oral and Maxillofacial Surgery Clinics of North America*, 12, 31–74.

Haack, J. and Papel, I.D., 2009. Caudal septal deviation. *Otolaryngology Clinics of North America*, 42 (3), 427–36.

Janis, J.E. and Rohrich, R.J., 2007. Rhinoplasty. In: C.H.M.Thorne, R.W. Beasely, S.J.Aston, S.P. Bartlett, G.C. Gurtner and S. Spear, eds. *Grabb and Smith's plastic surgery*. 6th ed. Philadelphia: Lippincott, Williams and Wilkins; Ch. 51.

Miloro, M., Ghali, G.E., Larsen, P.E. and Waite, P.D., 2012. *Peterson's principles of oral and maxillofacial surgery*. 3rd ed. Shelton, CT: PMPH-USA.

Numa, W., Johnson, C.M. and To, W.C. Primary open structure rhinoplasty. In: B. Azizzadeh, M.R. Murphy, C.M. Johnson and W.Numa, eds. *Master techniques in rhinoplasty*. Philadelphia: Saunders; pp. 55–77.

Nurse, L.A. and Duncavage, J.A., 2009. Surgery of the inferior and middle turbinates. *Otolaryngologic Clinics of North America*, 42, 295–309.

Oneal, R.M. and Beil, R.J., 1996. Surgical anatomy of the nose. *Clinics in Plastic Surgery*, 23 (2), 195–222.

Park, S.S., 2011. Fundamental principles in aesthetic rhinoplasty. *(Charlottesville, VA) USACEO Clinical and Experimental Otorhinolaryngology*, 4 (2), 55–66.

Rettinger, G., 2007. Risks and complications in rhinoplasty. *Current Topics in Otorhinolaryngology—Head and Neck Surgery*, 6, Doc08.

Tardy, M.E., 2004. Graduated sculpture refinement of the nasal tip. *Facial and Plastic Surgery Clinics of North America*, 12, 51–80.

Tardy, M.E., Jr., Dayan, S. and Hecht, D., 2002. Preoperative rhinoplasty: evaluation and analysis. *Otolaryngologic Clinics of North America*, 35, 1.

Tasman, A-J., 2007. Rhinoplasty—indications and techniques. *GMS Current Topics in Otorhinolaryngology—Head and Neck Surgery*, 6, Doc09.

Tebbetts, J., 2008. *Primary rhinoplasty*. Amsterdam: Elsevier; Ch. 8.

CHAPTER

Otoplasty

Curtis W. Gaball[1,2] and Matthew Keller[1]

[1]Department of Otolaryngology—Head and Neck Surgery, Naval Medical Center San Diego, San Diego, California, USA
[2]Uniformed Services of the Health Sciences University, San Diego, California, USA

Procedures aimed toward the correction of ear over- and underdevelopment and asymmetries.

Indications

1. Poorly developed or absent antihelical fold
2. Protruding ear (conchal cartilage overdevelopment or hypertrophy)
3. Significant asymmetry (i.e., unilateral protruding ear)

Contraindications

1. Incomplete ear growth (the ear is typically fully developed by age 6)
2. Unrealistic expectations of the patient or family
3. Patients unable to comply with strict postoperative instructions
4. Presence of active ear infection

Anatomy

The auricle is a complex combination of cartilage and skin with many involutions and folds. Its underlying structure is composed of fibroelastic cartilage. The auricle is composed of five critical elements: the concha, helix, antihelix, tragus, and lobule (Figure 43.1).

Initial Examination

The normal auricle protrudes 20–30° from the skull when viewed from the top of the head. The ideal conchomastoid and conchocephalic angles are 90°. The average length and width of the male auricle are 63.5 and 35.5 mm, respectively, compared to 59.0 and 32.5 mm in females. The average ear width should be approximately 60% of the ear length.

During the preoperative evaluation, measurements are typically made at three points (Figure 43.2) to identify ear deformities and asymmetries:

1. The mastoid-helical distance measured from the superior aspect of the helix (normal range: 10–15 mm) (Point A)
2. The mastoid-helical distance measured from the midpoint of the helix (normal range: 16–20 mm) (Point B)

3. The mastoid-helical distance as measured from the level of the lobule (normal range: 20–22 mm) (Point C).

Mustarde Technique (Conchascaphal Suturing): Correction of a Poorly Defined Antihelix

1. Preoperative photos and measurements are taken and are made available for intraoperative reference.
2. Sedation is performed with intravenous, laryngeal mask airway, or endotracheal anesthesia. Intravenous preoperative antibiotics are given based on patient weight. The patient is positioned supine on the operating room table, and ear wicks are placed bilaterally. The face, scalp, neck, and ear are prepped with Betadine or iodine (chlorhexidine may cause damage to the middle ear if a perforation of the tympanic membrane exists, and it can also damage the cornea).
3. Head drapes may be sutured or stapled to the scalp to prevent migration during surgery. Surgical drapes should be positioned to offer simultaneous visibility of both ears in addition to the entire face, and to allow the head to be turned easily from side to side during the procedure.
4. Local anesthetic in the form of 1% lidocaine with 1:100,000 epinephrine is injected horizontally across the lateral surface of the sternocleidomastoid muscle (SCM) at a level 6 cm below the tragus. This will block the greater auricular nerve as it courses superficial to the SCM and will provide anesthesia to the lower ear and lateral cheek. Additional local anesthetic is deposited just behind the postauricular sulcus to block the lesser occipital braches to the posterior pinna and within the areas of the auricle to be surgically manipulated, facilitating hydrodissection of the anterior and posterior skin–soft tissue envelope.
5. Using a #15 blade, a postauricular fusiform skin incision is placed within the postauricular sulcus (Figure 43.3). In planning the incision, account for the fact that the act of retracting the ear forward moves the skin overlying the sulcus laterally. The incision should be kept less

Atlas of Operative Oral and Maxillofacial Surgery, First Edition. Edited by Christopher J. Haggerty and Robert M. Laughlin
© 2015 John Wiley & Sons, Inc. Published 2015 by John Wiley & Sons, Inc.

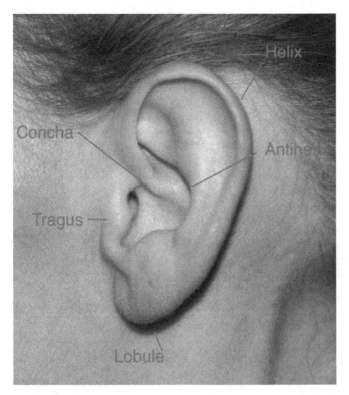

Figure 43.1. Normal external ear landmarks.

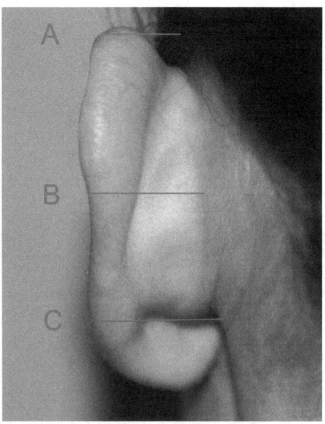

Figure 43.2. Measurements are made at point A, point B, and point C to determine ear deformities and asymmetries.

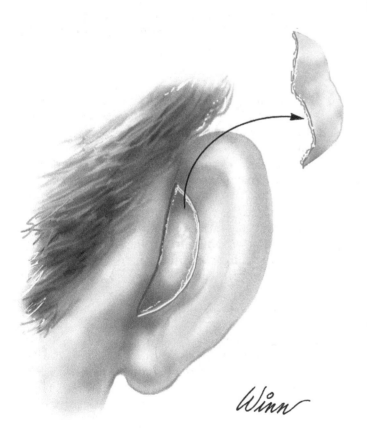

Figure 43.3. When using the Mustarde, Furnas, or combined techniques, a fusiform incision is hidden within the postauricular skin crease.

than 1 cm from the superior and inferior extent of the postauricular crease so that it remains hidden.

6. The postauricular skin over the concha, antihelix, and helical cartilage is undermined with a blunt elevator. The dissection typically does not extend to the helical rim, but can if necessary.

7. To determine the position of the new antihelix, the auricle is bent backward, and a line is marked along its summit. A 30-gauge needle is used to make through and through markings to assist with subsequent suture placement by marking out the arc of the desired antihelical fold along the posterior surface of the cartilage (Figure 43.4). The point at which the needle is protruding on the medial surface of exposed cartilage is marked with a standard marking pen. Alternatively, a 30-gauge needle dipped in Methylene blue dye may be used to mark the cartilage. Repeat along the entire arc of the desired antihelical fold.

8. Optionally, a small incision may be placed at the most cephalic end of the desired antihelical fold on the aurical's lateral surface, hiding the incision under the helical rim. A blunt elevator may be used to create a tunnel under the soft tissue envelope overlying the desired arc of the antihelical fold, and a rasp may be used to abrade the cartilage along this arc, thereby

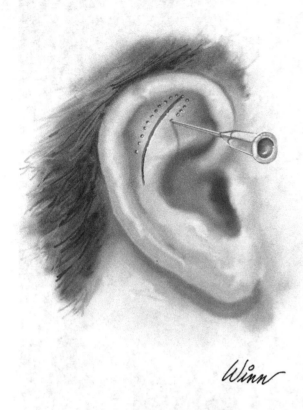

Figure 43.4. In patients with a poorly defined or absent antihelix, the ear is folded against the mastoid process, and the locations of the anticipated antihelical fold and Mustarde sutures are marked.

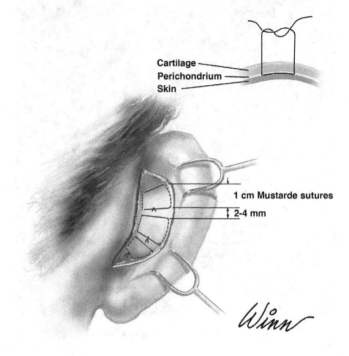

Figure 43.5. 1 cm wide Mustarde sutures are placed 2–4 mm apart and with 16 mm of separation between the outer and inner cartilage edges.

weakening the cartilage and increasing its pliability. Care should be taken to avoid cutting through the cartilage, which can result in an acute angulation and abnormal appearance of the antihelical fold.

9. Using the arc of dots along the posterior cartilaginous surface, 3–4 permanent 4-0 undyed Mersilene horizontal conchascaphal (Mustarde) sutures are used to secure the newly developed antihelical fold (Figure 43.5). It is important to use undyed sutures so that the sutures are not visible through the skin. The sutures should incorporate both the cartilage and perichondrium from the opposite surface. If the opposing perichondrium is not engaged, the suture is more likely to fail because ear cartilage is somewhat friable. Care is taken to not pierce the anterior skin during suture placement. As the Mustarde sutures are placed, lightly pull on the sutures to watch the ear's response to determine if suture placement is ideal, but refrain from tying the sutures at this point. This technique will allow for adjustment of the sutures in order to "fine-tune" the result. Attempt to minimize the number of suture passes, and try to make clean passes using the natural curve of the needle so as not to fracture the friable cartilage.

10. Sutures are not tied until all sutures are placed and their ideal location is verified. Plan for a slight overcorrection, perhaps 2 mm, as some relaxation will occur.

11. Prior to closure, confirm meticulous bipolar hemostasis while avoiding accidental thermal skin injury, ensure that the suture knots are free of hair, and assess surgical correction with preoperative photographs and goal measurements.

12. If performing **conchamastoid suturing (Furnas technique), do so at this point**.

13. Trim excess skin (only if necessary), and close the postauricular skin incision in a tension-free manner with 5-0 plain catgut sutures.

14. If performing surgery on the contralateral ear, ensure the freshly operated ear is carefully tucked while rotating the head so as not to avulse sutures. Furthermore, place a surgical sponge or gauze behind the auricle to prevent hematoma development and to support the ear. Leave a drainage port at the bottom of the incision to allow egress of any oozing while operating on the other side. Milk any blood out of the first side at the end of the case prior to dressing placement.

15. At the completion of the surgery, compare both sides for symmetry (especially from the frontal view, as this is often the most important view to the patient), and assess surgical correction with preoperative photographs and goal measurements. Measurements should be taken from both sides and should be within 2 mm of each other; otherwise, an asymmetry may be evident. Final adjustments are made if necessary.

16. Xeroform dressing is applied to the postauricular sulcus. Gauze is placed circumferentially around the auricle to ensure gentle pressure, especially over the areas of undermined skin dissection. If more exact molding is desired, cotton soaked in a 50:50 mixture of Betadine and mineral oil may be used, forming a soft cast-like dressing.

Furnas Technique (Conchamastoid Sutures): Conchal Setback to Correct Protruding or Prominent Ears

1. Steps 1–4 of the Mustarde technique are followed.
2. A cotton-tipped applicator is used to press the conchal bowl against the mastoid process to the point at which the ear is no longer prominent, typically in a posterior-superior vector. The junction where the concha meets the mastoid process is marked with a line along the posterior conchal wall.
3. An ellipse of postauricular skin is excised to expose the posterior surface of the auricular cartilage (Figure 43.3). The amount of skin excised is estimated using digital pressure to simulate the surgical repair. If uncertain about the amount of skin to remove, make a postauricular sulcus incision, and remove excess skin when closing.
4. Divide the posterior auricular muscle fibers and ligament using Bovie (unipolar) cautery. Care is taken to stay on the lateral surface of the mastoid.
5. The soft tissue overlying the lateral mastoid is debrided to expose a 1×2 cm area of the deep fascia overlying the mastoid process.
6. A full-thickness horizontal 4-0 undyed Merseline mattress suture is passed through the conchal cartilage and opposite perichondrium at the point identified in step 2. Light traction is applied to the suture to ensure the desired effect and to facilitate identification of the ideal point on the mastoid fascia to secure the suture. The vector of pull should be posterior and superior. The suture is passed through the mastoid fascia into the underlying periosteum. Ensure a solid "bite" of this mastoid suture, but do not tie the suture at this point. Place as many sutures as needed to achieve the desired result. Typically, a total of three conchamastoid sutures are required, depending on the character and position of the cartilage.

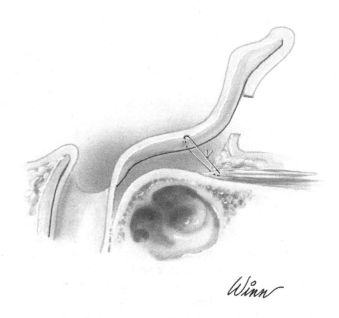

Figure 43.6. Furnas conchamastoid horizontal mattress sutures are passed through the conchal cartilage and anchored to the mastoid fascia in a slightly superior and posterior vector, thus correcting the protruding ear and opening the external auditory canal.

7. The suture knots are tied once all sutures have been placed. As the sutures are tied, ensure the anterior lip of the conchal bowl is not pulled anteriorly, resulting in a narrowed external auditory canal. This is caused by suture bites that are placed either too far anterior on the mastoid or too posterior on the concha, which may lead to stenosis of the external auditory canal. Appropriately placed sutures should pull the ear slightly up and back, thus opening the external auditory canal (Figure 43.6).
8. Steps 11–16 of the Mustarde technique are followed for closure.

Postoperative Management

1. Seven days of postoperative antibiotics with coverage of skin flora and pseudomonas are recommended.
2. A soft, but noncompressive sports headband is placed to protect the ears and to absorb drainage, but not to apply significant pressure to the ears.
3. The patient is seen on postoperative day 1 for dressing removal in order to inspect for hematoma formation. Thereafter, the sports headband is worn at night only for 2 weeks. For patients who may traumatize their ears (active young children), it may be appropriate to recommend more frequent and longer use of the headband according to the surgeon's judgment. Tucking gauze behind the ears while the headband is in

place early in the postoperative period helps minimize hematoma formation and supports the ears in a comfortable position.

4. The auricle may be lightly cleaned with a moist cotton-tip applicator after dressing removal.

5. The patient is reminded that the final postoperative appearance will not be finalized until 6 months postoperatively.

Complications

Early Complications

Hematoma: Hematomas are addressed immediately to minimize the development of infection, chondritis, and cartilage necrosis. Treatment involves opening the incision, evacuation of the hematoma, judicious cauterization of any active bleeding with bipolar cautery, pressure dressings, and frequent wound examinations to identify reforming hematomas.

Infection: Typically presents within the 3–4 days following surgery. Patients present with erythema to the surgical site, drainage, and purulence. Pain may or may not be present. Early infections are treated aggressively with improved wound care and antibiotics to minimize the development of chondritis or perichondritis.

Chondritis: Untreated chondritis may lead to cartilage necrosis and permanent ear deformity.

Skin and cartilage necrosis: Presents as discolored overlying tissue, pain, and auricular deformity. Typically occurs due to improper intraoperative handling of skin and cartilage, excessive use of cautery, damage to the subdermal plexus blood supply, failure to diagnose and evacuate postoperative hematoma, and an excessively tight postoperative pressure dressing.

Late Complications

Suture granuloma formation: Managed by making a small incision and removing the suture knot and as much of the offending suture as reasonably possible. In the author's experience, this does not result in recurrence of prominauris or interauricular asymmetry because it typically occurs weeks to months from the initial procedure after scarring and remodeling have occurred.

Suture extrusion: Typically results from incorrect suture placement, infection, or excessive tension during suture placement. Early suture extrusion with ear deformity is treated with revision surgery to replace the extruded suture. Late suture extrusions frequently require only the removal of the extruded suture provided there is no noticeable ear deformity.

Keloid and hypertrophic scar development: Results from surgery in individuals with darker skin pigmentation, incisions closed with excessive tension, and patients who develop postoperative infections. Keloids are treated with intralesional triamcinolone (40 mg/mL) injections. Hypertrophic scars can be treated with future scar revision surgery.

Postoperative aesthetic complications: Residual deformities, auricular asymmetry, distorted scaphoid fossa (resulting from poor suture placement or overtightening), distorted antihelical fold (resulting from poor suture placement or overtightening), telephone ear (relative prominence of the upper and lower poles of the ear caused by overcorrection of the midportion of the auricle), reverse telephone ear (relative prominence of the middle pole of the ear caused by an imbalanced correction), and overcorrection (ear too flat against head). Noticeable cases of postoperative aesthetic deformities require revision surgery to correct the specific deformity.

Key Points

1. Surgery is best performed when the cartilage has reached adequate consistency, size, and maturity, typically 6 years of age and older. Ideally, the repair is performed prior to the child becoming school aged to circumvent peer ridicule.

2. As a general rule, pediatric patients are typically managed with general anesthesia, whereas adult patients are typically managed with intravenous sedation with profound local anesthesia.

3. Otoplasty procedures are commonly performed to correct both an underdevelopment of the antihelix and a protruding auricle (overdevelopment of the conchal cartilage). If both Furnas and Mustarde procedures are performed, it is recommended that conchascaphal (Mustarde) suturing be performed first.

4. With pure suturing techniques (cartilage is not excised or incised), there are no irreversible changes, and the surgeon is free to adjust sutures until the desired result is achieved.

5. Cuts through cartilage, particularly when combined with suture recontouring, can result in noticeable contour deformities such as abnormal ridges or buckles.

6. It is important to achieve symmetry with the contralateral ear. The goal should be less than 0.5 cm difference between the sides when viewed anteriorly. The senior author tolerates a maximum of 2 mm difference intraoperatively to account for postoperative relaxation. A discussion is made with the patient or parents prior to surgery that absolute symmetry may not be achieved and that minor asymmetries are acceptable and rarely noticed.

Case Report 43.1. A 29-year-old female presents with a chief complaint of protruding ears bilaterally. Preoperative photos demonstrate a prominent middle and lower third of the ear caused by an excessive conchomastoid angle. The patient denied previous trauma to her auricles. The patients ear projection was measured at 25 mm at the middle third of the ear (point B) bilaterally with prominent conchal bowls. The patient had an

appropriately developed antihelix. The patient underwent a revision septorhinoplasty at the time of bilateral otoplasty. A cartilage graft was harvested from her left conchal bowl to assist with the septorhinoplasty. With her ear prominence predominantly affecting the middle third of her ear, she was treated with the Furnas technique (conchamastoid suture placement). (See Figures 43.7, 43.8, 43.9, and 43.10.)

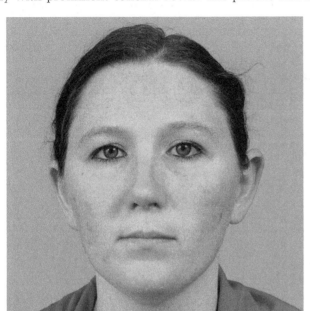

Figure 43.7.   Preoperative photograph illustrating bilateral excessively protruding ears.

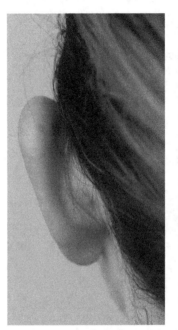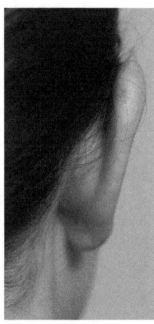

Figure 43.8.   Patient demonstrates bilateral conchal bowl hypertrophy with significant overgrowth of the middle third of the conchal cartilage.

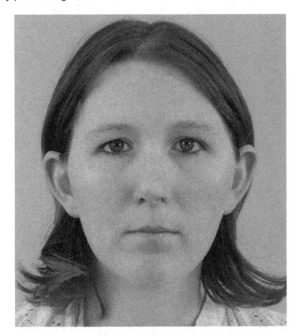

Figure 43.9.   Patient 1 year after bilateral otoplasty using the Furnas technique to correct her bilateral protruding ears.

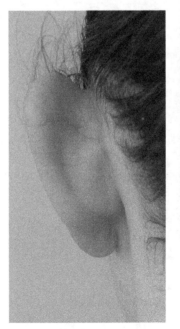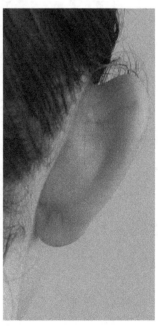

Figure 43.10.   1-year postoperative images depicting correction of bilateral conchal cartilage hypertrophy.

References

Adamson, P.A. and Litner, J.A., 2007. Otoplasty technique. *Otolaryngologic Clinics of North America*, 40 (2), 305–18.

Azuara, E., 2000. Aesthetic otoplasty with remodeling of the antihelix for the correction of the prominent ear. *Archives of Facial and Plastic Surgery*, 2 (1), 57–61.

Caouette-Laberge, L., Guay, N., Bortoluzzi, P. and Belleville, C., 2000. Otoplasty: anterior scoring technique and results in 500 cases. *Plastic and Reconstructive Surgery*, 105 (2), 504–15.

Dudley, W.H., Peet, A.L. and Flaggert, J.J., 1995. Otoplasty for correction of the prominent ear. *Journal of Oral and Maxillofacial Surgery*, 53, 1386–91.

Fritsch, M.H., 2009. Incisionless otoplasty. *Otolaryngologic Clinics of North America*, 42 (6), 1199–208.

Furnas, D., 1968. Correction of prominent ears by concha-mastoid sutures. *Plastic and Reconstructive Surgery*, 42(3), 189–93.

Furnas, D.W., 1978. Correction of prominent ears with multiple sutures. *Clinics in Plastic Surgery*, 5 (3), 491.

Handler, E.B., Song, T. and Shih, C., 2010. Complications of otoplasty. *Facial and Plastic Surgery Clinics of North America*, 21 (2103), 653–62.

Hoehn, J.G. and Ashruf, S., 2005. Otoplasty: sequencing the operation for improved results. *Plastic and Reconstructive Surgery*, 115 (1), 5e–16e.

Nachlas, N.E., 2008. Otoplasty. In: *Facial plastic and reconstructive surgery*. 3rd ed. New York: Thieme Medical Publishers; pp. 421–33.

Oswley, T., 2004. Otoplastic surgery for the protruding ear. *Atlas of Oral and Maxillofacial Surgery Clinics of North America*, 12 (1), 131–9.

Sclafani, A. and Mashkevich, G., 2006. Aesthetic reconstruction of the auricle. *Facial and Plastic Surgery Clinics of North America*, 14 (2), 103–16.

Sevin, K. and Sevin, A., 2006. Otoplasty with Mustarde suture, cartilage rasping, and scratching. *Aesthetic Plastic Surgery*, 30 (4), 437–41.

PART SEVEN

PATHOLOGY AND RECONSTRUCTIVE SURGERY

44

Benign Cysts of the Jaws

Christopher M. Harris[1] and Robert M. Laughlin[2]

[1]Department of Oral and Maxillofacial Surgery, Naval Medical Center Portsmouth, Portsmouth, Virginia, USA
[2]Department of Oral and Maxillofacial Surgery, Naval Medical Center San Diego, San Diego, California, USA

A cyst is defined as a space-occupying lesion with a connective-tissue outer wall and an inner wall (typically, epithelial tissues) lining. They are typically unilocular or multilocular radiolucencies with sclerotic borders. Cystic lesions of the jaws are divided into odontogenic cysts and non-odontogenic cystic lesions. Cysts typically have the following characteristics:

1. Epithelium lining and fluid filled
2. Occupy space, and displace or replace normal surrounding tissues
3. May resorb or displace adjacent teeth
4. May cause expansion of the bone
5. May cause neurosensory changes
6. Generally do not affect tooth vitality.

Odontogenic cysts arise from the enamel organ. The epithelial sources are the cell rests of Malassez, reduced enamel epithelium, and remnants of the dental lamina. Common non-odontogenic cystic lesions include the traumatic bone cavity, aneurysmal bone cysts, and nasopalatine cysts. All lesions should be treated individually based on their unique histopathology, aggressiveness, and clinical and radiographic presentation. *Please refer to Appendix 3 for further treatment guidelines.*

Odontogenic Cysts

Periapical Cysts

These cystic lesions arise from a necrotic dental pulp as a result of dental caries or trauma. Histologically, periapical cysts are inflammatory cysts with stratified squamous epithelial linings. Clinically, pulp testing should be completed to verify the presence of a necrotic pulp. Root canal therapy, apical surgery, or extraction of the offending tooth is required for necrotic pulps. Frequently, the authors have encountered cystic lesions associated with a root canal–treated tooth that are not periapical cysts histologically. Determination of tooth vitality is paramount to avoid unnecessary and costly endodontic therapy. Enucleation and curettage, as well as extraction or endodontic therapy of the offending tooth, are required for treatment. Small periapical cysts or granulomas (<1 cm) may resolve without surgical therapy. Recurrence after enucleation and curettage is not expected.

Dentigerous Cysts

Dentigerous cysts are believed to arise from an accumulation of fluid between the crown of an unerupted tooth. The epithelial origin is believed to be the reduced enamel epithelium of the dental follicle. Dentigerous cysts typically occur within the second and third decades of life. Radiographically, these lesions are associated with the crown of an unerupted tooth and are radiolucent. Dentigerous cysts vary in size and produce no calcified structures. Dentigerous cysts are treated by enucleation. Large dentigerous cysts may be treated with marsupialization, especially if wide surgical access is difficult to obtain. Recurrence is rare. Histologic studies of the entire lining are required due to the potential presence of a mural ameloblastoma.

Keratinizing Odontogenic Tumor (Odontogenic Keratocyst)

The odontogenic keratocyst (OKC) has been described by the World Health Organization as a keratinizing odontogenic tumor (KOT). This is primarily due to its aggressive behaviors, which more resemble those of an invasive tumor, and its high recurrence rates compared to a "benign" cyst. OKCs occur over a wide age range, peaking within the second and third decades of life. Histologically, the basement membrane is flattened and corrugated, and has basal palisading of the epithelial cells with parakeratin noted. Within the lumen, large amounts of keratin may be noted. Radiographically, OKCs can present as unilocular or multilocular radiolucencies and can present as small, non-expansile lesions or very large, expansile lesions (Figures 44.1, 44.2, and 44.3). OKCs have recurrence rates approaching 25–30%. Multiple OKCs may be seen in patients with nevoid basal cell syndrome (Gorlin's syndrome). Treatment for these lesions includes long-term decompression or marsupialization (with or without future enucleation and curettage), enucleation and curettage with adjunctive liquid nitrogen application, aggressive removal of adjacent cyst cavity bone (peripheral ostectomy), application of Carnoy's solution to the cystic cavity, and/or resection. Resection may be considered for large lesions that perforate the cortex,

Atlas of Operative Oral and Maxillofacial Surgery, First Edition. Edited by Christopher J. Haggerty and Robert M. Laughlin.

are difficult to access and visualize, and for recurrent lesions. Inadequate removal of cystic remnants may lead to a recurrence in an area of the maxillofacial region that is difficult or impossible to surgically treat (e.g., the posterior maxilla or ramus–condyle regions). Long-term follow-up is recommended due to the high percentage of recurrence, especially with enucleation and curettage.

Calcifying Odontogenic Cyst (Gorlin's Cyst)

The calcifying odontogenic cyst (COC) is unique in that it is the only odontogenic cyst that produces calcified structures. Radiographically, a COC can present as a mixed, radiolucent, or radiopaque lesion. These cysts have also been reported to arise in conjunction with other lesions, such as odontomas and ameloblastic fibro-odontomas. COCs are typically identified in adults through the third and fifth decades. Histologically, the cysts demonstrate an odontogenic epithelium, a palisaded basement membrane with reverse polarity, loose stellate reticulum–appearing cells, and eosinophilic "ghost cells." Ghost cells may calcify, leading to the calcified structures within radiographs. Rarely, these cysts can take on clinical and histologic characteristics of odontogenic tumors. COCs are treated with enucleation and curettage. Recurrence is uncommon. Histologic review of these lesions is required to rule out other more aggressive lesions associated with these cysts.

Non-odontogenic Cysts

Traumatic Bone Cyst (Idiopathic Bone Cavity)

Histologically, the traumatic bone cyst is not a true cystic lesion. The name suggests a traumatic origin, but there is little evidence to support this hypothesis. Traumatic bone cysts are commonly identified in adolescents and young adults. Teeth are generally vital and are not displaced. Traumatic bone cysts are unilocular radiolucencies that may scallop superiorly into the alveolus and between teeth roots. They may be expansile and are generally asymptomatic. Upon biopsy, an empty cavity is encountered without a discernible cystic lining. Curettage of the cavity stimulates bleeding into the cavity and generally causes bone formation. Typically, no further treatment is required. Serial films are obtained to ensure bone fill of the area. Recurrence is typically not seen.

Aneurysmal Bone Cyst

Like the traumatic bone cyst, this lesion is not a true cystic lesion. The mandible is the most common maxillofacial site involved. These lesions are typically unilocular radiolucencies and may be expansile and painful.

Teeth are vital. Tooth mobility, root displacement, and/or resorption may be seen. No bruit or thrill is appreciated. Aspiration may produce hemorrhagic fluid. On histopathologic exam, hemorrhagic tissue with endothelial cells, connective tissue, and possibly multinucleated giant cells may be seen. Treatment is curettage, typically done at the time of excisional biopsy. Large, destructive lesions may require resection. Bleeding is typically encountered upon opening of the region, but it is usually controlled with the removal of the lesion. Aneurysmal bone cysts can be considered a low-flow vascular lesion. Recurrence is rare with complete removal of the lesion. Serial radiographic follow-up is performed to ensure bone fill of the area.

Nasopalatine Duct Cyst

Nasopalatine duct cysts originate from the epithelial remnants of the nasopalatine duct, which typically disappears prior to birth. The cyst is located between the central incisors and may grow large enough to be palpable behind the central incisors on the palate. The teeth are vital. Radiographically, the cyst presents as a large radiolucency involving the incisive canal and central incisors. Small lesions are asymptomatic. Symptomatic nasopalatine duct cysts (i.e., those with pain and/or swelling) suggest an underlying infection. Pain, swelling, and/or continued enlargement warrant surgical excision. Recurrence is rare.

Procedure: Enucleation and Curettage

1. The patient is placed in a supine position. After endotracheal intubation, the patient is prepped and draped in a sterile fashion.
2. Local anesthetic containing a vasoconstrictor is infiltrated within the area of the lesion, and regional blocks may also be utilized.
3. The flap design should be such that allows for the final incision closure to be placed over supporting bone to prevent tension from the invagination of the tissues within the enucleated cavity, resulting in dehiscence of the site.
4. Wide surgical access can typically be obtained with a sulcular incision; care should be taken to avoid tearing the mucosal flap. If vertical releasing incisions are required, they should be designed such that the base of the flap is wider than the apex.
5. A full-thickness mucoperiosteal flap is elevated to expose the outer cortex of the lesion.
6. An 18-gauge needle should be inserted into the center of the lesion and aspirated (Figure 44.4). This allows the surgeon to determine if the lesion is of vascular origin.
7. A handpiece or Kerrison ronguer may be used to remove the outer cortex overlying the lesion.

8. Curettes are used to elevate the lesion off of the bony wall circumferentially (Figure 44.7). Care should be made not to tear or perforate the lesion.
9. The lesion is sent for final pathology (Figure 44.8).
10. The bone cavity should be painted with methylene blue to mark all aspects where the lesion and bone were in contact.
11. Using a diamond bur, a peripheral ostectomy (Figure 44.9) is performed on all marked surfaces. The peripheral ostectomy may also be performed with curettes.
12. The site is irrigated with copious amounts of sterile water to remove all debris from the surgical site.
13. Biological membranes may be used to overlay the surgical site or cavity.
14. The flap is repositioned and secured with individual horizontal mattress sutures interdentally with a resorbable suture. If vertical releasing flaps were used, they are closed in a standard fashion.
15. A periodontal pack dressing may be used to protect the surgical site. The dressing remains in place for approximately one week and is removed at the follow-up appointment.

Key Points

1. For large cysts, incisional biopsies are recommended so that the surgical approach and definitive treatment can be based on the aggressiveness and recurrence rates of the type of cyst involved.
2. Wide surgical access is key to successful enucleation in order to allow for adequate visualization of the entire cystic cavity.
3. Every attempt should be made to remove the cyst in its entirety to minimize recurrence. Aggressive cysts (odontogenic keratocysts) are treated with curettage and/or peripheral ostectomy (Figure 44.9) following enucleation.
4. Immediate reconstruction is warranted for lesions removed in their entirety and for lesions with low recurrence rates. Damaged adjacent structures (i.e., the nasal septum) should be repaired at the time of cyst enucleation.
5. For large cysts that have significantly weakened the surrounding bone, the placement of prophylactic rigid fixation is often necessary to prevent iatrogenic fracture of the mandible at the time of cyst removal or within the early postoperative period.

Case Report

Case Report 44.1. A 17-year-old male presents with a referral from his dentist for the evaluation and treatment of his third molars. An orthopantomogram demonstrated a grossly displaced tooth #1 and a fluid level within the right maxillary sinus (Figure 44.1). On questioning, the patient reported right-sided obstructed nasal breathing and congestion. A computed tomography scan was obtained that suggested a large cystic structure obliterating the right maxillary sinus with penetration into the right nasal cavity (Figures 44.2 and 44.3). Aspiration of the area produced a clear, straw-colored fluid (Figure 44.4). An incisional biopsy was performed through a lateral sinus approach (Figure 44.5), and a cystic lining was encountered and biopsied. Histopathological slide analysis suggested an odontogenic keratocyst. Due to the size, location, and recurrence rate of the cyst, wide surgical access was obtained via a Le Fort I osteotomy. Erich arch bars were placed, the osteotomy design was marked with a sterile pen, and mini-plates were secured to the uncut maxilla (Figure 44.6) prior to osteotomy. The mini-plates were removed, and the Le Fort I osteotomy was performed. The cyst was enucleated in its entirety (Figures 44.7 and 44.8), and a peripheral ostectomy was performed with a large round bur (Figure 44.9). The right inferior turbinate was in contact with the cyst and was removed with the specimen. A septoplasty and nasal antrostomy were also performed to improve nasal breathing. The patient was placed into maxillomandibular fixation, and the pre-bent mini-plates were secured to the maxilla using the predrilled screw holes. The Le Fort I osteotomy provided excellent access to the maxillary sinus and nasal cavity, allowed for repair of involved and damaged structures, and resulted in no external scars or changes in the patient's overall appearance (Figure 44.10).

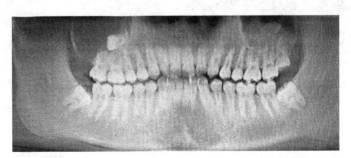

Figure 44.1. Orthopantomogram demonstrating a malpositioned tooth #1 and fluid level within the right maxillary sinus.

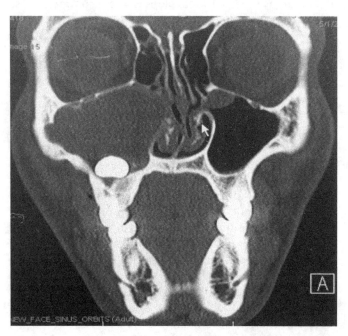

Figure 44.2. Coronal computed tomography scan demonstrating a mass obliterating the right maxillary sinus. The mass has penetrated through the lateral nasal wall and entered the right nasal cavity.

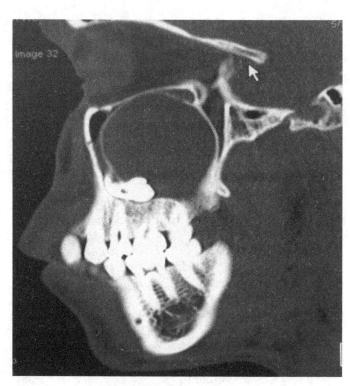

Figure 44.3. Sagittal computed tomography scan depicting a cystic mass within the maxillary sinus.

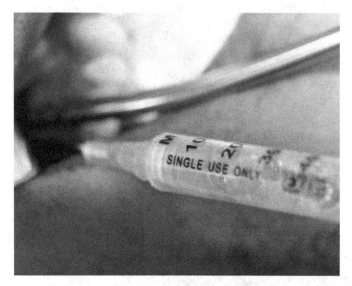

Figure 44.4. Aspiration of the mass produced a straw-colored fluid.

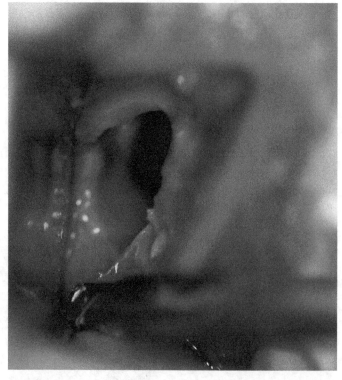

Figure 44.5. An incisional biopsy was performed through a lateral sinus window approach.

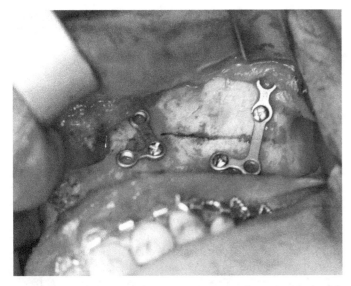

Figure 44.6.   The proposed Le Fort I osteotomy is marked and mini-plates are pre-bent and secured to the maxilla.

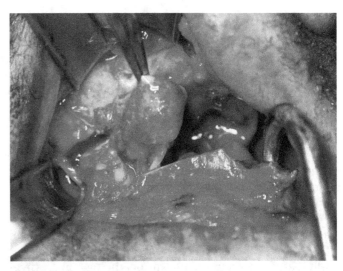

Figure 44.7.   The Le Fort I osteotomy provides wide surgical access to the maxillary sinus, nasal cavity, inferior turbinates, and nasal septum.

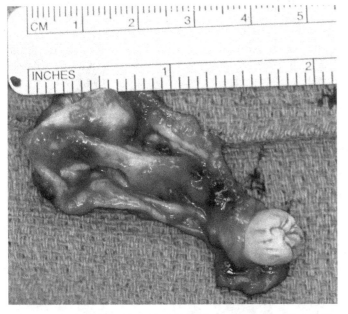

Figure 44.8.   The impacted tooth and the cystic lining removed in their entirety.

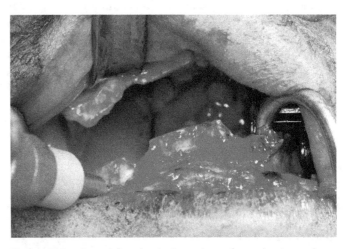

Figure 44.9.   A peripheral ostectomy is performed using a large round bur.

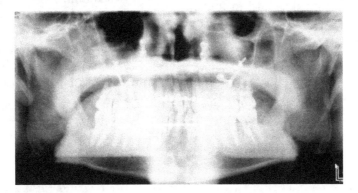

Figure 44.10.   Postoperative orthopantomogram.

Benign Tumors of the Jaws

Christopher M. Harris[1] and Robert M. Laughlin[2]
[1]Department of Oral and Maxillofacial Surgery, Naval Medical Center Portsmouth, Portsmouth, Virginia, USA
[2]Department of Oral and Maxillofacial Surgery, Naval Medical Center San Diego, San Diego, California, USA

Non-odontogenic Tumors

Non-odontogenic tumors include connective-tissue tumors, vascular lesions, reactive lesions, and neurogenic tumors. The clinical presentation and treatment of these lesions vary. This section will describe the general classification of common non-odontogenic tumors and highlight standard treatments. All lesions should be treated individually based on their unique histopathology, aggressiveness, and clinical and radiographic presentation. *Please refer to Appendix 3 for further treatment guidelines.*

Tumors of Connective Tissue

Osteomas

Osteomas are benign tumors of bone. They are commonly found within the skull, jaws, and sinuses. Osteomas are composed of cortical and cancellous bone in varying proportions. These lesions typically present as an asymptomatic mass, which can produce asymmetry of the jaw bones. Radiographically, these lesions appear as dense radiopaque projections of bone. Gardner's syndrome should be suspected in patients presenting with multiple osteomas. Gardner's syndrome is associated with multiple osteomas, polyps of the large intestine, multiple epidermal skin cysts, and multiple impacted teeth. The colon polyps in Gardner's syndrome are considered premalignant, and a referral to a colon and rectal surgeon is recommended due to the certain malignant transformation of these lesions. Treatment is with tumor excision. Recurrence is rare.

Osteoblastomas

Osteoblastomas are rare, benign tumors of bone. They commonly occur in the long bones and spinal column. They have a peak incidence within the third to fourth decades of life and occur more frequently in males. The mandible is the most commonly affected craniofacial bone. Osteoblastomas may be asymptomatic and found on routine exam. However, localized pain and swelling are commonly seen. Pain is unique in that in many cases it is relieved by aspirin. Radiographically, the osteoblastoma can resemble other benign and malignant tumors. Osteoblastomas are typically radiolucent (early) with radiopaque structures within the lesion (later). The lesions can be well defined or poorly defined. The lesions often have a radiolucent rim associated with them. Teeth may be displaced, and/or resorption of roots may be seen. Histologically, the osteoblastoma is similar to the osteoid osteoma. These are differentiated mainly by clinical features and size. Osteoblastomas demonstrate osteoid tissue and interconnected trabeculae of woven bone. These trabeculae are surrounded by a single layer of osteoblasts referred to as osteoblastic rimming. A fibrovascular stroma and osteoclasts are also seen. Aggressive osteoblastomas and low-grade osteosarcomas can look similar histologically. Treatment of osteoblastomas is with excision or aggressive curettage. Recurrence is uncommon with appropriate treatment. Recurrence is believed to arise from incomplete removal rather than inherent properties of the lesion. Aggressive osteoblastomas, however, have been reported to have higher recurrence rates and often require resection with definitive margins.

Chondromas

Chondromas are benign cartilaginous lesions of the jaws. They may occur centrally or peripherally. They are exceedingly rare in the head and neck. They are thought to arise in areas where embryonic cartilaginous cell rests are present. Therefore, the condyle, coronoid process, base of skull, and anterior maxilla are commonly involved sites. Radiographically, chondromas are well-demarcated radiolucencies. Local bone destruction should raise suspicion for malignancy. Chondromas have a peak incidence within the third and fourth decades of life and demonstrate an equal sex predilection. Histologically, they demonstrate mature hyaline cartilage. Treatment should be directed at total tumor excision due to the similarities of low-grade chondrosarcomas histologically.

Vascular and Reactive Lesions

Central Giant Cell Granulomas (CGCGs)

CGCGs are generally accepted to be nonneoplastic entities that behave like neoplasms. Whether these lesions are inflammatory, reactive, or true neoplasms is still debated.

Atlas of Operative Oral and Maxillofacial Surgery, First Edition. Edited by Christopher J. Haggerty and Robert M. Laughlin
© 2015 John Wiley & Sons, Inc. Published 2015 by John Wiley & Sons, Inc.

The lesions have been described as nonaggressive and aggressive. Aggressive lesions can cause pain, root resorption, cortical expansion and perforation, mucosal involvement, and higher recurrence rates after treatment. Nonaggressive lesions tend to be asymptomatic and do not have the above features. CGCGs have a peak incidence within the third, fourth, and fifth decades of life and have a higher predilection in females. Radiographically, these lesions can appear as unilocular or multilocular radiolucencies with noncorticated borders. Histologically, CGCGs demonstrate multinucleated giant cells (osteoclasts) scattered within a spindle cell background. Hemosiderin and erythrocytes may be seen. Fibrosis, osteoid, and bone may also be seen. Histological similarities to Brown tumors and aneurysmal bone cysts are noted. Hyperparathyroidism should be ruled out in these patients. Aneurysmal bone cysts may be a cystic variant of CGCGs. Cherubism also has similar histologic findings, but can usually be ruled out with clinical findings.

Various treatment modalities have been described in the current literature. Surgical curettage has a nearly 20% recurrence rate. Intralesional steroid injections have been used with mixed results. The protocol typically used includes a 50/50 mixture of lidocaine and triamcinolone, injecting 2 mL per 1 cm of lesion. Intralesional steroid injections are typically performed weekly for a total of 6 weeks. Calcitonin injections (100 μ/day) have been performed for up to 24 months with reported success. Subcutaneous interferon therapy has also been utilized. Nonsurgical treatments modalities frequently do not resolve the CGCG, but may allow for surgical intervention with less morbidity and cosmetic deformity and should be considered for large lesions. CGCGs that exhibit aggressive behavior, are recurrent or are refractory to intralesional steroid injections may be treated with peripheral ostectomy or resection with 5–10 mm margins.

Central Hemangiomas

Hemangiomas are benign proliferations of vascular tissues. It is debated whether hemangiomas are a proliferation of endothelium (true neoplasm) or a hamartomatous proliferation of mesoderm, which undergoes endothelial differentiation. Regardless of the etiology, they are potentially life-threatening entities. They are most commonly identified within the posterior mandible, but are otherwise rare within the jaws. They have a peak incidence within the first and second decades of life and a female predilection. Hemangiomas typically present as painless, firm swellings of the underlying bone. Patients may report a pulsation over the lesion. Teeth may be mobile with bleeding around the gingival margins. A bruit and thrill may be present. However, many hemangiomas are asymptomatic and present with none of the above findings. Radiographically, the lesions may be unilocular or multilocular radiolucencies. The multilocular variant has been described as the classic soap bubble or honeycomb appearance. Root resorption and cortical expansion with thinning may be seen, and phleboliths may be noted. There is no absolute pathognomonic radiographic finding for central hemangiomas; therefore, all lesions within the jaws should be initially treated as if they have a vascular component. Lesions that are suspicious for hemangiomas should undergo needle aspiration prior to biopsy. Aspirations that reveal frank blood are nearly pathognomonic for a vascular lesion. Angiography is required prior to any surgical manipulation of these lesions due to the potential for life-threatening hemorrhage and airway embarrassment. Angiography can demonstrate the borders of the lesion and afferent feeding vessels, and can be utilized for selective embolization prior to surgical removal. Embolization therapy with surgical removal (curettage or resection) the surgical ligation of afferent vessels, followed by surgical removal (curettage or resection), are the preferred therapies. Recurrence rates are low with complete removal of the lesion.

Fibrous Dysplasia (FD)

FD is a benign, non-encapsulated neoplasm characterized by cellular fibrous connective tissue and irregular islands of metaplastic bone replacing normal bone. FD occurs by mutations of the gene GNAS-1 (guanine nucleotide-binding protein, α-stimulating activity polypeptide-1). Postnatal mutations will cause localized monostotic disease. Mutations affecting stem cells in embryonic stages will cause systemic conditions (i.e., Jaffe–Lichenstein or McCune-Albright syndromes) characterized by defects in multiple cell lines resulting in multiple bone and cutaneous lesions, as well endocrine abnormalities.

FD commonly is discovered within the second decade of life. Sex predilection is equal. The lesions are typically nonpainful and expansile. Displacement of adjacent structures is common. Maxillary involvement is more prevalent than mandibular involvement. With maxillary involvement, other adjacent facial bones may be involved. This is described as craniofacial fibrous dysplasia. Growth generally ceases with skeletal maturation. Radiographs demonstrate an expansile "ground-glass" lesion with poorly defined borders. Histologically, the lesion is characterized by a cellular fibrous tissue with woven bone trabeculae that do not connect interspersed throughout this background. The bone trabeculae have been classically described as resembling "Chinese characters." The edges of the lesion fuse with the normal bone without a capsule. Treatment involves resection of small lesions. Surgical reduction and contouring are performed with larger lesions that cause functional or aesthetic concerns. In up to 50% of cases, repeated debulking procedures are necessary until growth ceases. Long-term surveillance is needed due to the possibility of malignant transformation.

Odontogenic Tumors

Odontogenic tumors arise from structures involved with tooth formation. Benign odontogenic tumors encompass a variety of lesions within the jaws. Odontogenic tumors vary significantly both histologically and with their clinical behavior. Many odontogenic tumors are true benign neoplasms, whereas others are extremely aggressive, locally destructive lesions. Malignant variants of these lesions are also encountered. This section will describe the general classification of these tumors and highlight *commonly* encountered lesions. All lesions should be treated individually based on their unique histopathology, aggressiveness, and clinical and radiographic presentation. *Please refer to Appendix 3A for further treatment guidelines.*

Benign odontogenic tumors can be characterized by the embryonic tissue of origin. Classifications include (i) odontogenic epithelium, (ii) odontogenic ectomesenchyme (primarily), and (iii) mixed odontogenic epithelium and ectomesenchyme. Ectomesenchymal tumors may have odontogenic epithelium histologically, but they are not believed to play a significant role in the pathogenesis. The classic odontogenic epithelial tumors are the ameloblastoma and the calcifying epithelial odontogenic tumor (CEOT). Ectomesenchymal tumors include the odontogenic myxoma and cementoblastoma. Mixed tumors include the ameloblastic fibroma and fibroodontoma or odontoma lesions.

Odontogenic Epithelial Tumors

Ameloblastomas

Ameloblastomas are one of the most commonly encountered benign odontogenic tumors. There are several histological variants and three major clinical variants. The major clinical variants include the multicystic or solid variant, the unicystic variant, and the peripheral ameloblastoma.

The multicystic or solid variant can be locally invasive and destructive. These lesions are typically slow growing and show little tendency to become aggressive (i.e., malignant). The most common location is within the posterior mandible, but they can occur in other locations of both jaws. One exception is the desmoplastic variant, which tends to occur within the anterior maxilla. Most cases occur in adulthood and are typically asymptomatic, exhibiting no neurosensory changes. Radiographically, these lesions are typically multilocular and expansile in nature. Radiopacities are not seen with ameloblastomas. The standard treatment is resection with 1 to 1.5 cm bony margins. For lesions that have perforated through the cortical plate and/or extended into adjacent areas, an intact anatomical boundary (i.e., periosteum) is included with the specimen. Recurrence is rare with definitive negative margins. Long-term follow-up is required.

The unicystic ameloblastoma is less common than the solid variant. The tumor's origin and whether it arises de novo or from neoplastic cystic transformation are still debated. Typically, these lesions occur in young adults within the posterior mandible. They are frequently associated with impacted third molars and can be mistaken for a cystic lesion (i.e., a dentigerous cyst or odontogenic keratocyst). Clinically, they may be asymptomatic or demonstrate a painless jaw swelling. Pain and neurosensory disturbance are not typical. Radiographically, unicystic ameloblastomas present as a unilocular radiolucency with or without expansion. The unicystic ameloblastoma varies in treatment depending on the histological findings of the tumor.

Three histological types are seen with unicystic ameloblastomas. These are the luminal, intraluminal, and mural ameloblastoma. These ameloblastic changes tend to support the concept of an evolving spectrum of neoplastic transformation of odontogenic cysts. Luminal unicystic ameloblastomas have ameloblastoma tumor confined within the cystic lining itself. Intraluminal variants have projections of ameloblastoma into the cystic lumen. Mural ameloblastomas have tumor that is within the cystic lining and invades the surrounding noncystic regions of the surrounding tissue. Treatment of the luminal and intraluminal unicystic ameloblastoma is typically complete with enucleation of the cyst. Marginal or segmental resections may be warranted for mural unicystic ameloblastomas due to the invasion of surrounding tissue. Long-term follow-up is recommended for all variants.

The peripheral ameloblastoma is histologically identical to the intraosseous ameloblastomas; however, they are alveolar mucosal lesions. They are typically small (<2.0 cm), non-ulcerated, nonpainful, and located within the posterior mandibular alveolar mucosa. Treatment consists of local excision with long-term follow-up as the recurrence rate is approximately 15%.

Calcifying Epithelial Odontogenic Tumors (Pindborg Tumors)

Calcifying epithelial odontogenic tumors (CEOT) behave as aggressive, benign lesions arising from odontogenic epithelium. Like the ameloblastoma, these lesions can be locally destructive and invasive. They are commonly identified within the posterior mandible, but can be found in other regions. Patients typically present with a painless expansion of the posterior mandible. Radiographically, CEOTs are typically multilocular and expansile, and demonstrate calcifications. Histologically, amyloid deposits with calcified ringlike structures called Liesgang rings are noted. Treatment of the CEOT is similar to the ameloblastoma with marginal or segmental resection with 1.0 cm margins. Recurrence rates have been reported at approximately 15%. Enucleation and curettage procedures are associated with higher recurrence rates.

Odontogenic Adenomatoid Tumors (OATs)

OATs are non-aggressive benign neoplasms arising from odontogenic epithelium. OATs occur more frequently in females with a peak incidence within the second decade of life, and they frequently involve an unerupted canine. OATs have been coined the two-thirds tumor: two-thirds occur in females, two-thirds occur in the maxilla, two-thirds are associated with unerupted teeth, and two-thirds are associated with canines. OATs can produce swelling if they are large; however, most are small, asymptomatic, and incidentally found on routine imaging. Radiographically, these lesions can be radiopaque or have small radiopaque structures within the lesion. The entire structure of an unerupted tooth is frequently involved. This differs from the dentigerous cyst, which tends to involve only the crown of the involved tooth. Large lesions may cause tooth displacement. Histologically, odontogenic epithelium is seen with ductlike structures possessing a lumen lined with a single row of low columnar cells with reverse polarization. Intraluminal eosinophilic material and scattered calcifications may also be seen. Clinically, OATs have a well-formed capsule with excision. Treatment is enucleation with the removal of the involved tooth. Recurrence rates are low.

Ectomesenchymal Tumors

Odontogenic Myxomas

Odontogenic myxomas are aggressive lesions that can arise in both jaws; however, mandibular involvement is more common. Patients may be asymptomatic or have a painless jaw swelling depending on the size of the lesion. Odontogenic myxomas have a peak incidence within the second and third decades of life and appear to have no sexual predilection. Radiographically, the lesions are typically multilocular with thin bone trabeculae noted. Expansion, cortical thinning, and tooth resorption or displacement are common. Impacted teeth are not necessarily seen with the lesion. Histologically, the lesion resembles dental pulp due to the mesenchymal tissue origin. Randomly arranged spindle cells within a loose myxoid stroma with minimal collagen fibrils scattered within are typical. Odontogenic epithelial rests and bone trabeculae are also noted. The lesions are not encapsulated and tend to penetrate bone further than their radiographic depiction. Due to this, the recommended treatment is marginal or segmental resection with 1.5 cm margins and an uninvolved anatomic boundary. Enucleation or curettage is reserved for only easily accessible and small lesions. Routine follow-up is recommended for enucleated lesions due to their propensity to recur.

Cementoblastomas

The cementoblastoma is a benign tumor of hamartomatous cementoblasts, which form a tumor of disorganized cementum. The lesion develops around the apical half of premolar and molar teeth, typically mandibular. Pain may be associated with the lesions. Radiographically, a radiopaque mass involving the roots of the teeth with a radiolucent border is seen. The involved teeth will typically test as vital with pulp testing. Areas of noncalcified tissue in the area of the radiolucent rimming are also seen. Histologically, cementum-like proliferation continuous with the tooth root is noted. Root resorption may be seen. Treatment consists of excision of the lesion and removal of the tooth. Recurrence is not expected.

Ossifying Fibromas (Cemento Ossifying Fibroma)

Ossifying fibromas are a type of benign fibro-osseous tumor. These lesions can arise in both jaws, but they have a predilection for the mandible. These lesions are thought to arise from the periodontal ligament. The premolar and molar regions are commonly affected. The lesions are slow growing, expansile, and typically not painful. Facial asymmetry is noted with larger lesions. Women are affected more frequently than men. Early lesions may appear completely radiolucent. With maturation, radiopacities appear, and the lesion will eventually become completely radiopaque with a radiolucent rim. The lesions are expansile in all directions and are therefore typically spherical in shape. Treatment is with enucleation and curettage for most lesions. Clinically, these lesions easily shell out of the affected bone. Larger lesions, which have significant expansion or aggressive growth features, may require resection. Recurrence is uncommon, but lifelong surveillance is recommended.

Mixed Odontogenic Tumors

Ameloblastic Fibromas

Ameloblastic fibromas can be classified as either a neoplasm or a hamartoma. The lesions typically arise within the posterior mandible, may be expansile, and are typically nonpainful. Radiographically, the lesion presents as a unilocular or multilocular radiolucent mass. Tooth displacement and/or root resorption may be seen. Patients are typically children between the ages of 6 and 10; however, lesions may be seen in older children and young adults. Histologically, the tumors demonstrate mesenchymal and epithelial components. Strands or islands of odontogenic, "ameloblastic-appearing" epithelium within a background connective tissue and myxoid stroma and a fibrous capsule are present. Treatment involves enucleation and curettage for all but very large lesions, which may require resection. Recurrence is rare with proper treatment. If recurrence occurs, ameloblastic fibrosarcoma should be considered within the differential diagnosis.

Odontomas

Odontomas are hamartomas of tissues of the developing tooth. Two types exist: compound and complex. Compound odontomas appear to be small, tooth-like structures. Complex odontomas present as a calcified mass not resembling teeth. These lesions are generally asymptomatic and found on routine radiographic examinations. Compound odontomas have a predilection for occurring in the anterior jaws, and complex odontomas in the posterior jaws. The lesions are typically found in patients younger than 25 years of age. Radiographically, they most often present as radiopacities, but they may be radiolucent or mixed depending on the progression of calcification of the lesions with time. Histologically, enamel, dentin, cementum, and pulpal tissue are seen. Treatment involves enucleation and curettage, and recurrence is rare.

Technique: Mandibular Resection

1. One must determine first if a transcutaneous (larger mandibular lesions with resultant continuity defects) or transoral (smaller mandibular lesions not resulting in continuity defects, and maxillary lesions) approach will be utilized.
2. The patient is placed in a supine position. After endotracheal intubation, the patient is prepped and draped in a sterile fashion.
3. Local anesthetic containing a vasoconstrictor is infiltrated within the area of the lesion, and regional blocks may also be utilized.
4. If performing a transcutaneous approach, the proposed incision should be placed within a natural skinfold, 1.5 to 2.0 cm below the inferior border, to minimize damage to the marginal mandibular branch of the facial nerve.
5. If performing a transoral approach, a sulcular incision with or without vertical releasing incisions is performed.
6. Transcutaneous incisions will follow sharp dissection through the skin, subcutaneous fat, and platysma muscle to the superficial layer of the deep cervical fascia (SLDCF). Within the region of the premasseteric notch, the marginal mandibular branch of the facial nerve and the facial artery and vein will be encountered deep to the SLDCF. Care is taken to isolate the marginal mandibular branch of the facial nerve. Once isolated, dissection can proceed either superior or inferior to the nerve.
7. Once the nerve is protected within the flap, dissection continues to the inferior border of the mandible. The facial vein and artery will be encountered. These vessels may be preserved depending upon the location of the lesion. In the event the vessels do not allow adequate surgical access, the vein and artery should be ligated and divided.
8. Wide exposure of the entire lesion (Figures 45.9, 45.10, and 45.11) through subperiosteal or supraperiosteal dissection is necessary. Depending on the type of the lesion and if cortical perforation has occurred, a supraperiosteal dissection may be required to allow for resection with an intact anatomical barrier.

9. A reconstruction plate may be pre-bent using a stereolithic model prior to surgical resection (Figures 45.6 and 45.8).
10. Osteotomies are performed using a reciprocating, oscillating, or giggly saw at the predetermined proximal and distal margins of the lesion (Figures 45.3, 45.10, and 45.11). The lesion is removed in its entirety and sent for final pathology (Figures 45.12 and 45.13). A small amount of cancellous bone may be harvested from the distal and proximal ends of the native bone and sent to pathology as frozen sections to identify atypical cells within the marrow.
11. Primary or secondary reconstruction (Figures 45.16 and 45.17) is performed based upon the surgeon's preference and the anticipated recurrence rate of the lesion.
12. The four-layer closure is performed to include the ptyergomasseteric sling–periosteum, platysma, subcutaneous tissues, and skin. A suction or passive drain may be inserted and secured to the overlying skin.

Key Points

1. A definitive diagnosis must be made prior to any definitive surgical procedure as lesions have different levels of aggressiveness and recurrence rates.
2. Adequate surgical exposure is necessary for both the resection and the reconstruction of pathological lesions.
3. Plain films may be utilized in the operating room for en bloc resection of bony lesions to evaluate peripheral margins.
4. Margins of the final specimen need to be evaluated on a microscopic level to ensure complete resection.
5. En bloc resections require a passively adapted reconstruction plate with at least three (preferably four or more) fixation screws on each side of the defect (Figure 45.15).
6. Teeth within or near the line of the planned osteotomy should be extracted in anticipation of 3–5 mm of bone dieback from the osteotomy site.
7. All pathologic resections should be planned with the final reconstruction (soft tissue, hard tissue, and prosthetic rehabilitation) in mind.

Case Report

Case Report 45.1. A 54-year-old presents with a chief complaint of left-sided mandibular pain, swelling, trismus, and weight loss for the past several months. On clinical examination, a significant swelling could be palpated extraorally along the left posterior aspect of the mandible, a maximum vertical opening of 5 mm was recorded, and there was severe pain to the area. On review of the cone beam computed tomography scan, a bony mass was identified within the patient's left posterior mandible. An incisional biopsy of the area was performed, and histopathological slides suggested an aggressive central giant cell granuloma. The patient was initially treated with serial steroid injections within the body of the mass to no avail. Due to the patient's trismus, pain, weight loss, refractory intralesional steroid injections, and request, an intraoral block resection was performed with 5 mm margins using Virtual Surgical Planning (VSP; Medical Modeling Inc., Golden, CO, USA). The pre-bent reconstruction plate was placed prior to creating the bone osteotomies. An inferior alveolar nerve pull-through was performed, and the reanastamosed nerve was tagged to the reconstruction plate with 2-0 Prolene sutures. Four months after definitive resection, the patient's continuity defect was reconstructed with an anterior iliac crest bone graft performed through an extraoral approach. The patient developed a partial return of sensation to the V3 distribution on the left side after nerve anastomosis. (See Figures 45.1 through 45.17.)

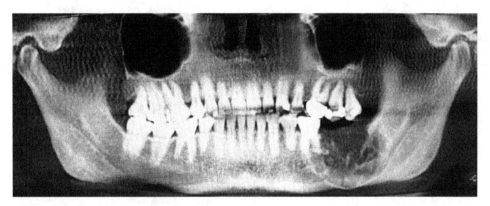

Figure 45.1. Radiograph demonstrating a multiloculated, aggressive, expansile hard tissue lesion located within the left posterior mandible with root resorption, and involvement of the inferior border of the mandible.

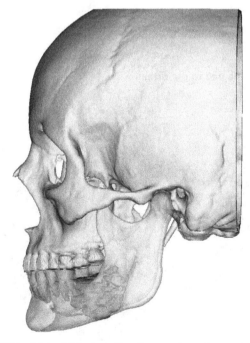

Figure 45.2. Virtual Surgical Planning workup demonstrating the anatomy of the craniofacial bones and teeth. The tumor and the inferior alveolar nerve are highlighted in red. Five-millimeter resection margins are measured from the tumor periphery.

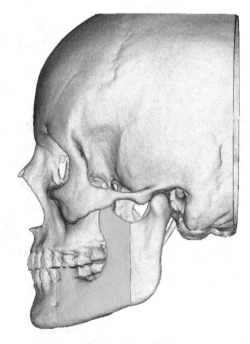

Figure 45.3. Based on the location of the mass, a vertical ramus osteotomy was outlined to resect the posterior margin.

411

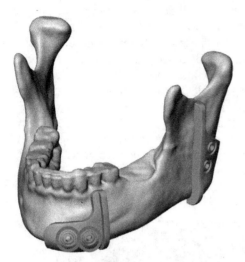

Figure 45.4. An intraoral cut guide is virtually designed. The dental occlusion will stabilize the anterior cut guide during the osteotomy. Predictive holes are marked in red and represent fixation points for both the guide and the pre-bent reconstruction plate.

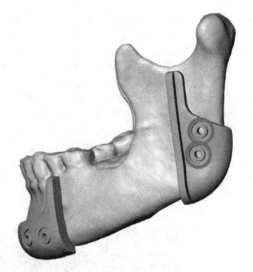

Figure 45.5. The posterior cut guide will articulate with the angle of the posterior mandible. Predictive holes are marked in red.

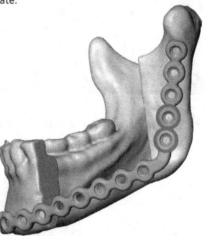

Figure 45.6. A reconstruction plate is virtual adapted to the virtual postoperative mandibular anatomy.

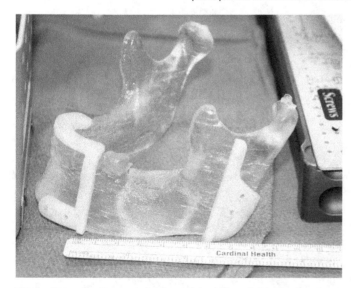

Figure 45.7. Sterile stereolithic model with cut guides in place.

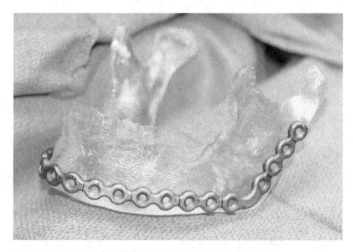

Figure 45.8. Sterile pre-bent reconstruction plate.

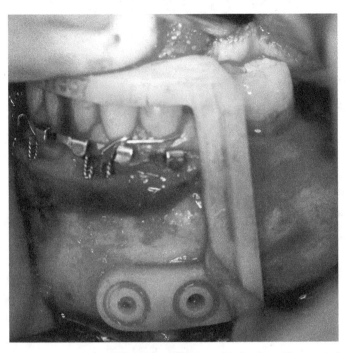

Figure 45.9.   Occlusal-based anterior cut guide in place. The mental nerve is retracted anteriorly with the cut guide.

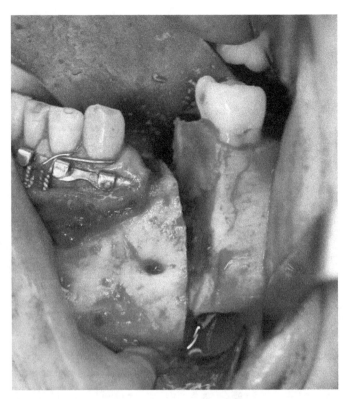

Figure 45.10.   The anterior resection is performed with a reciprocating saw utilizing the custom anterior cut guide. The premolar tooth anterior to the osteotomy is extracted in anticipation of 3–5 mm of bone die back post-osteotomy.

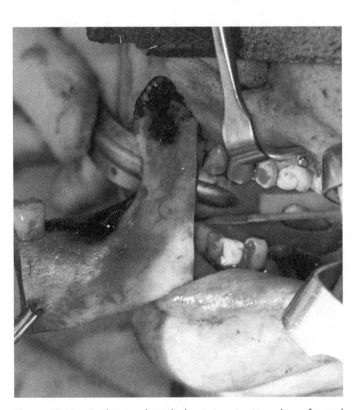

Figure 45.11.   An intraoral vertical ramus osteotomy is performed based on the Virtual Surgical Planning workup and utilizing the posterior cut guide. An inferior alveolar nerve pull-through was performed for this benign tumor.

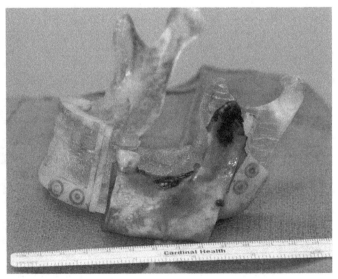

Figure 45.12.   En bloc resection compared to stereolithic model and cut guides.

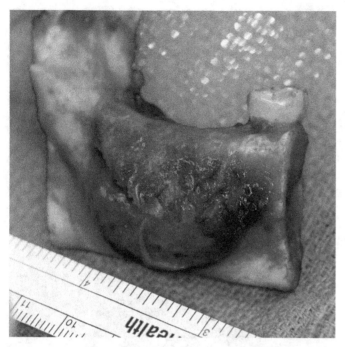

Figure 45.13. Due to the lingual cortical expansion of the mass, a cuff of periosteum was removed to serve as an anatomical barrier.

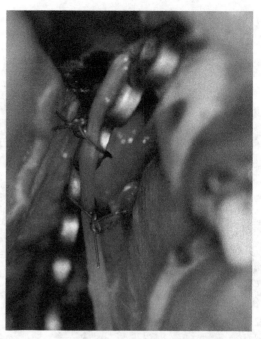

Figure 45.14. The transected inferior alveolar nerve was reapproximated with 7-0 Nylon sutures and secured to the reconstruction plate with 2-0 Prolene sutures.

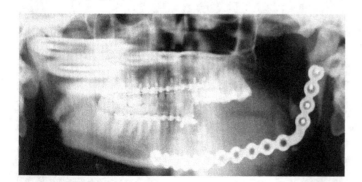

Figure 45.15. Immediate postoperative film depicting a well-positioned reconstruction plate with the condyle ideally seated within the glenoid fossa. The postoperative film correlated well with the Virtual Surgical Planning workup.

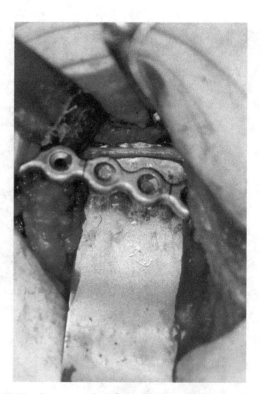

Figure 45.16. Four months after en bloc resection, an extraoral approach was utilized to expose the 4 cm mandibular continuity defect. The inferior alveolar nerve is identified and freed from surrounding scar tissue.

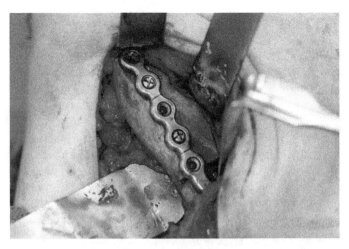

Figure 45.17. The defect was reconstructed with an anterior iliac crest corticocancellous graft secured to the reconstruction plate with fixation screws.

References

Ellis, E. and Zide, M.F., 2006. *Surgical approaches to the facial skeleton*. 2nd ed. Philadelphia: Lippincott, Williams & Wilkins.

Marx, R.E. and Stern, D., 2003. *Oral and maxillofacial pathology a rationale for diagnosis and treatment*. 2nd ed. Hnbover Park, IL: Quintessence.

Neville, B., Damm, D.D., Allen, C. and Bouquot, J., 2009. *Oral and maxillofacial pathology*. 3rd ed. Philadelphia: W.B. Saunders.

CHAPTER

46

Malignant Tumors of the Jaws

Christopher M. Harris[1] and Allen O. Mitchell[2]
[1]*Department of Oral and Maxillofacial Surgery, Naval Medical Center Portsmouth, Portsmouth, Virginia, USA*
[2]*Otolaryngology—Head and Neck Surgery, Naval Medical Center Portsmouth, Portsmouth, Virginia, USA*

Malignant tumors of the maxillofacial structures include oral and oropharyngeal cancers, salivary gland malignancies, skin cancers, and various types of non-oral epithelial malignancies (i.e., sarcomas, melanomas, and metastatic disease). Squamous cell carcinoma (SCCA) constitutes approximately 90% of all malignancies found in the oral cavity and oropharynx. This chapter will focus on the basic epidemiology, etiology, diagnosis, and staging of oral cancer lesions.

Epidemiology

Oral-cavity SCCA, when compared to all sites, is relatively uncommon in North America. However, worldwide oral and oropharyngeal carcinomas together represent the sixth most common cancer in the world. Approximately 40,000 new cases will be diagnosed this year, representing 3–4% of all new cancer cases in the United States. Compared to major cancer types, the incidence of oral cancer in all races is higher than leukemia and pancreatic cancer in the United States. The incidence is higher in other parts of the world, especially in South Central–East Asia, where 8–10% of new cancers are oral SCCA. The majority of patients, including all racial groups, presenting with new disease are males. The incidence rate is higher in African American males especially. The overall male incidence rate is approximately 2.5 times that of females of any racial group. However, overall there has been a decreasing incidence over the last 30 years. Historically, the higher male incidence rates have been associated with higher tobacco and alcohol use in comparison to women. Newer data demonstrate high adolescent tobacco usage among females. This changing trend, along with other risk factors such as human papilloma virus (HPV) exposure, may alter the male-versus-female incidence rates in the future.

Mortality rates in oral SCCA have recently fallen slightly compared to historical data. The factors for this decrease are thought to be better diagnostic modalities, and surgical and adjunctive therapies. However, a likely factor for such a small decrease in mortality over the past three decades is the continued presentation of the majority of patients with late-stage (e.g., stage III or IV) disease and continued use of tobacco products with and without heavy alcohol consumption. Logically, improved early disease diagnosis by better screening and minimization of highly modifiable risk factors (i.e., smoking and alcohol abuse) would likely make significant steps in decreasing incidence and mortality.

Etiology and Risk Factors

The etiology of oral and oropharyngeal cancers can primarily be attributed to tobacco and alcohol abuse. The overwhelming number of new cases can be linked to these two risk factors. Cigarette smoking has been associated with up to 90% of all oral cancers. The oral cancer risk in smokers is 2–12 times the risk in nonsmokers. Concurrent heavy alcohol use appears to synergistically increase the risk of cancer development in smokers by up to 30 times that of the nonsmoking population. Factors, such as HPV and other genetic issues, do play a role as well.

Cigarette smoking is the single most important etiologic factor associated with oral cancer. Cigarettes have over 50 known carcinogens in them. The most commonly found are nitrosamines and polycyclic aromatic hydrocarbons. The carcinogenic effects of alcohol have not been completely identified. However, alcohol's role as a solvent that may increase the cellular permeability of carcinogens is thought to be a major factor. Inhibition of genetic repair mechanisms and the role of alcohol in disrupting the immune response may be other ways it increases cancer risks.

Multiple genetic changes are required to alter normal mucosal epithelial cell lines to malignant cell lines. The primary mechanisms include the inactivation of tumor suppressor genes and activation of proto-oncogenes. The majority of genetic changes leading to malignancy are believed to occur early in mutagenesis and have a cumulative effect as the cell line progresses.

Viral-mediated changes have also been demonstrated in head and neck cancers as well, particularly those of the oropharynx. The viruses commonly associated with oral and oropharyngeal cancers are HPVs, in particular HPV 16. With HPV infection, the E6 and E7 viral oncoproteins result in the inactivation of tumor suppressor genes p53 and Rb. This can eventually lead to cellular immortalization, with continued accumulation of mutations that ultimately lead to carcinoma.

Atlas of Operative Oral and Maxillofacial Surgery, First Edition. Edited by Christopher J. Haggerty and Robert M. Laughlin.
© 2015 John Wiley & Sons, Inc. Published 2015 by John Wiley & Sons, Inc.

Early sexual contact and frequent sexual and orogenital sexual contacts have also been associated with HPV-related oral and oropharyngeal cancers, especially in younger populations who are nonsmokers. HPV-positive tumors tend to have earlier lymph node metastasis, yet also hold a better prognosis than HPV-negative tumors. HPV status is commonly reported with pathology specimens in most centers, but it plays no role currently in the staging of tumors.

These genetic changes do not directly correlate with clinical findings. The point of cellular transformation at which benignity becomes malignancy has yet to be elucidated and is typically thought to occur in a stepwise transition. The genetically altered cell lines cannot repair genetic damage and continue to accumulate genetic abnormalities with time. Eventually, the cell line transforms into a malignant phenotype, produces angiogenic factors to gain blood supply, evades immune surveillance, and extends beyond the basement membrane to become a clinical carcinoma.

Clinically, however, it is impossible to visually identify histological malignancy or this transformation period. For example, a leukoplakic lesion that may not make the clinician overly suspicious may in fact be a frank malignancy. A highly suspicious erythroleukoplakic lesion may only show dysplasia histologically. Several genetic changes could also likely be identified in histologically normal or dysplastic tissue that may not be present in a malignant lesion. The role of genetic alterations in the transformation of benign to malignant cell lines is an area of intense research and will hopefully yield better molecular- and genetic-level testing in the future, eventually giving surgeons better diagnostic and treatment modalities.

Premalignant Lesions

A premalignant lesion is a morphologically altered tissue with a higher likelihood of developing into a frank malignancy than normal tissue. Clinically, premalignant lesions are described as leukoplakia, erythroplakia, or erythroluekoplakia. Histologically, these premalignant lesions are described as dysplasia or carcinoma in situ.

Leukoplakia is defined as a white patch or plaque that cannot be removed by scraping or rubbing and cannot be characterized as another disease entity. Erythroplakia is a red plaque or patch that cannot be removed by scraping or rubbing and cannot be characterized as another disease entity. Leukoplakic lesions may be unifocal or multifocal, and they can occur anywhere in the oral cavity. Lesions located on the tongue (except the dorsal surface) and the floor of mouth are more worrisome, as more than 20% of tongue and lip lesions, and more than 40% of floor-of-mouth lesions, exhibit premalignant histologic features. Malignant transformation of leukoplakic lesions is poorly understood. Rates from less than 1% upward to 17.5%

have been reported. Erythroplakic lesions and erythroleukoplakic lesions are more serious lesions. The large majority of these lesions harbor some degree of histologic premalignancy or malignancy. Malignant transformation rates are thought to approach more than 20%.

There is no molecular marker, despite advances in research that can identify those lesions that will progress to malignancy. There is also no evidence that removal prevents the progression toward malignancy. Thus, there is debate about the management of leukoplakic premaligant lesions, with some practitioners advocating removal of the lesions, while some recommend close observations and biopsies as needed for clinical changes. Erythroleukoplakic lesions should be completely excised and sent for histopathologic evaluation.

Site Specific Lesions

The American Joint Committee on Cancer subdivides the oral cavity into distinct anatomical sites. These seven sites are an attempt to define the biological behavior and treatment modalities of the lesions within them. These sites are the mucosal lip, alveolar ridge (gingiva), buccal mucosa, floor of mouth, tongue (oral), retromolar region, and maxilla (hard palate).

Mucosal lip cancers are most commonly seen on the lower lip in elderly white male patients with a history of chronic sun exposure. This is one of the oral cancers whose primary etiology is not considered to be associated strongly with tobacco use. From 2% to 42% of oral cavity cancers have been reported on the mucosal lip. Lymphatic drainage is typically level I and level II nodes, perhaps bilaterally if the primary lesion is on or approaches the midline.

Alveolar ridge cancers, including gingival tumors, can be seen in the maxilla but predominantly involve the mandibular alveolar mucosa and gingiva. They range from 25% to 28% of all oral cancers, and approximately one-third involve the underlying bone. Typical nodal involvement occurs in level I and level II and occurs in approximately 25% of cases. These diagnoses of the lesions are frequently delayed due to misdiagnosis as periodontal lesions or traumatic and inflammatory gingival lesions.

Buccal mucosa cancers represent 2–10% of all oral cavity cancers. Lymphatic involvement is typically noted in level I and level II regions. Involvement of regional lymphatics occurs in up to 30% of presenting cases. There is some evidence arguing to electively treat the neck in many buccal mucosa lesions due to the high incidence of neck metastasis with even smaller lesions.

The floor of mouth is a common location for oral cancer. Approximately 25% of oral cancers are found in this area. Nearly one-half of all patients presenting with floor-of-mouth lesions will have regional metastasis. Tumor depth in this region is critical when evaluating the primary lesion. In patients with a tumor depth of >2 mm,

38% had nodal disease. Elective neck treatment for all but the smallest lesions is typically carried out. Selective neck dissection including levels I, II, and III (bilaterally, if a midline lesion is present) is the most common modality to manage the neck.

The oral tongue represents nearly 50% of all oral cancers diagnosed. Lateral and ventral tongue sites are the most common. Involvement of the dorsal surface is rare and, when present, is usually by extension of disease to the site. Lymphatic drainage includes levels I, II, III, and IV. Ipsilateral drainage is noted with lateral lesions; however, the tip and central portions of the tongue can lead to bilateral nodal drainage. Approximately 40% of all patients presenting with oral tongue cancer have regional metastatic disease.

The retromolar triangle, or retromolar pad, represents approximately 5% of presenting cases of oral cancer. Otalgia, odynophagia, and trismus can be seen. Trismus can be an ominous sign, as it may indicate tumor extension into the masticator space and pterygoid region, possibly indicating the skull base extension. Involvement of the posterior dentition and mandibular bone is also commonly seen. Levels I and II (including level IIb) are commonly involved first-echelon nodes. In reports, up to 56% of patients present with nodal involvement.

The maxilla, including the hard palate, is relatively uncommon. It makes up approximately 5% of all oral cancers. Soft palate lesions are seen in 75% of cases, and it is considered an oropharyngeal site. Lymphatic drainage to the palate is to level I and level II. Traditionally, elective neck dissection was not performed except for large lesions. There is more evidence that occult neck disease occurs more frequently than previously believed in smaller lesions and that selective neck dissection of levels I, II, and III may be beneficial.

Lymphatic Drainage of the Oral Cavity

The oral cavity has a predictable drainage pattern to the lymphatics of the neck. The standardized grouping of the more than 300 lymph nodes in the neck allows for clinicians to communicate with each other and define surgical or nonsurgical management decisions. There are six standardized levels that describe the groupings of neck lymphatics (level I through level VI); subdivisions exist within levels I, II, and V as well. These subdivisions were established due to established drainage patterns and allow for "superselective" dissections. For example, level IIb is rarely involved with metastatic disease, unless level II is involved, and there is increased morbidity from spinal accessory nerve damage with resultant shoulder dysfunction for no significant patient survival benefit.

Level I includes the submental and submandibular lymph nodes. The borders of level I are the inferior border of the mandible, the stylohyoid muscle, and the anterior digastric muscle. Level Ia is the submental triangle, which is defined by the anterior bellies of the digastric muscle and the hyoid bone. Level Ib is the submandibular triangle. All oral cancers can potentially drain into this level as a first-echelon node group. The submandibular gland, lingual and hypoglossal nerves, and multiple blood vessels are found in this region.

Level II includes the upper jugular lymph nodes. This region spans from the base of the skull to the inferior border of the hyoid bone. The anterior border is the sternohyoid muscle, and the posterior border is the sternocleidomastoid muscle. The internal jugular vein and spinal accessory nerve are found in this region. This region is subdivided into level IIa and level IIB by the course of the spinal accessory nerve. Level IIa is anterior and inferior to the spinal accessory, and level IIb is superior and posterior to the nerve. Oral cancers can potentially drain into this level as a first-echelon node group, but solitary level IIB involvement is rare. There is debate about the necessity of a level IIb dissection in the N0 neck due to the risk of spinal accessory nerve damage.

Level III includes the middle jugular lymph nodes. The region spans from the inferior border of the hyoid bone to the cricoid cartilage. The anterior border is the sternohyoid muscle, and the posterior border is the sternocleidomastoid muscle or cervical nerve branches. In the deep aspects of this level, the carotid and internal jugular vessels can be identified. Metastatic disease from oral cancer is commonly found in this region and can be seen in isolation. Commonly, levels I, II, and III are removed as a "selective" neck dissection for N0 oral cancers except the tongue.

Level IV includes the lower jugular lymph nodes. This region spans from the cricoid cartilage to the clavicle. The anterior border is the sternohyoid muscle, and the posterior border is the sternocleidomastoid muscle or cervical nerve branches. Metastatic disease from oral cancers can be found in this region, particularly tongue carcinomas and in N+ necks. Rarely are isolated metastatic nodes in the N0 neck found in level IV. Commonly, levels I, II, III, and IV are removed as a "selective" neck dissection for N0 tongue cancers.

Level V includes the posterior triangle lymph node group. Its borders are the posterior border of the sternocleidomastoid muscle, the anterior border of the trapezius muscle, and the clavicle. It can be subdivided at the level of the cricoid cartilage as level Va (superior) and level Vb (inferior). Level V is not considered a first-echelon node basin for oral cancer, but it can be involved with nodal disease. Surgeons' efforts to minimize damage to the spinal accessory nerve have lessened the frequency of elective dissection of this region. Level V nodal disease can be associated with oropharyngeal, nasopharyngeal, and posterior scalp tumors.

Level VI includes the central compartment nodes. This region lies between the carotid arteries, the hyoid bone, and the sternal notch. The larynx, supraglottic-pharynx regions, esophagus, and thyroid gland may drain here as a first-echelon nodal basin. The need for lymph node dissection of level VI is rare in oral cancers.

Diagnosis and Workup

The diagnosis of oral cancers primarily requires a thorough history, a clinical exam, a high index of suspicion, and a biopsy with histopathologic examination. A physical exam should also be undertaken. Particular attention should be directed at the family and social history to elucidate any familial diseases or patterns, and to determine a substance abuse history. Outside of the head and neck exam, a thorough exam of all systems should be performed. Particular emphasis should be placed on the cardiopulmonary system and vascular status of the patients. Many oral cancer patients have significant comorbidities that can impact their surgical and reconstructive treatment options.

The importance of accurately evaluating regional metastatic disease cannot be understated. A single lymph node with disease decreases the overall prognosis for cure by 50%. Extracapsular spread can reduce this again by another 50%. Historically, palpation of the neck was the gold standard for neck evaluation. However, inaccuracy in identifying nodes, estimating size, and interrater reliability has been noted with physical exam alone. The physical neck examination is still important, but imaging has essentially replaced the physical exam due to its increased accuracy, ability to localize disease relative to surrounding vital structures, and ability to reveal nonpalpable, occult disease.

The clinical examination should be standardized and include examination with visualization of all oral hard tissues and mucosa, and palpation of all areas of the oral cavity soft tissue and the neck. All removable dental appliances should be removed prior to the examination. The author's technique is to begin with visualization of skin of the head and neck to identify any dermatologic lesions. Palpation of the neck, salivary glands, temporomandibular joint region, and lips is performed, and then visualization of the anterior nasal cavity is performed. The intraoral exam then is performed and should involve visualization of *all* oral mucosa. The posterior and posterior-lateral tongue, as well as the posterior lateral floor of mouth, should be especially focused on as these are areas that are difficult to adequately visualize without manipulation by the clinician and can easily be missed on examination. Gingival lesions are frequently misdiagnosed as inflammatory or periodontal lesions and should be treated with a high index of suspicion if a failure to improve of 2–3 weeks is noted with therapy. Unilateral tonsil enlargement should be noted and is concerning.

A thorough dental examination with radiographs should also be undertaken. Poor oral hygiene, dental caries, and periodontal disease should be noted, and a discussion with the patient about the management of these issues should be carried out. Baseline laboratory studies are also recommended; these typically include an electrocardiogram, a complete blood count, chemistry panels, liver function tests, nutrition labs (e.g., albumin, prealbumin, and transferrin), and coagulation profiles. Appropriate consultation with medical colleagues to maximize the perioperative status of patients is also required.

The concept of *field cancerization* suggests that all carcinogen-exposed tissue of the upper aerodigestive tract has some genetic abnormalities. This condemned mucosa has been exposed to carcinogens and undergoes genetic changes that place the patient at higher risks for secondary mucosal upper-aerodigestive-tract tumors. The rates of synchronous upper-aerodigestive-tract tumors range from 2% to 16%. Identification of a secondary lesion can drastically alter the staging and overall treatment of the patient. Thus, the evaluation to rule out another lesion locally, regionally, and at a distant site is mandatory.

Historically, this evaluation has been done with *triple endoscopy* and imaging. Many institutions are moving away from panendoscopy as a routine procedure and are performing endoscopy of the upper aerodigestive tract only on a symptom-driven basis. Improvements in imaging techniques and the common use of flexible, in-office endoscopy have substituted for most of these procedures. It is the authors' opinion that flexible fiberoptic nasopharyngoscopy should be performed on all patients routinely during the workup to evaluate for other lesions in the region. Frequently, in our practice, the patient will have additional biopsies, dental extractions, dental implants placed, and an esophagogastroduodenoscopy with percutaneous endoscopic gastrostomy placement prior to the definitive surgical resection, or prior to radiotherapy or chemoradiation therapy when it is the primary treatment.

Imaging

Various imaging techniques have been utilized to evaluate the primary lesion and the extent of regional or distant disease. The standard imaging technique is typically a contrast computed tomography (CT) scan for better evaluation of the primary lesion and for regional metastasis. CT scans of the chest and upper abdomen to include the liver are also frequently used. Imaging artifacts from dental restorations frequently limit CT image quality. Magnetic resonance imaging is superior to evaluate the soft tissue extent of oral cancers. Panoramic radiographs and dental cone beam CT scanning have also been utilized to visualize the extent of bone involvement associated with the primary lesions as well. Standard chest radiography is used in some institutions to evaluate for pulmonary involvement. Positron emission tomography (PET) with or without CT scanning is routinely used in higher stage tumors that will likely require postoperative radiation or chemoradiation therapy. Ultrasound techniques have been used to evaluate the neck and suspicious masses, especially when neck disease needs to be confirmed and for evaluation of neck nodes after definitive chemoradiation, but they have not seen widespread use as the primary method for neck imaging in oral cancer.

Biopsy

Biopsy of suspicious lesions is warranted if the patient has significant risk factors and a history of a nonresolving lesion for greater than 2 weeks, or if the lesion itself is highly suspicious. Prior to biopsy, a description and measurement of the true size of the lesion are needed. Prior to the biopsy, careful attention to depth via palpation is needed, especially in areas such as the tongue, floor of mouth, and buccal mucosa. Frequently imaging is useful to determine the true extent of lesion depth. Extensive biopsies prior to imaging may alter the area and regional lymphatics via inflammation. This can potentially lead to altered staging, and thus overall treatment offered to the patient. It is the opinion of the authors that the surgeon who will be primarily managing the patient for the suspected malignancy should evaluate the patient, determine the need for imaging, and biopsy the lesion so that the presenting disease findings are not altered.

Biopsy techniques vary among practitioners. The most frequently used is an incisional biopsy. Excisional biopsies can be used for small lesions. Contrary to some teachings, oral pathologists do not require an adjacent section of "normal" tissue in the biopsy specimen. Tongue base, tonsil, and laryngeal cancers are frequently biopsied with small cupped forceps during a diagnostic laryngoscopy, and the diagnosis is accurately made from these small pieces of malignant tissue without adjacent "normal" mucosa. Biopsies can hopefully provide two pieces of information: (1) a tissue diagnosis, and (2) the depth of the lesion if malignant. Tissue punches are commonly used for incisional biopsies primarily due to the ease of use and uniform specimen size and depth. Tumor depth is evaluated by clinical exam, imaging, and biopsy specimen. Tumor depth of invasion is an important factor in some oral cancer sites in the decision to treat or observe the node-negative neck in oral cancers.

Staging

Once the patient has had a clinical exam, imaging, laboratory studies, and biopsies performed, the tumor is clinically staged according to the American Joint Committee on Cancer (AJCC) guidelines. All available information is utilized to stage the patient. Clinical examination alone can be inaccurate; thus, all available information, including clinical and imaging modalities should be utilized to preliminarily stage the primary lesion and neck. Questionable yet suspicious neck masses can undergo ultrasound-guided fine-needle aspiration to assist with neck staging. Staging is based on the TNM system: primary tumor size and invasion (T), the extent of nodal disease (N), and the presence of distant metastatic disease (M). Staging is final at this point if the patient is undergoing nonsurgical therapy, as no additional tissue aside from the biopsy is recovered. Patients who undergo surgical therapy can have staging (clinical TNM, or cTNM) altered based on the histopathologic examination. Clinical and imaging size measurements of tumor size are typically not changed due to tissue shrinkage in fixed histological specimens of up to 25%. Nodal disease status, based on histological examination, can be upstaged or downstaged depending on these findings. The pathologic stage (pTNM) is reported, which may alter the final stage of the tumor. Pathologic reports may also discover negative prognostic factors such as perineural invasion, vascular invasion, frank bone invasion, extracapsular extension of tumor within a lymph node, or close or positive margins. The presence of these factors may require further surgical therapy (i.e., a close or positive margin), or they are indications for postoperative radiotherapy or chemoradiotherapy.

Key Points

1. The oral cavity has a predictable drainage pattern to the lymphatics of the neck. An understanding of the lymphatic drainage patterns is crucial in the treatment and care of oral cancers. The standardized grouping of the more than 300 lymph nodes in the neck allows for clinicians to communicate and define surgical or nonsurgical management decisions.

2. A complete workup of patients with a high index of suspicion for oral cancer is essential. Elements include a thorough history, clinical examination, biopsy with histopathologic examination, and imaging studies. Prior to surgery, a chest CT or chest films should be obtained as well as an electrocardiogram, complete blood count, chemistry panels, liver function tests, nutrition labs (i.e., albumin, prealbumin, and transferrin), and coagulation profiles. Additional consultations may be needed depending on the patient's comorbidities.

3. Patients should be presented to a formal multidisciplinary tumor board.

4. Lesions of the lateral and ventral surfaces of the tongue should have a high level of suspicion for malignancy.

5. Lymphatic drainage of the tongue includes levels I, II, III, and IV. Ipsilateral drainage is noted with lateral lesions; however, the tip and central portions of the tongue can lead to bilateral nodal drainage. When performing lymphadenectomy for lateral lesions of the tongue, dissection should include level IV due to the potential for skip metastasis.

Case Report 46.1. A 46-year-old male presents to the oral and maxillofacial surgery service with an erosive, solitary lesion of the left mandible. Biopsy demonstrated osteosarcoma. Further metastatic workup yielded several enlarged nodes within the left neck. The AJCC classification for osteosarcoma was $T_2N_1M_0G$. The patient underwent wide local incision of the lesion with left neck dissection levels I–V. The soft tissue defect was reconstructed with a latissimus dorsi flap. The continuity defect was treated secondarily utilizing a free vascularized fibula flap. (See Figures 46.1 through 46.9.)

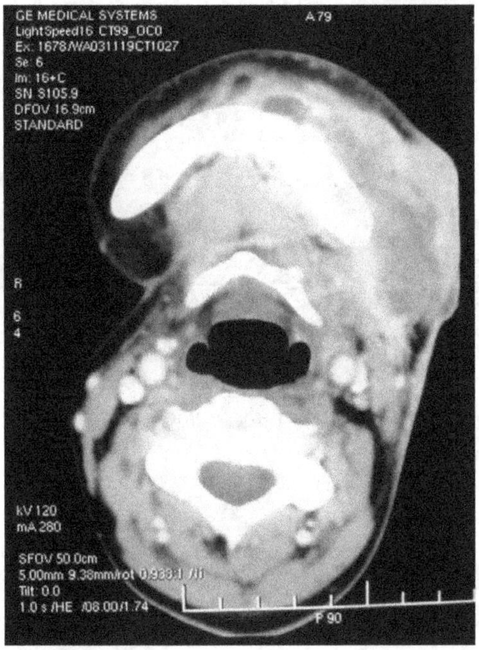

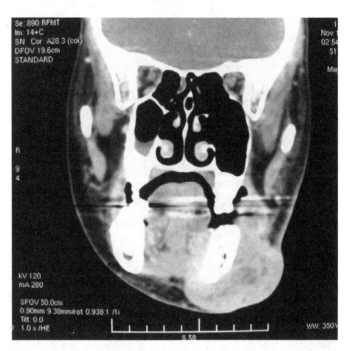

Figure 46.1. Axial computed tomography scan depicting a large osteosarcoma of the left mandible.

Figure 46.2. Coronal computed tomography scan depicting an osteosarcoma of the left mandible.

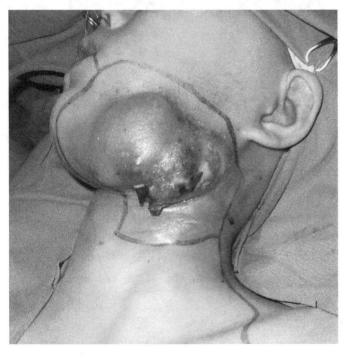

Figure 46.3. Osteosarcoma of the left mandible extending into the skin.

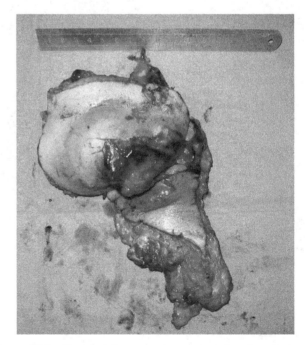

Figure 46.4. Resected tumor and corresponding lymphadenectomy.

421

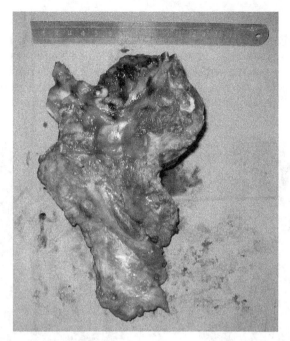

Figure 46.5.   Resected tumor with continuity radical neck dissection.

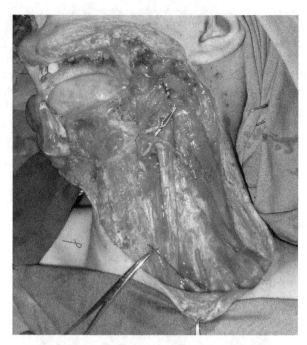

Figure 46.6.   Resultant defect after tumor ablation.

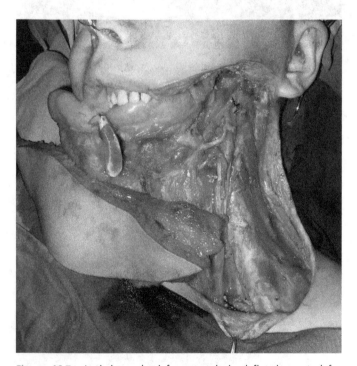

Figure 46.7.   Latissimus dorsi free vascularized flap harvested for reconstruction.

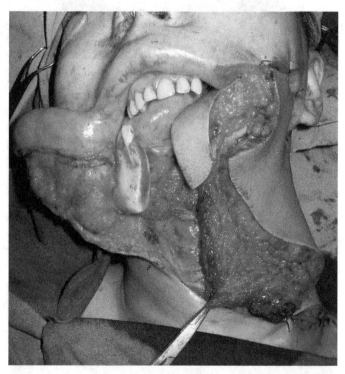

Figure 46.8.   Serial inset of latissimus dorsi flap after anastamosis.

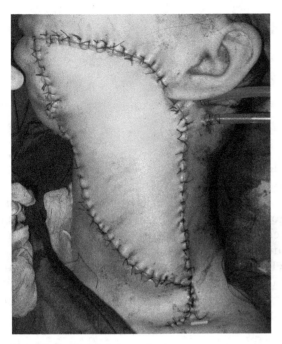

Figure 46.9.   Fully inset latissimus dorsi.

References

Edge, S., Byrd, D.R., Compton, C.C. and Fritz, A.G., eds., 2011. *AJCC cancer staging manual*. 7th ed. New York: Springer.

Myers, E.N., Suen, J.Y., Myers, J.N. and Hanna, E.Y.N., 2003. *Cancer of the head and neck*. 4th ed. Philadelphia: Saunders.

Shah, J., 2003. *Head and neck surgery and oncology*. 3rd ed. St.Louis, MO: Mosby.

47

Surgical Management of the Neck

Anthony B.P. Morlandt[1] and Jon D. Holmes[2]
[1]Department of Oral and Maxillofacial Surgery, University of Florida Health Science Center, Jacksonville, Florida, USA
[2]Clark Holmes Oral and Facial Surgery; and Department of Oral and Maxillofacial Surgery University of Alabama, Birmingham, Alabama, USA

Indications for Neck Dissection

A complex cervical lymphovascular system, containing approximately 300 lymph nodes (40% of the body's estimated 800 nodes), drains the head and neck region. Cervical lymph node involvement in head and neck tumors is the single most important prognostic indicator, resulting in a 50% decreased overall survival and immediate classification as stage 3 or 4. Timely and appropriate management of at-risk cervical lymphatics therefore serves two critical purposes: to remove disease (macroscopic or microscopic) and to properly stage the neck, guiding adjuvant therapies based on histopathologic features. Neck dissection is indicated in nearly all cases of oral cavity cancer, although the extent and levels of dissection have evolved over the past four decades. In contemporary practice, neck dissections may be classified into two broad categories based on the therapeutic intent or purpose:

1. **Elective neck dissection** is the removal of at-risk cervical nodal basins in a patient *without* clinically or radiographically evident cervical metastases.
2. **Therapeutic neck dissection** is the removal of at-risk node-bearing tissues in the patient *with* clinically or radiographically evident neck disease.

Neck Dissection Classification

The first widely used classification system was presented in 1991 by the American Society of Head and Neck Surgery and was adopted by the American Academy of Otolaryngology—Head and Neck Surgery. This system was revised in 2002 and clarified in 2008 with respect to boundaries between sublevels. In 2011, Ferlito *et al.* proposed an updated, concise classification system based on three parts:

1. Symbol *ND* with laterality indicated
2. Specific lymphatic levels *removed* (Ia/b, IIa/b, III, IV, Va/b, VI, and VII)
3. Specific nonlymphatic structures *removed* (sternocleidomastoid muscle [SCM]; internal jugular vein [IJV]; cranial nerve [CN] XII [hypoglossal nerve]; CN XI [spinal accessory nerve]; skin [SKN]; external carotid artery [ECA], etc.). (See Table 47.1.)

Relevant Anatomy

Neck dissection requires detailed knowledge of the anatomy of the entire neck, extending from the mandible to the clavicle and from the midline to the trapezius muscle. Selective neck dissection of levels I, II, and III (Figure 47.3) demands understanding the fascial layers enveloping the neck contents and the maneuvers necessary to "unwrap" the muscles to deliver an intact specimen. Levels and key structures include the following (Figures 47.1 and 47.2):

1. **Level I**
   - **Ia (submental)**: Extends from the mandible superiorly to the hyoid bone inferiorly, and is bounded laterally by the anterior bellies of the digastric muscles bilaterally. The submental artery will be encountered and must be preserved if the submental island flap is planned.
   - **Ib (submandibular)**: Bounded by the mandible superiorly to the anterior and posterior bellies of the digastric muscle anteroinferiorly, and the stylohyoid muscle posteriorly. The perifacial lymph nodes, facial artery and vein, and submandibular gland are encountered, as well as the marginal mandibular, lingual, and hypoglossal nerves.

2. **Level II (upper jugular)**
   - **IIa**: Includes the tissues bounded by the skull base superiorly, inferiorly by the hyoid bone radiographically and carotid bifurcation surgically, the stylohyoid muscle anteriorly, and posteriorly by the spinal accessory nerve. The jugulodigastric node (i.e., the principal node of Kuttner), the retromandibular vein, hidden in the tail of the parotid gland, is commonly encountered and ligated.
   - **IIb ("submuscular recess")**: The posterosuperior extension of level IIa and IIb is delineated anteriorly by a vertical line at the level of the spinal accessory nerve and posteriorly by the posterolateral edge of the SCM. The superoinferior boundaries are identical to those of level IIa.

Atlas of Operative Oral and Maxillofacial Surgery, First Edition. Edited by Christopher J. Haggerty and Robert M. Laughlin.
© 2015 John Wiley & Sons, Inc. Published 2015 by John Wiley & Sons, Inc.

Table 47.1.   Neck dissection classification systems

Robbins *et al.* (1991)	Robbins *et al.* (2002/2008)	Ferlito *et al.* (2011)
Radical neck dissection	Radical neck dissection	ND (I–V, SCM, IJV, CN XI)
Modified radical neck dissection (preservation of CN XI)	Modified radical neck dissection (preservation of CN XI)	ND (I–V, SCM, IJV)
Selective (supraomohyoid) neck dissection	Selective neck dissection (SND I–III)	ND (I–III)
Selective (lateral) neck dissection	Selective neck dissection (SND II–IV)	ND (II–IV)
Extended neck dissection with removal of skin and hypoglossal nerve	Extended neck dissection with removal of skin and hypoglossal nerve	ND (I–V, SCM, IJV, CN XI, SKN, CN XII)

Note: SCM, sternocleidomastoid muscle; IJV, internal jugular vein; CN, cranial nerve; CN XII, hypoglossal nerve; CN XI, spinal accessory nerve; SKN, skin; ECA, external carotid artery.

3. **Level III (midjugular)**: Level III is bounded superiorly by the inferior aspect of level II, anteriorly by the sternohyoid muscle, and posterolaterally by the posterolateral edge of the SCM. The inferior edge is demarcated by the omohyoid muscle surgically and cricoid cartilage radiographically. The jugulo-omohyoid node is contained in level III.

4. **Level IV (lower jugular)**: Extends from the inferior border of level III superiorly to the clavicle inferiorly, and from the lateral border of the sternohyoid muscle anteriorly to the posterolateral edge of the SCM. Level IV contains the transverse cervical artery and, in the left neck, the thoracic duct. A smaller accessory thoracic duct may be encountered in the right neck.

5. **Level V (posterior triangle)**: Extends from the posterior edge of the SCM to the anterior edge of the trapezius muscle, and inferiorly to the clavicle. Level V contains the spinal accessory nerve as it penetrates the SCM, coursing posteroinferiorly to innervate the trapezius muscle on its deep surface.

6. **Level VI (central compartment)**: Bounded by the hyoid bone superiorly and the suprasternal notch inferiorly, and extending to the carotid sheaths bilaterally, level VI contains the pretracheal (Delphian), prelaryngeal, and paratracheal lymph nodes.

7. **Level VII (superior mediastinal)**: Extends from the suprasternal notch superiorly to the level of the innominate artery inferiorly, and bounded laterally by

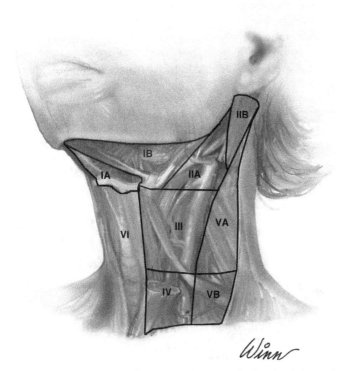

Figure 47.1.   Schematic illustration depicting the levels of the neck.

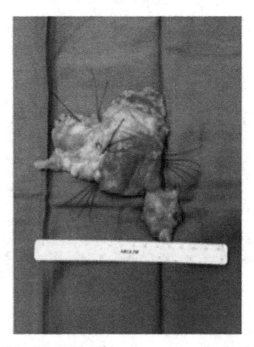

Figure 47.2.   Sutures identifying the corresponding levels of the neck after lymphadenectomy.

the carotid sheaths. Although often considered outside the boundaries of the neck, the definition of level VII nodes as an inferior extension of paratracheal lymph nodes into the superior mediastinum persists in contemporary literature and is included here in the interest of completeness.

Surgical Technique

Selective Neck Dissection, Levels I–III

1. With the patient in the supine position, a vertically oriented shoulder roll is placed, allowing the scapulae to drop and spread laterally, exposing the anterolateral neck. Using monopolar electrocautery (or a scalpel blade), a curvilinear incision is made in a natural skin crease from the mastoid process to the midline at the level of the cricoid cartilage. If unilateral neck dissection is planned, the incision must be carried past the midline to allow sufficient exposure of level Ia with retraction of the platysmal flaps.

2. The incision is carried through skin and subcutaneous tissues using electrocautery until the platysma muscle is exposed along the length of the incision. Skin hooks or Lahey clamps may be used to aid in skin retraction.

3. The platysma is incised along its length, and subplatysmal flaps are raised superiorly to the inferior of the mandible and inferiorly to just above the clavicle. The platysma is deficient in the midline and posteriorly, and in these areas skin flap elevation is in the subcutaneous plane. Keeping the greater auricular nerve and external jugular vein down on the SCM at this step indicates that elevation is proceeding in the proper plane. Superior traction with skin hooks or finger grip and countertraction with a Kittner or

sponge facilitate expeditious subplatysmal flap elevation in a relatively avascular plane (Figure 47.4).

4. The neck dissection may proceed in an anterior-to-posterior direction, starting in level Ia with elevation of the fibrofatty node-bearing contents off of the anterior bellies of the digastric muscles bilaterally, the mandibular symphysis superiorly, and the mylohyoid muscle on the deep aspect. The submental artery will be encountered The specimen is brought inferiorly to the level of the hyoid bone, then slightly posterior as the strap muscles are encountered to elevate the fascia and nodal tissue from the surface of the sternohyoid muscle.

5. The specimen is then freed sharply from the underlying musculature using monopolar electrocautery and carried posteriorly, crossing the digastric tendon, until the posterior edge of the mylohyoid muscle is encountered in level Ib. The inferior border of the mandible is cleaned superiorly, taking care to control vessels in this area with vascular clips or suture ligatures.

6. Attention is then directed to the submandibular gland, which may be appreciated as a bulge just beneath the superficial layer of deep cervical fascia. The fascia is incised at the inferior aspect of the gland, approximately 2 cm below the inferior border of the mandible, and elevated (Figure 47.5). Care is taken to protect the marginal mandibular nerve from injury, which may be visualized coursing through the fascia.

7. The facial artery and vein are dissected, ligated, and divided. Further protection to the facial nerve may be afforded by keeping the superior ties on the facial vein long and retracting superiorly.

8. The posterior edge of the mylohyoid muscle is retracted superomedially using an army-navy

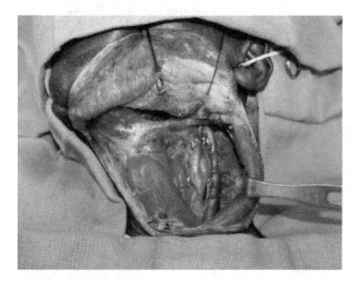

Figure 47.3. Selective neck dissection Levels I, II, and III.

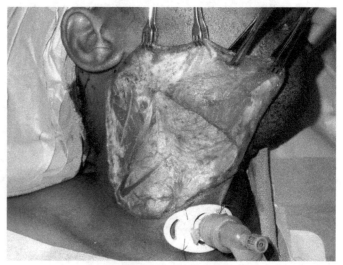

Figure 47.4. Subplatysmal flap elevation exposing the superficial layer of the deep cervical fascia.

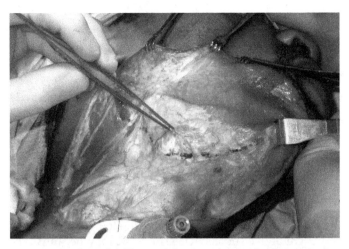

Figure 47.5. Superficial layer of the deep cervical fascia is incised at the inferior aspect of the submandibular gland and the fascia is elevated. Care must be taken to protect the marginal mandibular nerve from injury, which may be visualized coursing through the fascia.

retractor, which is applied in a sweeping motion to expose the lingual nerve. An Allis clamp may be used to retract the submandibular gland and remaining specimen inferoposteriorly.

9. The submandibular duct is then ligated and divided, as are numerous Ranine veins. Failure to adequately control venous bleeding in this region increases the risk of injury to the underlying hypoglossal nerve and deep aspect of the facial artery. A small arterial branch to the mylohyoid muscle will likewise be encountered here and is controlled with vascular clips.

10. The deep aspect of the facial artery is then dissected free from the submandibular gland and ligated. If microvascular reconstruction is anticipated, careful dissection with bipolar electrocautery is advised to avoid thermal injury to the vessels with subsequent increased risk of thrombosis. An additional 1 to 2 cm of length may be gained by freeing the artery from the medial aspect of the gland until the first major branch point is encountered. This maneuver is often necessary when upper or midface reconstruction is planned, and it may avoid the need for vein grafts.

11. Level Ib dissection is completed by retracting the specimen posteroinferiorly and cleaning the posterior belly of the digastric and stylohyoid muscles inferiorly and the mandible superiorly. Care must be taken to avoid dissection on the deep aspect of the muscles, which exposes the hypoglossal nerve and great vessels to injury. Dissection is then carried posteriorly across the tail of the parotid gland, where the retromandibular vein is ligated and divided. Excision of the parotid tail leads to significantly increased postoperative edema; therefore, its judicious removal is advised when it is clinically uninvolved with disease.

12. Attention is then directed to the midline, where dissection proceeds from along a broad front, from level Ia superiorly to the inferior belly of the omohyoid muscle inferiorly. Fascia is bluntly undermined with tonsil hemostats and divided with electrocautery. The superior laryngeal and superior thyroid arteries and the common facial vein will be encountered and are preserved. The carotid artery will come into view with further reflection of the specimen in a posterior direction. The internal jugular vein is identified at this point and may be cleaned; however, transitioning from a posterior to anterior approach is an option.

13. At this point, attention is directed to the medial edge of the SCM. The external jugular vein is ligated and divided, again protecting length in anticipation of immediate or future microvascular anastomosis. Fascia is reflected off the muscle, starting laterally and proceeding medially. Numerous muscular vessels are controlled with vascular clips or cautery.

14. At the junction of the upper one-third and lower two-thirds of the muscle, the spinal accessory nerve is identified by bluntly dissecting in a superomedial to postero-inferior direction and mobilized in anticipation of IIb dissection. The nerve is cleaned of overlying specimen in a superomedial direction until the internal jugular vein is encountered. The upper edge of the vein may be cleaned of specimen at this point to prevent subsequent injury.

15. Level IIb is then cleaned of nodal contents by placing army-navy or appendiceal retractors at 90° angles, retracting the SCM laterally and the posterior belly of the digastric muscle superiorly. It is recommended to start the dissection laterally, incising until the fascia overlying the splenius capitus muscle is encountered deeply, and carry the specimen inferomedially. A branch of the occipital artery, when inadvertently divided here, may lead to troublesome bleeding. Care must be taken to identify and protect the internal jugular vein and spinal accessory nerve medially. Following sufficient mobilization of the nerve, the IIb nodal contents are then brought under the nerve in continuity with the remainder of the specimen.

16. With the spinal accessory nerve protected superiorly, monopolar cautery is used to define the posterior extent of the dissection at the posterolateral edge of the SCM. Medial retraction of the specimen with Allis or Babcock clamps and posterolateral retraction of the muscle with army-navy retractors aid in visualization as the deep surface is cleaned. The cervical plexus rootlets are encountered deeply and serve as an important early landmark, as maintaining the plane of dissection superficial to the nerves will ensure integrity of the scalene fascia and minimize

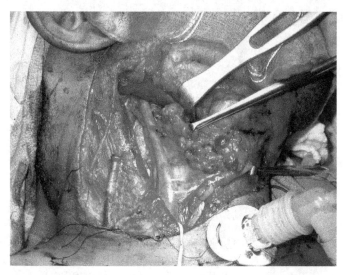

Figure 47.6. Exposure of the internal jugular vein. The deep jugular nodes are retracted anteriorly.

risk of injury to the underlying brachial plexus and phrenic nerve as dissection proceeds anteriorly.

17. With the omohyoid muscle retracted inferiorly, the inferior edge of the specimen is defined, taking care to avoid injury to the transverse cervical artery and thoracic duct lying inferiorly in level IV. A high-riding subclavian vein may also be encountered, which when inadvertently injured presents significant risk of cervical as well as intrathoracic hemorrhage. If level IV dissection is performed, the omohyoid muscle may be divided to aid in exposure without significant functional deficits.

18. The entire specimen is then carried medially along a broad front, tracing the cervical plexus rootlets anteriorly to the internal jugular vein and the deep jugular chain lymph nodes. With the specimen retracted laterally, the vein is retracted medially with a moistened laparotomy sponge. Kittner dissecting sponges are useful at this step to bluntly dissect the vein from the carotid sheath fascia (Figure 47.6). Branching tributary veins are controlled with silk ligatures. The shrewd ablative surgeon will leave several millimeters of stump attached to the jugular vein in case of the need for future flap anastomosis. Dissection is carried out carefully as the specimen is essentially "unwrapped" from the vein at this step.

19. The specimen is delivered intact and oriented for permanent section.

20. Closure is achieved in layers over closed suction drains.

Radical Neck Dissection

1. The steps that differ from the selective neck dissection steps described in this chapter are outlined here, namely, the sacrifice of the internal jugular vein, spinal accessory nerve, and SCM.

2. The incision to expose levels I through IV may be the same as for the selective neck dissection; however, exposure to level V is limited. Visualization is improved by dropping a Schobinger or Lahey releasing incision inferolaterally toward the clavicle.

3. Superior and inferior skin flaps are elevated as in steps 2–3 of the "Selective Neck Dissection, Levels I–III" section. The external jugular vein and greater auricular nerves are divided superiorly and inferiorly in anticipation of SCM resection.

4. Levels I and II are dissected as in steps 4–15 in the "Selective Neck Dissection, Levels I–III" section.

5. The anterior aspect of the trapezius muscle is then identified, and the SCM is divided approximately 2 cm above the clavicle. The SCM may be transfixed with heavy silk sutures to prevent postoperative ooze.

6. The omohyoid muscle is then identified, traced to level V, and divided posteriorly. Care is taken to identify and protect the phrenic nerve and brachial plexus deep to the scalene fascia at this point, as well as to suture ligate the thoracic duct to prevent postoperative chyle leak.

7. The anterior edge of the trapezius is cleaned from inferiorly to superiorly, defining the posterior extent of the dissection. Blunt finger dissection at this step is a valuable aid. The spinal accessory nerve in level V is divided. The superior edge of the SCM is then divided and ligated with silk transfixion sutures.

8. Dissection is then carried along the posterior belly of the digastric muscle until the internal jugular vein is encountered.

9. With the specimen retracted anteriorly, dissection is carried along a broad front, again taking care to maintain the scalene fascia intact, avoiding injury to the phrenic nerve and cervical plexus. Cervical nerve rootlets are divided.

10. The carotid sheath is approached, and the specimen is returned to its anatomic position. The internal jugular vein is then isolated inferiorly and double suture ligated (one circumferential, one transfixion). The remaining specimen is then divided at the level of the clavicle and retracted superiorly. The ansa cervicalis is divided.

11. With the carotid artery and vagus nerve in view, the specimen is elevated superiorly toward the posterior belly of the digastric muscle.

12. With the posterior belly of the digastric muscle retracted superiorly, the hypoglossal nerve is identified and the descendens hypoglossi divided. Multiple ranine veins of the hypoglossal plexus are controlled with vascular clips and ties.

13. The superior aspect of the internal jugular vein is double suture ligated and divided. The anterosuperior aspect of the spinal accessory nerve is divided deep to the digastric muscle, and the specimen is delivered.

14. Closure is achieved in layers over closed suction drains.
15. The specimen is oriented and submitted for permanent section. One practice is to identify the lymph node levels with sutures: one suture in level I, two sutures in level II, and so on.

Complications and Postoperative Management

Neurologic Injury

Spinal accessory nerve: The division of CN XI with resultant shoulder weakness and pain syndrome has been the basis of many of the modifications to the radical neck dissection. Preserving the nerve results in improved outcomes, although function remains compromised in many cases. Level IIb may be preserved with decreased risk of shoulder dysfunction in the absence of macroscopic disease. Physical therapy is indicated for patients with postoperative complaints.

Phrenic nerve: May be injured if the deep layer of deep cervical fascia is violated. This may occur when defining the inferior and deep boundaries of the dissection at the point where the nerve lies on the anterior scalene muscle, deep in level IV. Postoperative elevation of the affected hemi-diaphragm with decreased lung volumes may be appreciated; however, adverse sequelae are limited in the absence of preexisting pulmonary disease.

Facial nerve: The marginal mandibular branch of the facial nerve may be injured when dissecting level Ib. Visualization of the nerve when dissecting the perifacial lymph nodes and along the inferior border of the mandible is helpful in decreasing risk of injury. Use of the Hayes–Martin maneuver may also minimize, but not absolutely prevent, injury to the nerve.

Hypoglossal nerve: Risk of injury to CN XII is increased in patients requiring dissection of level Ib, as hemorrhage from the neighboring Ranine plexus of veins may obscure visualization of the nerve. Careful dissection is key with vascular control using clips or ties. Unilateral injury is manifested postoperatively by deviation of the tongue to the affected side; bilateral injury may result in oral phase dysphagia.

Chyle Leak

Chylous leakage is reported in 1–2.5% of radical neck dissections, and it commonly occurs on the left side (75–92% of cases) when dissecting deep into level IV. To prevent injury, the nodal specimen in this region should be ligated prior to division. Intraoperatively, clear or milky fluid egress may be appreciated; the opacity of the fluid depends on the concentration of lipids in the patient's preoperative diet and duration of NPO (*nil per os*, i.e., no food or fluids) status. The anesthesiologist may assist in identifying a leak by maintaining positive pressure briefly, increasing intrathoracic pressure and venous return. Oversewing using nonresorbable sutures may be attempted to repair a leak, with topical application of a fibrin sealant. Management of chylous leakage is critical to minimize electrolyte derangement and hypoalbuminemia.

Management: Chyle leakage noted postoperatively will be most noticeable when tube feeding is initiated. Options for conservative management include maintaining closed suction drains, applying a pressure dressing (contraindicated in free tissue transfer and if skin flaps demonstrate vascular compromise), and administering a medium-chain triglyceride diet. Daily needle aspiration of low-output fistulae (<1000 mL/day) following suction drain removal and/or negative pressure wound therapy at −50 mmHg may offer resolutions. If conservative measures fail to resolve the leak in a timely fashion, surgical exploration is indicated, although identification of the injured duct may be difficult due to fibrin debris. Oversewing the region of injury and coverage with vascularized tissue are recommended to improve success rates and avoid delays in adjuvant radiation therapy.

Bleeding

Intraoperative injury to the great vessels of the neck must be managed expediently to minimize blood loss and operative morbidity. The use of monopolar cautery in immediate proximity to the vein must be performed with caution, as charring of the adventitial layer may predispose the patient to late vessel wall rupture and exsanguinating hemorrhage several days or even weeks postoperatively.

In the rare case of internal jugular injury, the defect must be immediately occluded to avoid air embolism. To provide exposure for repair, finger tamponade of the vein above and below the laceration is maintained by the assistant, expressing blood from that portion of the vein while the rent is repaired with fine nonresorbable vascular sutures on a tapered needle.

Late bleeding due to carotid blowout is associated with radiation therapy and is more common following radical neck dissection with minimal overlying vessel coverage. A high rate of mortality is associated with this untoward event.

Key Points

1. If tracheostomy is performed with neck dissection, subplatysmal flap elevation should avoid extension into the tracheostomy site. Maintain the surgical sites as two separate compartments to avoid contamination and infection of the neck dissection wound.
2. The posterior belly of the digastric muscle is an important landmark. Known as the "resident's friend" in neck dissection, maintaining it in view minimizes risk

to major structures (carotid artery, internal jugular vein, vagus nerve, and hypoglossal nerve).

3. The use of gentle finger dissection along the scalene fascia cannot be underestimated.

4. Have the anesthesiologist apply intraoperative Valsalva while examining deep level IV under loupe magnification to identify an early thoracic duct injury with chyle leak.

5. Application of appropriate traction and countertraction is essential when identifying fascial planes, as it facilitates dissection while minimizing blood loss.

References

Andersen, P.E., Warren, F., Spiro, J. and Burningham, A., 2002. Results of selective neck dissection in management of the node-positive neck. *Archives of Otolaryngology—Head and Neck Surgery*, 128 (10), 1180–4.

Brandwein-Gensler, P.S.M., 2011. *Lymph nodes of the neck, in head and neck imaging*. Philadelphia: Mosby.

Byers, R.M., Weber, R.S., Andrews, T., McGill, D., Kare, R. and Wolf, P., 1997. Frequency and therapeutic implications of "skip metastases" in the neck from squamous carcinoma of the oral tongue. *Head and Neck*, 19 (1), 14–19.

Calearo, C.V. and Teatini, G, 1983. Functional neck dissection: anatomical grounds, surgical technique, clinical observations. *Annals of Otology, Rhinology, and Laryngology*, 92 (3 Pt. 1), 215–22.

Carter, R.L., Tsao, S.W., Burman, J.F., Pittam, M.R., Clifford, P. and Shaw, H.J., 1983. Patterns and mechanisms of bone invasion by squamous carcinomas of the head and neck. *American Journal of Surgery*, 146 (4), 451–5.

Crile, G., 1906. Excision of cancer of the head and neck with special reference to the plan of dissection based upon one hundred thirty-two operations. *JAMA*, 47, 1780–86.

Crile, G., 1905. On the surgical treatment of cancer of the head and neck. *Transactions of the Southern Surgical and Gynecological Association*, 18, 109–27.

Davidson, B.J., Kulkarny, V., Delacure, M.D. and Shah, J.P., 1993. Posterior triangle metastases of squamous cell carcinoma of the upper aerodigestive tract. *American Journal of Surgery*, 166 (4), 395–8.

de Gier, H.H., Balm, A.J., Bruning, P.F., Gregor, R.T. and Hilgers, F.J., 1996. Systematic approach to the treatment of chylous leakage after neck dissection. *Head and Neck*, 18 (4), 347–51.

Fakih, A.R., Rao, R.S., Borges, A.M. and Patel, A.R., 1989. Elective versus therapeutic neck dissection in early carcinoma of the oral tongue. *American Journal of Surgery*, 158 (4), 309–13.

Ferlito, A., Johnson, J.T., Rinaldo, A., Pratt, L.W. and Fagan, J.J., 2007. European surgeons were the first to perform neck dissection. *Laryngoscope*, 117 (5), 797–802.

Ferlito, A., Rinaldo, A., Robbins, K.T. and Silver, C.E., 2006. Neck dissection: past, present and future? *Journal of Laryngology and Otology*, 120 (2), 87–92.

Ferlito, A., Robbins, K.T., Shah, J.P., Medina, J.E. and Silver, C.E., 2011. Proposal for a rational classification of neck dissections. *Head and Neck*, 33 (3), 445–50.

Fischel, E., 1933. Surgical treatment of metastases to cervical lymph nodes from intraoral cancer. *American Journal of Roentgenology*, 29, 237–40.

Holmes, J.D., 2008. Neck dissection: nomenclature, classification, and technique. *Oral and Maxillofacial Surgical Clinics of North America*, 20 (3), 459–75.

Howlader, N., Noone, A.M., Krapcho, M., Garshell, J., Neyman, N., Altekruse, S.F., Kosary, C.L., Yu, M. and Ruhl, J., eds., 2013. *SEER cancer statistics review, 1975–2010*. Bethesda, MD: National Cancer Institute.

Kligerman, J., Lima, R.A., Soares, J.R., Prado, L., Dias, F., Freitas, E.Q. and Olivatto, L.O., 1994. Supraomohyoid neck dissection in the treatment of T1/T2 squamous cell carcinoma of oral cavity. *American Journal of Surgery*, 168 (5), 391–4.

Kocher, T., 1880. Ueber Radicalheilung des Krebses. *Deutsche Zeitschrift für Chirurgie*, 13, 134–66.

Lindberg, R., 1972. Distribution of cervical lymph node metastases from squamous cell carcinoma of the upper respiratory and digestive tracts. *Cancer*, 29 (6), 1446–9.

Martin, H., Del Valle, B. and Ehrlich, H., 1951. Neck dissection. *Cancer*, 4 (3), 441–99.

Medina, J.E., 1989. A rational classification of neck dissections. *Otolaryngology—Head and Neck Surgery*, 100 (3), 169–76.

Myers, E.N. and J.J. Fagan, 1998. Treatment of the N+ neck in squamous cell carcinoma of the upper aerodigestive tract. *Otolaryngology Clinics of North America*, 31 (4), 671–86.

Robbins, K.T., Clayman, G., Levine, P.A., Medina, J., Sessions, R., Shaha, A. and Som, P., 2002. Neck dissection classification update: revisions proposed by the American Head and Neck Society and the American Academy of Otolaryngology—Head and Neck Surgery. *Archives of Otolaryngology—Head and Neck Surgery*, 128 (7), 751–8.

Robbins, K.T., Medina, J.E., Wolfe, J.T., Levine, P.A., Sessions, R. and Pruet, C.W., 1991. Standardizing neck dissection terminology. Official report of the Academy's Committee for Head and Neck Surgery and Oncology. *Archives of Otolaryngology—Head and Neck Surgery*, 117 (6), 601–5.

Robbins, K.T., Shaha, A.R., Medina, J.E., Califano, J.A., Wolf, G.T., Ferlito, A. and Som, P.M., 2008. Consensus statement on the classification and terminology of neck dissection. *Archives of Otolaryngology—Head and Neck Surgery*, 134 (5), 536–8.

Rouviere, H., 1938. *Anatomy of the human lymphatic system* (Trans. M.J. Tobies). Ann Arbor, MI: Edwards Brothers.

Shah, J., 2012. *Jatin Shah's head and neck surgery and oncology*. Philadelphia: Elsevier Mosby.

Shah, J.P., Medina, J.E., Shaha, A.R., Schantz, S.F. and Marti, J.R., 1993. Cervical lymph node metastasis. *Current Problems in Surgery*, 30 (3), 1–335.

Skolnik, E.M., Yee, K.F., Friedman, M. and Golden, T.A., 1976. The posterior triangle in radical neck surgery. *Archives of Otolaryngology*, 102 (1), 1–4.

Suen, J.Y. and Goepfert, H., 1987. Standardization of neck dissection nomenclature. *Head and Neck Surgery*, 10 (2), 75–77.

Ward, G.E. and Robben, J.O., 1951. A composite operation for radical neck dissection and removal of cancer of the mouth. *Cancer*, 4 (1), 98–109.

48 Surgical Management of Lip Cancer

Terence E. Johnson,[1] Michael Grau, Jr.,[2] Craig Salt,[3] and Robert M. Laughlin[2]
[1]Department of Otolaryngology, Naval Medical Center San Diego, San Diego, California, USA
[2]Department of Oral and Maxillofacial Surgery, Naval Medical Center San Diego, San Diego, California, USA
[3]Department of Plastic Surgery, Naval Medical Center San Diego, San Diego, California, USA

Lip Switch Flaps: Abbe and Estlander Flaps

A method of achieving immediate reconstruction of lip resections with primary reconstruction of the upper or lower lips utilizing tissue from the opposite lip.

Abbe flap: A segment of the opposing (donor) lip is rotated to reconstruct the resected (recipient) lip. The Abbe flap is primarily utilized for resections not involving the oral commissure. There are numerous variations of the Abbe flap.

Estlander flap: Similar to the Abbe flap, but involves rotating the opposing (donor) lip around the oral commissure to reconstruct the resected (recipient) lip. Utilized for resections involving the oral commissure. Frequently requires a secondary commissuroplasty.

Indications

1. Defects of one-half to two-thirds of the upper or lower lip as a result of pathology or trauma
2. The Abbe (Sabattini) flap is utilized for medial defects
3. The Abbe flap can also be used during secondary reconstruction of the philtrum in bilateral cleft lip patients
4. The Estlander flap is utilized for lateral defects with commissure involvement. This area is difficult to reconstruct due to the complex muscle interdigitations and functional importance

Contraindications

1. Patient who is unable to tolerate closure of lips for 2–3 weeks
2. Cases with evidence of damage to the proposed vascular pedicle
3. Defects of the lip greater than two-thirds of the total lip length

Flap Anatomy

The labial artery serves as the pedicle of the interpolated flap and venous drainage is provided by small veins parallel with the labial artery.

Surgical Technique: Abbe Flap

1. The patient is positioned supine on the operating table. The surgical site is prepped and draped in a sterile fashion.
2. The height and width of the defect are measured. A flap is designed on the opposite lip directly adjacent to the defect. The height of the flap will be 1:1, and the ratio of the width of the flap will be 1:1/2 of the defect.
3. Pertinent surgical anatomy and flap design are marked with methylene blue and a 30-gauge needle. Key areas to mark include the vermillion borders on both sides of the defect and both sides of the donor site. This will allow for the correct reapproximation of the donor site after flap harvest and inset of the flap to the defect.
4. Local anesthetic containing epinephrine is injected within the surgical site. Local anesthetic is only injected after the defect is measured, and the donor flap has been designed to avoid distortion to the tissues.
5. A full-thickness flap is developed from the donor site. The labial artery is visualized and divided only on one side of the flap (typically the lateral side, preserving the medial side).
6. The flap is elevated from the donor site, maintaining the vascular pedicle and a small cuff of muscle.
7. The flap is rotated into the defect. Care must be taken to ensure the vascular pedicle does not kink or occlude arterial flow to the flap. Adequacy of the arterial flow may be verified by Doppler ultrasound.
8. The donor site is closed in three layers from the inside out (mucosa, muscle, and skin). Vermillion border alignment is critical. The use of the previously marked vermillion border with methylene blue may assist with proper alignment.
9. The flap is then serially inset, in a three-layer closure, paying close attention to accurately align the vermillion border.
10. The vascular pedicle is left attached for 2–3 weeks to establish sufficient collateral vascularity prior to final division of the pedicle.

Atlas of Operative Oral and Maxillofacial Surgery, First Edition. Edited by Christopher J. Haggerty and Robert M. Laughlin
© 2015 John Wiley & Sons, Inc. Published 2015 by John Wiley & Sons, Inc.

11. After a minimum of 14 days, the pedicle is isolated and temporarily occluded with a vascular tie. The flap should be observed for venous congestion and/or vascular insufficiency. If no congestion or insufficiency is noted, the pedicle is ligated and transected under local anesthesia. Minor trimming may be required to provide optimal aesthetic contour.

Surgical Technique: Estlander Flap

1. For the Estlander flap, the same sequence is utilized as with the Abbe flap.
2. Care must be taken to ensure the vascular pedicle does not kink or occlude arterial flow to the flap. The adequacy of arterial flow may be verified by Doppler ultrasound.
3. A secondary commissuroplasty is often required after the procedure to reestablish a normal-appearing commissure.

Postoperative Management

Care must be taken to ensure minimal oral opening to limit or minimize tension on the vascular pedicle. The patient may be placed in maxillomandibular fixation with Erich arch bars, Ivy loops, orthodontic brackets, or internal maxillomandibular fixation screws. The use of chin dressings extending to the cheeks, or jaw bras, may also be useful to limit opening.

Complications

1. **Vascular compromise**: Either venous congestion and/or vascular insufficiency.
2. **Asymmetry of the lips**: Results from inadequate or excessive donor flap harvest.
3. **Significant notching of the lips**: Results from misalignment of the orbicularis oris.

Key Points

1. Care must be taken during dissection to preserve the vascular pedicle. A small muscle cuff around the artery helps to preserve the venous system.
2. The flap width is designed on the unaffected lip to be approximately one-half the width of the defect to preserve lip proportions. The height of the flap should approximate the height of the defect.

3. As the flap rotates approximately 180° on its pedicle, care must be taken to ensure that vascular compromise has not been introduced from torsion of the pedicle.
4. The flap should remain in place and attached for 2–3 weeks (14–21 days) to establish sufficient collateral vascularity prior to final division of the pedicle.
5. Patient's opening should be limited during initial healing to avoid tension on the pedicle.

References

Baker, S.R., 2007. *Local flaps in facial reconstruction*. St. Louis, MO: Mosby/Elsevier.
Butler, C., *Procedures in reconstructive surgery: head and neck reconstruction*. Philadelphia: Saunders/Elsevier, 2009.
Papel, I.D., 2002. *Facial plastic and reconstructive surgery*, 2nd ed. New York: Thieme.
Stauch, B., 2009. *Grabb's encyclopedia of flaps, head and neck*. 3rd ed. Philadelphia: Lippincott, Williams & Wilkins.

Full-thickness Wedge Resection (V Shaped, V-Y Shaped, and W Shaped)

Full-thickness wedge resection for ablative treatment of lip cancer with immediate reconstruction utilizing primary closure.

Indications

1. Full-thickness defects of less than one-third of the upper or lower lip as a result of pathology or trauma
2. Full-thickness wedge resections are typically used for midline or para-midline defects, but may be utilized in the lateral region of the lip with minor design modifications

Contraindications

1. Defects of the lip greater than one-third
2. Areas where non-full-thickness resections were performed

Flap Anatomy

The labial artery serves as the primary blood supply to the lips. Venous drainage is provided by small veins in parallel with the labial artery. The layers of the lips are the epithelium of the skin, subcutaneous tissues including the deep dermis, orbicularis oris, and mucosa.

Surgical Technique: Full-thickness V Shaped Wedge Resection

1. The patient is positioned supine on the operating table. The surgical site is prepped and draped in a sterile fashion.
2. The height and width of the defect are measured.
3. The flap is designed to extend from the complete height of the lip from the vermillion border to the labio-mental fold. The apex of the V-shaped design should be centered directly over the center of the lesion to be resected (Figure 48.1 [all figures appear in Case Report 48.1]). For lesions within the lateral lip region, the design should be slightly skewed to better parallel the natural skin tension lines in this region.
4. Pertinent surgical anatomy may be marked with methylene blue and a 30-gauge needle. Key areas to mark include the surgical margins and the vermillion borders on both sides of the anticipated surgical defect in order to allow for the correct reapproximation of the vermillion border after the resection is completed.
5. Local anesthetic containing epinephrine is injected within the surgical site. However, local anesthetic should only be injected after the defect is measured and marked and the proposed flap design is outlined, to avoid any distortion of the tissues.
6. A full-thickness resection of the lesion is performed (Figure 48.2) and sent for final pathology (Figure 48.3).
7. Adequate hemostasis is achieved through bipolar electrocautery.
8. The orbicularis muscle is identified on both medial and lateral aspects of the surgical defect. The mucosa and the subcutaneous tissues are sharply dissected off the muscle for approximately 1 cm to allow for isolation of the orbicularis muscle.
9. The orbicularis muscle is reapproximated with resorable sutures in an interrupted fashion. Alignment of the muscle is critical, as misalignments and improper approximation may result in notch defects.
10. The vermillion border is aligned with either resorbable or nonresorbable sutures. Accurate alignment of the vermillion is critical for postoperative aesthetics. The remaining layers (the mucosa, subcutaneous tissue and skin) are closed in a standard layered fashion.

Postoperative Management

1. Care must be taken to ensure minimal oral opening to limit or minimize tension to sutures.
2. Antibiotic ointments are recommended for skin incisions for a period not to exceed 3 days.

Complications

1. **Asymmetry of the lips**: Typically results from inadequate or excessive tissue removal, incorrect alignment of the vermilion border and/or failure to accurately reapproximate any of the 4 layers (skin, subcutaneous tissue, orbicularis oris muscle or mucosa) upon closure of the surgical site.
2. **Significant notching of the vermillion**: Results from misalignment of the orbicularis oris muscle.

Key Points

1. Care must be taken during dissection to preserve the orbicularis oris muscle. Approximately 1 cm of muscle length should be visualized to ensure correct realignment.
2. The vertical arms for the V shape and lateral arms for the W-shaped designs should extend to the labio-mental fold and should parallel the resting skin tension lines.
3. A meticulous reapproximation of all four layers—mucosa, muscle, subcutaneous tissues, and skin—is paramount to providing an optimal aesthetic outcome.
4. Lip defects that involve less than one-half of the original length of the lip are frequently treated with either V- or W-shaped full-thickness wedge resections and closed primarily. Defects one-half to two-thirds of the original lip length may be reconstructed with Abbe (not involving the oral commissure) and Estlander (involving the oral commissure) flaps.

References

Baker, S.R., 2007. *Local flaps in facial reconstruction*. St. Louis, MO: Mosby/Elsevier.

Butler, C., *Procedures in reconstructive surgery: head and neck reconstruction*. Philadelphia: Saunders/Elsevier, 2009.

Papel, I.D., 2002. *Facial plastic and reconstructive surgery*, 2nd ed. New York: Thieme.

Case Report

Case Report 48.1. A 29-year-old male presents with a chief complaint of a nonhealing ulceration to his lower lip. On exam, the mass measured 1.8 cm in its greatest dimension and was located along the vermillion border. The commissure was uninvolved. An incisional biopsy was performed that revealed a well-differentiated squamous cell carcinoma of the lower lip. The mass was classified as a T1N0M0. A full-thickness V-shaped resection was performed with 1.0 cm margins. All frozen margins taken intraoperatively were negative, and the resection was primarily reconstructed with a layered closure. (See Figures 48.1, 48.2, 48.3, 48.4, and 48.5.)

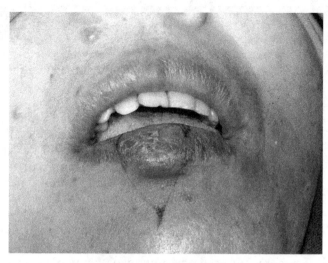

Figure 48.1.   The resection design is marked prior to the administration of local anesthetic to avoid distortion of the tissues. The apex of the resection extends to the submental crease.

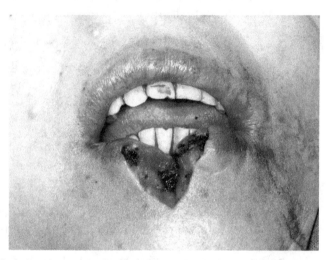

Figure 48.2.   A full-thickness V-shaped wedge resection with 10 mm margins is performed. Hemostasis is achieved with bipolar cautery, and frozen margins are taken from the periphery of the defect site.

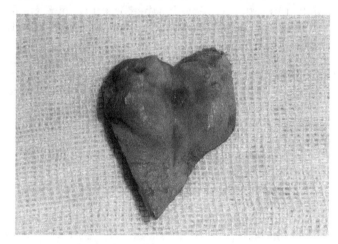

Figure 48.3.   The final specimen is sent to pathology.

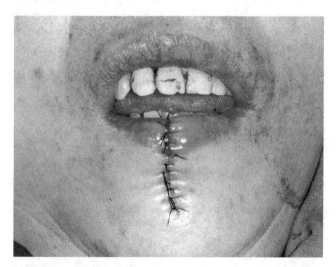

Figure 48.4.   The defect is repaired primarily with a layered closure. Care is taken to align the vermilion border for optimal aesthetics and to reapproximate the orbicularis oris muscle to minimize notch defects.

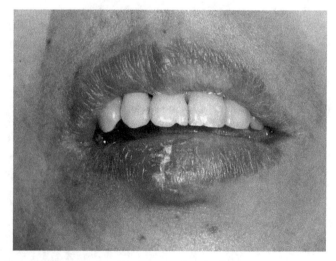

Figure 48.5.   Four-month postoperative result.

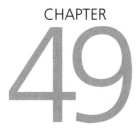

Salivary Gland Pathology

Michael Grau, Jr.,[1] **Markus S. Hill,**[1] **Billy Turley,**[1] **Vincent Slovan,**[1]
Christopher J. Haggerty[2], **and Robert M. Laughlin**[1]

[1]*Department of Oral and Maxillofacial Surgery, Naval Medical Center San Diego, San Diego, California, USA*
[2] *Private Practice, Lakewood Oral and Maxillofacial Surgery Specialists, Lees Summit; and Department of Oral and Maxillofacial Surgery, University of Missouri–Kansas City, Kansas City, Missouri, USA*

Mucocele (Mucous Extravasation Phenomenon) Excision

Local excision of a damaged minor salivary gland and associated soft tissue.

Indications

1. Soft tissue swelling associated with damage or rupture of a minor salivary gland duct

Contraindications

1. Significant medical comorbidities (i.e., anticoagulated patients)

Anatomy

Mucocele: A damaged or ruptured minor salivary gland duct leading to extravasation of mucus within the surrounding soft tissue.

Technique

1. Local anesthesia is administered specific to the location of the mucocele. For lower lip mucoceles, bilateral mental nerve or inferior alveolar nerve blocks are performed.
2. An elliptical excision of the mucocele, with its associated overlying mucosa and glandular tissue/damaged minor salivary gland, is performed down to the muscle layer (Figure 49.3). Care is taken to preserve the integrity of the vermillion border of the lip, to remove the entire involved minor salivary gland, and to minimize iatrogenic damage to adjacent minor salivary glands.
3. Deep 4-0 Vicryl sutures are placed depending on the size and depth of the surgical defect.
4. Interrupted 4-0 chromic sutures are used to reapproximate the mucosa (Figure 49.4). Care is taken to not deform the lower lip with inappropriate suture placement.

Postoperative Management

1. Pain medication is prescribed based on the invasiveness of the procedure.

2. If the lower lip is the site of excision, ice is applied to the affected area off and on for the first 24 hours.
3. A 2-week follow-up is advised to assess the healing of the site and to review the pathology results with the patient.

Complications

1. **Lower lip asymmetry**: Results from inappropriate suture placement. If identified at the time of the procedure, the asymmetry may be corrected with suture removal and resuturing of the lower lip. If identified late, the asymmetry may require revision surgery.
2. **Recurrence**: Due to incomplete removal of the involved minor salivary gland or from damage to adjacent minor salivary glands. Prior to the procedure, the possibility of recurrence should be discussed with the patient.

Key Points

1. Although mucoceles may occur at any location containing minor salivary glands (i.e., the soft palate, retromolar pad, ventral tongue, floor of mouth, and buccal mucosa), over 80% of mucoceles are found within the lower lip.
2. The majority of mucoceles occur within the first three decades of life.
3. Mucoceles typically present as a blue, purple, gray, or normal-colored painless, soft, fluid-filled vesicle on the lower lip. Mucoceles may undergo a fibrotic transformation from chronic inflammation and lip biting.
4. Mucoceles infrequently exceed 1.0 cm in their greatest dimension.
5. Drainage of mucoceles or incomplete excision of the damaged gland will result in a recurrence of the mucocele.
6. Recurrence rates of mucoceles are related to incomplete excision of the involved minor salivary gland and/or damage to adjacent minor salivary glands during the excisional procedure.
7. All removed tissue is sent for pathological examination.

Atlas of Operative Oral and Maxillofacial Surgery, First Edition. Edited by Christopher J. Haggerty and Robert M. Laughlin
© 2015 John Wiley & Sons, Inc. Published 2015 by John Wiley & Sons, Inc.

References

Chi, A.C., Lambert, P.R., Richardson, M.S. and Neville, B.W., 2011. Oral mucoceles: a clinicopathologic review of 1,824 cases, including unusual variants. *Journal of Oral and Maxillofacial Surgery*, 69, 1086–93.

Huang, I.Y., Chen, C.M., Kao, Y.H. and Worthington, P., 2007. Treatment of mucoceles of the lower lip with carbon dioxide laser. *Journal of Oral and Maxillofacial Surgery*, 65, 855–8.

Case Report

Case Report 49.1. A 24-year-old patient presents with a chief complaint of a slow-growing, painless mass to his lower lip. On examination, the patient presents with a 1.0 cm, pink, asymptomatic, fluid-filled mass to the left lower lip. (See Figures 49.1, 49.2, 49.3, 49.4, and 49.5.)

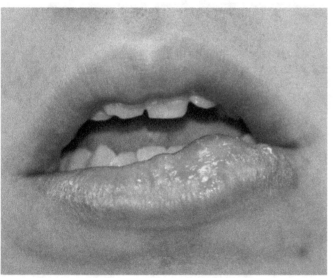

Figure 49.1.   Asymptomatic mass to the lower lip.

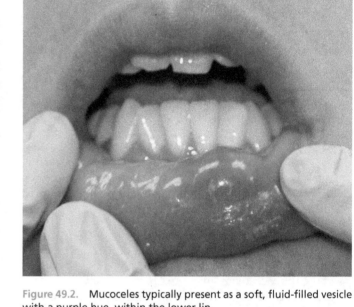

Figure 49.2.   Mucoceles typically present as a soft, fluid-filled vesicle with a purple hue, within the lower lip.

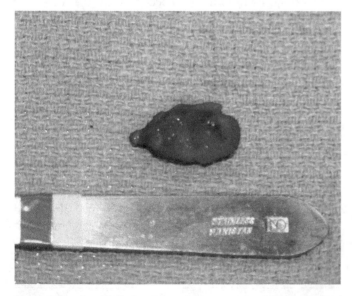

Figure 49.3.   An elliptical excision of the mucocele with its associated overlying mucosa and glandular tissue/damaged minor salivary gland.

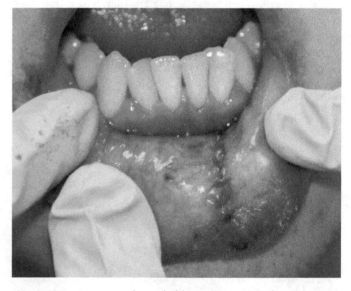

Figure 49.4.   Interrupted resorbable sutures are used to reapproximate the mucosa.

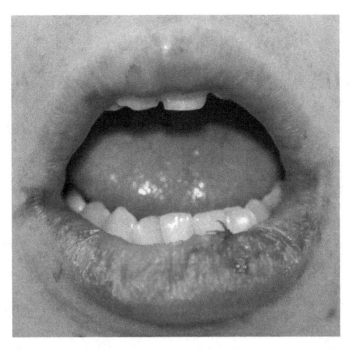

Figure 49.5. The lip is checked for asymmetries. Any asymmetries are corrected with suture removal and resuturing of the lip.

Sublingual Gland Excision

A surgical method for excising an infected or pathologic sublingual gland with or without an associated ranula.

Indications

1. Ranula formation
2. Sialadenitis
3. Sublingual pathology

Contraindications

1. Significant medical comorbidities
2. Relative contraindication: active infection

Anatomy

Ranulas: Extravasation mucoceles that arise from the sublingual gland due to damage or rupture of a main duct or the acini after obstruction.

Plunging ranulas: A ranula that extends through the mylohyoid muscle and extends into the neck, with or without intraoral swelling.

Sublingual gland: The sublingual gland is the smallest of the major salivary glands and produces 3–5% of the total salivary flow to the oral cavity. The sublingual saliva exits the gland via small ducts of Rivinas. These ducts may empty directly into the floor of the mouth, join Wharton's duct directly, or coalesce into a larger, common sublingual (Bartholin's) duct before joining the submandibular duct.

Lingual nerve: A large, flat nerve that is located within the lateral floor of mouth, superior to the submandibular gland. The lingual nerve descends from the mandibular division of the trigeminal nerve near the lingula, and it courses from lateral to medial as it nears the tongue. During its descension, the lingual nerve loops underneath the submandibular duct, first crossing from the lateral side, and then again passing the duct as the nerve ascends on the medial side to innervate the dorsal tongue.

Technique: Intraoral Ranula and Sublingual Gland Excision

1. The procedure may be performed with local anesthesia alone, intravenous sedation, or general anesthesia with endotracheal intubation.
2. Local anesthesia is administered in the form of bilateral nerve blocks and local infiltration. A lacrimal probe is inserted into Wharton's duct (Figure 49.7) to allow for the identification and retraction of the duct. Traction sutures may be placed within the periphery of the tongue to aid in retraction.
3. An elliptical incision is made around the periphery of the ranula through the oral mucosa only. Care is taken to not perforate the ranula itself.
4. Blunt dissection with a fine hemostat is used to identify the associated sublingual gland (Figure 49.7). During dissection, the surgeon should be cognizant of the location of Wharton's duct (easily identifiable if a lacrimal probe was placed) and the lingual nerve medial to the sublingual gland.

5. An Allis clamp is used to grasp and elevate the sublingual gland as it is freed from its surrounding tissue with blunt dissection (Figure 49.8).
6. The site is copiously irrigated, and the lacrimal probe is removed. The defect is evaluated for hemostasis.
7. The mucosal defect may be reapproximated with interrupted resorbable sutures or may be left open to granulate secondarily (Figure 49.10).

Technique: Intraoral Sublingual Gland Excision without Associated Ranula

1. Follow steps 1–2 of the "Technique: Intraoral Ranula and Sublingual Gland Excision" section.
2. A lingual gingival sulcular incision is initiated along the posterior teeth. The incision may be carried to the midline if additional exposure of the floor of the mouth is necessary.
3. A subperiosteal tissue plane is developed, and a full-thickness tissue flap is developed along the lingual aspect of the body or ramus of the mandible.
4. The sublingual gland is palpated medial to the periosteal reflection, superior to the mylohyoid muscle. The periosteum overlying the sublingual gland is penetrated with blunt dissection, and the sublingual gland is identified.
5. The ensuing sublingual gland removal is described in steps 4–6 of the "Technique: Intraoral Ranula and Sublingual Gland Excision" section.
6. The incision is closed primarily with interrupted interproximal resorbable sutures.

Technique: Transcutaneous Plunging Ranula and Sublingual Gland Excision

1. The approach to the submandibular triangle is described in steps 1–6 of the "Submandibular Gland Excision" section.
2. Once the ranula is identified, blunt dissection is used to mobilize the ranula from its surrounding tissue. Blunt dissection and mobilization continue superiorly until the plunging ranula is freed from the anterior and posterior bellies of the digastric muscles, the hyoglossus muscle, and the herniation through the mylohyoid muscle is identified.
3. The dehiscence through the mylohyoid muscle is enlarged, and the attachment of the plunging ranula to the ipsilateral sublingual gland is identified. Blunt dissection is used to free the sublingual gland from its associated tissue. Care is taken to avoid iatrogenic damage to the lingual nerve and Wharton duct medial to the gland.
4. The plunging ranula and the associated sublingual gland are delivered through the transcutaneous incision. The dehiscence in the mylohyoid muscle is repaired with interrupted resorbable sutures.

5. The incision is irrigated, hemostasis is confirmed, and the wound is closed in a layered fashion. Drains are placed dependent on the size of the plunging ranula excised.

Postoperative Management

1. Broad-spectrum antibiotics are prescribed for 5 days postoperatively.
2. Saline rinses are begun the day after surgery and continued until the complete mucosalization of the defect or incision site.
3. Analgesics are prescribed based on the invasiveness of the procedure.
4. Follow-up appointments are typically at 1 week, 3 weeks, and 6 weeks to assess surgical site healing and to assess lingual nerve and Wharton's duct function.

Complications

Hematoma formation: Minimized with meticulous dissection and careful inspection of the surgical site prior to procedure completion. Managed with hematoma evacuation with or without drain placement.

Damage to the lingual nerve (CN V3): Iatrogenic damage to this structure as it courses medial to the sublingual gland will result in a sensory disturbance to the tongue. Most injuries are stretch injuries and improve with time. Witnessed nerve transections should be repaired primarily at the initial surgery.

Damage to Wharton's duct: Minimized by cannulation of Wharton's duct with a lacrimal probe prior to surgical exploration of the floor of the mouth. Damage to Wharton's duct may lead to stenosis, obstructive sialadenitis, and sialocele formation. Observed transections or lacerations are treated with intraoperative sialodochoplasty or intraoral cannulation with plastic tubing. The tubing should be left in place for several weeks to promote epithelialization around the stent to reestablish duct continuity (Figures 49.24 and 49.25).

Ranula recurrence: Recurrence rates are directly related to the procedure performed. Complete sublingual gland excision has the lowest recurrence rate, whereas marsupialization alone is associated with the highest recurrence rate.

Key Points

1. Multiple treatment modalities exist for ranula management. Surgical treatments and associated recurrence rates are listed in descending order: complete excision of the ranula and the associated sublingual gland, partial sublingual gland resection, and marsupialization. Recurrence rates are highly variable within the literature.

2. The approach selection for plunging ranulas is based on the size of the ranula. Smaller plunging ranulas may be surgically excised via an intraoral approach alone. Larger plunging ranulas may be resected with an extraoral approach, with or without a combined intraoral approach. The type of extraoral approach is determined by the extension (submandibular, cervical, and/or parapharyngeal) and the size of the ranula.

3. Combined transcutaneous and intraoral approaches are required for plunging ranulas with intraoral extension or when the sublingual gland cannot be identified through an extraoral approach.

4. Early identification of the lingual nerve and Wharton's duct along the medial aspect of the sublingual gland is key to minimizing postoperative complications associated with these structures. Cannulation of Wharton's duct prior to floor-of-mouth dissection will minimize iatrogenic damage to this structure and allow for its retraction from the surgical field.

References

Galloway, R.H., Gross, P.D., Thompson, S.H. and Patterson, A.L., 1989. Pathogenesis and treatment of ranula: report of three cases. *Journal of Oral and Maxillofacial Surgery*, 47, 302–6.

Sigismund, P.E., Bozzato, A., Schumann, M., Koch, M., Iro, H. and Zenk, J., 2013. Management of ranula: 9 years' clinical experience in pediatric and adult patients. *Journal of Oral and Maxillofacial Surgery*, 71, 538–44.

Skouteris, C.A. and Sotereanos, G.C., 1987. Plunging ranula: report of a case. *Journal of Oral and Maxillofacial Surgery*, 45, 1068–72.

Zhao, Y.I., Jia, J. and Jia, Y.L., 2005. Complications associated with surgical management of ranulas. *Journal of Oral and Maxillofacial Surgery*, 63, 51–54.

Case Report

Case Report 49.2. A 24-year-old patient presents with a chief complaint of a soft, painless mass within the right floor of his mouth that has been present for over 12 months. On examination, the patient has a 2.5 cm × 1.3 cm fluctuant, nontender soft tissue mass located along the right lingual gutter. The location and appearance of the mass had a high clinical suspicion for a ranula. The patient was treated with general anesthesia via nasotracheal intubation and an in continuity excision of the right sublingual gland and overlying ranula. The final histopathology revealed a ranula with extravasation of mucus from the included sublingual gland. (See Figures 49.6, 49.7, 49.8, 49.9, and 49.10.)

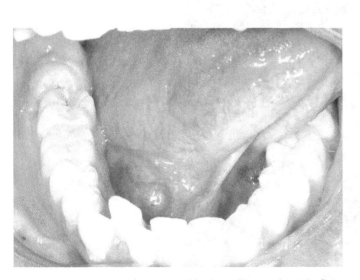

Figure 49.6.   A 2.5 cm soft, painless, bluish swelling to the right floor of the mouth.

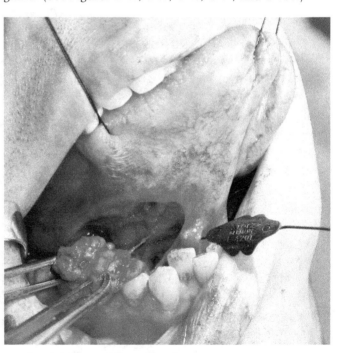

Figure 49.7.   Traction sutures and lacrimal probe in place. An elliptical incision was made over the ranula to allow for excision of the ranula and sublingual gland in continuity.

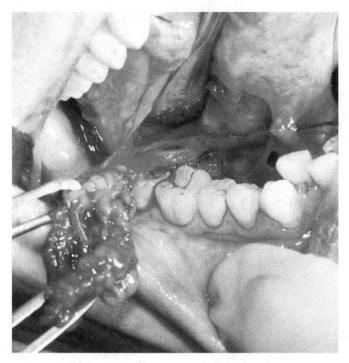

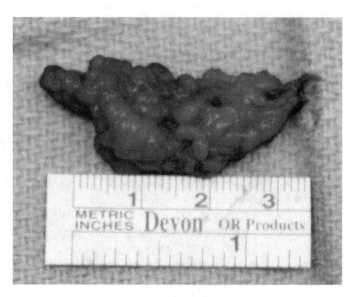

Figure 49.9.   Excised right sublingual gland.

Figure 49.8.   Allis clamps are used to grasp the sublingual gland. Blunt dissection is used to free the gland from its surrounding tissue. Wharton's duct is identified along the medial aspect of the dissection.

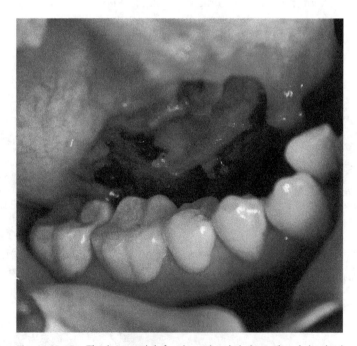

Figure 49.10.   The intraoral defect is copiously irrigated and checked for hemostasis. The mucosa surrounding the defect may be reapproximated with interrupted resorbable sutures or allowed to heal secondarily.

Submandibular Gland Resection

A surgical method for transcutaneously excising a non-functional, hyperfunctional, or pathologic submandibular gland.

Indications

1. Recurrent or chronic sialadenitis
2. Obstructive sialocholithiasis
3. Benign or malignant neoplasms
4. As part of a neck dissection to remove lymph nodes in level Ib

Contraindications

1. **Suspicion of tumor**: Removal of the gland should not be done as a biopsy to rule out tumor, whether benign or malignant. A formal level I neck dissection, rather than a "shelling out" of the gland, should be performed unless the evaluation clearly points to a non-neoplastic indication for gland removal
2. **Significant medical comorbidities precluding the use of general anesthesia**: For patients unable to tolerate general anesthesia, the gland may be removed under local anesthesia if indicated
3. Hematologic disorders
4. Sialolithiasis within the distal portion of Wharton's duct

Anatomy

Submandibular gland: The submandibular gland is located within the submandibular triangle (level 1b) of the neck. The superficial part of the gland is immediately deep to the platysma and is encapsulated by the investing layer of the deep cervical fascia. The gland is bilobed, forming a C shape around the posterior margin of the mylohyoid muscle. The superficial lobe can be found above the mylohyoid muscle within the lateral sublingual space, while the larger deep lobe is located inferior to the mylohyoid muscle. Medially, the submandibular gland is intimately associated with the stylohyoid, digastric, and styloglossus muscles.

Wharton's duct: Arises from multiple branches on the medial side of the deep lobe of the submandibular gland. Wharton's duct courses forward, superior, and medial to the mylohyoid muscle and in close proximity to the lingual nerve. As the duct moves forward, it travels medial to the sublingual gland. The submandibular duct advances anteriorly and medially until its orifice opens at the summit of small papilla on the side of the frenulum linguae, called the lingual caruncle. Not only is the course of the submandibular duct tortuous, but it is also the longest salivary duct at approximately 5 cm. Therefore, salivary secretions have more time in transit before being discharged into the mouth. The duct possesses two bends, the first at the posterior border of the mylohyoid muscle and the second near the duct orifice. In addition, the duct partially courses from inferior to superior, forcing the flow of saliva against gravity and increasing the risk of retrograde movement. The calcium concentration of the saliva produced by the submandibular gland is twice that of the parotid gland, and the saliva is more viscous and alkaline. These factors promote salivary stasis and sialolith formation within the submandibular duct. 90% of submandibular duct stones are radiopaque, whereas 90% of parotid gland stones are radiolucent. Stones anterior to the first molar can often be seen on an occlusal film and are more amenable to treatment via an intraoral incision and sialodochoplasty.

Marginal mandibular nerve: At risk of injury as it runs within the investing (superficial) layer of deep cervical fascia overlying the gland. The marginal mandibular nerve may be located up to 3 cm below the inferior border of the mandible. It consists of up to four parallel branches that cross the facial artery and vein before ascending to innervate the depressor anguli oris.

Hypoglossal nerve: Enters the submandibular triangle posteroinferiorly and medial to the stylohyoid muscle and the posterior belly of the digastric. After entering the submandibular triangle, it travels in an anterosuperior direction against the lateral surface of the hyoglossus muscle. The nerve ultimately passes above the posterior border of the mylohyoid muscle prior to entering the musculature of the tongue.

Surgical Technique

1. Preoperative intravenous antibiotics are initiated pre-incision.
2. The patient is induced with short-acting paralytics to allow for monitoring of the marginal mandibular branch of the facial nerve during dissection. General anesthesia is typically obtained via oral endotracheal intubation.
3. The patient is placed in a supine position, the neck is hyperextended, and the head is rotated to the contralateral side. The patient is prepped and draped in a sterile fashion. The ipsilateral commissure of the mouth should be prepped and readily visible.
4. A natural skin crease at least 3 cm below the inferior border of the mandible or at the level of the hyoid bone, extending anteriorly from the anterior border of the sternocleidomastoid (SCM) muscle, is located and marked (Figure 49.11). 2% lidocaine with 1:100,000 epinephrine may be infiltrated into the subcutaneous tissues in the region of the proposed incision to aid with hemostasis.

5. The incision is carried through skin and subcutaneous tissue to the level of the platysma muscle. A subplatysmal flap is developed superiorly to the inferior border of the mandible to expose the investing (superficial) layer of the deep cervical fascia and the superficial aspect of the submandibular gland (Figure 49.12). A nerve stimulator is used to assist in the identification of marginal mandibular nerve during dissection to the submandibular gland.

6. The submandibular capsule is incised inferiorly. A subcapsular dissection is performed to expose the gland. Care must be taken during this step to keep the dissection subcapsular to avoid damage to the marginal mandibular nerve. Alternatively, the marginal mandibular nerve may be exposed as the nerve crosses the facial vessels. The nerve may then be retracted superiorly within the subplatysmal flap.

7. The facial artery and vein are divided and ligated. The anterior margin of the gland is freed from the anterior belly of the digastric muscle with blunt dissection or electrocautery. The dissection continues in a posterior direction, elevating the gland from the lateral surface of the mylohyoid muscle. The mylohyoid vessels are divided and ligated to allow access to the mylohyoid muscle.

8. The posterior free margin of the mylohyoid is identified. Care must be taken to avoid damage to the hypoglossal nerve, the venous comitans of the hypoglossal, and the lingual nerve, which are exposed and vulnerable to injury immediately posterior to the mylohyoid muscle. Retracting the posterior free margin of the mylohyoid anteriorly and with careful finger dissection, the lingual nerve, submandibular ganglion, and submandibular duct come into view. An index finger is passed in the well-defined interfascial plane between the gland and submandibular ganglion laterally and the fascia covering the hypoglossal nerve and venous comitans medially.

9. After the hypoglossal nerve has been identified, one may safely clamp, divide, and ligate the submandibular duct and divide the lingual nerve from the submandibular ganglion. Bipolar electrocautery should be utilized at the junction of the lingual nerve and the ganglion prior to division. Care must be taken not to damage the lingual nerve. The gland is reflected inferiorly, and the facial artery is identified, ligated, and divided where it exits from behind the posterior belly of the digastric. The gland is freed from the tendon and posterior belly of the digastric and removed (Figure 49.13). The gland is sent for final pathology (Figure 49.14).

10. The view of the surgical field following resection demonstrates the hypoglossal nerve, the venous comitans, the lingual nerve, and the transected Wharton's duct all on the lateral aspect of the hyoglossus muscle (Figure 49.15). Deep to the hyoglossus muscle lies the lingual artery within Little's triangle.

11. The wound is irrigated with copious amounts of sterile saline. The surgical site is closed in layers. A suction drain or passive drain may be utilized (Figure 49.16).

Postoperative Management

1. Patients are typically admitted for 24-hour observation.
2. Broad-spectrum intravenous antibiotics (e.g., Cefazolin) are administered during the hospital course, followed by 1 week of oral antibiotic therapy.
3. The head of bed is elevated 30°, and a gentle pressure dressing is placed on the anterior neck.
4. The suction drain is removed at 36 hours postoperatively or when three consecutive 8-hour shifts produce less than 30 mL cumulative output.

Complications

1. **Injury to the hypoglossal nerve**: Damage to this nerve results in deviation of the tongue toward the injured side upon tongue protrusion.
2. Injury to the lingual nerve
3. Injury to the marginal mandibular nerve
4. Surgical site infections
5. Bleeding or hematoma formation

Key Points

1. Ensure the use of short-acting paralytics during induction to allow for facial nerve monitoring.
2. The incision should be placed within a natural skin fold to prevent an unaesthetic postoperative scar.
3. The marginal mandibular nerve must be identified in all cases.
4. If removal of the gland is indicated because of tumor, ensure the entire gland is removed and an enucleation is not performed.

References

Chen, W., Yang, Z., Wang, Y., Huang, Z. and Wang, Y., 2009. Removal of the submandibular gland using a combined retroauricular and transoral approach. *Journal of Oral and Maxillofacial Surgery*, 67, 522–7.

Pruess, S.F., Klussmann, J.P., Wittekindt, C., Drebber, U., Beutner, D. and Guntinas-Lichius, O., 2007. Submandibular gland excision: 15 years of experience. *Journal of Oral and Maxillofacial Surgery*, 65, 953–7.

Rapidis, A.D., Stavrianos, S., Lagogiannis, G. and Faratzis, G., 2004. Tumors of the submandibular gland: clinicopathologic analysis of 23 patients. *Journal of Oral and Maxillofacial Surgery*, 62, 1203–8.

Case Report 49.3. A 26-year-old male presents with a chief complaint of a 1-year history of recurrent pain and intermittent swelling to the right mandibular region. Physical examination revealed a firm mass isolated to the right submandibular triangle. No salivary flow was appreciated from the right submandibular duct. A contrasted computed tomography (CT) scan was obtained that revealed a marginated homogeneous mass within the right submandibular gland with no associated lymphadenopathy. Fine-needle aspiration (FNA) results suggested pleomorphic adenoma. The patient underwent a right submandibular gland resection with a definitive diagnosis of a pleomorphic adenoma. (See Figures 49.11 through 49.16.)

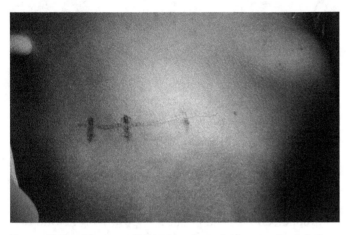

Figure 49.11. The proposed incision is marked approximately 3 cm below the inferior border of the mandible, extending anterior to the anterior border of the sternocleidomastoid muscle.

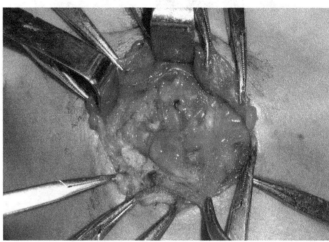

Figure 49.12. The initial incision is through skin, subcutaneous tissues, and platysma.

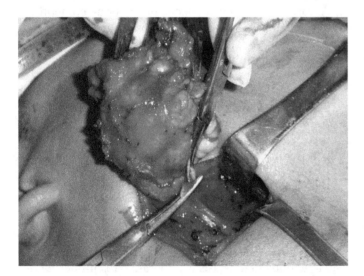

Figure 49.13. The diseased gland is freed from all attachments. The duct and vessels are divided and ligated. The lingual nerve retracts superiorly after division from the ganglion.

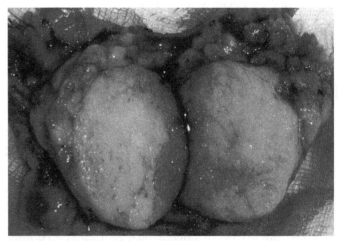

Figure 49.14. The diseased gland is examined prior to being sent for final pathology. Classic "cut-potato" appearance of a pleomorphic adenoma.

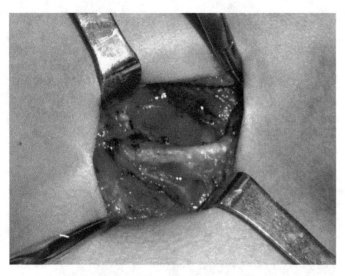

Figure 49.15. View of the surgical field after resection. Note the mylohyoid muscle and digastric tendon.

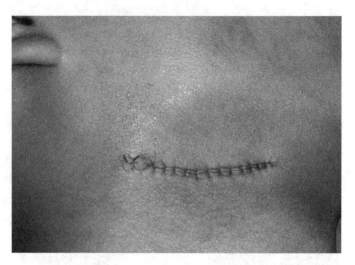

Figure 49.16. Surgical site is closed in layers. A passive Penrose drain is in place.

Sialodochoplasty

A ductotomy to reposition and widen the salivary duct orifice.

Indications

1. Chronic or recurrent sialolithiasis or sialadenitis
2. Evidence of distal ductal dilatation, obstruction, or stenosis on ultrasonography, computed tomography, or magnetic resonance sialography
3. Traumatic or iatrogenic violation of Stenson's, Wharton's, or Bartholin's ducts
4. Adjunct to salivary calculi removal via sialolithectomy or extracorporeal shock wave lithotripsy (ESWL)
5. Distal ductal pathology
6. Excessive sialorrhea (drooling)

Contraindications

1. Proximal obstruction of salivary duct or gland
2. Salivary gland pathology or dysfunction

Anatomy

Sialolithiasis: The formation of salivary calculi (sialoliths) within the major salivary glands or ducts. Sialoliths (salivary stones) are typically single, calcium-rich crystallized minerals; however, multiple stones may be present. Approximately 85% of sialoliths occur within the submandibular duct (Wharton's duct). Only 5–10% occur within the parotid gland due to the short and straight course of Stenson's duct and lower viscosity serous saliva. The ducts of Rivinus and Bartholin's ducts are usually unaffected, with less than 5% of cases within the sublingual or minor salivary glands.

Technique

1. The patient is placed under general anesthesia and prepped and draped to allow exposure of the oral cavity. Local anesthesia is administered with blocks and/or infiltration with care to avoid anatomical distortion of the floor of the mouth by excessive local anesthetic infiltration.
2. A vasodilator such as lidocaine without epinephrine may be injected within the region of the duct opening to aid in the dilation and identification of the duct orifice. Once identified, serial lacrimal probes are used to dilate the duct for later stent placement. The expected site of the stone or of the obstruction is identified via gentle retrograde probing.
3. A 2-0 silk suture is placed distal to the stone and around the duct to prevent retrograde migration of the stone toward the hilum of the gland (Figure 49.17). This suture may then be used for elevation and retraction.
4. If necessary, additional sutures may be passed through the tongue to aid with retraction.
5. The superficial floor-of-mouth mucosa directly overlying the stone or site of stricture is excised via sharp dissection, incising parallel to the duct (Figure 49.21). Meticulous hemostasis is imperative for proper identification of floor-of-mouth contents. Once the duct and lingual nerve are clearly identified, a ductotomy is performed to remove the sialolith or site of stenosis.
6. The injured duct should be cleanly transected and the cut end sutured to the adjacent floor-of-mouth mucosa with 5-0 Vicryl (Figure 49.25) or chromic sutures. If dissection needs to be continued proximally, it is recommended to "suture as you go" with one stitch per 0.5 cm of transected duct.

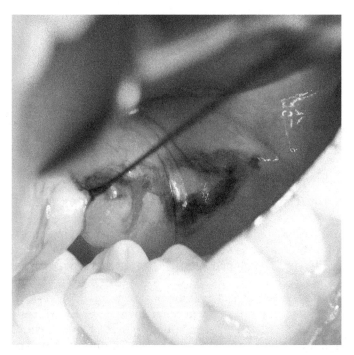

Figure 49.17. The location of the palpable stone is marked in purple. A 2-0 silk suture is placed distal to the stone and around the duct to prevent retrograde migration of the stone toward the hilum of the gland.

7. Copious sterile saline irrigation should be used to flush out any additional stones and dilute any purulence or inflammatory mediators.
8. Stent or gauze strip placement is optional in the neo-osteum. Alternatively, the duct may be closed entirely with a distally placed catheter or stent to maintain the original patency (Figures 49.24 and 49.25). If placed, the stent should remain in place for a minimum of 14 days in order to allow epithelialization around the stent to reestablish duct continuity.

1. Nonsteroidal anti-inflammatory drugs are used for both their anti-inflammatory and analgesic properties.
2. Conservative therapies such as hydration, warm compresses, and gentle glandular massage aid in minimizing stasis and subsequent infection.
3. Sialologues, such as pilocarpine, may or may not be prescribed in addition to the slow consumption of sour candies to stimulate salivary secretion.
4. Postoperative antibiotics are optional for elective cases, but they are recommended and routinely prescribed for cases with symptomatic sialadenitis.
5. Diet should begin with clear liquids post anesthesia and may be advanced to a full mechanical diet as tolerated.
6. Patients may resume their normal activities the next day as tolerated.

Early Complications

1. **Bleeding**: Postoperative bleeding is rare. The translucent mucosa allows easy visualization of sublingual vasculature, and any compromise would likely be identified immediately. In patients with an underlying coagulopathy, a slow bleed or hematoma can present as a medical emergency with potential airway compromise. It is important to warn patients in advance with regards to floor-of-mouth edema/hematoma formation and subsequent airway compromise to hasten their return to the hospital after outpatient treatment.
2. **Lingual nerve damage**: The lingual nerve lies in close proximity to the submandibular duct, as described in this chapter, and careful scrutiny is imperative to avoid damaging the nerve.
3. **Stent dislodgement**: If a surgical stent or gauze strip is left in place, it must be secured adequately to prevent dislodgment by mastication or parafunctional habits. Early failure may lead to restenosis of the neo-osteum.
4. **Infection**: Rare. If an infection is present, appropriate cultures followed by empirical antibiotic therapy should be initiated. Amoxicillin–clavulanate is recommended or clindamycin for penicillin-allergic individuals, in addition to oral rinses such as 0.12% chlorhexidine gluconate (Peridex). Incision and drainage are indicated, and the patency of the duct and neo-osteum should be verified.

Late Complications

1. **Impaired glandular function**: Salivary gland function typically returns following sialodochoplasty; however, clinically impaired function may warrant further workup for xerostomia or glandular studies via sialogram, magnetic resonance imaging (MRI), or ultrasound assessment.
2. **Recurrent sialolithiasis**: Individuals prone to sialolith formation may have stone recurrence with or without obstruction. The shortened path and enlarged opening after sialodochoplasty may allow natural stone passage without additional treatment.
3. **Restenosis and recurrent sialadenitis**: If obstruction and inflammation recur, retreatment may be justified. Alternatively, gland removal may be considered. The risk of neo-ostium stenosis is 2%.

1. The most common cause of salivary gland enlargement is benign inflammatory disease secondary to ductal outflow obstruction. This may be due to sialolithiasis, strictures, polyps, mucous plugs, mass effect, or other

pathology causing stasis and retrograde salivary flow. All of the above may lead to an inflammatory response within the salivary acini and glandular enlargement with or without a bacterial infection. The submandibular (Wharton's) duct is the most common site for sialolithiasis.

2. *Sialodochoplasty* refers to salivary duct repair. This may be performed in conjunction with sialolithectomy in order to prevent restenosis of the ductal system. The duct may be simply stitched open or packed with a gauze strip, or it may require a stent to be left in place for 7–10 days in order to heal properly.

3. The goal of sialodochoplasty is to posteriorly reposition the duct orifice. This reduces the duct length and eliminates the most common site of obstruction in the distal duct. Stones located within the distal submandibular duct are usually superficial and may be removed easily via a transoral approach under local anesthesia. Conversely, proximal or glandular stones may require more invasive treatment with removal of the affected salivary gland and its duct.

4. In addition to medical management, recent technical innovations and literature encourage the utilization of non-invasive techniques such as sialendoscopy and ESWL to remove or break up sialoliths. Sialodochoplasty may be completed in conjunction with the above procedures or as a second line of treatment after failure or recurrence.

5. Sialodochoplasty after sialolithectomy via a transoral technique is frequently unnecessary.

References

Bailey, B.J. and Johnson, J.T., 2006. *Head and neck surgery—otolaryngology*. 4th ed. Philadelphia: Lippincott Williams & Wilkins.

Capaccio, P., Torretta, S., Ottavian, F., Sambataro, G. and Pignataro, L., 2007. Modern management of obstructive salivary diseases. *Acta otorhinolaryngologica Italica: organo ufficiale della Società italiana di otorinolaringologia e chirurgia cervico-facciale* 27 (4), 161–72.

Fonseca, R., Barber, D., Powers, M. and Frost, D., 2012. *Oral and maxillofacial trauma*. 4th ed. Philadelphia: Saunders.

Hupp, J., Ellis, E. and Tucker, M., 2008. *Contemporary oral and maxillofacial surgery*. 5th ed. St. Louis, MO: Mosby Elsevier; pp. 398, 407–9.

Miloro, M. and Schow, S., 2003. Diagnosis and management of salivary gland disorders. *Contemporary Oral and Maxillofacial Surgery*, 442.

Park, J., Kim, J., Lee, Y., Oh, C., Chang, H. and Lee, S., 2012. Long-term study of sialodochoplasty for preventing submandibular sialolithiasis recurrence. *Clinical and Experimental Otorhinolaryngology*, 5 (1), 34–8.

Pogrel, M.A., 1987. Sialodochoplasty—does it work? *International Journal of Oral and Maxillofacial Surgery*, 16 (3), 266–9.

Roh, J.L. and Park, C.I., 2008. Transoral removal of submandibular hilar stone and sialodochoplasty. *Otolaryngology Head and Neck Surgery*, 139 (2), 235–9.

Rontal, M. and Rontal E., 1987. The use of sialodochoplasty in the treatment of benign inflammatory obstructive submandibular gland disease. *Laryngoscope*, 97, 1417–21.

Zenk, J., Constantinidis, J., Al-Kadah, B. and Iro, H., 2001. Transoral removal of submandibular stone. *Archives of Otolaryngology Head and Neck Surgery*, 127, 432–6.

Case Report

Case Report 49.4. A 37-year-old patient presents with a chief complaint of a mass to the floor of her mouth and recent-onset pain while eating. The patient reports that the mass has been there for years, but that pain on eating has developed over the past several weeks. On examination, the patient has a indurated, mobile, and tender mass to the left floor of the mouth. No cervical lymphadenopathy was noted. On review of her cone beam CT scan, a 23 mm (length) by 12 mm (width) sialolith was identified (Figures 49.18 and 49.19). The patient's submandibular gland appeared normal on exam and on review of additional radiographs. The patient underwent sialolithectomy and sialodochoplasty of the left submandibular (Wharton's) duct. (See also Figures 49.20 through 49.25.)

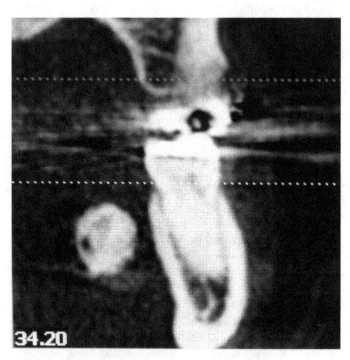

Figure 49.18. Coronal cone beam computed tomography scan demonstrating a radiolucent mass associated with the soft tissue of the left floor of the mouth.

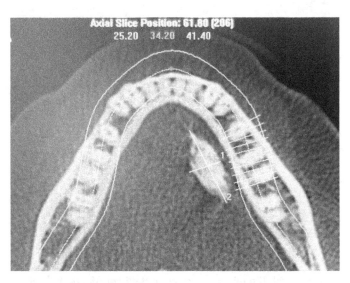

Figure 49.19.   Axial cone beam computed tomography scan demonstrating a 23 mm (length) by 12 mm (width) sialolith located within the left submandibular (Wharton's) duct.

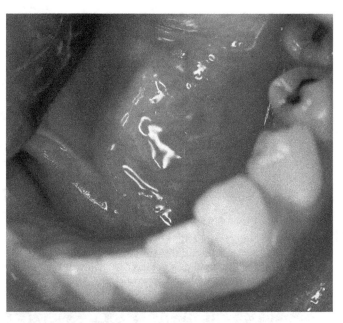

Figure 49.20.   Obvious floor-of-mouth mass. Wharton's duct was found to be functional.

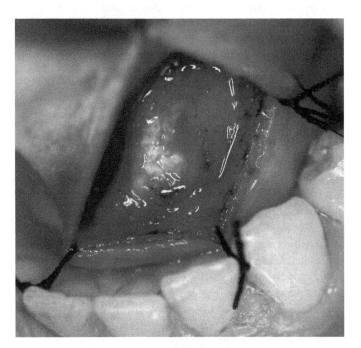

Figure 49.21.   The superficial floor-of-mouth mucosa directly over the stone is transected via sharp dissection incising parallel to the duct. Traction sutures are placed to aid in visualization.

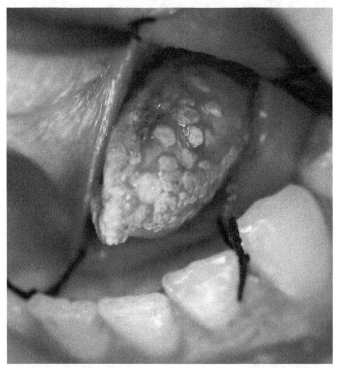

Figure 49.22.   The sialolith is delivered from the left submandibular duct.

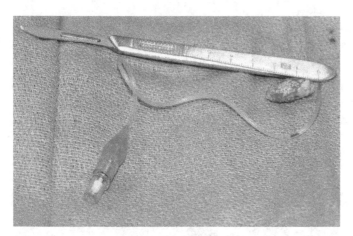

Figure 49.23.   The 23 mm × 12 mm sialolith and the sterile tubing from an endotracheal tube cuff. The sterile tubing from the endotracheal tube cuff will be used as a catheter to maintain the original patency of the damaged submandibular duct.

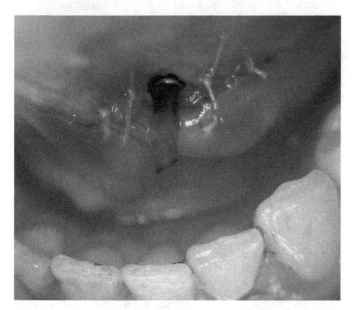

Figure 49.25.   The orifice of the duct is sewn to the floor-of-mouth tissues.

Superficial Parotidectomy

The removal of the superficial (or lateral) lobe of the parotid gland with preservation of the facial nerve due to pathology within the gland.

Indications

1. Biopsy of parotid mass
2. Definitive treatment of an intraparenchemal parotid mass
3. Excision of benign to low-grade malignancy within the superficial lobe of the parotid gland
4. Treatment of chronic sialodenitis (parotitis) refractory to conservative therapy and medical management

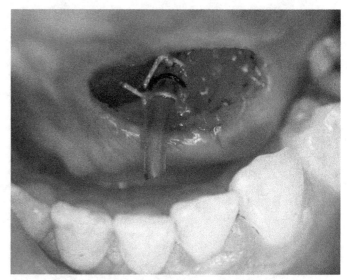

Figure 49.24.   Sterile tubing is positioned within the dilated submandibular duct and passively inserted to the hilum of the submandibular gland. The tubing is secured to the floor-of-mouth tissues.

5. Symptomatic chronic sialolithiasis
6. In conjunction with lymphadenectomy and/or local tissue excision for malignancy
7. To ensure sufficient margins for cheek resections involving malignancies (e.g., melanoma and squamous cell carcinoma)
8. Cosmesis for neoplasm-like conditions of the parotid (i.e. Sjögren's syndrome and benign lymphoepithelial cysts)

Contraindications

1. Treatment of high-grade parotid neoplasms: Requires total parotidectomy with adjunctive procedures
2. Neoplasm involving extension into or near the deep lobe of the parotid

Anatomy

Parotid gland: The largest of the major salivary glands and primarily a serous salivary gland. The parotid is invested by the anterior or superficial layer of the deep cervical fascia (SDCF), also known as the investing fascia. This layer surrounds the entire neck, with attachments starting posteriorly at the spinous process of the vertebrae and splitting to invest the trapezius and SCM muscles. The SDCF is continuous across the midline without interruption. The structures of the parotid fascia are deep to the superficial fascia of the neck, and superficial to the middle (pretracheal) layer of the deep cervical fascia.

Facial nerve: Exits the stylomastoid foramen approximately 2 cm deep from the surface of the overlying skin. The bifurcation of the main trunk is 1.5–2.8 cm inferior from the inferior-most portion of the bony external auditory canal. The main trunk bifurcates into the temporo-facial and cervico-facial divisions within the parotid parenchyma, with the cervico-facial division running more superficial within the gland than the temporo-facial division. The five main branches of the facial nerve include the temporal, zygomatic, buccal, marginal mandibular, and cervical branches. The main branches of the facial nerve have a wide variability as they course through the parotid parenchyma with variable anastamosis between the branches (Figures 49.26, 49.27, and 49.32).

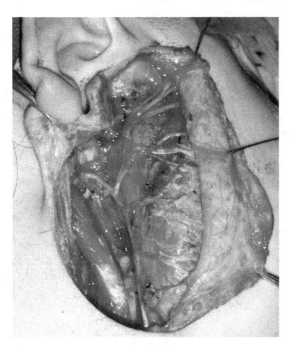

Figure 49.26. Exposure of the facial nerve after removal of the superficial lobe of the parotid.

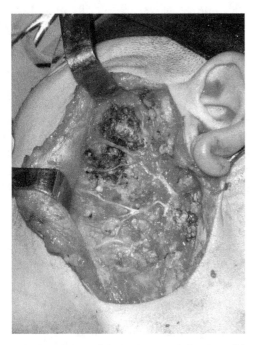

Figure 49.27. Variability of the anastomosis between branches of the facial nerve (compare Figure 49.27 to Figures 49.26 and 49.32).

Surgical Landmarks to Identify the Main Nerve Trunk (MNT) of the Facial Nerve

1. **Tympanomastoid suture line (fissure)**: The tympanomastoid suture line is located between the mastoid and the tympanic bones. The MNT lies 6–8 mm distal to the endpoint of this fissure.
2. **Tragal pointer**: The MNT lies 1.0–1.5 cm deep and slightly anterior and inferior to the tip of the external ear canal cartilage.
3. **Posterior belly of the digastric muscle**: The MNT lies 1.0 cm deep to the medial attachment of the posterior belly of the digastric muscle to the digastric groove (mastoid notch) of the mastoid bone.
4. **Mastoid process**: The MNT can be identified in the mastoid bone by mastoidectomy and followed peripherally. This approach is typically reserved for intratympanic or large tumors.

Procedure: Superficial Parotidectomy

1. Preoperative intravenous antibiotics (e.g., Cefazolin) are initiated pre-incision.
2. The patient is induced with short-acting paralytics to allow for monitoring of the branches of the facial nerve during dissection. General anesthesia is obtained via endotracheal intubation.
3. The patient is placed in a supine position, the neck is hyperextended with the placement of a shoulder roll and the head is turned to the opposite side of the involved parotid. The ispilateral eye is lubricated with ophthalmic ointment and is protected with either a corneal shield or a tarsorrhaphy stitch.
4. A modified-Blair incision is marked with a sterile marking pen, and 2% lidocaine with epinephrine is injected within the subcutaneous tissues of the proposed surgical incision. The patient is prepped and draped in a sterile fashion to allow for direct observation of the ipsilateral muscles of facial expression.
5. The skin incision begins in the pre-auricular region, extending posteriorly under the lobe of the ear, and retaining an adequate cuff of skin to prevent tethering of the lobule and a pixie-ear deformity. The incision continues for a variable distance posteriorly over the mastoid process. The incision may be extended into the hairline for cosmesis or curved inferiorly and anteriorly within a natural neck crease, allowing for transition into cervical lymphadenectomy if needed (Figure 49.28).
6. An anterior subplatysmal/subsuperficial musculoaponeurotic system (SMAS) flap is developed using the natural plane on the surface of the parotid gland. Dissection continues anteriorly within a tissue plane just superficial to the parotid fascia. Numerous filaments of connective tissue pass from the skin to the parotid fascia, which may resemble nervous tissue. The branches of the facial nerve, however, will only be found at the

anterior and peripheral extent of the gland. The flap is carried beyond the extent of the tumor to completely expose the parotid fascia anterior to the tissue to be removed (Figure 49.29).

7. A posterior skin flap may be developed to free the parotid tissue located posterior to the incision line or when combined with a neck dissection. If needed, the posterior flap is raised at the level of the SCM fascia. The greater auricular nerve branch and the external jugular vein are identified as they traverse the SCM, and the plane of dissection is developed superficial to these structures.

8. Low-pressure clamps are used to grasp the exposed posterior glandular tissue, and a skin rake is used to retract the tragus in a superior and posterior direction. Scissors or hemostats paralleling the cartilaginous portion of the external auditory canal are used to dissect free the parotid fascia. Multiple small veins may be encountered within this region. Minimizing venous ligation, however, will help to reduce venous congestion to the tissues, which will improve surgical visualization of the gland. Dissection continues to the level of the mastoid process.

9. The parotid tissue is carefully dissected from the mastoid region, paying special attention as dissection continues inferior to the mastoid tip, because the main nerve trunk (MNT) of the facial nerve is located slightly deep and anterior to this region. A broad front of dissection is now used in the areas of the cartilaginous external auditory ear canal, mastoid tip, and posterior belly of the digastric muscle to progressively separate and free the parotid tissue. The cartilaginous pointer (tragal pointer) may be used to aid in identification of the bifurcation of the facial nerve trunk. Surgical assistants should pay close attention for any facial muscle twitching. Ligation of any bleeding vessels should be delayed until definitive identification of the MNT is achieved.

10. The MNT will be identified as a 2–4 mm diameter shiny white cord-like structure (Figure 49.30). Once the temporo-facial and cervico-facial branches are identified, systematic dissection of the overlying parotid tissue is completed from a posterior-to-anterior direction, ensuring instrumentation is parallel to the motor nerve fibers (Figures 49.31 and 49.32). Attempts should be made to preserve anastomoses if possible. No long-term facial nerve deficit should result from transaction of these anastomotic fibers as long as the main nerve branches remain intact and undisturbed.

11. Once the anterior aspect of the gland is reached, Stenson's duct may be identified and ligated. Final release of the anterior aspect of the superficial lobe completes the removal.

12. Bipolar electrocautery can be used to control hemorrhage. A flat Jackson Pratt (JP) drain to bulb suction is placed through a stab incision within the tissue of the neck. The anterior and posterior flaps are repositioned and closed in layers. For large parotid tumors, a wedge of tissue may be removed to facilitate an aesthetic closure (Figure 49.33).

Postoperative Management

1. Postoperative broad-spectrum antibiotics are prescribed for 5 days.
2. Local wound care is performed with a mixture of half hydrogen peroxide and half sterile saline, triple-antibiotic ointment, and a loose dressing.
3. Drains are removed between 48 and 72 hours, or when they become nonproductive.
4. Patients are followed indefinably for tumor recurrence.

Complications

1. **Facial nerve injury**: Facial nerve injury can be minimized by early identification of the main nerve trunk of the facial nerve, appropriate flap plane development, dissection parallel to the anticipated direction of the motor nerve fibers, the use of a nerve stimulator during dissection, and judicious use of cautery. Witnessed transections are repaired primarily.

2. **Gustatory sweating (Frey syndrome)**: Anomalous (misdirected) innervation of postganglionic parasympathetic salivary nerves with cutaneous sweat glands results in a localized flushing and sweating during mastication and salivation. Treatment involves topical application of antiperspirant, botulinum toxin injection, and the surgical interposition of tissue (e.g., superficial temporal fascia or free fat) or implantable materials between the skin flap and the underlying parotid bed.

3. **Salivary leakage**: May lead to the development of a sialocele and/or a salivary fistula. Treatment of sialoceles involves drainage and pressure dressings. Salivary fistulae are treated with local wound revision if low-flow leakage is present. Adjunctive botulinum toxin injections may be used to block the release of acetylcholine from postganglionic parasympathetic fibers and decrease salivary flow. Recalcitrant salivary leakage typically necessitates surgical reexploration.

4. **Ear numbness**: Hypoesthesia in the distribution of the greater auricular nerve is common and typically lessens over time.

5. **Flap necrosis**: Appropriate flap design and adequate flap thickness will minimize distal flap necrosis. Small defects are conservatively managed with standard wound care techniques. Larger defects may require additional surgical intervention to correct.

6. **Tumor recurrence**: Often related to the type of tumor excised.

Key Points

1. Parotid neoplasms include pleomorphic adenoma, Warthin's tumor, mucoepidermoid carcinoma, and adenoid cystic carcinoma. Parotid masses typically

undergo FNA and MRI to obtain a working diagnosis prior to definitive surgical therapy.

2. For smaller benign tumors, extracapsular dissection (subtotal parotidectomy) may be preferable to complete removal of the superficial lobe of the parotid.

3. Total parotidectomy (superficial and deep lobe) indications include a malignant condition within the deep lobe of the parotid, metastasis to parotid lymph nodes, and tumors with underlying bone invasion.

4. The cartilaginous (tragal) pointer can be used as a guide for the location of the bifurcation of the main trunk of the facial nerve. The cartilaginous pointer follows the course of the inferior one-third of the helix of the ear, which points in an antero-inferior direction to the region of the facial nerve bifurcation.

5. Identification and preservation of the facial nerve are essential for preventing inadvertent facial nerve injury. Careful observation for facial muscle twitching, from light mechanical stimulation or using a handheld nerve stimulator, will elicit muscle contracture.

6. Dissection directed from a posterior to anterior direction with blunt instrumentation will help minimize nerve damage.

7. The parotid capsule should be closed after removal of the involved portion of the gland. If closure is not feasible, an interposing tissue or implantable biologic material should be considered between the exposed gland and the skin to prevent postganglionic parasympathetic fibers from cross-innervating facial sweat glands, resulting in gustatory sweating (Frey syndrome).

References

de Bree, R., van der Waal, I. and Leemans, C.R., 2007. Management of Frey syndrome. *Head and Neck*, 29 (8), 773–8.

Dias, F.L., Lima, R.A. and Pinho, J., 2008. Practical tips to identifying the main trunk of the facial nerve. In C.R. Cernea, F.L. Dias, D. Fliss, R.A. Lima, E.N. Myers and W.I. Wei, eds. *Pearls and pitfalls in head and neck surgery*. Basel: Karger; pp. 106–7.

Ellies, M., Gottstein, U., Rohrbach-Volland, S., Arglebe, C. and Laskawi, R., 2004. Reduction of salivary flow with botulinum toxin: extended report on 33 patients with drooling, salivary fistulas, and sialadenitis. *Laryngoscope*, 114 (10), 1856–60.

Myers, E.N., Suen, J.Y., Myers, J.N. and Hanna, E.Y.N., 2003. *Cancer of the head and neck*. 4th ed. Philadelphia: Saunders.

Motamed, M., Laugharne, D. and Bradley, P.J., 2003. Management of chronic parotitis: a review. *Journal of Laryngology and Otology*, 117 (7),521–6.

Shah, S., 2003. *Head & neck surgery and oncology*. 3rd ed. St. Louis, MO: Mosby.

Case Report

Case Report 49.5. A 35-year-old male presents with a chief complaint of a slow growing right-sided facial mass. Examination revealed a firm, nonmobile mass within the right preauricular area extending inferiorly. The patient exhibited mild to moderate weakness to all five branches of the right facial nerve. MRI imaging was consistent with partial compression of the right main nerve trunk with a large mass confined to the superficial lobe of the parotid gland. FNA was suggestive of pleomorphic adenoma. The patient underwent a superficial parotidectomy with facial nerve preservation, and a definitive diagnosis of a pleomorphic adenoma was made. (See Figures 49.28 through 49.33.)

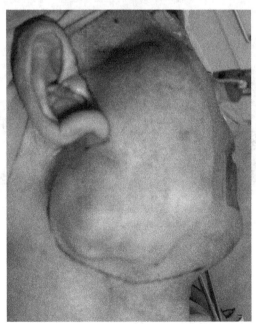

Figure 49.28.   Modified-Blair incision is marked.

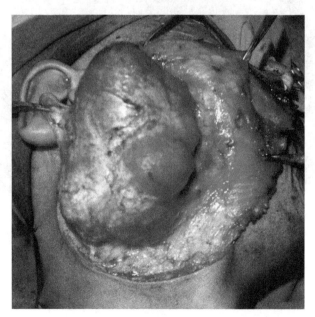

Figure 49.29.   The anterior skin flap is extended beyond the tumor margin.

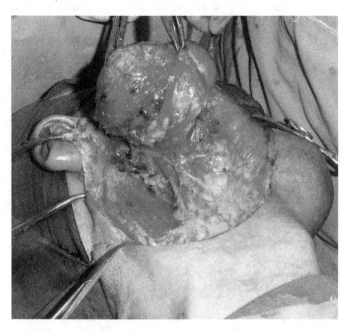

Figure 49.30.   The main nerve trunk of the facial nerve and subsequent branches are identified.

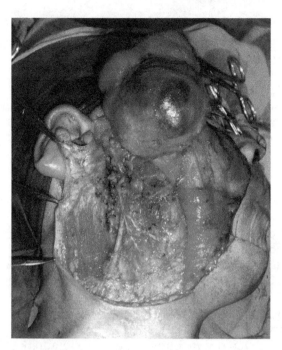

Figure 49.31.   The tumor is dissected free of the facial nerve divisions (branches).

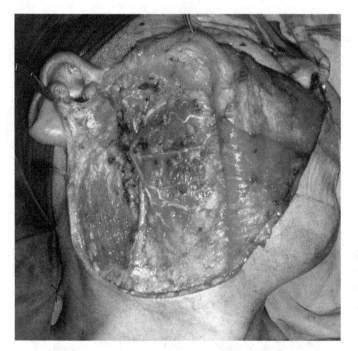

Figure 49.32.   All five branches of the facial nerve are exposed.

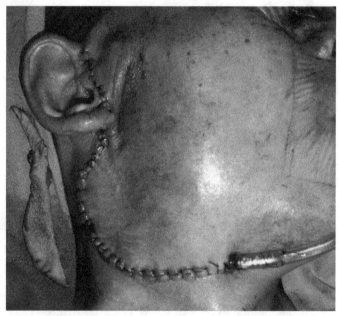

Figure 49.33.   Closure of surgical site. Note the removal of excess tissue due to the expansive nature of the tumor.

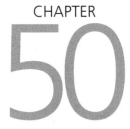

CHAPTER

50

Neck Pathology

Anil N. Shah[1] and Matthew T. Brigger[2]

[1]Department of Otolaryngology—Head and Neck Surgery, Naval Medical Center San Diego, and San Diego, California, USA

[2]Department of Otolaryngology—Head and Neck Surgery, Naval Medical Center San Diego; and Uniformed Services of the Health Sciences University, San Diego, California, USA

Midline Neck Pathology

Differential Diagnosis

Thyroglossal duct cyst (TGDC)
Dermoid or epidermoid cyst
Lipoma
Submental lymphadenopathy
Thyroid masses or goiter
Vascular malformations (hemangioma)
Teratoma
Ectopic thyroid (lingual thyroid)

Procedure: Excision of Midline Neck Mass

A midline neck mass, prior to excision, must be differentiated from a thyroid gland mass and normal thyroid tissue should be confirmed, generally through imaging, to ensure that excision will not result in complete removal of functioning thyroid tissue from an ectopic location. Standard imaging modalities include ultrasound, computed tomography (CT) scan, and magnetic resonance imaging (MRI). Fine-needle aspirate (FNA) cytology is recommended prior to an open biopsy of midline and lateral neck masses.

Indications

1. Excisional biopsy to determine the diagnosis when prior cytologic evaluation was nondiagnostic
2. Aesthetic correction of biopsy proven benign mass within the neck (i.e., lipoma)
3. Prior history of infection within the anterior neck
4. Relative risk of malignancy originating in a thyroglossal duct cyst

Contraindication

1. Acute infection or inflammation at the surgical site (relative contraindication)

Anatomy

The thyroid anlage originates as a thickening of cells at the foramen cecum, which is located on the dorsum of the tongue posteriorly at the apex of the V-shaped sulcus formed by the circumvallate papillae. Fusion of the second branchial arch anlage in the midline may result in entrapment of the thyroglossal duct by the hyoid bone.

Neck layers:

1. Skin
2. Subcutaneous tissue
3. Platysma muscle
4. Superficial (investing) layer of deep cervical fascia
5. Midline linea alba with laterally located strap muscles
6. Middle (pretracheal) layer of the deep cervical fascia
7. Pretracheal space, which contains the thyroglossal duct cyst

Sistrunk Procedure for Thyroglossal Duct Cyst (TGDC) Excision

1. Preoperative antibiotics are administered. Short-acting paralytics are utilized to allow for facial nerve testing. The patient is intubated with the endotracheal tube directed cephalically or toward the contralateral side of the mass.
2. The patient is placed in cervical extension using a shoulder roll. Prominent landmarks (midline mandible, hyoid bone, and thyroid and cricoid cartilage) are marked using a sterile marking pen.
3. A transverse incision is marked in the midline in a skin crease within the upper part of the neck overlying the mass. If there is evidence of a draining sinus, then an elliptical incision should be made to include the involved skin.
4. The marked incision is injected with 1% lidocaine with 1:100,000 epinephrine within the subdermis just superficial to the platysma.
5. The patient is prepped and draped from the mandible to a point several centimeters below the sternal notch. Use of a split drape will allow for manual palpation of the base of tongue through the mouth during the final stages of the dissection if needed.
6. The initial incision is made with a #15 blade through skin, dermis, and subcutaneous fat. Once the platysma is identified, dissection proceeds through the platysma layer, and superior and inferior subplatysmal flaps are elevated. Of note, the platysma is often deficient in the immediate midline in the region of the midline

Atlas of Operative Oral and Maxillofacial Surgery, First Edition. Edited by Christopher J. Haggerty and Robert M. Laughlin

raphe. It is more important to elevate the superior flap due to the course of dissection compared to the inferior flap. Deep to the platysma are the right and left anterior jugular veins, which can either be ligated or elevated within the superior subplatysmal flap.

7. Once the strap muscles are identified, they are retracted laterally at the midline raphe without division. However, a portion of the sternohyoid, at the level of the hyoid, may have to be excised with the specimen depending on the proximity of the walls of the cyst to the strap muscles.

8. The mass (Figure 50.1) is dissected free from the surrounding strap musculature, thyroid cartilage, and thyrohyoid membrane using a combination of blunt and sharp dissection up to the hyoid bone. It is absolutely critical to identify and confirm the location of the thyroid notch and cartilage prior to making cuts within the hyoid bone. This will prevent inadvertent damage to the thyroid cartilage, which is in close proximity to the hyoid bone in the pediatric population.

9. The muscles, soft tissue, and periosteum are dissected off of the hyoid bone on both sides in order to remove the middle one-third of the hyoid bone with the specimen. Bone-cutting ronguers or heavy scissors should be used to cut the hyoid bone.

10. As the hyoid bone is elevated anteriorly, dissection can proceed up to the base of tongue, and an ellipse of tissue is taken with the specimen. Placing a new glove on the surgeon's hand will allow manual palpation of the base of tongue and position the foramen cecum into the dissection plane.

11. A 2-0 silk ligature is used at the deep aspect of the dissection upon removal of the mass to induce scarring within the wound bed and to ensure closure of any remaining duct remnant (Figure 50.2).

12. If the vallecula or oropharynx is entered, the defect should be closed with interrupted non-absorbable sutures through the transcervical incision.

13. The wound bed should be copiously irrigated and inspected for signs of hemorrhage. A passive drain is placed in most cases, although some cases may require active drainage.

14. The wound is closed in a layered fashion with 3-0 Vicryl sutures for the deep fascia, 4-0 Vicryl for the superficial fascia and deep dermis, followed by a running 5-0 Monocryl subcuticular skin closure.

15. The skin incision is covered with a thin layer of antibiotic ointment, and a light pressure dressing (i.e., fluffed gauze and tegaderm) is applied.

Postoperative Management

1. Patients are given intravenous (inpatient) and oral (outpatient) antibiotics for 5 days postoperatively.
2. Analgesics are prescribed.

3. Drains are typically removed after 48 hours or when nonproductive.
4. Follow-up is based on the nature of the mass excised.

Complications

1. **Recurrence of TGDC**: Minimized with resection of the midline portion of the hyoid bone with a Sistrunk procedure. A history of a prior infection increases the risk of recurrence, especially infections within 6 months of definitive treatment and requiring incision and drainage. Recurrence is likely after re-excision and may be due to the presence of accessory ducts and diverticula from the main duct and pharyngeal mucosa that was not removed at the initial surgery. Re-excision should be performed with wide dissection of a generous core of muscle between the superior aspect of the hyoid bone and the base of the tongue as well as an additional portion of the hyoid bone.

2. **Iatrogenic hypothyroidism**: Secondary to removal of functional thyroid tissue within the thyroglossal duct cyst. Preoperative imaging should be performed to verify the presence of a descended thyroid gland.

3. **Nerve injury**: Injury to the hypoglossal and superior laryngeal nerves may occur during re-excision of a scarred TGDC or when cysts are located lateral to the midline.

Key Points

1. Obtain preoperative radiological confirmation of normal thyroid gland tissue prior to excision of TGDC. This will allow for preoperative counseling and postoperative management in cases where the TGDC contains functioning ectopic thyroid tissue.

2. In order to adequately excise a thyroglossal duct cyst, the middle one-third of the hyoid bone and a core of tissue from the hyoid upward toward the foramen cecum should be removed in continuity (Sistrunk procedure). Failure to excise the central core of the hyoid bone has been associated with an increased rate of recurrence of up to 38%, whereas the Sistrunk procedure has a reported recurrence rate of 1.5% to 7%.

3. Always clearly identify the thyroid notch prior to excising the central core of the hyoid, particularly in children.

4. Although rare, TGDCs may contain a malignancy. The presence of calcifications on preoperative imaging should raise suspicion for malignancy.

References

Brereton, R.J. and Symonds, E., 1978. Thyroglossal cysts in children. *British Journal of Surgery*, 65, 507–8.

Gourin, C.G. and Eisele, D.W., 2009. Complications of thyroid surgery. In: D.W. Eisele and R.V. Smith, eds. *Complications in head and neck surgery*. Philadelphia: Mosby Elsevier; pp. 505–11.

Hawkins, D.B., Jacobsen, B.E. and Klatt, E.C., 1982. Cysts of the thyroglossal duct. *Laryngoscope*, 92, 1254–8.

Hoffman, M.A. and Schuster, S.R., 1988. Thyroglossal duct remnants in infants and children: Reevaluation of histopathology and methods for resection. *Annals of Otology, Rhinology and Laryngology*, 97, 483–6.

Myers, E.N., 2008. Thyroglossal duct cyst. In: E.N. Myers, ed. *Operative otolaryngology: head and neck surgery*. Philadelphia: Saunders Elsevier.

Richardson, M.A. and Rosenfeld, R.M., 2002. Congenital malformations of the neck. In: C.D. Bluestone and R.M. Rosenfeld, eds. *Surgical atlas of pediatric otolaryngology*. Hamilton, ON: B.C. Decker; pp. 491–5.

Sistrunk, W.E., 1920. The surgical treatment of cysts of the thyroglossal tract. *Annals of Surgery*, 71, 121–6.

Case Report

Case Report 50.1. A 30-year-old patient presents with a 2-year history of a midline neck mass that originally arose in the setting of an upper respiratory infection. The mass was noted to be tender and the patient reported that the mass had not changed in size since it initially developed. The patient reports no loss of neck range of motion and denies hemoptysis, fever, chills, or unintentional weight change. On physical examination, the mass is noted to be 6 cm in size, oval, firm, and slightly to the left of midline. The mass is intimately associated with the hyoid bone and elevates with tongue protrusion and swallowing. There were no skin changes overlying the mass. The patient initially underwent ultrasound, which characterized the cystic mass superficial to the normal-appearing thyroid gland. A computed tomography scan of the neck with contrast was performed, which demonstrated a 6 cm × 3.4 cm × 3.2 cm peripheral enhancing mass just to the left of midline with central low fluid attenuation. The patient underwent a successful Sistrunk procedure to excise their thyroglossal duct cyst. (See Figures 50.1 and 50.2.)

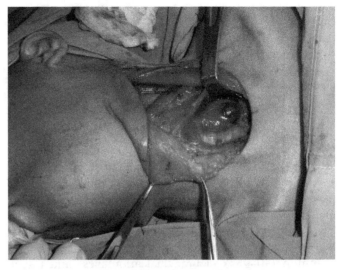

Figure 50.1. Surgical exposure of a thyroglossal duct cyst.

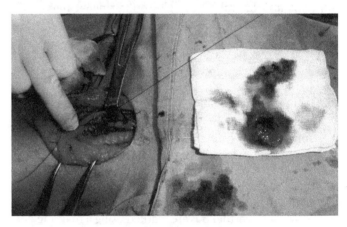

Figure 50.2. A silk ligature is used along the deep aspect of the dissection after removal of the mass to induce scarring within the wound bed, as well as to ensure closure of any remaining duct remnants.

Lateral Neck Pathology

Differential Diagnosis

Inflammatory cervical lymphadenopathy

Primary tumors (malignant and benign)

Nodal metastasis from a distant site (i.e., squamous cell carcinoma)

Branchial cleft remnant (cyst, sinus, and fistulae)

Vascular malformations (hemangioma)

Lymphatic malformations (cystic hygroma)

Laryngocele

Lipoma

Dermoid or epidermoid cysts

Infection or inflammatory (tuberculosis, HIV, sarcoid, Epstein–Barr virus, staphylococcus, cat scratch disease, etc.)

Lymphoma

Salivary pathology (adenocarcinoma, pleomorphic adenoma, and Sjögren's syndrome)

Carotid pathology

Excision of Lateral Neck Mass

Preoperative fine-needle aspiration and imaging are essential in determining a working diagnosis of the lesion, the extent of the lesion, and to allow for preoperative surgical planning.

Indications

1. Excisional biopsy to determine the diagnosis when prior cytologic evaluation was nondiagnostic
2. Aesthetic correction of biopsy proven benign mass within the neck (i.e., lipoma)
3. Prior history of infection within the lateral neck

1. Acute infection or inflammation at the surgical site (relative contraindication)

Anatomy

Branchial cleft remnants can be divided into cysts, sinuses, or fistulae and may be located anywhere along the development of the branchial clefts (from the preauricular region to the supraclavicular fossa, lateral to the midline and medial to the sternocleidomastoid muscle [SCM]). Cysts are lesions that are contained within the neck and have no opening to the skin or pharynx. Sinuses are blind pouches that have tracts to the skin or pharynx. Fistulae are abnormal connections between the skin and pharynx. The second branchial cleft remnant is by far the most common (90–95% of branchial anomalies) and travels between the internal and external carotid arteries and superior and lateral to the glossopharyngeal nerve (CN IX) and hypoglossal nerve (CN XII).

Surgical Technique: Excision of Lateral Neck Mass (Branchial Remnant)

1. Preoperative antibiotics are administered. Short-acting paralytics are utilized to allow for facial nerve testing. The patient is intubated with the endotracheal tube directed cephalically or toward the contralateral side of the mass.
2. Cervical extension is employed, and the head is rotated away from the side of the neck mass. Prominent landmarks (the angle of the mandible, cricoid cartilage, SCM, and mastoid tip) are marked using a marking pen.
3. A transverse incision is planned and outlined within a cervical skin crease overlying the mass. Incision planning should include orientation to allow for more extensive excision (i.e., neck dissection) in the future. If there is evidence of a sinus tract, an elliptical incision is planned around the tract.
4. The marked incision is injected with 1% lidocaine with 1:100,000 epinephrine within the subdermis, just superficial to the platysma.
5. If a fistula is suspected, cannulating the tract from the pharynx may aid in the identification of the tract during the approach from the cervical neck. The palatine tonsil should be inspected and palpated first, followed by the piriform sinus.
6. The patient is prepped and draped from the mandible to a point several centimeters below the sternal notch on the side of the lesion. The use of a split drape will allow for entry into the oral cavity for cases involving a suspected pharyngeal fistula.
7. If a sinus tract is present, a lacrimal probe can be gently placed into the sinus tract to help identify the course of the tract without creating a false passage. Additional options to help identify a tract include using a Fogarty

catheter (3–5 French) with or without slight balloon dilation or a Prolene suture to cannulate the tract.
8. The initial incision is made with a #15 blade through skin, dermis, and subcutaneous fat.
9. Dissection proceeds through the platysma layer. Subplatysmal flaps should be elevated superiorly and inferiorly in order to protect the marginal mandibular branch of the facial nerve if the location of the mass places the nerve at risk. The nerve can be found within the neck between the angle of the mandible and up to 2 cm inferior.
10. The external jugular veins are located perpendicular to the incision and may be ligated if needed. The greater auricular nerve is located along the SCM and should be identified and spared.
11. The deep cervical fascia should be incised, and the lesion elevated from its fascial attachments.
12. Once the mass is identified, it should be circumferentially dissected free from surrounding attachments, and any tracts should be followed cranially (Figure 50.4). The spinal accessory nerve may be identified deep to the SCM and should be identified and preserved when retracting the SCM laterally.
13. During superior dissection in the case of a branchial remnant, the lingual venous plexus may be encountered, and care must be taken to not inadvertently ligate the hypoglossal or superior laryngeal nerve. After passing the carotid artery (the second branchial remnant will be located between the internal and external carotid arteries; the third branchial remnant will be posterior to the internal carotid artery), the tract will pass deep to the posterior belly of the digastric.
14. As the dissection proceeds cranially, it may be necessary to create a second stair-step incision in order to access it along its deeper surface. This can be performed by passing a dissector into the tract along its deepest surface and palpating the dissector from the skin. A transverse incision can be made into the skin overlying the dissector (level of hyoid bone), and the tract can be brought out through the skin for ease of dissection.
15. Once the tract is followed to either the oropharynx (Figure 50.5) or piriform sinus, the tract can be clamped at the mucosal border, and a 2-0 silk suture can be used as a tie around the stump.
16. The wound bed should be copiously irrigated and inspected for signs of hemorrhage. A passive drain is placed in most cases, although some cases may require active drainage.
17. The wound is closed in a layered fashion with 3-0 Vicryl sutures for the deep fascia, 4-0 Vicryl for the superficial fascia and deep dermis, followed by a running 5-0 Monocryl subcuticular skin closure.
18. The skin incision is covered with a thin layer of antibiotic ointment, and a light pressure dressing (i.e., fluffed gauze and tegaderm) is applied.

Postoperative Management

See Steps 1–4 of postoperative management in the "Midline Neck Pathology" section.

Complications

1. **Bleeding**: Hematoma formation typically occurs within 24 hours after surgery. Treatment consists of exploration of the surgical wound to decompress and evacuate the hematoma, and to identify and ligate any sources of active bleeding.
2. **Seroma formation**: May occur if a large dead space is present after surgical excision. Managed with needle aspiration, the placement of a closed-suction drain, drainage through the wound, or management with observation as gradual resorption of a seroma is expected.
3. **Wound infection**: Occurs more frequently if the branchial cleft cyst has been previously infected or is infected at the time of surgery, if a large amount of dead space is left after excision, or if there is a break in sterile technique.
4. **Salivary fistula**: May occur if the pharynx is entered and there is a persistent gap within the pharyngeal suture line or incomplete imbrication of the mucosal lining. Minimized with layered wound closure technique. Initial treatment is conservative with a pressure dressing and limiting oral intake. Wound exploration and fistulectomy are necessary if a chronic fistula develops.
5. **Recurrence of the branchial cleft cyst either as a mass or as a deep neck abscess**: There is an increased risk of recurrence if there is a history of prior infection requiring incision and drainage, current infection, or a failure to completely identify a tract that enters the pharynx. Recurrence of the cyst as an abscess or mass should alert the surgeon to the possibility of a pharyngeal fistula, and imaging should be obtained to confirm that finding prior to re-excision of the tract.

Key Points

1. Branchial anomalies comprise 20% of pediatric congenital head and neck masses, with 95% of branchial anomalies involving the second branchial cleft.
2. Seventy-five percent of lateral neck masses in patients over 40 years of age are malignant.
3. Fine-needle aspiration cytology is an accurate, sensitive, inexpensive, and rapid technique that aids in the evaluation and diagnosis of central and lateral neck masses and adenopathy.

References

Chandler, J.R. and Mitchell, B., 1981. Branchial cleft cysts, sinuses, and fistulas. *Otolaryngology Clinics of North America*, 14, 175–86. (This article discusses the embryology of branchial cleft cysts.)

Edmonds, J.L., Girod, D.A., Woodroof, J.M. and Bruegger, D.E., 1997. Third branchial anomalies: avoiding recurrences. *Archives of Otolaryngology—Head and Neck Surgery*, 123, 438–41.

Gleeson, M., Herbert, A. and Richards, A., 2000. Management of lateral neck masses in adult. *BMJ*, 320, 1521–4.

Goff, C.J., Allred, C. and Glade, R.S., 2012. Current management of congenital branchial cleft cysts, sinuses, and fistulae. *Current Opinion in Otolaryngology & Head and Neck Surgery*, 20 (6), 533–9.

Inglis, A.F. and Richardson, M.A., 2009. Complications of pediatric head and neck surgery. In: D.W. Eisele and R.V. Smith, eds. *Complications in head and neck surgery*. Philadelphia: Mosby Elsevier 2009; pp. 67–77.

Myers, E.N., 2008. Branchial cleft cysts and sinuses. In: E.N. Myers, ed. *Operative otolaryngology: head and neck surgery*. Philadelphia: Saunders Elsevier.

Richardson, M.A. and Rosenfeld, R.M., 2002. Congenital malformations of the neck. In: C.D.Bluestone and R.M.Rosenfeld, eds. *Surgical atlas of pediatric otolaryngology*. Hamilton, ON: B.C. Decker; pp. 499–514.

Case Report

Case Report 50.2. A 29-year-old patient presents with an intermittent history of a painful swelling to her left lateral neck. The patient denies stridor, dyspnea, dysphonia, fever, chills, and night sweats. On clinical examination, a single, smooth, fluctuant, tender mass was identified along the anteromedial border of the sternocleidomastoid muscle. No fistula formation was noted. A computed tomography scan demonstrated a well-demarcated, non-enhancing cystic mass. A fine-needle aspiration (FNA) was performed with multiple passes with a 25-gauge needle. FNA revealed a straw-colored fluid aspirate with squamous cells consistent with a branchial cleft cyst. The patient underwent an excisional biopsy of the branchial cyst with ligation of its residual oropharyngeal tract. (See Figures 50.3, 50.4, 50.5, 50.6, and 50.7.)

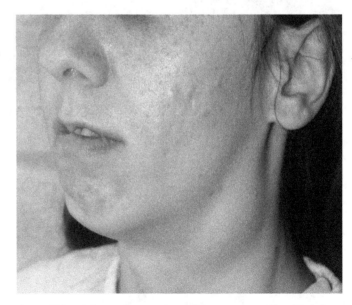

Figure 50.3. A 6 cm × 6 cm tender and fluctuant mass identified along the anteromedial border anterior of the sternocleidomastoid muscle.

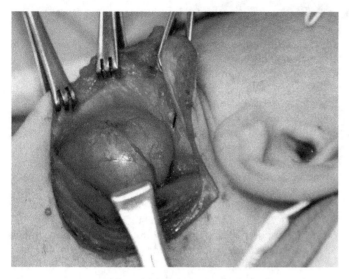

Figure 50.4.   Second branchial cleft cyst located anterior to the SCM and dissected free from its surrounding tissue. Care is taken to not rupture the cyst, as this makes its complete removal more difficult.

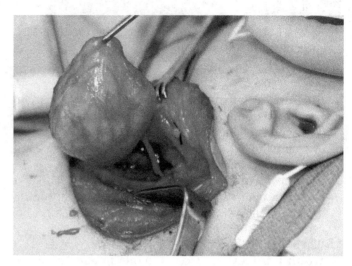

Figure 50.5.   Residual oropharyngeal tract is identified at the deep border of the branchial cyst. The tract is dissected free from its surrounding tissue and ligated with two 2-0 silk suture ties.

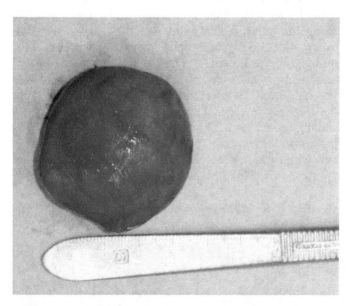

Figure 50.6.   Second branchial cleft cyst removed in its entirety without rupture.

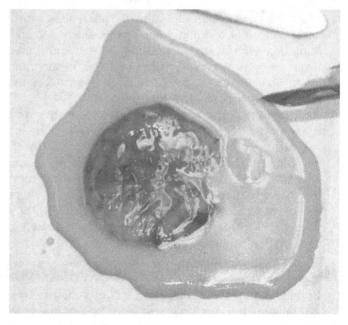

Figure 50.7.   Rupture of the cyst reveals a brown fluid, which is pathognomic for a branchial cleft cyst.

51 Pectoralis Major Myocutaneous Flap

Eric R. Carlson and Andrew Lee

Department of Oral and Maxillofacial Surgery, University of Tennessee Medical Center, University of Tennessee Cancer Institute, Knoxville, Tennessee, USA

A soft tissue reconstructive surgical procedure that provides oral lining and facial cover of soft tissue defects. Referred to as the *workhorse flap* of head and neck reconstruction.

Indications

1. Immediate reconstruction of oral lining (floor of mouth, buccal mucosa, and mandibular gingiva) and lower third facial/neck cover in patients undergoing ablative cancer surgery of the oral and maxillofacial region
2. Delayed reconstruction of oral lining and facial/neck cover tissue in patients who have experienced avulsive trauma of the oral and maxillofacial region
3. Reconstruction of oral lining and facial/neck cover in patients undergoing surgical treatment of radiation tissue injury of the oral and maxillofacial region
4. Immediate muscular coverage of the carotid artery in patients who have undergone radical and modified radical neck dissections
5. Salvage reconstructive surgery for failed free microvascular flap reconstruction of the oral and maxillofacial region
6. Primary method of reconstruction of the oral and maxillofacial region where systemic medical comorbidity (i.e., uncontrolled diabetes, cardiopulmonary failure, or renal insufficiency) precludes the execution of a microvascular flap for reconstruction

Contraindications

1. Excessive trauma sustained by the subclavian artery during the placement of a central venous catheter, whereby the integrity of the thoracoacromial artery has been compromised. Preoperative angiography is indicated when an injury is suspected to this primary pedicle that might result in inadequate vascularity to the pectoralis major muscle if myocutaneous flap development were performed
2. Midfacial, upper third facial, and maxillary soft tissue defects where the arc of rotation and length of the pectoralis major myocutaneous flap are insufficient
3. Excessively large skin paddle required to perform the reconstruction. Women are able to undergo pectoralis major myocutaneous flap development with larger skin paddles than men due to the redundancy of the female breast. Skin grafting the chest wall is not advisable in the event of inability to achieve primary closure of the chest wall due to the likely development of postoperative costochondritis

Anatomy of the Pectoralis Major Muscle

Pectoralis Major Muscle

A broad, flat, fan-shaped muscle that covers the pectoralis minor, subclavius, serratus anterior, and intercostal muscles on the anterior thoracic wall.

The muscle originates from the medial one-half to two-thirds of the clavicle, the lateral portion of the entire sternum and the adjacent cartilages of the first six ribs, and the bony portions of the fourth, fifth, and sixth ribs. The muscle inserts on the greater tubercle of the humerus.

Three major segmental subunits of the pectoralis muscle have been described: a clavicular segment, a sternocostal segment, and a laterally placed external segment. The clavicular segment arises from the midclavicular area, receives its blood supply from the deltoid branch of the thoracoacromial artery, and is innervated by branches of the lateral pectoral nerve. The sternocostal segment accounts for most of the pectoralis major muscle and receives its blood supply from the pectoral branch of the thoracoacromial artery with its nerve supply from the medial and lateral pectoral nerves. The external segment has a variable blood supply with contributions from the lateral thoracic and thoracoacromial artery.

The motor action of the pectoralis major muscle is to medially rotate and adduct the humerus. The muscle is innervated by the medial and lateral pectoral nerves that develop from the brachial plexus. Development of the pectoralis major myocutaneous flap is of little functional ill consequence as the latissimus dorsi muscle compensates for otherwise lost adductor activity.

Thoracoacromial Artery

The muscle's primary blood supply is from the thoracoacromial artery that arises as the second branch of the

---

Atlas of Operative Oral and Maxillofacial Surgery, First Edition. Edited by Christopher J. Haggerty and Robert M. Laughlin.

axillary artery coming off the subclavian artery. Secondary pedicles include the lateral thoracic and superior thoracic arteries.

Deltopectoral Groove

This represents the anatomic junction of the deltoid and pectoralis major muscles through which the cephalic vein passes.

Bony landmarks of importance in the development of the pectoralis major myocutaneous flap include the clavicle and the manubrial notch and xiphoid process that demarcate the midline of the chest wall.

Soft tissue landmarks of importance in the development of the pectoralis major myocutaneous flap include the nipple and, in the case of a woman, the inframammary crease.

Pectoralis Major Myocutaneous Flap Surgical Technique

1. Development of the recipient tissue bed prior to the development of the myocutaneous flap is paramount in the performance of reconstruction with the pectoralis major myocutaneous flap. In the case of immediate reconstruction of an ablative soft tissue defect (Figure 51.5), the delivery of the cancer specimen (Figure 51.4) permits a quantitative measurement of the defect with the subsequent design of this exact skin paddle size on the chest wall. In the case of an avulsive traumatic defect, the release of scar tissue in the recipient tissue bed permits a more accurate appreciation and measurement of the skin paddle requirement and subsequent design of this exact skin paddle size on the chest wall. Simultaneous recipient and donor site surgeries may result in the development of a skin paddle that is of insufficient size to adequately reconstruct the defect.

2. Following the determination of the required skin paddle size, the skin paddle is designed medial and inferior to the nipple on the chest wall. The required skin paddle size is slightly overestimated when designing the skin paddle on the chest wall so as to reduce tension on the closure at the recipient site, thereby reducing possible dehiscence at the recipient site (Figure 51.6). In the case of a woman, the inferior aspect of the skin paddle is designed in the inframammary crease.

3. A curvilinear incision is designed that connects the medial aspect of the skin paddle to the region approximating the greater tubercle of the humerus.

4. The dissection is initiated by incising the skin and subcutaneous tissues about the proposed incision. The deeper dissection is performed with the electrocautery unit to the level of the pectoralis major muscle fascia that is maintained on the ventral aspect of the muscle (Figure 51.7). This dissection is carried superiorly to the region of the clavicle, supero-laterally to the deltopectoral groove, infero-laterally to the free margin of the pectoralis major muscle, and medially to the region of the lateral aspect of the sternum.

5. In the area of the skin paddle, the deep dissection is performed so as to not undermine the skin paddle and risk its viability. The circumferential dissection of the skin paddle is completed down to the pectoralis fascia superiorly and down to the rectus abdominus fascia inferiorly. Often, the inferior dissection will divulge that the skin paddle is not supported by underlying pectoralis major muscle. This realization does not jeopardize the skin paddle's viability. The skin paddle is temporarily sutured to the underlying pectoralis major fascia and possibly to the inferiorly located rectus abdominus fascia.

6. The elevation of the myocutaneous flap is initiated by elevating the rectus abdominus fascia off of its muscle that inserts on the inferior aspect of the sixth rib. The entirety of the pectoralis major muscle is elevated off the ribs' superficial surfaces as well as the intercostal muscles that are encountered thereafter. This technique is continued from the free margin of the pectoralis major muscle laterally to the origination of the muscle medially. In general, approximately 1 cm of pectoralis major muscle is maintained on the lateral aspect of the sternum in the development of the myocutaneous flap. Further superior dissection will identify the pectoralis minor muscle. In addition, as the myocutaneous flap is mobilized superiorly, the axial vessels will be identified within the deep surface of the muscle. Retraction of the muscle during its elevation is important to avoid inadvertent trauma to the primary and secondary pedicles of the flap.

7. Perforators from the intercostal artery coursing through the intercostal muscles and perforators from the internal mammary artery coursing in the parasternal region should be identified and properly coagulated or ligated during the dissection to prevent postoperative bleeding.

8. The insertion of the pectoralis major muscle at the greater tubercle of the humerus will be identified supero-laterally. The cephalic vein is identified in the deltopectoral groove. The disinsertion of the pectoralis major muscle is performed in an incremental fashion with the electrocautery unit (Figure 51.8). Complete disinsertion is typically required to realize an effective arc of rotation of the myocutaneous flap into the recipient tissue bed (Figure 51.9).

9. A bipedicled neck flap is required so as to pass the myocutaneous flap into the neck and ultimately into the oral cavity. This bipedicled neck flap serves to communicate the dissection of the neck with that

of the chest wall. It is created deep to the platysma muscle and superficial to the sternocleidomastoid muscle and clavicle. The bipedicled neck flap is created in this surgical plane from the neck approach as well as from the chest wall approach, after which the communication is created that must have the breadth of five fingers so as to not constrict the flap's vasculature.

10. The myocutaneous flap is passed deep to the bipedicled neck flap and into the oral cavity (Figure 51.10). The previously placed skin paddle sutures are removed prior to initiating the closure of the skin paddle to the oral mucosa to complete the reconstruction (Figure 51.11).

11. Two suction drains are placed in the chest wall donor site. One is typically oriented vertically toward the disinsertion, and one is placed in a dependent horizontal fashion. The chest wall is closed in anatomic layers with staples placed at the skin surface.

12. Two suction drains are commonly placed in the neck. If a neck dissection was performed, one drain will be placed in the carotid sheath area, and one drain will be placed in the submental triangle. The neck is closed in anatomic layers with sutures placed at the skin surface.

Postoperative Management

1. Following pectoralis major myocutaneous flap reconstruction, patients typically maintain their endotracheal intubation and ventilator support for at least 12 hours postoperatively due to the magnitude of these surgeries.

2. Intravenous antibiotics are routinely ordered postoperatively for a time period determined by the preference of the surgeon.

3. Perioperative corticosteroid administration is of benefit to patients due to the excessive swelling that otherwise occurs. If significant, oral swelling can prolong the time required to maintain the endotracheal tube postoperatively and may increase the likelihood of postoperative tracheotomy.

4. Suction drains are maintained until trends in their drainage identify the ability to remove the drains. This is typically 10 days.

5. The skin staples are typically removed in 10 days.

6. Patients are typically fed via a nasogastric feeding tube that is maintained until acceptable healing without signs of infection or wound breakdown is realized within the oral cavity. This is commonly a 2-week period postoperatively.

Early Complications

1. **Bleeding**: May result from ineffective coagulation or ligation of perforators from the intercostal or internal mammary vessels. In addition, ineffective coagulation

of the disinsertion site at the greater tubercle of the humerus can lead to significant postoperative bleeding. When a postoperative hematoma is identified, a return to the operating room is required for evacuation of the hematoma and proper coagulation of the offending vessel(s).

2. **Infection**: Minimized with meticulous adherence to sterile techniques, the use of perioperative antibiotics, and copious irrigation of the oral cavity, neck, and chest wall. Treatment is via drainage with culture-directed antibiotic therapy.

3. **Dehiscence**: this complication is commonly noted and probably related to movement of the oral tissues during function. Wound dehiscence is managed with conservative measures, including local wound care. Complete healing is realized as long as exposure of the underlying reconstruction bone plate does not occur. Placing a skin paddle of slightly larger size than is required will decrease tension on the closure and decrease the likelihood of dehiscence postoperatively.

Late Complications

1. **Skin paddle necrosis**: Marginal or complete skin paddle necrosis is occasionally observed. Most cases occur in women with pendulous breasts, whereby a significant volume of fat separates the skin paddle and underlying muscle of the myocutaneous flap.

2. **Lip incompetence**: The weight of the myocutaneous flap is such that inferior migration of the lower lip may occur during healing. As such, maintenance of the marginal mandibular branch of the facial nerve during neck dissection is beneficial to maintain motor innervation of the lower lip. The loss of motor innervation of the lower lip and the weight of the myocutaneous flap will discourage lip competence in the postoperative period. Failure to maintain lip competence compromises the patient's ability to successfully take an oral diet. This problem becomes clinically noticeable with the resolution of surgical edema and the development of scar tissue in the recipient tissue bed.

3. **Recurrent disease**: The bulk of the pectoralis major muscle may hide early recurrence in the neck that might otherwise be readily detectable by palpation. As such, obtaining computed tomograms might be indicated in patients who underwent the placement of a pectoralis major myocutaneous flap whose neck dissection specimens showed microscopic evidence of metastatic nodal disease with or without extracapsular extension.

Key Points

1. The pectoralis major myocutaneous flap is supplied primarily by the pectoral branch of the thoracoacromial

artery and secondarily by the lateral thoracic artery and the superior thoracic artery. The incorporation of primary and secondary pedicles in the myocutaneous flap reduces the complication of partial or total loss of the skin paddle. This is a departure from the originally described technique for the development of this myocutaneous flap that was based exclusively on the pectoral branch of the thoracoacromial artery.

2. The skin paddle of the pectoralis major myocutaneous flap is able to reconstruct oral lining and facial cover, or it can be split to simultaneously reconstruct both.

3. The pectoralis major myocutaneous flap is ideally suited to reconstruct oral soft tissue in the floor of mouth, ventral tongue, mandibular gingiva, and inferior buccal mucosa and skin in the lower third of the face. This flap does not practically possess an acceptable arc of rotation or length to reconstruct oral mucosa in the maxillary gingiva or palate or the skin of the upper two-thirds of the face.

4. A quantitative assessment of the ratio of the chest wall length to the neck length is also important to determine preoperatively when considering the selection of a myocutaneous flap for oral and maxillofacial reconstruction. It is important to ensure that the distance from the proposed skin paddle to the clavicle exceeds the distance from the recipient tissue bed to the clavicle before committing to the use of the pectoralis major myocutaneous flap. A long neck and relatively shorter chest wall length will impair the arc of rotation of this flap into the recipient tissue bed.

5. The pectoralis major myocutaneous flap has added value in its ability to cover the carotid artery when performed in conjunction with a radical or modified radical neck dissection where exposure of the carotid artery occurs.

6. The skin color of the chest wall is generally not favorable compared to the upper neck and facial skin, such that a color mismatch will occur when performing a pectoralis major myocutaneous flap for facial/neck cover reconstruction.

Case Report

Case Report 51.1. An 81-year-old male (Figure 51.1) presented for evaluation of a squamous cell carcinoma of the right mandibular gingiva (Figure 51.2). Clinical and radiographic evaluation (Figure 51.3) identified a 3 cm cancer of the right mandibular gingiva and underlying mandible with no evidence of cervical lymph node metastases, indicative of a T4N0M0 cancer. The patient underwent a composite resection of the right mandibular gingiva, mandible, and prophylactic neck dissection (Figure 51.4). The resultant soft tissue defect of the oral mucosa measured 6 cm × 3.5 cm (Figure 51.5). The proposed skin paddle was designed on the chest wall with slight overcorrection, 7 cm × 4 cm (Figure 51.6). The dissection was performed at the donor site while maintaining the pectoralis fascia on the pectoralis major muscle (Figure 51.7). The muscle was disinserted at the greater tubercle of the humerus, and the cephalic vein can be seen in the deltopectoral groove (Figure 51.8). The myocutaneous flap was mobilized superiorly (Figure 51.9) based on the pectoral branch of the thoracoacromial artery as well as the superior thoracic and lateral thoracic arteries. The flap was passed through the bipedicled neck tunnel (Figure 51.10) and ultimately into the oral cavity, where a primary closure was accomplished in a single-layer fashion (Figure 51.11). Postoperative evaluation of the patient shows acceptable facial form and the obvious prominence of the pectoralis major muscle in the neck (Figure 51.12). A well-healed skin paddle is noted in the oral cavity (Figure 51.13).

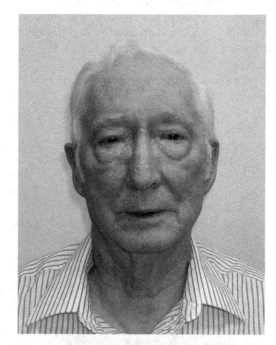

Figure 51.1. An 81-year-old patient presents with a chief complaint of a mass of his right lower jaw.

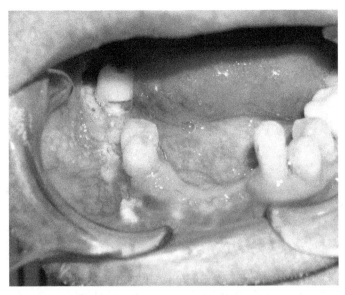

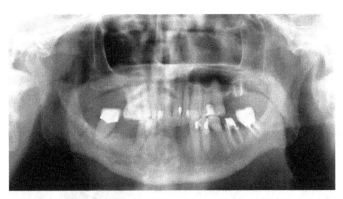

Figure 51.3.   Orthopantogram demonstrates bony involvement of the right posterior mandible.

Figure 51.2.   3 cm biopsy proven SCCA of the right mandibular gingiva and underlying mandible. There was no evidence of cervical lymph node on physical or radiographic examinations. The SCCA was classified as a T4N0M0 based on the TNM classification by the AJCC.

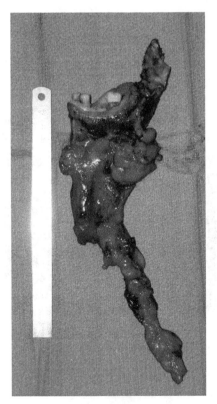

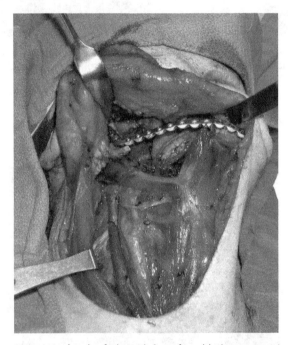

Figure 51.5.   Hard and soft tissue defect after ablative surgery. An oral soft tissue defect of 6 cm × 3.5 cm is present after composite resection.

Figure 51.4.   Medial aspect of composite resection specimen of the right mandibular gingiva, mandible, and elective neck dissection.

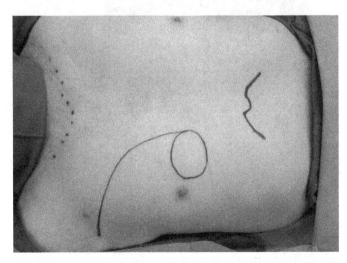

Figure 51.6.   Proposed skin paddle designed on the chest wall with slight overcorrection, 7 cm × 4 cm.

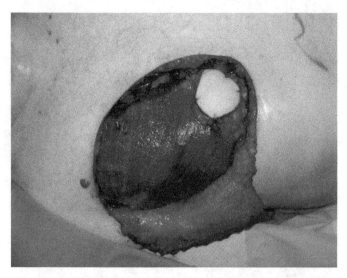

Figure 51.7. The dissection was performed at the donor site while maintaining the pectoralis fascia on the pectoralis major muscle.

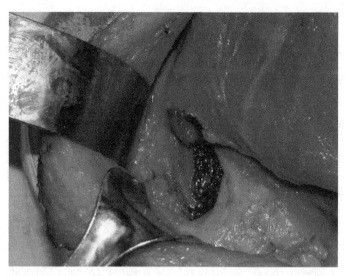

Figure 51.8. The muscle is disinserted at the greater tubercle of the humerus, and the cephalic vein can be seen in the deltopectoral groove.

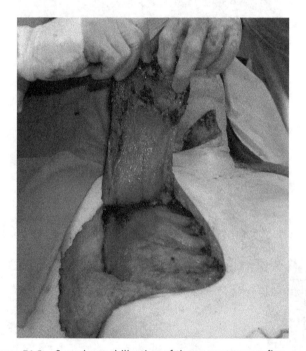

Figure 51.9. Superior mobilization of the myocutaneous flap.

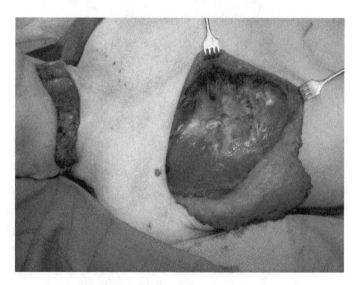

Figure 51.10. Flap passed through the bipedicled neck tunnel and ultimately into the oral cavity.

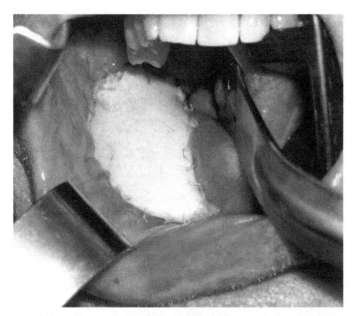

Figure 51.11. Oral defect primarily reconstructed with the skin paddle from the pectoralis major myocutaneous flap.

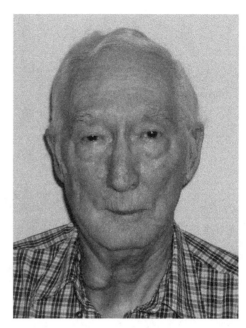

Figure 51.12. Postoperative evaluation of the patient shows acceptable facial form and the obvious prominence of the pectoralis major muscle in the neck.

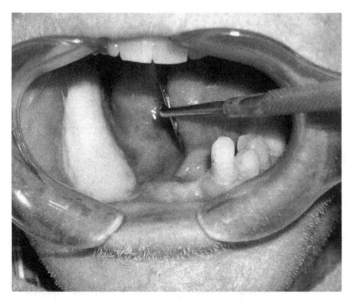

Figure 51.13. Well-healed skin paddle to intraoral defect.

References

Ariyan, S., 1979. Further experiences with the pectoralis major myocutaneous flap for the immediate repair of defects from excisions of head and neck cancers. *Plastic and Reconstructive Surgery*, 64, 605–12.

Ariyan, S., 1979. The pectoralis major myocutaneous flap: a versatile flap for reconstruction in the head and neck. *Plastic and Reconstructive Surgery*, 63, 73–81.

Carlson, E.R., 2003. Pectoralis major myocutaneous flap. *Oral and Maxillofacial Surgery Clinics of North America*, 15, 565–75.

Carlson, E.R. and Layne, J.M., 1997. The pectoralis major myocutaneous flap for reconstruction of soft tissue oncologic defects. *Atlas of Oral and Maxillofacial Surgery Clinics of North America*, 5, 15–35.

Chiummariello, S., Iera, M., Domatsoglou, A. and Alfano, C., 2010. The use of pectoralis major myocutaneous flap as "salvage procedure" following intraoral and oropharyngeal cancer excision. *Il Giornale di Chirurgia*, 31, 191–6.

Hsing, C.Y., Wong, Y.K., Wang, C.P., Wang, C.C., Jiang, R.S., Chen, F.J. and Liu, S.A., 2011. Comparison between free flap and pectoralis major pedicled flap for reconstruction in oral cavity cancer patients—a quality of life analysis. *Oral Oncology*, 47, 522–7.

Kekatpure, V.D., Trivedi, N.P., Manjula, B.V., Mathan Mohan, A., Shetkar, G. and Kuriakose, M.A., 2012. Pectoralis major flap for head and neck reconstruction in era of free flaps. *International Journal of Oral and Maxillofacial Surgery*, 41, 453–7.

Marx, R.E. and Smith, B.R., 1990. An improved technique for development of the pectoralis major myocutaneous flap. *Journal of Oral and Maxillofacial Surgery*, 48, 1168–80.

McLean, J.N., Carlson, G.W. and Losken, A., 2010. The pectoralis major myocutaneous flap revisited: a reliable technique for head and neck reconstruction. *Annals of Plastic Surgery*, 64, 570–3.

Moloy, P.J. and Gonzales, F.E., 1986. Vascular anatomy of the pectoralis major myocutaneous flap. *Archives of Otolaryngology—Head and Neck Surgery*, 112, 66–9.

Ossoff, R.H., Wurster, C.F., Berktold, R.E., Krespi, Y.P. and Sisson, G.A., 1983. Complications after pectoralis major myocutaneous flap reconstruction of head and neck defects. *Archives of Otolaryngology*, 109, 812–14.

Shah, J.P., Haribhakti, V., Loree, T. and Sutaria, P., 1990. Complications of the pectoralis major myocutaneous flap in head and neck reconstruction. *American Journal of Surgery*, 160, 352–5.

465

52

Closure of Oral-Antral Communications

Brent B. Ward
Department of Oral and Maxillofacial Surgery, University of Michigan Hospital, Ann Arbor, Michigan, USA

A method of obtaining closure of oral-antral communications (OAC) and oral-antral fistulae (OAF).

Indications

1. OAC over 4 mm in dimension noted intraoperatively
2. OACs or OAF that persist postoperatively

Contraindications

1. Defects smaller than 4 mm. Defects smaller than 4 mm frequently close with conservative treatment consisting of sinus precautions, antibiotics, and decongestants
2. OAC or OAF with signs and symptoms of active infection
3. Obstruction of the osteomeatal complex. Evaluation of the osteomeatal complex with a sinus computed tomography (CT) is warranted, especially in the case of recurrent fistulae. If the osteomeatal complex is obstructed, functional endoscopic sinus surgery (FESS) prior to OAF closure is indicated

General Considerations for Fistulectomy

1. Circumferential fistula excision is paramount to resolution of chronic fistula formation. With care, the fistula may be excised and the medial edges approximated with sutures as a first-layer sinus closure (Figure 52.1).
2. Additional tissue may be advanced for an additional one or two layers of closure, based on the size of the defect and the planned reconstructive technique.
3. Suture tissue into place in an interrupted fashion.
4. Consider a protective splint as indicated.

Specific Surgical Techniques for Oral-Antral Communications and Oral-Antral Fistulae

1. Primary closure
2. Buccal advancement flap
3. Palatal rotation advancement flap
4. Buccal fat pad flap
5. Bone graft
6. Temporalis muscle flap
7. Temporoparietal galea flap

Primary Closure

Used only when tissue can be closed without tension (not specifically described).

Buccal Advancement Flap

Indication

1. First-line treatment when insufficient soft tissue is available for primary closure

Contraindication

1. Buccal vestibular tissue that cannot be adequately mobilized and advanced to obtain primary closure due to scarring or size of defect

Technique: Buccal Advancement Flap

1. A full-thickness mucoperiosteal tissue flap is raised, and anterior and posterior releasing incisions are incorporated into the flap design (Figure 52.6). The divergent releasing incisions allow for the creation of a wide flap base and additional tissue advancement over the defect.
2. Additional periosteal releasing incisions (Figure 52.7) may be incorporated as needed for enhanced flap mobility to achieve a tension-free closure.
3. Adjunctive alveoplasty may be necessary to remove sharp bony ridges and to reduce the buccal plate in order to allow for additional flap advancement.
4. The buccal flap is advanced over the defect to obtain primary closure (Figure 52.10). Closure is obtained with resorbable sutures such as polyglactin (i.e., Vicryl, Ethicon Inc., Somerville, New Jersey, USA), which will maintain strength during healing.

Palatal Rotation Advancement Flap

Indication

1. Secondary alternative for closure of defects with insufficient soft tissue available for primary closure
2. Previously failed closure with a buccal advancement flap

Atlas of Operative Oral and Maxillofacial Surgery, First Edition. Edited by Christopher J. Haggerty and Robert M. Laughlin
© 2015 John Wiley & Sons, Inc. Published 2015 by John Wiley & Sons, Inc.

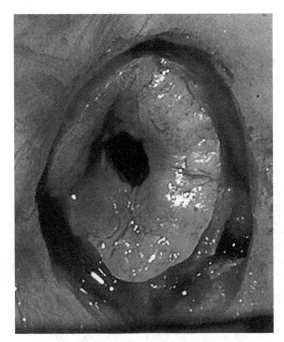

Figure 52.1. Circumferential fistula excision is performed to allow involution and closure of the fistula, and to establish closure of the nasal mucosa.

Contraindications

1. When the thick palatal tissue cannot be adequately mobilized for defect coverage due to scarring or large defect size
2. Relative contraindication: Where previous surgeries or trauma have disrupted the blood supply of the greater palatine artery. However, random pattern flaps of the palate have been reported successful in most cases

Surgical Anatomy

The palatal flap is a full-thickness axial flap based on the greater palatine artery, which exits the greater palatine foramen. The artery courses along the lateral aspect of the palate and anastomosis with the incisive and contralateral artery, allowing the entire palate to be elevated based on a single greater palatine arterial supply. The palate consists of oral mucosa, submucosa, and periosteum, which attaches to the hard palate by Sharpey's fibers. The soft palate consists of the tensor veli palatine, levator veli palatini, and uvula muscularis muscles. The tensor muscles pass around the hamulus, insert into the palatal aponeurosis, and may tether flap rotation.

Technique: Palatal Rotation Advancement Flap

1. The greater palatine foramen and neurovascular bundle are identified by manual palpation.
2. The necessary pedicle length is measured from the buccal aspect of the defect to the greater palatine foramen. The flap design is outlined with a sterile marking pen (Figure 52.2).
3. A full-thickness incision is made lateral to the neurovascular bundle and carried anteriorly, up to the palatal mucosa of the central incisors, or extended to the contralateral side as necessary for the defect size and location.

   A. At least 1 mm of mucosa apical to the gingival sulcus is preserved.
   B. In the edentulous patient, the incision may extend just palatal to the alveolar crest.
   C. Unilateral flaps may be rotated up to 180°, allowing the flap to be positioned with the mucosal side oral or nasal.
   D. A full palate flap has the additional flexibility of 360° rotation, allowing the flap to fold back onto itself for oral and nasal coverage when necessary.
   E. When elevating a full palatal flap, the neurovascular bundle of the incisive canal must be severed and cauterized or tied.

4. The full-thickness mucoperiosteal flap is raised from anterior to posterior and rotated into place (Figure 52.3). Care is taken to preserve the vascular supply of the flap.
5. The flap is sutured in place with 3-0 resorbable sutures to obtain a tension-free closure (Figure 52.4).
6. If further laxity is necessary to obtain passive approximation, the hamulus can be fractured, which will provide additional length to the flap. Alternatively, an island flap can be created with a circumferential incision, leaving the pedicle as the only anchor of the flap.
7. A soft plastic surgical stent may be placed over the flap and denuded palate for patient comfort. Care should be taken to avoid any pressure on the pedicle. The stent is removed 7 to 10 days after surgery.
8. Separation of the pedicle is usually required for small lateral defects when the flap bridges normal palatal tissue to reach the surgical site. This can be performed at 3 weeks. Prior to separation of the pedicle, verification of sufficient collateral supply can be assessed by tightly fastening a suture around the pedicle. If sufficient collateral blood supply is present, the flap will remain pink and well perfused. The pedicle may then be taken down, excess tissue trimmed, and inset at the new margin.

Case Report 52.1. A 58-year-old patient presents with a chief complaint of a bump to her right posterior maxilla. On examination, an 8 mm × 5 mm mass was identified within the right posterior maxilla. An incision biopsy was performed that rendered a diagnosis of a clear cell adenocarcinoma. A definitive resection was performed with wide local excision. The resulting oro-antral communication was primarily reconstructed with a palatal rotation advancement flap.

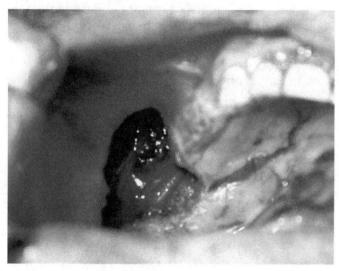

Figure 52.2. Oro-antral communication (OAC) following posterior maxillary resection of clear cell adenocarcinoma with palatal flap outlined.

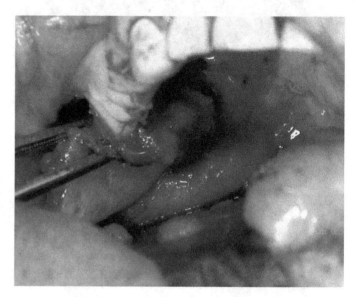

Figure 52.3. Palatal flap elevated and rotated into place.

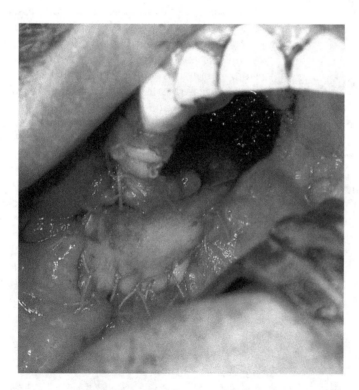

Figure 52.4. Flap inset and closure of the recipient site with resorbable Vicryl sutures in a tension-free manner. Denuded palatal bone is visualized at the flap donor/harvest site.

Buccal Fat Pad Advancement

Indications

1. Used alone or in conjunction with buccal or palatal advancement flaps as an additional layer of closure
2. Useful for persistent fistulae or as a local flap where adjacent tissue is inadequate for closure. The described technique may be used in defects up to 6 cm in diameter

Contraindications

1. Prior buccal fat surgery, trauma, or harvest
2. Defect sizes greater than 6 cm

Anatomy

The buccal fat pad serves as a gliding pad during masticatory and facial muscle contraction. It consists of the main body and three lobes: anterior, intermediate, and posterior. The main body lies on the anterior border of the masseter muscle, extends deeply to lie on the posterior maxilla, and extends forward along the buccal vestibule. The buccal extension is intimately related to Stenson's duct, and the buccal and zygomatic branches of the facial nerve, and gives fullness to the cheek. Each lobe is separated by investing connective tissue and has its own blood supply. This necessitates disruption of the septa to allow delivery of the fat pad, but it must be done carefully to prevent disruption of the blood supply.

Technique: Buccal Fat Pad Advancement

1. An incision is made through the periosteum elevated with the full-thickness mucoperiosteal flap and lateral to the maxillary tuberosity (Figure 52.6).
2. Metzenbaum scissors or fine hemostats are directed posterior and lateral, inserted with the beaks closed to puncture through the periosteum, and gently spread to provide access to the buccal fat pad and to gently disrupt the interlobular septa (Figure 52.8).
3. The fat pad is gently teased out with a pair of toothed Gerald forceps. Pressure may be placed within the temporal region to assist in delivering the fat pad. Minimal traction should be placed on the fat pad, as excessive tension will disrupt the blood supply. If the operator is having difficulty achieving sufficient fat pad release, the Metzenbaum scissors or fine hemostats are reinserted and spread to free the fat from its surrounding connective tissue.
4. The fat pad is draped across the OAC and passively sutured in place (Figure 52.9).
5. When used as a second layer of closure, the buccal fat is anchored to bone or sewn to submucosa to allow primary mucosal closure above the level of the buccal fat flap (Figure 52.10). The pedicled buccal fat pad flap undergoes complete epithelialization within 2–3 weeks.

Case Report

Case Report 52.2. A 36-year-old male with autism and seizure disorder presents requiring extraction of teeth #14 and 15. After removal of tooth #15, an oral-antral communication (OAC) with a 1 cm bony defect was appreciated. The OAC was repaired with a buccal fat pad advancement and a buccal tissue advancement flap. (See Figures 52.5 through 52.10.)

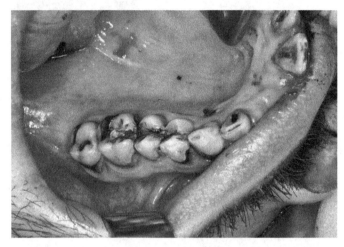

Figure 52.5.   Preoperative image of patient undergoing extraction of teeth #14 and #15 due to extensive decay and pain.

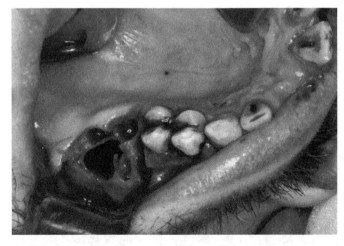

Figure 52.6.   Oro-antral communication following extraction of teeth #14 and #15. A full-thickness mucoperiosteal tissue flap with releasing incisions is created to enable acess to the buccal fat pad and for buccal advancement flap closure.

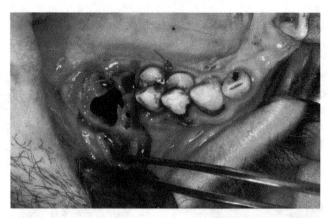

Figure 52.7.   Mobilization of the buccal flap and scoring of the periosteum to allow for increased flap mobility and buccal advancement.

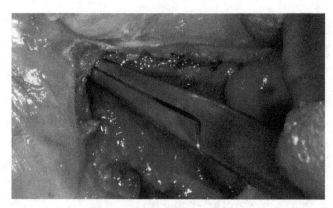

Figure 52.8.   Insertion of hemostats within the area of the buccal fat pad (lateral, posterior, and superior to the maxillary tuberosity). Gentle traction is used to deliver the buccal fat pad after disrupting the interlobular septa by spreading the hemostats.

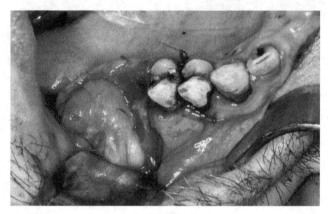

Figure 52.9.   Buccal fad pad is advanced into the oral-antral communication and secured to the submucosa with interrupted resorbable sutures.

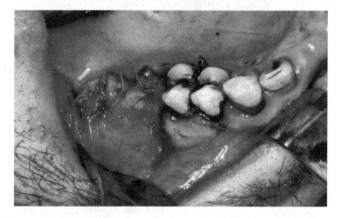

Figure 52.10.   A sliding buccal advancement flap is sutured above the buccal fat pad advancement to provide a layered closure of the OAC defect.

Bone Graft

Indications

1. Where future implant placement is planned and separation of the sinus and oral mucosa can be achieved
2. Previously failed closure of an OAC or OAF

Contraindications

1. Defect size too large to allow stable bone graft placement
2. Alveolar ridge atrophy too severe to allow graft placement or fixation
3. Previously failed bone graft

Technique: Bone Graft

1. The bony defect of the maxillary sinus is standardized with a trephine bur just large enough to create a round defect.
2. When possible, the sinus mucosa is closed.
3. A block bone graft is obtained from the donor site of choice, often the mandibular ramus or mental region. A monocortical bone graft is harvested with a second

trephine bur with an inner diameter matching the outer diameter of the trephine bur used to define the defect.
4. Gentle pressure is used to press fit the bone graft to the defect with care not to displace the block of bone into the sinus. If primary stability is not achieved, a miniplate or bone screw may be used to provide fixation.
5. A second-layer closure is then achieved, utilizing the oral mucosa described in the buccal advancement flap.
6. Three months following closure, the sinus may be reentered for a sinus lift. Any previously placed plates and screws may be removed at this time.

Temporalis Muscle Flap

Indication

1. Large, persistent defect requiring closure

Contraindications

1. Defects amenable to less invasive therapies
2. Previous surgery or trauma disrupting the blood supply of the anterior and posterior deep temporal arteries or middle temporal artery

3. Relative: Balding hair patterns with inability to hide surgical scars and the appearance of temporal wasting

Anatomy

It is of utmost importance that the surgeon is able to identify the layers of the face and their contents. The temporal branch of the facial nerve extends from the zygomaticotemporal branch, anteriorly and superior, below a line from the tragus to a point 2 cm lateral and 3 cm superior to the superior orbital rim. Care must be taken in flap harvesting to avoid injury to the facial nerve.

The blood supply to the temporalis muscle flap is derived from the anterior and posterior deep temporal arteries supplying the anterior and middle thirds, and the posterior portion of the muscle is supplied primarily by the middle temporal artery. The venous drainage and innervation follow the arterial supply.

The temporalis fascia, or deep temporal fascia, covers the superficial portion of the temporalis muscle. Two centimeters superior to the zygomatic arch, the fascia splits into the deep and superficial temporalis fascia, which surrounds the temporal fat pad and attaches to the medial and lateral surfaces of the zygomatic arch.

The temporalis muscle lies within the temporal fossa. The temporalis muscle varies in thickness from 5 to 15 mm.

The temporalis muscle flap can be divided to create a bilobed flap by preserving both the anterior and posterior deep temporal arteries using a one-third anterior and two-thirds posterior rule.

Technique: Temporalis Muscle Flap

1. The patient is prepped and draped in a sterile fashion. A corneal shield is placed on the ipsilateral side, and the hair overlying the incision is banded or shaved to allow access to the incision site.
2. A standard pre-auricular or modified endaural incision is outlined with a marking pen. The superior aspect of the pre-auricular marking is extended into the scalp sufficient to develop a flap of adequate length, identify the vascular supply, and provide a sufficient arc of rotation of the pedicled flap, while preserving the temporal branch of the facial nerve. After marking, 0.5% lidocaine with epinephrine is injected within the proposed incision site as a tumescent.
3. The incision begins above the helix of the ear. Skin hooks are utilized to retract the subcutaneous tissue laterally. The incision is extended through the temporoparietal fascia to the deep temporal fascia, which is recognizable by the glistening white fascia.
4. The pre-auricular or modified endaural incision is continued inferior to the helix of the ear and follows the cartilage of the external auditory canal to the base of the zygomatic arch.
5. An incision is made through the temporalis fascia at a 45° angle extending anterosuperiorly from the root of the zygoma, exposing the temporalis muscle. Subperiosteal dissection is started over the arch of the zygoma with a #9 periosteal elevator, lifting the superficial temporal fascia and protecting the facial nerve.
6. The temporalis muscle may be divided into two flaps consisting of the anterior one-third and posterior two-thirds (Figure 52.13). The anterior one-third may be passed over the zygomatic arch into the oral cavity. If needed, an osteotomy of the zygoma may be used to lengthen the pedicle and reach of the flap. The posterior two-thirds are rotated anteriorly to prevent a cosmetic defect (Figure 52.14). Alternatively, an alloplastic temporal implant may be used for the same purpose.
7. The donor site is closed in a layered fashion. To minimize postoperative hematoma and seroma, a postauricular suction drain may be placed.

Case Report

Case Report 52.3. A 74-year-old patient referred from an outside institution presents with a chief complaint of halitosis, fluid communication to the right sinus, and chronic right-sided sinus pain and obstruction. The patient reports a previous history of a resected right posterior maxillary gingival squamous cell carcinoma and multiple failed attempts at sinus closure. On examination, the patient has a large right oral-antral fistula with signs and symptoms of a sinus infection. On review of the sinus computed tomography scan (Figure 52.11), a large bony defect was noted along the right posterior maxilla, and obstruction of the osteomeatal complex was identified. The patient underwent FESS prior to OAF closure with a temporalis muscle flap advancement. (See also Figures 52.12, 52.13, and 52.14.)

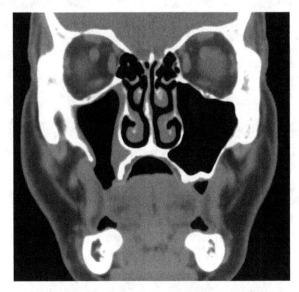

Figure 52.11. Coronal view of computed tomography demonstrating the oral-antral fistula. Note the obstructed osteomeatal complex on the right side and the patent osteomeatal complex on the left side.

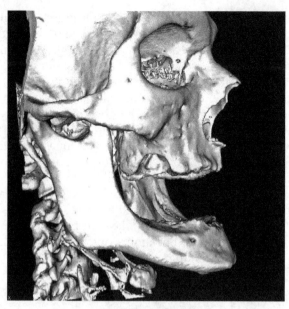

Figure 52.12. 3D reconstruction of maxillofacial computed tomography demonstrating the oro-antral communication.

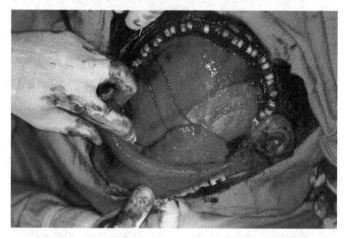

Figure 52.14. The anterior one-third of the temporalis flap is used to close the intraoral oral-antral fistula after fistulectomy. The posterior two-thirds of the temporalis flap is repositioned anteriorly to prevent a cosmetic defect.

Temporoparietal Galea Flap

Indications

1. Large maxillary defects not amenable to closure with less invasive local flaps

Contraindications

1. Adequate treatment achievable by less invasive means
2. Trauma or surgery of the temporal region placing the tissues at risk of ischemia or necrosis

Anatomy

The temporoparietal galea flap is derived from the temporoparietal tissues, which are the continuation of the

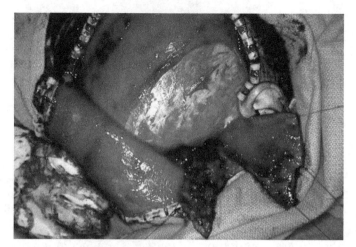

Figure 52.13. The temporalis muscle flap is elevated and split into an anterior one-third and a posterior two-thirds.

subcutaneous musculoaponeurotic system (SMAS) above the zygomatic arch. Superficially, the galea is adherent to the subcutaneous layer of the overlying skin. This plane must be surgically created at a level of the dermal appendages. The deep surface is easily separated from the temporalis fascia and pericranium.

The temporoparietal galea flap is 2–4 mm thick, up to 20 cm in length (when based off the posterior branch of the superficial temporal artery and vein), and described to have up to 180 cm^2 of surface area. The superficial temporal artery divides into anterior and posterior branches between 2 and 4 cm above the zygoma. The posterior branch curves posteriorly within a 2 cm strip above the external auditory canal (EAC). 10 cm above the EAC, the superficial temporal artery ascends to the subdermal plexus. Care must be taken to avoid damaging the vascular supply in flaps designed to include this area.

The venous drainage is noted to consistently lie posterior and superior to the artery and is at risk for vascular compromise. As mentioned for the temporalis muscle flap, the ability to identify the facial layers and protect the facial nerve is of greatest importance. The temporal branch of the facial nerve extends anteriorly and superiorly below a line from the tragus to a point 2 cm lateral and 3 cm superior to the superior orbital rim.

Technique: Temporoparietal Galea Flap

1. The patient is prepped as described for the temporalis muscle flap.
2. The superficial temporal artery can be found approximately 2 cm anterior to the external auditory canal. Doppler or palpation and marking can be beneficial in preservation of the vascular pedicle. Shaving the hair is not necessary. Sterile lubricant may be applied to part the hair and staple it down with the drapes.

3. A pre-auricular or endaural incision is extended superiorly into a hemicoronal incision.

4. The incision is brought to a subcutaneous depth at the level of the dermal appendages. This dissection is difficult, as a natural plane does not exist. Appropriate depth is achieved when successfully elevating and visualizing the hair follicles, but preserving the dermal plexus and subcutaneous fat with the galea. The superficial temporal vein is located rather superficially; if dissection is too deep, both the subdermal plexus and vein may be compromised, and both are essential for flap viability. However, it is inevitable to leave some hair follicles with the galea, or take some subdermal fat with the skin flap at times. Generally, dissection is started posteriorly, with care to preserve the posterior branch of the superficial temporal artery.

5. The flap is designed with a 2–3 cm wide pedicle to protect the vessels, and a length is measured that will achieve the appropriate arc of rotation to reach the OAC/OAF. Once the flap has been designed, dissection is deepened to the loose areolar tissue overlying the pericranium and temporalis. The flap is easily elevated with blunt scissors along the belly of the temporalis muscle and is brought down to the level of the zygomatic arch (Figure 52.15). The anterior branch of the superficial temporal artery will be encountered and require ligation. Transillumination may prove useful in identification and preservation of the pedicle. If additional length is necessary, the pedicle can be dissected inferior to the tragus at the level of the parotid gland.

6. A tunnel to the oral cavity is created by subcutaneous dissection, superficial to the SMAS until the anterior border of the masseter is identified. A right-angled hemostat works well for penetration to the oral cavity. The tunnel should be large enough to prevent strangulation, and care should be made to avoid damage to the facial nerve and Stenson's duct.

7. The flap is gently passed into the oral cavity and sutured in place (Figure 52.16), with care to prevent flap rotation, which will occlude the pedicle.

8. Hemostasis may be achieved with electrocautery, but care must be taken not to compromise the thin remaining skin. A Penrose or suction drain may be used along with a pressure dressing superior to the base of the flap to prevent hematoma and seroma, and to obliterate potential dead space. It is important if a pressure dressing is utilized to not apply pressure directly over the vascular pedicle.

Case Report

Case Report 52.4. A 64-year-old patient presents after resection of posterior maxillary squamous cell carcinoma with a large residual oral-antral fistula. The patient was treated with fistulectomy, which resulted in a 6 cm × 4 cm oral-antral communication. The patient underwent successful reconstruction with a temporoparietal galea flap inset to the intraoral defect. (See Figures 52.15 and 52.16.)

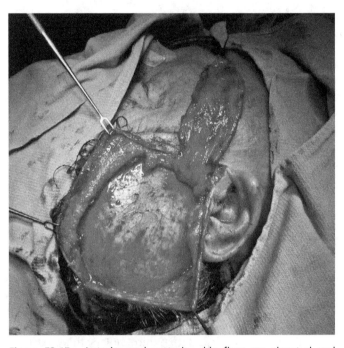

Figure 52.15. Anterior and posterior skin flaps are elevated and retracted with the temporoparietal galea flap elevated and draped across the face to demonstrate the reach of the flap. The temporalis muscle and overlying temporalis fascia remain in place.

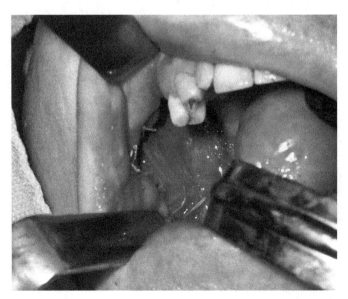

Figure 52.16. The temporoparietal galea flap is inset to the intraoral defect.

Postoperative Management

1. Antibiotics to target sinus and oral flora
2. Nasal decongestants
3. Sinus precautions

   a. No nose blowing
   b. Sneeze with mouth open
   c. Avoid pressure differential between the sinus and mouth
   d. No smoking

4. Diet based on flap choice and closure method

   a. **Flaps with primary mucosal closure**: Clear liquids, advancing to a soft diet as tolerated, then a regular diet at 7 days
   b. **Flaps with secondary intention healing**: Clear liquids, advancing to a full liquid diet for 3 days and then a soft diet until secondary intention healing is complete (3–4 weeks)

Complications

1. Infection, including sinusitis
2. Bone graft failure
3. Partial flap necrosis
4. Recurrent oral-antral fistula

Key Points

1. Oral-antral communications are most frequently seen in extraction of maxillary molars, with greatest incidence in the first, second, and then third molars; this is particularly true in older patients due to pneumatized sinuses.
2. Local anesthesia may be used for local tissue advancement, while general anesthesia should be considered for larger surgical procedures.
3. Critical size defect:

   a. A communication of 4 mm or less may heal well with minimal intervention and can be treated with primary closure or a buccal advancement flap.
   b. A communication greater than 4 mm is at greater risk of failing primary closure.

4. Small defects are amenable to buccal advancement and palatal rotation flaps. Defects up to 6 cm may be closed with buccal fat pad advancement. Larger defects may be more amenable to a temporalis muscle flap or temporoparietal galea flap.
5. Preoperative evaluation of osteomeatal complex patency should be considered, especially if a previous closure has failed. If the osteomeatal complex is obstructed, Functional Endoscopic Sinus Surgery (FESS) should be pursued to obtain proper drainage prior to closure of the oral-antral communication.
6. Appropriate antibiotic coverage should be considered for any procedure involving the sinus. Bacteriology of the oral cavity and sinus often include alpha and beta hemolytic *Streptococcus*, *Haemophilus*, *Proteus*, and *Escherichia coli*.

References

Amin, M.A., Bailey, B.M.W., Swinson, B. and Witherow. H., 2005. Use of the buccal fat pad in the reconstruction and prosthetic rehabilitation of oncological maxillary defects. *British Journal of Oral and Maxillofacial Surgery*, 43 (2), 148–54.

Cesteleyn, L., 2003. The temporoparietal galea flap. *Oral and Maxillofacial Surgery Clinics of North America*, 15 (4), 537–50.

Dym, H. and Wolf, J., 2012. Oroantral communication. *Oral and Maxillofacial Surgery Clinics of North America*, 24 (2), 239–47.

Haas, R., Watzak, G., Baron, M., Tepper, G., Mailath, G. and Watzek, G., 2003. A preliminary study of monocortical bone grafts for oroantral fistula closure. *Oral Surgery, Oral Medicine, Oral Pathology, Oral Radiology, and Endodontology*, 96 (3), 263–6.

Hanazawa, Y., Itoh, K., Mabashi, T. and Sato, K., 1995. Closure of oroantral communications using a pedicled buccal fat pad graft. *Journal of Oral and Maxillofacial Surgery*, 53 (7), 771–5; discussion, 775–6.

Loukas, M., Kapos, T., Louis, R.G., Jr., Wartman, C., Jones, A. and Hallner, B., 2006. Gross anatomical, CT and MRI analyses of the buccal fat pad with special emphasis on volumetric variations. 2006 Mar 10;28(3):254–60.

Rothamel, D., Wahl, G., d'Hoedt, B., Nentwig, G-H., Schwarz, F. and Becker, J., 2007. Incidence and predictive factors for perforation of the maxillary antrum in operations to remove upper wisdom teeth: Prospective multicentre study. *British Journal of Oral and Maxillofacial Surgery*, 45 (5), 387–91.

Sindet-Pedersen, S., Skoglund, L.A., Hvidegaard, T. and Holst, E., 1983. A study of operative treatment and bacteriological examination of persistent oro-antral fistulas. *International Journal of Oral Surgery*, 12 (5), 314–8.

von Wowern, N., 1973. Correlation between the development of an oroantral fistula and the size of the corresponding bony defect. *Journal of Oral Surgery*, 31 (2), 98–102.

Ward, B.B., 2003. The palatal flap. *Oral and Maxillofacial Surgery Clinics of North America*, 15 (4), 467–73.

Ward, B.B., 2007. Temporalis system in maxillary reconstruction: temporalis muscle and temporoparietal galea flaps. *Atlas of Oral and Maxillofacial Surgery Clinics*, 15 (1), 33–42.

Zhang, H-M., Yan, Y-P., Qi, K-M., Wang, J-Q. and Liu, Z-F., 2013. Anatomical structure of the buccal fat pad and its clinical adaptations. *Plastic and Reconstructive Surgery*, 109 (7), 2509–18; discussion, 2519–20.

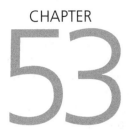

53 Anterior Iliac Crest Bone Graft

Michael Carson
Department of Oral and Maxillofacial Surgery, Naval Medical Center Portsmouth, Portsmouth, Virginia, USA

A surgical procedure for harvesting a cortical, cancellous, or corticocancellous block graft from the anterior ilium.

Indications

1. When autogenous grafting is desired that requires a high ratio of cancellous to cortical bone (a high volume of osteocompetent cells)
2. Hard tissue maxillofacial defects requiring 50 mL or less of cancellous bone

Contraindications

1. Reconstruction of maxillofacial defects requiring more than 50 mL of cancellous bone
2. Patients with previous head and neck radiation involving the graft recipient site

Anatomy

Anterior ilium: Located between the anterior iliac spine and the ilium tubercle. The ilium serves as a site for numerous muscular attachments responsible for normal gait and core stability.

Anterior superior iliac spine: Serves as the attachment of the external abdominal oblique muscle medially and the tensor fascia lata laterally.

Tensor fascia lata: Originates at the anterior superior iliac spine and the antero-lateral portion of the anterior iliac crest, and inserts into the iliotibial tract of the lateral thigh. The iliotibial tract (band) continues inferiorly and inserts along the lateral condyle of the tibia. Damage or excessive retraction of this muscle is the most common cause of postoperative gait disturbances.

Iliacus muscle: Originates along the superior half of the iliac fossa (medial iliac crest). The iliacus muscle joins the psoas major muscle and inserts along the lesser trochanter of the femur.

Sensory cutaneous nerves (3):

Iliohypogastric nerve (L1, L2): The lateral cutaneous branch of the iliohypogastric nerve is located overlying the ilium tubercle and is the most commonly injured nerve during an anterior iliac crest bone graft (AICBG). The iliohypogastric nerve provides sensory innervation to the skin of the pubis and lateral aspect of the buttock.

Lateral branch of the subcostal nerve (T12, L1): Located overlying the anterior superior iliac spine. The subcostal nerve is located medial to the iliohypogastric nerve and provides sensory innervation to the lateral buttock.

Lateral femoral cutaneous nerve: Located between the psoas major and the iliacus muscle, medial to the subcostal nerve. In 2.5% of the population, the lateral femoral cutaneous nerve can be found within 1 cm of the anterior superior iliac spine. The lateral femoral cutaneous nerve provides sensory innervation to the skin of the anterior and lateral thigh. Damage to this nerve may result in a meralgia paresthetica.

Anterior Iliac Crest Bone Graft (AICBG) Harvesting Technique (Medial Approach)

1. Preoperative intravenous antibiotics are administered. The patient is intubated and positioned supine on the operating room table. A hip roll is placed under the pelvis to accentuate the anterior iliac crest anatomy. Surgical markings are made to include the locations of the anterior superior iliac spine, the ilium tubercle, and the anterior iliac crest (Figure 53.1).
2. A hand is used to place medial (toward the abdomen) pressure, and the anticipated incision line is marked 2–4 cm lateral to the height of the anterior iliac crest (Figure 53.1). Incisions placed directly overlying the anterior ilium will cause postoperative pain along the beltline. Local anesthetic containing a vasoconstrictor is injected within the area of the proposed skin incision within the subcutaneous tissue.
3. The patient is prepped and draped in a sterile fashion. An iodoban antimicrobial incise drape (3M, St. Paul, MN, USA) may be used if desired.
4. A 4–6 cm skin incision is made with a #10 blade 1 cm posterior to the anterior superior iliac spine and terminating 1–2 cm anterior to the ilium tubercle.
5. The dissection proceeds through the subcutaneous tissue until Scarpa's fascia is reached. A 4 × 4 sterile gauze is used to bluntly dissect Scarpa's fascia (Figure 53.2) from the overlying subcutaneous fat. Prior to transversing Scarpa's fascia, electrocautery

Atlas of Operative Oral and Maxillofacial Surgery, First Edition. Edited by Christopher J. Haggerty and Robert M. Laughlin.
© 2015 John Wiley & Sons, Inc. Published 2015 by John Wiley & Sons, Inc.

is used to control all hemorrhaging subcutaneous vessels.

6. A #15 blade is used to transect Scarpa's fascia. A hypovascular tissue plane is identified overlying the anterior iliac crest between the insertions of the tensor fascia lata laterally and the external and transverse abdominal muscles medially. Elevating within this hypovascular tissue plane will minimize bleeding and postoperative pain or gait disturbances. The periosteum is released, and dissection proceeds within a subperiosteal tissue plane over the medial (inner) iliac cortical plate. The iliacus muscle is identified and reflected to expose the medial iliac crest (iliac fossa).

7. A blunt retractor (i.e., a Bennett retractor) is placed to retract the musculoperiosteal layer and to protect the intra-abdominal contents during the medial approach to the anterior ileum.

8. Osteotomies are made utilizing combinations of saws, burs, and chisels based on the type of graft required (corticocancellous block or cancellous graft) and the size of the defect requiring reconstruction. Regardless of the osteotomy design, it is imperative to preserve the attachments to the anterior superior iliac spine and to maintain a minimum safe distance of 1 cm from the anterior superior iliac spine and 1–2 cm from the ilium tubercle.

9. For standard medial (inner) AICBG harvest, the author marks the proposed osteotomy site with either a sterile marking pen or electrocautery (Figure 53.3). A reciprocating saw with copious irrigation is used to outline the osteotomy (Figure 53.4). If only cancellous bone is required, the medial cortical plate is outfractured with a chisel, marrow is removed with curettes and bone gouges, and the medial plate is repositioned (clamshell technique). If a corticocancellous block graft is required, the inferior aspect of the medial cortical plate (just superior to the fusion of the inner and outer iliac plates) is scored with either a reciprocating or a sagittal saw, and a sharp chisel is used to outfracture the medial plate (Figures 53.5). The chisel is directed against the outer (lateral) cortical plate to maximize the amount of cancellous bone attached to the inner (medial) cortical bone (Figures 53.6 and 53.7). Additional marrow is removed with curettes and bone gouges to increase the amount of graft material and to minimize marrow oozing.

10. After the harvest is completed, the wound site is irrigated copiously and inspected for hemostasis. Marrow bleeding is minimized with the removal of all bone marrow from the harvest site and with the placement of hemostatic agents (i.e., microfibrillar collagen, gelfoam, bone wax, and topical thrombin). If minor to moderate marrow oozing is present that is refractory to marrow removal and hemostatic agents, a drain may be placed within the bony defect, placed to low suction, and monitored closely postoperatively.

11. Meticulous layered closure is required to minimize postoperative hematoma and seroma formation.

12. A long-lasting local anesthetic agent may be infiltrated within the soft tissues overlying the donor site, and/or an ON-Q C-bloc continuous nerve block system (I-Flow Corporation, Lake Forest, CA, USA) (Figure 53.8) may be placed.

13. A thin layer of antibiotic ointment is placed over the wound, and an external dressing is placed.

Postoperative Management

1. Nonsteroidal anti-inflammatory drugs and narcotics are utilized postoperatively. A pain-controlled analgesia pump (PCA) may be required in the immediate postoperative period.

2. Drains are typically removed when they become nonproductive for a 24-hour period.

3. Antibiotics are recommended for 5–7 days.

4. Ambulation is initiated within 24 hours postoperatively. Ambulation should be closely monitored with the assistance of a physical therapist and nursing support prior to discharge from the hospital. Ambulation aids (cane and walker) may be required for short periods of time postoperatively.

5. Moderate- to high-impact physical activity is restricted for a period of 6 weeks.

Complications

Early Complications

1. **Pain and gait disturbances**: Minimized with preservation of the muscular attachments to the anterior superior iliac spine (tensor fascia lata and external abdominal oblique) and the lateral iliac crest (tensor fascia lata and gluteus medius).

2. **Nerve injury**: Involved areas are dependent on the specific nerve(s) injured (i.e., iliohypogastric, subcostal, and lateral femoral cutaneous).

3. **Hematoma formation**: Minimized with meticulous dissection, hemostasis prior to wound closure, and the use of local hemostatic agents and drains when applicable.

4. **Infection**: Infections rates from AICBG harvests coincide with infection rates from similar orthopedic procedures (1–3%). Appropriate preoperative antibiotic administration, proper site preparation, maintenance of a sterile field, and meticulous wound closure will minimize infection occurrences. Infection

management is aimed toward incision and drainage procedures, with antibiotic coverage based on culture and sensitivity results.

5. **Cosmetic deformity**: Avoided by taking split-thickness grafts (avoiding harvesting of both the medial and lateral cortical plates) and maintaining an intact supero-lateral rim of the anterior iliac crest.

6. **Peritoneal perforation**: Minimized by maintaining an intact musculoperiosteal layer during medial reflection, using blunt abdominal retractors (i.e., a Bennett retractor), avoiding excessive retraction, and judiciously using periosteal elevators and electrocautery during initial dissection of the medial crest (iliac fossa).

7. **Fracture**: Minimized by maintaining a minimum safe distance of 1 cm from the anterior superior iliac spine and 1–2 cm from the ilium tubercle, and by avoidance of moderate- to high-impact activity for 6 weeks postoperatively. Treatment typically consists of bed rest followed by activity restriction and assisted ambulation.

8. **Meralgia paresthetica**: Numbness and/or pain to the outer thigh caused by injury to the lateral femoral cutaneous nerve.

Key Points

1. When evaluating a maxillofacial defect prior to definitive reconstruction, typically 10 mL of uncompressed bone is required to reconstruct a 1 cm bony defect. For mandibular continuity defects where a reconstruction plate will be placed or has already been placed, each screw hole span is roughly 1 cm. A mandibular continuity defect with a four–screw hole span would require a minimum of 40 mL of uncompressed marrow to appropriately reconstruct the defect.

2. AICBGs are ideal for segmental and marginal defects in which less than 50 mL of bone are required.

3. For continuity defects spanning greater than 5 cm and for patients who have undergone previous head and neck radiation therapy, microvascular reconstruction is recommended.

4. The harvest of AICBG can be performed in a two-team manner for most oral and maxillofacial reconstructions. Using a second team to harvest the AICBG decreases the overall procedure time significantly.

5. The overall infection rate of the recipient site can be decreased by minimized contamination with oral microbes. For secondary reconstruction of mandibular continuity defects, transcervical approaches should be utilized when possible.

6. The defect/recipient site should always be exposed prior to harvesting the AICBG. For reconstructing mandibular continuity defects through an extraoral

approach, large intraoral perforations often preclude the placement of the graft. Small intraoral perforations may be treated with a tension-free watertight closure (4-0 Vicryl interrupted horizontal mattress sutures) and copious irrigation prior to graft placement.

7. The size of the graft harvested or the osteotomy design is based on the defect size. The maximum size of the graft is limited anteriorly-posteriorly by maintaining a minimum safe distance of 1 cm from the anterior superior iliac spine and 1–2 cm from the ilium tubercle. The maximum vertical height is traditionally 4–5 cm and coincides with the fusion of the medial and lateral cortical plates.

8. The graft harvest to recipient placement time should be minimized in order to preserve the viability of osteocompetent cells.

9. For pediatric patients, the cartilaginous cap overlying the iliac crest is bisected longitudinally, preserved, and reapproximated with suture after completion of bone harvesting.

Case Report

Case Report 53.1. A 34-year-old female presents for the secondary reconstruction of a 4 cm continuity defect to the right posterior mandible from a previous ameloblastoma resection. (See Figures 53.1 through 53.9.)

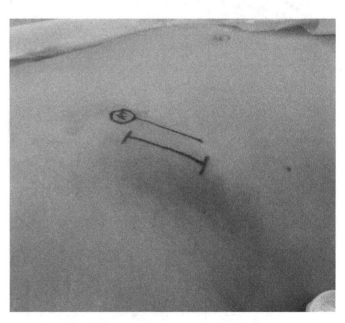

Figure 53.1. After palpation of the anterior superior iliac spine and the ileum tubercle, the anterior iliac crest is palpated and drawn. The inferior-lateral marking represents the location of the proposed skin incision (inferior and lateral to the anterior iliac crest) to minimize postoperative pain along the beltline.

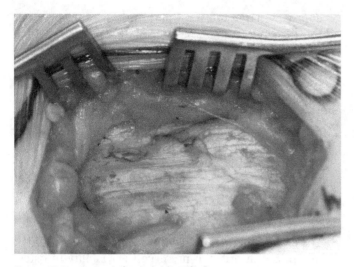

Figure 53.2.   Scarpa's fascia is identified.

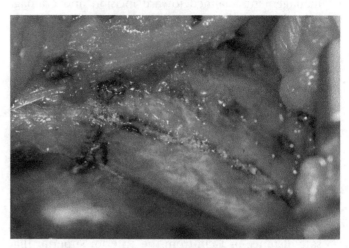

Figure 53.3.   A subperiosteal dissection is performed to expose the medial (inner) cortical plate of the anterior ilium. Electrocautery is used to outline the osteotomy design and to maintain a minimum safe distance of 1 cm from the anterior superior iliac spine and 1–2 cm from the ilium tubercle.

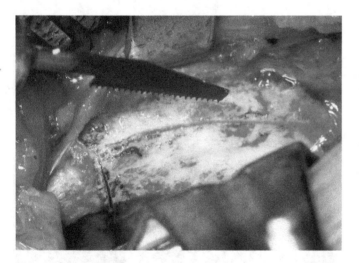

Figure 53.4.   A reciprocating saw is used to create osteotomies along the medial aspect of the anterior iliac crest.

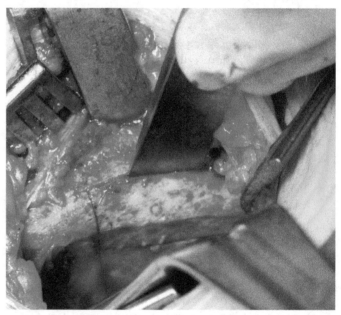

Figure 53.5.   A sharp, broad osteotome is used to carefully initiate the osteotomy.

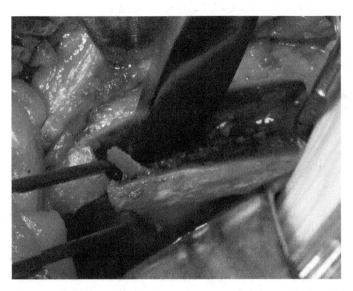

Figure 53.6. The osteotome is used to separate the corticocancellous block graft from the outer (lateral) cortical plate.

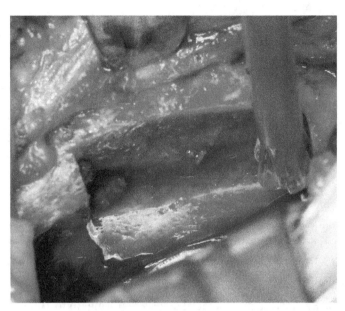

Figure 53.7. The corticancellous block graft is removed, and the remaining marrow is curetted.

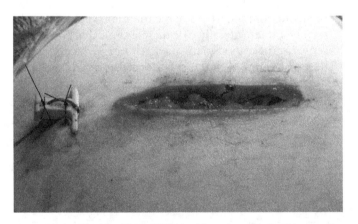

Figure 53.8. The deep layers are closed, and an On-Q C-bloc continuous nerve block system (I-Flow Corporation, Lake Forest, CA, USA) catheter is inserted prior to closure of the subcutaneous layer and skin.

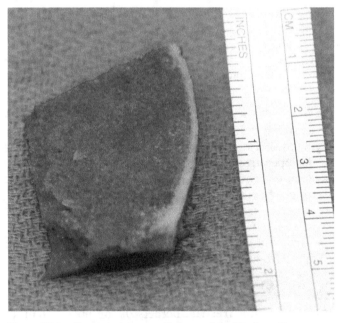

Figure 53.9. Harvested 4 cm corticocancellous block graft.

References

American Association of Oral and Maxillofacial Surgeons (AAOMS), 1994. *OMFS knowledge update*. Vol. 1. Rosemont, IL: AAOMS.

Kademani, D. and Keller, E., 2006. Iliac crest grafting for mandibular reconstruction. *Atlas of Oral and Maxillofacial Surgery Clinics of North America*, 14, 161.

Maus, U., 2008. How to store autogenous bone graft perioperatively. *Archives of Orthopedic Trauma Surgery*, 128, 1007–11.

Wilk, R.M., 2004. Bony reconstruction of the jaws. In: M. Miloro, G.E. Ghali, P. Larsen and P. Waite, eds. *Peterson's principles of oral and maxillofacial surgery*. 2nd ed. Shelton, CT: PMPH-USA.

54

Posterior Iliac Crest Bone Graft

Patrick B. Morrissey,[1] Robert A. Nadeau,[2] and Eric P. Hoffmeister[3]

[1]Department of Orthopedic Surgery, Naval Medical Center, San Diego,California, USA
[2]Department of Oral and Maxillofacial Surgery, University of Missouri–Kansas City Schools of Medicine and Dentistry, Kansas City, Missouri, USA
[3]Department of Orthopedic Surgery, Naval Medical Center San Diego; and Uniformed Services University of the Health Sciences, San Diego, California, USA

A method of obtaining large amounts of cortical, cancellous, or corticocancellous autogenous bone from the posterior ilium.

Indications

1. When autogenous grafting is desired that requires a high ratio of cancellous to cortical bone (a high volume of osteocompetent cells)
2. Hard tissue maxillofacial defects requiring up to 100 mL of uncompressed bone or 5 cm of structural cortical graft
3. The presence of a bone void unable to be filled with local tissue-grafting techniques
4. The need for augmentation of biologic healing capability (transfer of osteocompetent cells) to fracture or osteotomy sites
5. The need for additional osseous structural stability within traumatic or surgical defects

Contraindications

1. Local infection at, or adjacent to, the harvest site
2. Relative: The obese population is at increased risk for postoperative complications
3. Relative: The smoking population is at increased risk for postoperative complications
4. Relative: Osteoporotic and osteopenic patients are more likely to sustain intraoperative or postoperative fracture at the site of harvest. The procedure should be approached with caution in this population

Anatomy of the Posterior Ilium

Osseous structure: The borders of the posterior ilium are the iliac crest superiorly, the posterior superior iliac spine (PSIS) posteriorly, and the greater sciatic notch inferiorly. The bone is slightly concave on its lateral surface with three distinct ridges comprising the posterior, anterior, and inferior gluteal lines.

Musculature and fascia: The outer surface of the ilium serves as the broad attachment site for the gluteus minimus (between the anterior and inferior lines), the gluteus medius (between the anterior and posterior lines), and the gluteus maximus (from the posterior line to the iliac crest). The gluteus medius and minimus comprise the hip abductors and are innervated by the superior gluteal nerve. The gluteus maximus functions to extend and externally rotate the hip and is innervated by the inferior gluteal nerve. The medial edge of the posterior iliac crest is the attachment site for the lumbodorsal fascia.

Vasculature: The superior gluteal vessels arise from the posterior division of the internal iliac system and run adjacent to the cortex in the superior aspect of the sciatic notch. They supply the gluteal musculature and are located an average of 63 mm anteroinferiorly from the PSIS and 37 mm inferior to a line drawn perpendicular to the vertical axis at the level of the PSIS.

Neurologic structures: The superior cluneal nerves originate from the L1–L3 nerve roots and cross directly over the posterior iliac crest. The superior cluneal nerves supply sensory innervation to the superior two-thirds of the buttocks and are located an average of 68 mm anterosuperiorly from the PSIS. The middle cluneal nerves originate from the S1–S3 nerve roots and course from the sacral foramen laterally. The middle cluneal nerves supply sensory innervation to the medial buttock. Excessive traction or laceration to the superior and/or middle cluneal nerves can lead to numbness or symptomatic neuromas.

The greater sciatic notch contains the following nerves: the sciatic, superior and inferior gluteal, internal pudendal, posterior femoral cutaneous nerves, the nerve to quadratus femoris, and the nerve to obturator interuns. The greater sciatic notch is located 6–8 cm inferior to the posterior iliac crest and must not be violated during the surgical approach to the posterior ilium.

Posterior Iliac Crest Bone Graft (PICBG) Harvesting Technique

Posterior Iliac Approach

1. Harvesting from the posterior iliac region can be performed with the patient positioned either prone or in the lateral position. For harvesting in a prone position, the patient is intubated supine and then positioned prone, with 210° of reverse hip flexion.

---

2. Anatomical landmarks are palpated and marked, and include the posterior iliac crest, the posterior superior iliac spine (PSIS), the sacral midline and the site of the proposed incision (Figure 54.3). Local anesthetic containing a vasoconstrictor is injected at the surgical site. The patient is prepped and draped in a sterile fashion.

3. A 6–8 cm oblique or curvilinear skin incision (Figure 54.1) originating 3–4 cm lateral to the midline and 1 cm lateral to the posterior superior iliac spine is placed overlying and following the arc of the palpable bony prominence of the posterior iliac crest. The dissection proceeds through skin and subcutaneous tissue until the prominent dorsolumbar (i.e., lumbodorsal or thoracolumbar) fascia is encountered. The dorsolumbar fascia is transected, and dissection continues to the posterior iliac crest. A full-thickness flap, including the dorsolumbar fascia, gluteus maximus muscle, and periosteum, is elevated 1 cm lateral to the PSIS to expose the outer cortex of the posterior ilium (Figure 54.4). Preserving the continuity of this single, stout layer will greatly facilitate closure of the surgical site once the graft is obtained and will minimize postoperative complications. Preserving the PSIS and its attachments (sacroiliac ligaments) will minimize postoperative pelvic instability and will aid in maintaining a safe distance from the sacroiliac joint.

4. Subperiosteal elevation continues lateral to the PSIS and inferior to the posterior iliac crest for approximately 4–6 cm, depending on the size of the graft to be harvested. Care is taken with inferior reflection of the tissues to minimize damage to the structures within the sciatic notch and to the superior gluteal vessels.

Corticocancellous (Unicortical) Harvesting

1. After exposure of the grafting–donor site, the osteotomy design is contrived (Figure 54.2). The osteotomy size is dependent on the amount of bone required by the recipient site. The medial aspect of the osteotomy should originate 1 cm lateral to the PSIS, should extend no more than 5 cm inferior to the iliac crest, and should be directed perpendicular to the crest–iliac rim to avoid undermining the PSIS, to orient the medial osteotomy distal to the sacroiliac joint, and to reduce the potential for a future stress fracture of the posterior ilium.

2. The location of the lateral (distal) osteotomy is placed 4–6 cm lateral (distal) to the medial osteotomy. The inferior osteotomy should extend no more than 5 cm inferior to the posterior iliac crest–iliac rim. The superior osteotomy may be designed to incorporate the iliac rim or may be performed just inferior to the iliac rim (a rim-sparing osteotomy) (Figures 54.2 and 54.6). The deep aspect of the osteotomy should extend just into the marrow cavity. The osteotomies may be performed with combinations of chisels and saws (i.e., reciprocating and oscillating).

3. The outer cortical table of the posterior ilium may be harvested in strips or as a whole, depending on the reconstruction needs of the recipient site. The outer cortical table is elevated with a combination of a chisel and a freer. Care is taken to orient the chisel away from the sacroiliac joint and sciatic notch–superior gluteal vessels to minimize iatrogenic damage to these key structures (Figure 54.2).

4. Once the outer table has been removed, cancellous bone (Figure 54.6) may be harvested from the underlying marrow space. Care is taken to not undermine the PSIS and to avoid penetration of the inner table. Cancellous bone is harvested utilizing large curved and straight curettes in a two-handed, controlled maneuver, ensuring the inner table is not violated.

Cancellous-Only Harvesting: The Trapdoor Technique

1. In this technique, the lateral soft tissue attachments are not stripped from the ilium.

2. After exposure of the grafting site, an incision is made through the lateral rim of the cortex of the iliac crest using osteotomies. The crest is reflected medially, ensuring that all medial and lateral musculature remains intact.

3. Once exposed, cancellous bone can be curetted through the "trapdoor," in which three sides of the rectangular block are cut and hinged opened on the fourth side. The harvest should only extend lateral (distal) to the PSIS, and care should be taken to avoid perforating the inner table of the ilium.

4. Once the cancellous bone harvest is complete, the trapdoor is closed and gently secured into place with a bone tamp.

Closure

1. After bone harvesting is complete, all exposed cancellous surfaces are copiously irrigated and covered with bone wax or Gelfoam to obtain hemostasis at the graft site and to minimize postoperative hematoma formation.

2. Meticulous hemostasis should be obtained as soft tissues are closed. Drains are not required if wound hemostasis is achieved.

3. Any subperiosteally dissected musculature should be repaired to its origin on the iliac crest utilizing heavy, absorbable sutures (i.e., 0-0 Vicryl).

4. The wound is closed in a layered fashion. The full-thickness deep flap (dorsolumbar fascia, gluteus maximus muscle, and periosteum) is reapproximated with 2-0 Vicryl sutures. The subcuticular layer is closed with a running 3-0 Monocryl suture. Skin tension is achieved with surgical skin glue or steri-strips with an island dressing overlay.

5. Judicious infiltration on local anesthetic both superficially and deep will assist in postoperative pain control.

Postoperative Management

1. Analgesics should be prescribed as necessary. Nonsteroidal anti-inflammatory drugs (NSAIDs) should be avoided as their use may slow the bone-healing process.
2. Up to 24 hours of prophylactic intravenous antibiotics may be utilized on an individualized basis.
3. The patient can begin weight bearing as tolerated immediately following surgery.
4. The wound should remain sterilely dressed for 5 days prior to showering. Complete submergence of the wound should be avoided until the wound is sealed and healed at about 4 weeks postoperatively.

Complications

1. **Donor site pain**: Reported to occur in 3–40% of individuals (highly variable). Pain at the graft site will often decrease with time, but some individuals develop a persistent low-grade pain that may last for months to years.
2. **Superficial infection**: The rate of superficial infection is similar to that of most orthopedic procedures (ranging from 0.5% to 5%). Superficial infections are treated with or without antibiotics based on the clinical presentation.
3. **Deep infection**: The rate of deep infection is 1–2.5%. Deep donor site infections are addressed by surgical irrigation and debridement with antibiotics as indicated based on the clinical situation.
4. **Cluneal nerve injury**: May occur if dissection is carried too far laterally from the PSIS (more than 6 cm). If damaged, the patient may experience numbness, dysesthesias, or chronic neuroma pain in the upper two-thirds (superior cluneal) or medial aspect (middle cluneal) of the buttocks.
5. **Sacroiliac joint disruption**: May occur if bone harvesting is undertaken in close proximity to the joint or if the joint is undermined with inappropriate osteotomy design. Disruption of this joint will predispose the patient to sacroiliac joint pain, instability, and early-onset arthritis.
6. **Abductor weakness**: Muscle weakness can occur without appropriate repair of the lateral musculature dissected free from the ilium. This will result in a patient with a Trendelenburg gait, which is characterized by a drop in the contralateral pelvis during the stance phase of the affected limb. The patient will compensate by leaning their body over the affected side during the stance phase.
7. **Major vessel injury**: The superior gluteal vessels run against the cortex of the superior portion of the greater sciatic notch and can be injured if aggressive retraction, dissection, or harvest extends into the notch.
8. **Major nerve injury**: The sciatic and superior gluteal nerves run within the greater sciatic notch and can be damaged with errant violation of this space.

Key Points

1. The posterior iliac region can provide a large amount of cortical and cancellous bone graft (up to 100 mL of uncompressed bone).
2. Preoperative counseling regarding the likelihood of donor site pain is an important part of setting realistic expectations for the patient undergoing this procedure and will increase patient satisfaction even if pain is encountered.
3. When performing posterior iliac crest bone-grafting procedures in the prone position, care is taken to ensure the endotracheal tube is adequately secured and to appropriately cushion the patient to prevent pressure ulcerations and to provide adequate space for respiratory function.
4. Appropriate incision location, osteotomy design, and procurement of the posterior iliac bone graft will minimize postoperative complications such as vessel, nerve, and muscle injury; damage and instability of the sacroiliac joints; and fracture (Figures 54.1 and 54.2).
5. Meticulous subperiosteal dissection and packing of cancellous graft sites with bone wax or Gelfoam will minimize significant hemorrhage and lessen the likelihood of postoperative complications secondary to hematoma formation and infection. Postoperative drains may be required if hemostasis cannot be achieved with local measures.
6. If additional particulate graft is required, a bone mill may be used to convert cortical bone into uniform-sized particulate bone (Figure 54.7).
7. Care should be taken to avoid injury to the superior gluteal artery. If lacerated, local control and cauterization should be attempted immediately. If the vessel retracts into the pelvis, the area should be packed with laparotomy sponges, and an approach to the vessel should be made in a retroperitoneal or transperitoneal fashion. Additionally, catheter embolization is advised when local control cannot be obtained.
8. In patients with known osteopenia or osteoporosis, graft harvesting should be undertaken with caution. These patients are more likely to sustain a fracture intraoperatively and postoperatively. Additionally, the amount of bone available for harvest may be insufficient. A computed tomography scan of the pelvis may be of benefit during preoperative planning to assess the amount of bone available for harvest.
9. In patients with symptomatic sacroiliac joints, the graft harvest should be performed on the symptomatic side to avoid iatrogenic injury to the asymptomatic joint.

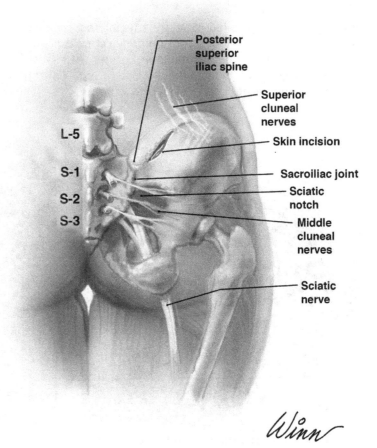

Figure 54.1. Anatomy of the posterior ilium and incision location for posterior iliac crest bone graft harvest.

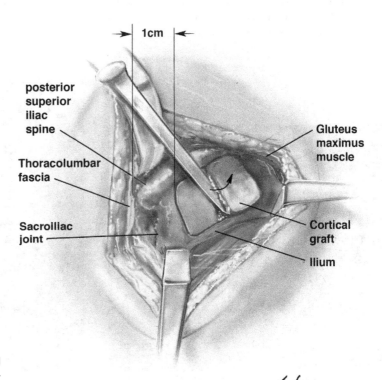

Figure 54.2. The osteotomy is designed 1 cm lateral (distal) to the posterior superior iliac spine and perpendicular to the iliac crest–iliac rim to avoid undermining the sacroiliac joint.

Case Report 54.1. A 54-year-old male presents for the secondary reconstruction of a 10 cm continuity defect to the right posterior mandible 4 months status post continuity resection of an aggressive ameloblastoma. Due to the length of the defect and the desire to bridge the continuity defect with both cortical and cancellous bone, the decision was made to harvest bone from the posterior iliac crest for the secondary reconstruction. (See Figures 54.3 through 54.8.)

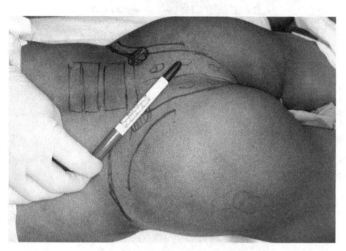

Figure 54.3.   The patient is positioned prone with 210° of reverse hip flexion, and anatomical landmarks are marked to include the posterior iliac crest, the posterior superior iliac spine, and the site of the proposed 6–8 cm curvilinear or oblique skin incision.

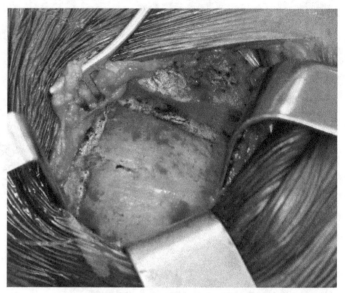

Figure 54.4.   A full-thickness flap, including the dorsolumbar fascia, gluteus maximus muscle, and periosteum, is elevated to expose the outer cortex of the posterior ilium.

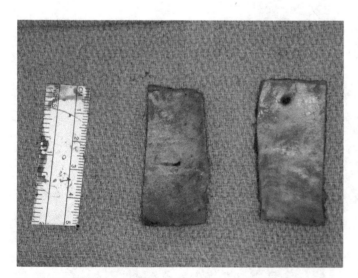

Figure 54.5.   Two 5 cm × 2.5 cm cortical struts are harvested from the outer table of the posterior ilium.

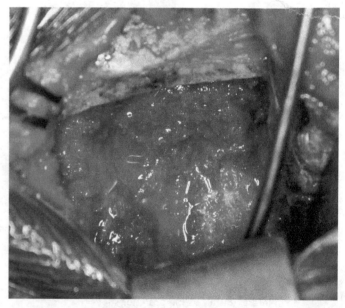

Figure 54.6.   Cancellous bone is harvested utilizing large curved and straight curettes in a two-handed, controlled maneuver, ensuring the inner table is not violated.

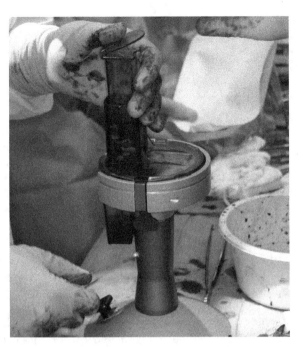

Figure 54.7. A bone mill may be utilized if additional particulate graft is required.

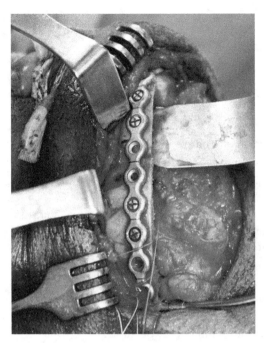

Figure 54.8. The right posterior mandible continuity defect is reconstructed with two, 2.5 cm × 5 cm cortical struts. Additional particulate grafting was performed along the medial aspect of the defect.

References

Ebraheim, N.A., Elgafy, H. and Xu, R., 2001. Bone-graft harvesting from iliac and fibular donor sites: techniques and complications. *Journal of the American Academy of Orthopaedic Surgeons*, 9 (3), 210–18.

Kademani, D. and Keller, E., 2006. Iliac crest grafting for mandibular reconstruction. *Atlas of Oral and Maxillofacial Surgery Clinics of North America*, 14, 161.

Mazcock, J.B., Schow, S.R. and Triplett, R.G., 2003. Posterior iliac crest bone harvest: review of technique, complications, and use of an epidural catheter for postoperative pain control. *Journal of Oral and Maxillofacial Surgery*, 61, 1497.

Myeroff, C. and Archdeacon, M., 2011. Autogenous bone graft: donor sites and techniques. *Journal of Bone and Joint Surgery (American Volume)*, 93 (23), 2227–36. doi:10.2106/JBJS.J.01513

Sittitavornwong, S., Falconer, D.S., Shah, R., Brown, N. and Tubbs, R.S., 2013. Anatomic considerations for posterior crest bone procurement. *Journal of Oral and Maxillofacial Surgery*, 71, 1777.

Westrich, G.H., Geller, D.S., O'Malley, M.J., Deland, J.T. and Helfet, D.L., 2001. Anterior iliac crest bone graft harvesting using the corticocancellous reamer system. *Journal of Orthopaedic Trauma*, 15 (7), 500–6.

Xu, R., Ebraheim, N.A., Yeasting, R.A. and Jackson, W.T., 1996. Anatomic considerations for posterior iliac bone harvesting. *Spine*, 21(9), 1017–20.

55 Proximal Tibial Bone Graft

Nathan Steele[1] and J. Michael Ray[2]

[1]Private Practice, Cheyenne Oral and Maxillofacial Surgery, Cheyenne, Wyoming, USA
[2]Private Practice, DFW Facial and Surgical Arts, Dallas, Texas, USA

A surgical procedure for harvesting cancellous bone from the proximal tibia.

Indications

1. The need for autogenous bone in a quantity greater than can be harvested intraorally
2. Hard tissue maxillofacial defects requiring 30 mL or less of cancellous bone

Contraindications

1. Reconstruction of maxillofacial defects requiring more than 30 mL of cancellous bone
2. Severe peripheral vascular disease
3. Total knee arthroplasty
4. Skeletally immature patient

Anatomy

Gerdy's tubercle: The lateral tubercle on the proximal metaphysis of the tibia, which serves as the insertion of the iliotibial tract superiorly and the anterior tibialis muscle inferiorly

Technique: Lateral Approach to the Proximal Tibia

1. Preoperative intravenous antibiotics are recommended. The procedure may be performed with general endotracheal intubation or with intravenous sedation dependent on the patient's anxiety level and the invasiveness of the coinciding reconstructive procedure.
2. The patient is positioned supine with a knee bump (i.e., towels, a sand bag, or an intravenous fluid bag) placed under the ipsilateral knee, providing a medial rotation of the tibia.
3. The surgical site is prepped and draped in a sterile fashion. Pertinent anatomy is marked to include the patella, the patellar tendon, Gerdy's tubercle, the tibial tuberosity, the fibular head, and the planned incision (Figure 55.1).
4. Local anesthetic containing a vasoconstrictor is infiltrated subcutaneously and deep to the periosteum.

5. A 2–3 cm length oblique incision is placed overlying Gerdy's tubercle. The incision initially extends through skin and subcutaneous tissue (Figure 55.2). A Weitlaner retractor may be placed to assist in the retraction of the supraperiosteal tissues (Figure 55.3).
6. The periosteum is incised, and a subperiosteal dissection is performed to expose Gerdy's tubercle. A 701 bur with copious irrigation is used to remove the cortical bone overlying Gerdy's tubercle. The cortical bone should be removed en bloc so that it may be used at the recipient site (Figure 55.4).
7. Gouges or curettes are used to remove cancellous bone from the tibial plateau and the proximal portion of the shaft. The amount of cancellous bone harvested is dependent on the size of the proximal tibia. Typically, 10 to 30 mL of uncompressed cancellous bone can be harvested (Figure 55.5).
8. Once the graft harvest is complete, the surgical site is irrigated with normal saline (Figure 55.6), and microfibrillar collagen is placed within the surgical site to aid in hemostasis.
9. The incision site is closed in a layered fashion (Figure 55.7). The periosteum is reapproximated with 3-0 polylactic acid sutures. The subcutaneous tissues are reapproximated with 4-0 polylactic sutures. The skin can be closed with either a running subcuticular or standard skin-suturing technique.
10. Antibiotic ointment is applied to the wound, and a sterile compressive dressing is placed (Figure 55.8).

Postoperative Management

1. Opioid analgesics are recommended for pain control.
2. Antibiotics are generally not required.
3. Patient may begin to ambulate as tolerated the day after surgery.
4. Although typically not necessary, ambulation may be assisted with a rolling walker or cane as needed.

Complications

1. **Seroma or hematoma formation**: Rare, but possible in patients with peripheral vascular disease and especially in the obese patient.

Atlas of Operative Oral and Maxillofacial Surgery, First Edition. Edited by Christopher J. Haggerty and Robert M. Laughlin
© 2015 John Wiley & Sons, Inc. Published 2015 by John Wiley & Sons, Inc.

2. **Infection**: Typically caused by not adhering to sterile technique or by poor postoperative Management. Treatment consists of drainage, cultures, and oral antibiotics.
3. **Wound dehiscence**: Caused by inappropriate closure technique (i.e., not performing a layered closure, or closure under tension).
4. **Pain and gait disturbance**: Common during the first 2 weeks after surgery. Typically resolves with time.

Case Report

Case Report 55.1. A 68-year-old male presents with a chief complaint of loss of numerous maxillary teeth. On examination and on review of the patient's cone beam computed tomography scan, the patient has posterior left maxillary edentulism and moderate sinus pneumonization. The patient also exhibited a large

Key Points

1. A thorough understanding of the pertinent anatomy and proper patient selection are vital in minimizing potential intraoperative and postoperative complications.
2. This procedure can be predictably performed in an office setting with intravenous sedation and local anesthesia.
3. A medial approach to the proximal tibia may also be performed. Both the lateral and the medial approaches to the proximal tibia have thin overlying tissue with a relative lack of neurovascular structures.

anterior maxilla defect. The patient was treated with a tibial cortical onlay graft to the anterior maxillary defect and a left-sided sinus augmentation using cancellous bone from the proximal tibia. Implants were placed after 5 months of graft consolidation. (See Figures 55.1 through 55.8.)

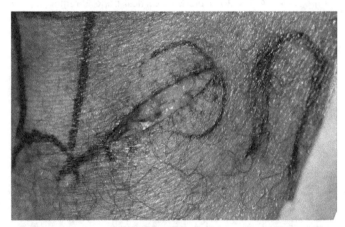

Figure 55.2. Incision through skin and subcutaneous tissue.

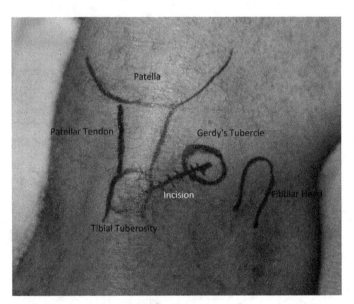

Figure 55.1. Preoperative surgical markings include the patella, the patellar tendon, Gerdy's tubercle, the tibial tuberosity, the fibular head, and the planned incision. Gerdy's tubercle is palpated between the tibial tuberosity and fibular head. The incision is marked obliquely from Gerdy's tubercle to the tibial tuberosity.

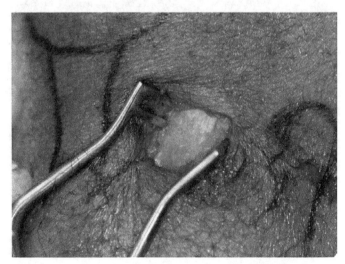

Figure 55.3. The periosteum overlying Gerdy's tubercle is exposed. Self-retracting devices (i.e., a Weitlaner retractor) aid in tissue reflection.

487

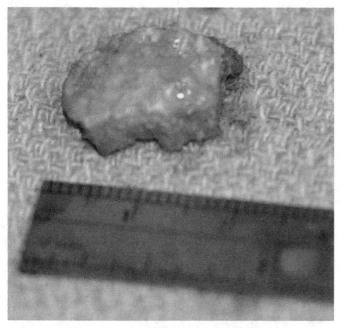

Figure 55.4. A 1 × 2 cm block of cortical bone is removed from Gerdy's tubercle to expose the marrow space of the proximal tibia. The cortical bone may be used as a small onlay graft or may be milled into particulate bone.

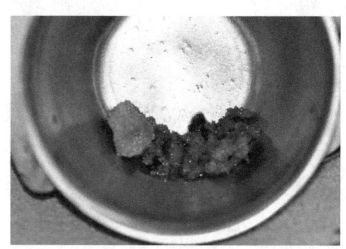

Figure 55.5. Cancellous bone is removed from the proximal tibia with curettes and gouges. The proximal tibia typically yields 10–30 mL of uncompressed marrow.

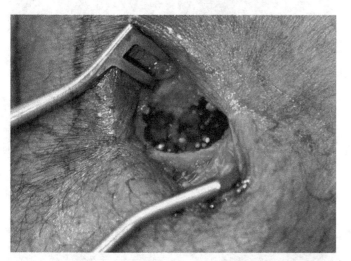

Figure 55.6. Defect after bone harvest. Local hemostatic agents (i.e., microfibrillar collagen) may be placed to enhance hemostasis.

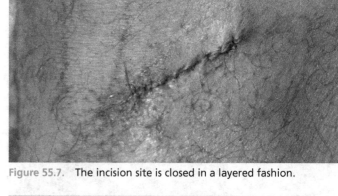

Figure 55.7. The incision site is closed in a layered fashion.

References

Galano, G.J. and Greisberg, J.K., 2009. Tibial plateau fracture with proximal tibia autograft harvest for foot surgery. *American Journal of Orthopedics (Belle Mead, NJ)*, 38 (12), 621–3.

Herford, A.S. and Dean, J.S., 2011. Complications in bone grafting. *Oral and Maxillofacial Surgery Clinics of North America*, 23 (3), 433–42.

Mazock, J.B., Schow, S.R. and Triplett, R.G., 2004. Proximal tibia bone harvest: review of technique, complications, and use in maxillofacial surgery. *International Journal of Oral and Maxillofacial Implants*, 19 (4), 586–93.

Michael, R.J., Ellis, S.J. and Roberts, M.M., 2012. Tibial plateau fracture following proximal tibia autograft harvest: case report. *Foot Ankle International*, 33 (11), 1001–5.

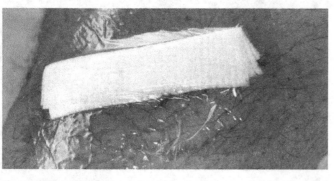

Figure 55.8. Antibiotic ointment is applied over the incision site, and a compressive dressing is placed.

56 Parietal Bone Graft

Christopher J. Haggerty

Private Practice, Lakewood Oral and Maxillofacial Surgery Specialists, Lees Summit; and Department of Oral and Maxillofacial Surgery, University of Missouri–Kansas City, Kansas City, Missouri, USA

A means of obtaining membranous bone for the reconstruction of hard tissue craniomaxillofacial defects.

Indications

1. Reconstruction of the nasal dorsum in patients requiring augmentation rhinoplasty (saddle nose deformity) or naso-orbito-ethmoid (NOE) fractures (loss of bony support)
2. Reconstruction of orbital wall and floor defects (correction of posttraumatic enophthalmos)
3. Reconstruction of alveolar process defects prior to implant placement
4. Reconstruction of craniomaxillofacial defects caused by tumor ablative surgery
5. Reconstruction of alveolar clefts
6. Reconstruction of skull defects or cranioplasty

Contraindications

1. Harvest can be complicated in older patients due to a lack of diploe space and/or thin dura
2. Anticoagulated patients
3. Patients with suspected intracranial injuries
4. Minimal or no diploe space identified on computed tomography (CT) or magnetic resonance imaging (MRI)
5. Venous lacunae identified on CT or MRI
6. Anatomical aberration identified on CT or MRI
7. Less than 6 mm of parietal bone thickness
8. When cancellous bone is required

Anatomy

The superior sagittal sinus (SSS) originates anteriorly from the crista galla of the ethmoid bone and empties posteriorly into the torcular Herophili at the internal occipital protuberance.

The superior temporal line serves as the superior attachment of the temporalis fascia. The inferior temporal line serves as the superior attachment of the temporalis muscle.

The thickness of the parietal bone ranges from 3–12 mm.

Split-Thickness Parietal Bone Graft Harvest Procedure

1. Preoperative antibiotics are administered to provide coverage for skin and scalp flora. Preoperative ster-

oids are administered to minimize postoperative soft tissue edema.

2. The patient is placed under general anesthesia and positioned supine within a Mayfield headrest. The patient is prepped and draped to include the area of parietal bone harvest and the recipient site for the graft (ie. the orbit or NOE region). A linear band of hair is either shaved or parted in the area of the proposed scalp incision. The scalp incision is marked with a sterile marking pen, and a mixture of local anesthetic with a vasoconstrictor is injected into the subgaleal plane to aid in hemostasis and for hydrodissection of the tissue.
3. Exposure of the parietal bone can be achieved either with a linear incision in the location of the parietal bone or via a coronal incision. If a linear incision is utilized, the length of the incision and the extent of the exposure correlate with the amount of parietal bone to be harvested. Alternatively, a coronal incision can be utilized if additional exposure is required to areas such as the orbital rims, the dorsum of the nose, and the frontal sinus.
4. Vertical dissection should proceed through the scalp layers until the pericranium is reached. Lateral dissection should begin within the subgaleal plane, preserving the attachment of the pericranium to the calvarium. The pericranium is sharply incised, reflected, and preserved dependent on the amount of parietal bone graft required and the adjunctive procedures performed.
5. The graft site should be a minimum of 2 cm lateral to the midline sagittal suture and should avoid crossing other sutures (coronal, lambdoid, and squamous).
6. The area of the graft is marked either with a sterile marking pen or with electrocautery. If the exact size of the defect is known, a template made of sterile foil, sterile paper, or bone wax can be used.
7. A reciprocating saw, round bur, or fissured bur is used to outline the area of the parietal bone to be harvested (Figure 56.4). The bur or saw is taken to the depth of the outer cortex until the diploe space is entered. The author prefers the use of either a round bur or a fissured bur due to the improved tactile feel once the diploe space is entered.
8. Depending on the nature of the graft, the bur or saw may be used to outline numerous linear strips of calvarian bone or a single larger segment to harvest.

Atlas of Operative Oral and Maxillofacial Surgery, First Edition. Edited by Christopher J. Haggerty and Robert M. Laughlin.

9. A bur is used to bevel two edges of the graft—typically, the lateral and the superior margin of the graft. The bevel will allow for the insertion of an osteotome into the diploe space. A thin spatula osteotome is initially used to enter the diploe space from a beveled edge, and then a larger curved osteotome is used to elevate the outer table (Figure 56.5). The osteotome blade should be moved sequentially along the two beveled edges of the graft site. The blade of the osteotome should be sharp, and it should be directed parallel to the diploe space (Figure 56.1B). If numerous side-by-side segments (strips) of bone are to be removed, after the removal of the initial segment, the osteotome can be laid parallel to the diploe space to facilitate additional parietal bone segment harvest (Figure 56.8).

10. Once the outer table is removed, the marrow of the diploe space should be removed with a curette in order to decrease bleeding and to expose the inner table to check for fractures and cerebrospinal fluid (CSF) leakage. The site is copiously irrigated, and if bleeding persists, a thin layer of bone wax is applied to bleeding areas with a Freer elevator.

11. A layer of surgicel can be placed within the outer table defect, and the incision is closed in a layered fashion. Larger graft sites or sites with non-ideal hemostasis will require drain placement.

Postoperative Management

1. A pressure dressing is applied.
2. Pain is controlled by either intravenous (IV) or oral analgesics depending on the discourse of the patient.
3. IV or oral antibiotics are used for 7 days postoperatively.
4. If placed, the drain is removed at postoperative day 3 or when output is minimal.
5. For larger cranial harvests, the patient is kept for overnight observation.

Complications

1. **Hemorrhage of the superior sagittal sinus (SSS)**: Entry into the SSS can lead to life-threatening hemorrhage, severe neurological deficits, rapidly increased intracranial pressure (ICP), air emboli, and death. SSS injury can be avoided by maintaining a distance of at least 2 cm, preferably 3 cm, from the midline sagittal suture during osteotomy placement and by judicious use of osteotomes.
2. **Dural lacerations**: May lead to the formation of CSF leak or persistent CSF fistula formation
3. Subcutaneous hematoma or seroma formation
4. Infection
5. Epidural abscess formation
6. Meningitis
7. Damage to underlying brain
8. Damage to underlying cerebral vessels
9. Coup or contrecoup brain injury due to osteotome usage
10. Fracture of the graft being harvested
11. Intracranial bleed (intracerebral, subdural, or epidural)

Key Points

1. Typically, left-handed surgeons will harvest bone from the patient's left side and vice versa. Others advocate harvesting the graft from the patient's nondominant hemisphere.
2. Vertical linear scalp incisions are preferred to horizontal incisions as they potentiate less scalp paresthesia.
3. It is imperative to stay at least 2 cm lateral to the midline sagittal suture during the harvest of the parietal bone. The author prefers to stay 3 cm lateral to the sagittal suture and to harvest bone from the middle and posterior aspect of the parietal bone graft. The graft should be harvested medial to the superior temporal line to minimize patient discomfort and temporal wasting (Figure 56.1A).
4. Avoid crossing other sutures (coronal, lambdoid, and squamous) during bone harvest.
5. Utilizing a fissured bur or a round bur will give the surgeon more control and a better tactile sensation of when the diploe space is reached than when using a oscillating or reciprocating saw.
6. The surgeon can feel when the diploe space is entered by the change in tactile sensation and by the increased bleeding of the diploe space.
7. While separating the outer table from the diploic layer, the osteotome should be used with a gentle tapping motion to minimize the possibility of damage to the cranial contents. The osteotome should be directed parallel to the diploic layer to minimize the chance of fracture of the inner table (Figure 56.1B). Osteotomes should be kept sharp to avoid excessive force to the calvarian and to minimize the potential for graft fracture.
8. Depending on the amount of bone that needs to be harvested, the bone may be harvested in a single segment or taken in numerous linear segments (strips). It is difficult to remove a segment larger than 40 mm without fracturing the segment. If longer spans of cranial bone are required, two or more segments of parietal bone can be joined and fixated with plates and screws.
9. Do not leave excessive bone wax in the parietal bone harvest site. Only use enough bone wax to obtain hemostasis.
10. Be cognizant of CSF leaks. CSF leakage typically necessitates entering the cranial cavity and repairing the damaged dura.
11. Closure of the scalp in a layered fashion will help to minimize postoperative infection and hematoma and seroma formation. Closure of the scalp with Vicryl sutures instead of staples will cause less postoperative patient discomfort and will decrease future postoperative appointment time.

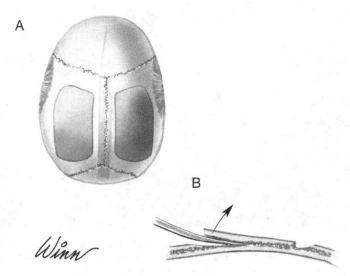

Figure 56.1. Schematic drawing demonstrating the ideal location of parietal bone harvest. (A) The medial osteotomy should be placed at a minimum of 2 cm (preferably 3 cm) lateral to the midsagittal suture to avoid damage to the superior sagittal sinus. (B) When separating the diploic layer, the osteotome is directed parallel to the diploic layer to minimize the chance of fracture or inadvertent entry of the inner table.

Case Report

Case Report 56.1. A 42-year-old female presents status post significant blunt trauma resulting in multiple facial fractures and a severely displaced naso-orbital-ethmoid fracture (NOE) with significant deformation of the nasal bridge. A coronal approach was utilized to reduce the NOE fractures and permitted the harvesting of strips of the parietal bone for reconstruction of the depressed nasal bridge. (See Figures 56.2 through 56.12.)

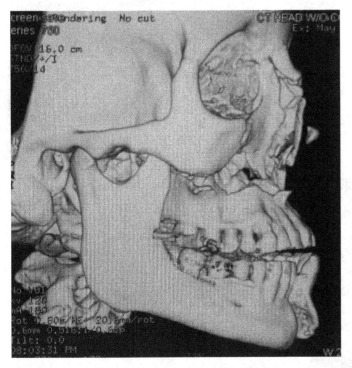

Figure 56.2. Sagittal 3D reconstruction demonstrating displaced naso-orbital-ethmoid fracture with depression of the nasal dorsum.

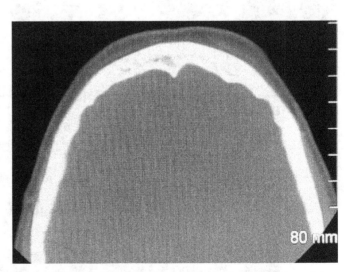

Figure 56.3. Axial computed tomography demonstrating 7–8 mm of parietal bone thickness at the middle and posterior aspect of the left parietal bone.

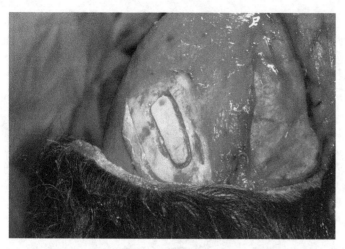

Figure 56.4. Coronal flap reflected and a 10 mm × 35 mm calvarian graft is outlined and beveled with a 703 fissured bur. The harvest site is located within the middle and posterior portion of the parietal bone, cephalic to the superior temporal line and at least 2 cm lateral to the midline sagittal suture.

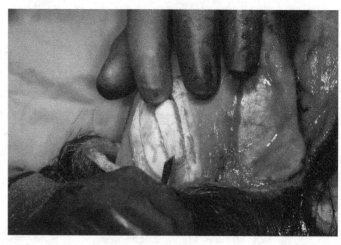

Figure 56.5. A curved osteotome is directed into the diploic bone at the beveled side of the graft. The osteotome blade is oriented as parallel to the diploic space as possible.

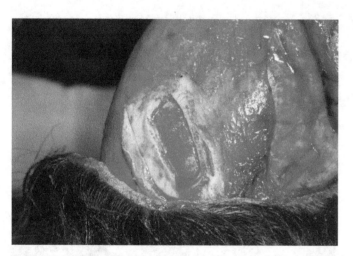

Figure 56.6. The calvarian graft has been harvested. The bleeding diploic bone and intact inner cortex are visible.

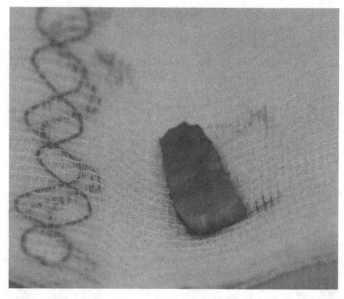

Figure 56.7. A 10 mm × 35 mm segment of harvested outer table parietal bone.

Figure 56.8. Once the initial segment of calvarian bone has been harvested, the removal of subsequent segments is much easier.

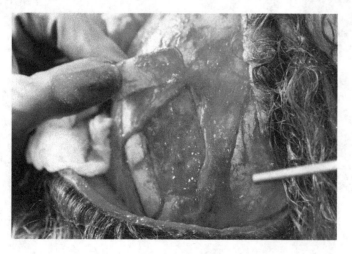

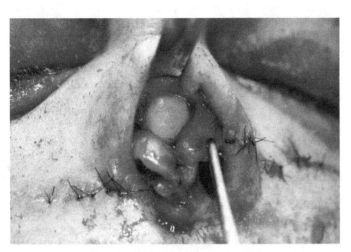

Figure 56.9. The calvarian graft is shaped to function as a nasal strut and fixated to the frontal bone. An open septorhinoplasty was performed in order to accurately position the proximal segment of the strut and to reposition the displaced lower lateral cartilages.

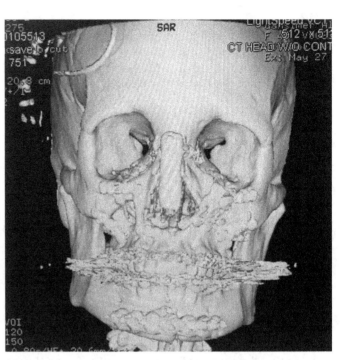

Figure 56.10. Coronal postoperative 3D reconstruction showing position of the cranial graft.

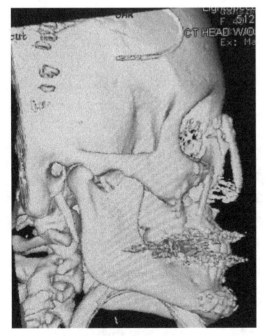

Figure 56.11. Sagittal postoperative 3D reconstruction demonstrating nasal projection with the calvarial strut graft.

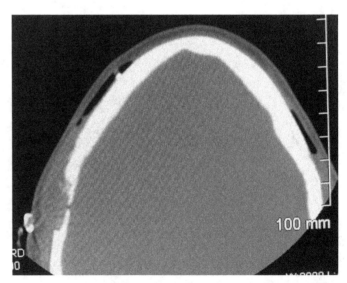

Figure 56.12. Postoperative axial head computed tomography demonstrating the harvest site with an intact inner cortex and no intracranial bleeds, pneumocephalus, or anomalies.

References

Cannella, D.M. and Hopkins, L.N., 1990. Superior sagittal sinus laceration complicating an autogenous calvarial bone graft harvest: report of a case. *Journal of Oral and Maxillofacial Surgery*, 48, 741–3.

De Ceulaer, J., Swennen, J., Abeloos, C. and De Clercq C., 2012. Presentation of a cone-beam CT scanning protocol for pre-prosthetic cranial bone grafting of the atrophic maxilla. *International Journal of Oral and Maxillofacial Surgery*, 41, 863–6.

Fernandes, A.C., Neto, A.I., Freitas, A.C. and Moraes, M., 2011. Dimensional analysis of the parietal bone in areas of surgical interest and relationship between parietal thickness and cephalic index. *Journal of Oral and Maxillofacial Surgery*, 69, 2930–5.

Jaskolka, M.S. and Olavarria G., 2010. Reconstruction of skull defects. *Atlas of Oral and Maxillofacial Surgery Clinics of North America*, 18, 139–49.

Laure, B., Geais, L., Tranquart, F. and Goga, D., 2011. Mechanical characterization and optoelectronic measurement of parietal bone thickness before and after monocortical bone graft harvest: design and validation of a test protocol. *Journal of Craniofacial Surgery*, 22, 113–7.

Laure, B., Tranquart, F., Geais, L. and Goga, D., 2010. Evaluation of skull strength following parietal bone graft harvest. *Plastic and Reconstructive Surgery*, 126, 1492–9.

Markowitz, N.R. and Allan, P.G., 1989. Cranial bone graft harvesting: a modified technique. *Journal of Oral and Maxillofacial Surgery*, 47, 1113–5.

Schortinghuis, J., Putters, T.F. and Raghoebar, G.M., 2012. Safe harvesting of outer table parietal bone grafts using an oscillating saw and a bone scraper: a refinement of technique for harvesting cortical and "cancellous"-like calvarial bone. *Journal of Oral and Maxillofacial Surgery*, 70, 963–5.

Tessier, P., 1982. Autogenous bone grafts taken from the calvarium for facial and cranial applications. *Clinics in Plastic Surgery*, 9, 531–41.

Tessier, P., Kawamoto, H., Posnick, J., Raulo, Y., Tulasne, J.F. and Wolfe, S.A., 2005. Taking calvarial grafts, either split in situ or splitting of the parietal bone flap ex vivo-tools and techniques: V. A 9650 case experience in craniofacial and maxillofacial surgery. *Plastic and Reconstructive Surgery*, 116, 54S–71S.

Tessier, P., Kawamoto, H., Posnick, J., Raulo, Y., Tulasne, J.F. and Wolfe, S.A., 2005. Complications of harvesting autogenous bone grafts: a group experience of 20,000 cases. *Plastic and Reconstructive Surgery*, 116, 72S–73S.

Wilk, R.M., 2004. Bony reconstruction of the jaws. In: M. Miloro, ed. *Peterson's principles of oral and maxillofacial surgery*. Hamilton, ON: B.C. Decker; pp. 783–801.

57

Costochondral Graft

Brian W. Kelley[1] and Christopher J. Haggerty[2]

[1]*Private Practice, Carolinas Center for Oral and Facial Surgery, Charlotte, North Carolina; and Department of Oral and Maxillofacial Surgery, Louisiana State University Health Sciences Center, New Orleans, Louisiana, USA*
[2]*Private Practice, Lakewood Oral and Maxillofacial Surgery Specialists, Lees Summit; and Department of Oral and Maxillofacial Surgery, University of Missouri–Kansas City, Kansas City, Missouri, USA*

A means of obtaining autogenous, nonvascularized bone for the reconstruction of hard tissue defects and for the replacement of mandibular condyles. A means of obtaining a hyaline cartilage graft for the reconstruction of cartilaginous maxillofacial defects.

Indications

1. Temporomandibular joint (TMJ) replacements in pediatric patients with active growth centers to reconstruct condylar processes defects caused by trauma, neoplasms, infections, congenital dysplasias, growth abnormalities, ankyloses, and rheumatoid arthritis
2. TMJ reconstruction in adult patients due to idiopathic condylar resorption, osteoarthritis, and rheumatoid arthritis when other methods (alloplastic joint replacement) are contraindicated
3. Reconstruction of craniomaxillofacial defects caused by loss of hard tissue
4. Reconstruction of skull defects or cranioplasty
5. Reconstruction of nasal dorsum defects or saddle nose deformities (costochondral cartilage)
6. Reconstruction of the helical framework of the ear (costochondral cartilage)

Contraindications

1. History of restrictive lung disease
2. History of recent pulmonary infection
3. History of cardiopulmonary instability

Anatomy

Hyaline cartilage can withstand the stresses of the TMJ and also has an active growth center, allowing for spontaneous growth in the pediatric patient.

The first seven vertebrosternal ribs (true ribs) are attached to the sternum and the manubrium directly by means of costal cartilage.

Vertebrochondral ribs 8,9, and 10 (false ribs) are attached to the vertebrosternal ribs above by means of costal cartilage.

Vertebral ribs 11 and 12 (floating ribs) have no attachment to the sternum.

Costochondral Graft (CCG) Harvest Technique

1. The anterior chest wall is prepped and draped, allowing for visualization of the sternum, clavicle, nipple, and umbilicus.
2. The ribs are counted and marked with a marking pen.
3. A sterile marking pen is used to outline a 6–8 cm line within the inframammary crease of female patients (Figure 57.1) or at the level of the sixth or seventh rib in male patients. In pediatric female patients, the incision is placed in the anticipated future location of the inframammary crease.
4. Local anesthetic containing a vasoconstrictor is used to infiltrate the subcutaneous tissue overlying the rib to be harvested.
5. Digital pressure is used to identify the fifth, sixth, or seventh rib and the costochondral spaces. A 6–8 cm skin incision is made with a #15 blade directly over the superior aspect of the rib to be harvested. The incision transverses skin, subcutaneous tissue, and pectoralis muscle (Figure 57.2) down to the periosteum directly overlying the rib.
6. A #9 periosteal elevator is used to dissect circumferentially around the rib. A tissue plane is developed between the rib's periosteum–perichondrium and the thin parietal pleura (Figure 57.3). The subperiosteal dissection continues laterally as far as is needed and medially until the costochondral junction is reached. It is important to stay subperiosteal in order to avoid injury to the vascular bundle on the inferior portion of the rib.
7. At the costochondral junction, dissection proceeds in a supraperichondrial plane so as not to detach the hyaline cartilaginous cap from the medial aspect of the rib.
8. A guillotine rib cutter is used to transect the lateral portion of the rib.

Atlas of Operative Oral and Maxillofacial Surgery, First Edition. Edited by Christopher J. Haggerty and Robert M. Laughlin
© 2015 John Wiley & Sons, Inc. Published 2015 by John Wiley & Sons, Inc.

9. Either a Doyen retractor or a silk suture (Figure 57.4) is used to elevate the rib and to check the deep margin for tissue–muscle adherence.
10. A malleable retractor is placed deep to the medial aspect of the rib. A #10 blade is used to cut the medial aspect of the rib preserving a 5–10 mm cartilaginous cap. The malleable retractor will prevent the #10 blade from cutting into the underlying parietal pleura.
11. The harvested costochondral graft is placed within a sterile, saline-soaked gauze until the recipient site is prepared.
12. Once the rib or ribs are removed, sterile water is placed over the anterior chest wall defect, and the anesthesiologist is asked to provide positive pressure in order to inspect the harvest site for pleural perforations. If no air bubbles are present, then the harvest site is closed in layers. If minor air bubbles are present, pleural tears can be closed primarily with interrupted sutures. If large air bubbles are present, then a thoracotomy tube is placed.
13. After closure of the surgical site in a layered fashion, steri-strips are applied to provide additional skin tension. Generally, a drain is not required.

Postoperative Management

1. A postoperative chest film is taken to evaluate for pneumothorax.
2. Patients are placed on weight-appropriate analgesics and antibiotics for one week.

Complications

Immediate or Early Complications

1. **Pleural tears, pneumothorax, and pleuritis**: Prevented or lessened with meticulous dissection of the periosteum overlying the deep portion of the rib and cartilage cap. Large pleural tears are treated with thoracotomy tube placement.
2. **Infection**: Infections are rare and typically result from contamination of the surgical site at surgery or contamination of the wound in the postoperative period.
3. **Hematoma or seroma formation**: Minimized with closure of the harvest site in a layered fashion. Hemostasis should be attained prior to closure of the surgical site. Treatment involves exploration and drain placement.
4. **Injury to the intercostal neurovascular**: Avoided by maintaining a subperiosteal dissection plane and by placing the incision over the midbody or superior aspect of the rib.

5. **Fracture at the bone–cartilage interface of the CCG**: The longer the length of the cartilaginous cap, the more mechanically unstable the bone–cartilage interface of the costochondral graft.

Late Complications

1. **Chest concavity**: Occurs when multiple, adjacent ribs are harvested.
2. **Scar formation over the breast in female patients**: Incisions in female patients should be placed in either the inframammary crease or in the area of the anticipated future inframammary crease. At no point should the incision be placed over the developing breast mound or near the areolas.
3. **Areola retraction**: Occurs when the incision is placed near the areolas.

Key Points

1. The main advantage of CCGs over other forms of autogenous bone grafts is the ability of continued growth in the pediatric and adolescent patient population. The continued growth is a result of the growth center located within the hyaline cartilage cap and makes the main use of the CCG TMJ reconstruction in the prepubescent population.
2. Most surgeons prefer to harvest CCGs from the contralateral side of the recipient site. The rationale is that the contralateral rib has a more ideal curvature and will adapt more desirably to the lateral surface of the recipient ramus. Others prefer to harvest CCGs from the right side due to a concern that left-sided chest pain from the harvest site may mimic or be confused with cardiogenic pain.
3. In female patients, the location of the incision (inframammary crease, or anticipated inframammary crease in pediatric patents) often determines the rib to be harvested.
4. Once the rib is isolated, care is taken to maintain the rib–cartilage junction. Because this junction (especially in pediatric patients) is inherently weak and is easily fractured, maintaining a small cuff of periosteum or perichondrium around the rib–cartilage interface will enhance the structural integrity of this area and will help prevent its fracture during both harvest and placement.
5. Longer lengths of cartilage create a lever arm that is more prone to fracture at the bone-cartilage interface (junction). A 10 mm or less cartilaginous cap is sufficient for tempomandibular reconstruction procedures.

Case Report 57.1. A 14-year-old female patient presents with an ameloblastoma involving the right posterior ramus with extension to the condyle. Due to the patient's age, the decision was made for immediate reconstruction of the ablative defect utilizing a contralateral costochondral graft. (See Figures 57.1 through 57.6.)

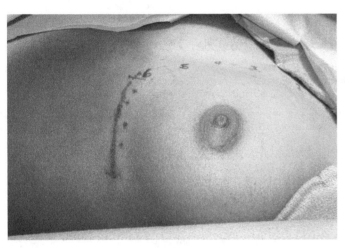

Figure 57.1. A 6 cm incision is marked corresponding to the anticipated location of the inframammary crease, which corresponds to rib #6.

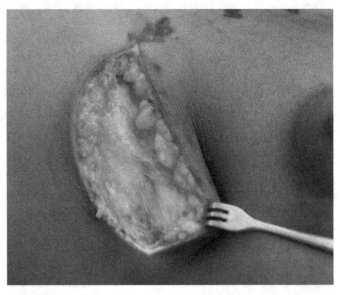

Figure 57.2. Dissection directly over the superior aspect of the rib to be harvested. The incision transverses skin, subcutaneous tissue, and pectoralis muscle.

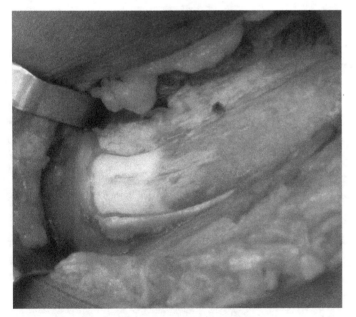

Figure 57.3. A #9 periosteal elevator is used to dissect circumferentially around the rib. A tissue plane is developed between the rib's periosteum–perichondrium and the thin parietal pleura.

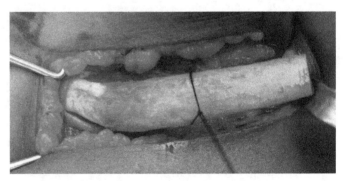

Figure 57.4. A silk suture is used to elevate the rib and to check the deep margin for tissue–muscle adherence after osteotomy of the lateral margin.

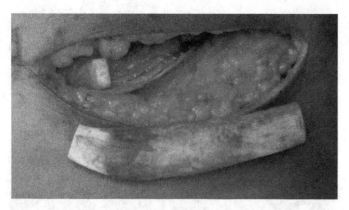

Figure 57.5.   Once the rib is removed, the anterior chest wall cavity is inspected for any bleeding or signs of pneumothorax. Sterile water can be placed over the anterior chest wall defect, and positive pressure is provided in order to inspect for pleural perforations.

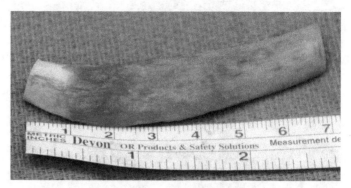

Figure 57.6.   A portion of the cartilaginous cap is left attached to the medial aspect of the harvested rib in order to serve as a growth center and to function against the native disc or glenoid fossa.

References

Fernandes, R., Fattahi, T. and Steinberg, B., 2006. Costochondral rib grafts and mandibular reconstruction. *Atlas of Oral and Maxillofacial Surgery Clinics of North America*, 14, 179.

Frodel, J.L., 2002. Grafts and free flaps. In: B.J. Bailey and K.H. Calhoun, eds., *Atlas of head and neck surgery-otolaryngology*. 2nd ed. Philadelphia: Lippincott Williams & Wilkins.

Ko, E.W., Huang, C.S. and Chen, Y.R., 1999. Tempomandibular joint reconstruction in children using costochondral grafts. *Journal of Oral and Maxillofacial Surgery*, 57, 789.

Nelson, C.L. and Buttrum, J.D., 1989. Costochondral grafting for posttraumatic tempomandibular joint reconstruction: a review of six cases. *Journal of Oral and Maxillofacial Surgery*, 47, 1030.

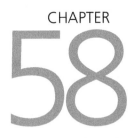

Microvascular Principles

Christopher M. Harris,[1] Allen O. Mitchell,[2] and Robert M. Laughlin[3]

[1]Department of Oral and Maxillofacial Surgery, Naval Medical Center Portsmouth, Portsmouth, Virginia, USA

[2]Otolaryngology—Head and Neck Surgery, Naval Medical Center Portsmouth, Portsmouth, Virginia, USA

[3]Department of Oral and Maxillofacial Surgery, Naval Medical Center San Diego, San Diego, California, USA

Indications for Microvascular Reconstruction of Maxillofacial Defects

1. Composite mandibular reconstruction
2. Moderate to large soft tissue reconstruction in malignancy (i.e., hemiglossectomy and buccal carcinomas)
3. Reconstruction of stage III osteoradionecrosis (bone and/or composite defects)
4. Reconstruction of large soft tissue defects and soft tissue radionecrosis
5. Large maxillectomy defects where obturation is unsuitable reconstruction
6. Orbitomaxillary defects
7. Benign, anterior mandibular defects with or without soft tissue deficiency

Contraindications for Microvascular Reconstruction of Maxillofacial Defects

1. Medical status unsuitable for prolonged surgical procedure (advanced age alone is not a disqualifier)
2. Medical history of hypercoaguable state (e.g., sickle cell anemia, Factor V Leiden, antiphospholipid syndrome, myeloproliferative disorders, or morbid obesity)
3. Significant peripheral vascular disease

Microvascular Principles and Technique

A thorough preoperative evaluation is undertaken prior to performing any vascularized tissue flap. A complete medical history and physical exam are undertaken, including laboratory and imaging studies as indicated. Many patients presenting with oral cancers have significant medical comorbidities (e.g., chronic obstructive pulmonary disorder, polysubstance abuse, diabetes, and cardiovascular disease) that require evaluation and optimization prior to surgery.

Accurate assessment of the planned ablative defect and its consequences on flap selection, as well as the final prosthetic rehabilitation planning, must be performed prior to surgical therapy. Choosing the donor site is based on the types of tissues to be replaced, the prosthodontic requirements, and the quality of the donor site. The surgeon's familiarity and success with the flap choice are also considered. For example, in our practice, most oral cancer defects are reconstructed with radial forearm, anterolateral thigh, and fibula free flaps. The reliability with these flaps is likely to be much higher, and the complication rate much lower, than a flap that is rarely utilized. When treatment planning any microvascular reconstruction, a "backup" reconstructive plan is also devised in the event that the primary flap choice is unusable or inadequate.

Specialized equipment is required to perform microvascular procedures. Equipment typically includes microvascular surgical instruments, microsurgical anastomotic couplers, surgical loupes, an operating microscope, microsurgical sutures and vascular clamps, Doppler ultrasound (external and internal), and warmed, heparinized irrigation fluids. Microsurgical instruments should be lightweight and made of titanium, measure 10–18 cm in length, and have low closing pressures. Magnetization of nontitanium instruments can increase the difficulty of positioning microsurgical needles. All instruments should be carefully inspected prior to the start of any case, and a reserve set should be available. It is a common occurrence to discover a bent instrument that needs to be replaced. A typical microsurgical instrument set consists of multiple jeweler's forceps (curved and straight), microsurgical adventitial scissors (curved and straight), microsurgical suture scissors, vein dilator forceps, vascular clamp applying forceps, and microsurgical needle holders. The vascular clamp set contains multiple arterial and venous, single and double approximating clamps with or without frames of varying size. Clamps can be disposable or reusable, depending on the surgeon's preference. Requirements for clamp pressures depend on vessel size and type; the pressure should be light enough to prevent leakage and damage to the vessel walls.

Venous anastomotic coupler devices are being used routinely in many institutions for venous anastomosis (Figures 58.1, 58.10, and 58.11). Studies have demonstrated an equivalent patency rate when compared to hand-sewn anastomoses, with significantly shorter anastomosis times and higher anastomosis strength. The Synovis™

Atlas of Operative Oral and Maxillofacial Surgery, First Edition. Edited by Christopher J. Haggerty and Robert M. Laughlin
© 2015 John Wiley & Sons, Inc. Published 2015 by John Wiley & Sons, Inc.

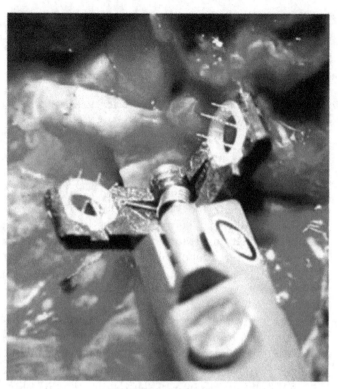

Figure 58.1. Synovis™ microvascular anastomotic coupling device.

anastomotic coupler (Birmingham, Alabama, USA) (Figure 58.1) is routinely used at our institution. The device can be used with vessel sizes from 1.0 mm to 4.0 mm. Arterial coupling is also possible with this device. The anastomotic coupler consists of two polyethylene rings in which several stainless-steel pins are embedded. The vessels are measured for the appropriate size, the vessels are passed through the rings, and the walls are everted over the steel pins. The coupler is closed, and the venous walls are sealed together by piercing the opposing ring.

The flap and pedicle should be routinely irrigated to prevent desiccation. Warmed lactated Ringer's solution is adequate. Heparinized normal saline (10 u/mL) is used to irrigate the vessel lumens during anastomosis. A 24-gauge angiocatheter is used for delivery. Ophthalmic cellulose wick spears can be used to absorb excess fluid or blood if needed. Papverine solution or plain 4% lidocaine can also be utilized to help minimize vasospasm if required. Epinephrine solutions should not be used.

Magnification is required during flap harvest. Typically, surgical loupes with 2.5× or greater magnification are utilized by the surgeons. Magnification for vascular anastomosis is performed with a surgical microscope. The surgical microscope should be dual headed, have a variable focal length, provide controls for focus and zoom for the two surgeons, and be ergonomic. The scope should be adjustable in order to allow for the procedure to be performed while sitting or standing.

Recipient vessel selection is a critical aspect of successful microvascular surgery. The reconstructive surgeon must impress this point on the ablative surgeon prior to the procedure. Unnecessary removal of usable recipient veins can make the reconstructive process difficult and prolong the surgical time. In most maxillofacial reconstructions, the facial vessels can be utilized for anastomosis (Figure 58.3). The external and internal jugular veins are also used frequently, as are other easily accessible branches of the external carotid. Frequently, in maxillofacial reconstruction, the end-to-end anastomosis method is utilized; however, the end-to-side anastomosis method can also be used, particularly if the internal jugular is the recipient vein. The end-to-end is a technically simpler procedure.

Preparation for anastomosis begins with maximizing exposure to the recipient vessels. Determination of recipient and flap vessel geometry is then ascertained. Proper geometry should prevent twisting, kinking, or tension on the pedicle (Figure 58.4). In most cases, a partial inset of the flap is performed prior to anastomosis. Bone contouring and placement on a reconstruction plate are typically undertaken prior to pedicle division and flap transfer to the maxillofacial region, where only minor adjustments are needed for final inset. Flaps should be positioned prior to anastomosis to ensure that proper pedicle geometry and length are available.

The vessels are positioned to allow for an end-to-end, tension-free anastomosis. Single vascular clamps are placed on the arteries and veins. Flow is verified from the recipient artery. The adventitia is removed for approximately 1–1.5 mm from the cut edge of each vessel with adventitial scissors (Figure 58.5). The cut edge is inspected to ensure no irregularities are present, and the lumen is inspected for intimal damage, separation, plaques, and clots (Figure 58.6). If needed, the vessel can be recut and the process repeated until adequate. Double approximating clamps are applied, and the vessel ends are brought into close approximation (Figure 58.7). A background material is placed under the vessels to aid in visualization. Heparinized normal saline is used frequently to keep the vessel lumens open and free from debris. A 9-0 or 10-0 nylon suture on a tapered needle is used for the anastomosis. The anastomotic coupler may also be used.

The authors typically perform the arterial anastomosis first. Two sutures, 180° apart, are placed and suspended on a frame or tucked under adjacent tissue to provide slight tension (Figure 58.8). Three more sutures are placed, halving the remaining distance. The clamp is turned over, and the anastomosis is inspected to verify proper placement of the sutures and recognize any back wall injuries. The same process is completed on the back side of the anastomosis (Figure 58.9). The double approximating clamp is removed. The veins can be hand sewn in the same manner, or a venous coupler can be utilized (Figures 58.10 and 58.11).

The single vascular clamps are removed, venous side first, and the anastomoses are inspected for any significant leaks. Small areas of leakage will typically resolve, whereas larger ones may need an additional suture. The minimum number of sutures possible should be used to perform the anastomosis. Strip testing of the venous anastomosis is used to verify blood flow out of the flap. The flap is allowed to perfuse, irrigated with warmed fluid, and inspected for adequate revascularization. Once revascularization is confirmed, the remainder of the inset is performed. Prior to closure of the wound, the anastomosis is inspected, and an implantable Doppler ultrasound transducer is secured to monitor the venous (and arterial) side (Figure 58.12). This is particularly useful to monitor bone flaps without a skin paddle, which are commonly used in benign, mandibular defects.

Postoperative management of the patient begins in the operating room. There must be clear communication between the anesthesiologist and surgeon regarding the extubation plans for the patient. It is not unusual for many patients, especially those with tracheostomies, to be admitted to the intensive care unit (ICU) with mechanical ventilator support postoperatively. Extubation is then performed, usually within 24 hours. Many patients with benign defects do not require elective tracheostomies and are extubated in the operating room. Extubation is performed in a calm, gentle manner. Significant increases in blood pressure and excessive patient movement may cause wound bleeding, hematoma formation, and/or damage to the vascular anastomosis.

The nursing staff in the ICU must be educated about patient care and flap monitoring. The patient should be well hydrated; have adequate levels of analgesia; be well oxygenated; have a stable, nonlabile blood pressure; and remain calm. The use of constrictive tracheostomy ties is prohibited. The use of vasopressors should be avoided, and sedation may be needed to manage anxiety and restlessness. Prophylaxis for alcohol withdrawal should be utilized in patients whose history warrants it or if signs manifest regardless of history.

Anticoagulants or antiplatelet agents should be started on admission to the ICU. Multiple agents have been used for this, and they vary depending on the institution. 325 mg aspirin daily and low-molecular-weight heparin injections (deep vein thrombosis prophylaxis dose) are commonly used. There is no consensus as to which method is the best agent. These agents can increase the risk of postoperative hematoma formation and hemorrhage. Postoperative antibiotic coverage is surgeon dependent but typically continues for 72 hours. Routine laboratory measurements are surgeon dependent.

A member of the surgical team should assess the patient and inspect the flap at a minimum of every 4 hours for the first 72 hours. Most vascular issues with the flap will

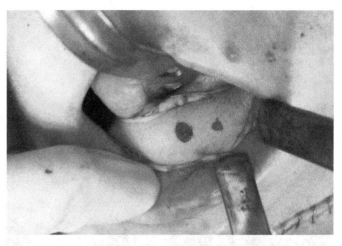

Figure 58.2.   Radial forearm free flap covering a large soft tissue defect resulting from resection of a T4N2bM0—stage IVa gingival carcinoma. The flap demonstrates good vascularity, and the perforator is marked and bleeding from a 27-gauge needle stick.

appear within this period, although late problems can rarely be seen. Donor sites should have vascular checks and drain outputs monitored at least every 2 hours. Nursing staff should inspect the flap and verify a Doppler signal (external or internal) every hour during this period. A prominent perforator can be marked on the skin paddle for easy location for the nursing staff when using an external Doppler (Figure 58.2). Notification of any changes in flap appearance or Doppler signals should be relayed to the surgeon. Rates of successful salvage of flaps are high with early intervention. Signs of vascular issues may include pallor, congested-bluish or cold skin paddle, formation of neck swelling or hematoma, poor capillary refill, rapid capillary refill, and loss or decrease in Doppler signals. The use of implantable Doppler probes for buried flaps can cause false negatives and false positives that may result in unnecessary return visits to the operating room for flap inspection. Without complications, the typical ICU stay is 72 hours, and the total hospital course is approximately 7–10 days before the patient is ready for discharge.

Key Points

1. Microvascular reconstructions often permit single-stage ablative and reconstructive surgeries and allow the ability to reconstruct 3D defects (skin, deep soft tissue, and bone) of significant size.
2. Microvascular reconstructions typically demonstrate a success rate approaching 95% within the head and neck region.
3. Microvascular reconstructions of continuity defects of the maxilla and mandible allow for the placement of endosteal dental implants with a high success rate, shortened prosthetic treatment times, and early return to function.

Case Report 58.1. A 29-year-old male presents with a chief complaint of a slow-growing mass to his right mandible. Maxillofacial computed tomography scans demonstrated an 8 cm radiolucent mass located within the right mandible. The mass demonstrated a multilocular appearance, cortical expansion, and scalloped margin. An

incision biopsy was performed, and a definitive diagnosis of an ameloblastoma was made. The patient was treated with mandibular resection with 1 cm margins and immediate reconstruction with a free vascularized fibula. (See Figures 58.3 through 58.13.)

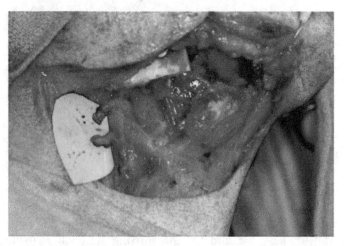

Figure 58.3. After resection of the amleloblastoma, the recipient facial vessels are identified, isolated and prepared.

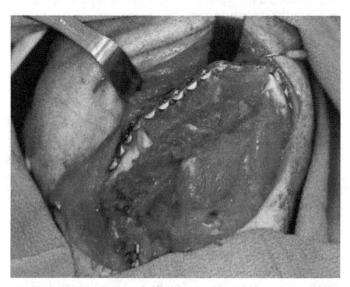

Figure 58.4. Inset of fibula free flap with pedicle geometry aligning well with recipient vessels to prevent twisting and kinking of the vasculature.

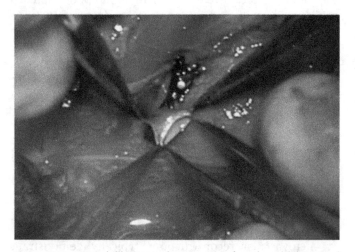

Figure 58.5. Vessel dilation and preparation for adventitial removal Care must be taken to ensure there is no damage to the endothelium.

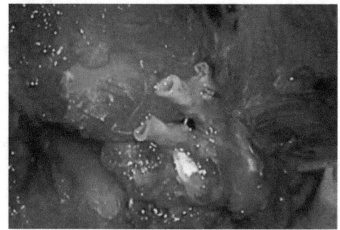

Figure 58.6. Pedicle vessels with adventitia removed and vessel dilation.

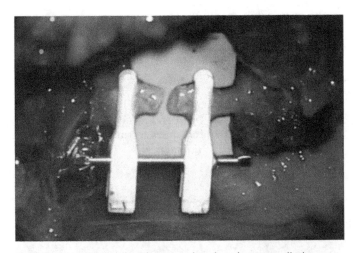

Figure 58.7.   Arterial double approximating clamps applied.

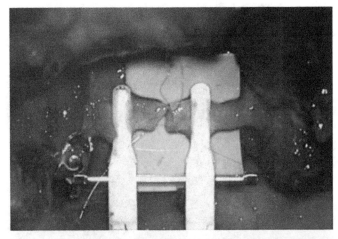

Figure 58.8.   First sutures placed 180° apart and tucked to provide tension.

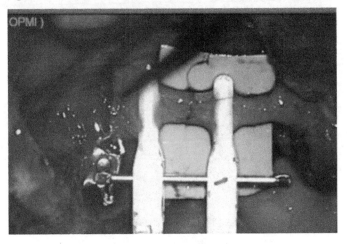

Figure 58.9.   Completed arterial anastomosis.

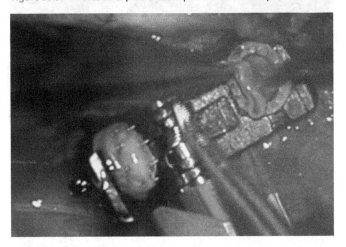

Figure 58.10.   Pulling of vein through anastomotic coupler ring. Note the recipient vein is already positioned.

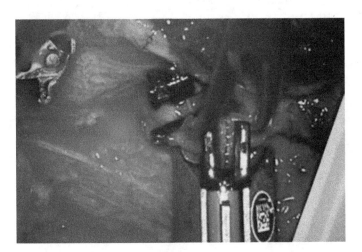

Figure 58.11.   Closure of anastomotic coupler. Hemostat secures rings firmly.

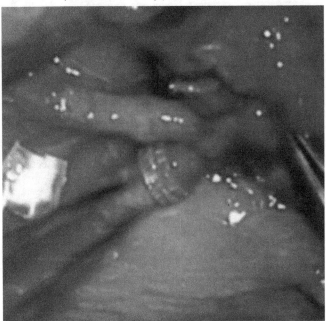

Figure 58.12.   Implantable Doppler probe being placed. Note finished arterial and venous anastomosis.

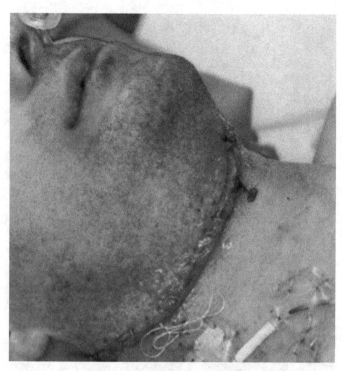

Figure 58.13. Doppler transducer wires (arterial and venous) secured with staples to the supraclavicular area.

References

Hoffman, G.R., Islam, S. and Eisenberg, R.I., 2012. Microvascular reconstruction of the mouth, jaws and face: experience of an Australian oral and maxillofacial surgery unit. *Oral and Maxillofacial Surgery*, 70, e371–7.

Mucke, T., Ritschl, L.M., Balasso, A., Wolff, K.D., Mitchell, D.A. and Liepsch, D., 2014. Open end-to side technique for end-to-side anastomosis and analyses by an elastic true-to scale silicone rubber model. *Microsurgery*, 34, 28–36.

59

Free Vascularized Fibula and Graft Harvest

Robert M. Laughlin[1] and Christopher M. Harris[2]

[1]Department of Oral and Maxillofacial Surgery, Naval Medical Center San Diego, San Diego, California, USA
[2]Department of Oral and Maxillofacial Surgery, Naval Medical Center Portsmouth, Portsmouth, Virginia, USA

The harvest of a free vascularized fibula for the reconstruction of combined hard and soft tissue maxillofacial defects.

Indications

1. Reconstruction of surgical defects following oncologic ablative surgery, traumatic defects, and congenital anomalies requiring cutaneous and/or osseous vascularized tissue
2. Segmental continuity defects of the maxilla and mandible greater than 5 cm. A long segment of bone up to approximately 25 cm is available for harvest. The skin paddle has proven to be dependable if care is taken to preserve the fasciocutaneous perforators. Innervation of the flap is possible, and the flap has adequate bone stock to accept endosseous dental implants

Contraindications

1. Medical conditions that would not be compatible with extended operative procedures
2. Hypercoagulable states
3. Relative contraindications:

   A. Vasculitis
   B. Connective tissue disorders
   C. Peripheral vascular disease
   D. Venous insufficiency
   E. Congenital anomalies of the peroneal artery
   F. Other disorders that may impact coagulation and wound healing

Note: Evaluation of the patient's physiologic status is more important than the chronologic age of the patient in determining the appropriateness of a free tissue transfer procedure.

Preoperative Studies

1. Bilateral lower extremity angiogram or magnetic resonance angiography. The arteriogram should demonstrate normal three-vessel runoff of the right and left popliteal artery with normal patency of the anterior, posterior, and peroneal vessels bilaterally.
2. Palpation of the dorsalis pedis (anterior tibial artery) and posterior tibial pulses.

Flap Anatomy

1. Dominant-peroneal artery

   Length: 2.0 cm (2–4 cm)
   Diameter: 1.5 mm (1–2.5 mm)

2. Minor-periosteal and muscular branches

   Length: 1.2 mm (0.8–1.7 mm)
   Diameter: 1.0 mm (0.8–1.7 mm)

Typically, 4–8 cutaneous arteries arise from the peroneal artery. These typically are septal or septo-muscular cutaneous perforators coursing through the posterior crural (lateral) septum.

Surgical Anatomy

The lower leg can be viewed as four compartments:

Lateral compartment: Bordered by the posterior crural septum and the anterior crural septum and contains the peroneus longus and peroneus brevis muscles.

Anterior compartment: Bordered by the anterior crural septum and the interosseous membrane and contains the extensor digitorium longus and extensor hallucis longus muscles. The anterior tibial vasculature and deep peroneal nerve lie on the superficial aspect of the interosseous membrane in the anterior compartment.

Superficial posterior compartment: Bordered by the interosseous membrane and the intermuscular membrane of the flexor hallucis longus and soleus muscles. The peroneal vessels lie on the deep aspect of the interosseous membrane and course distal along the fibula. The posterior tibial vessels are deep to the tibialis posterior muscle.

Deep posterior compartment: Bordered by the intermuscular membrane of the flexor hallucis longus and soleus muscles and the posterior crural septum; it contains the lateral aspect of the soleus muscle.

Atlas of Operative Oral and Maxillofacial Surgery, First Edition. Edited by Christopher J. Haggerty and Robert M. Laughlin
© 2015 John Wiley & Sons, Inc. Published 2015 by John Wiley & Sons, Inc.

Preoperative Preparation

1. A bump may be placed under the ipsilateral hip to aid in access to the lateral surface of the lower extremity.
2. A heel bump (i.e., a 5 lb. sandbag or 1 L IV fluid bag) is placed on the operating room table that allows the lower extremity to maintain 90° of flexion at the knee; it will aid in the graft harvest.
3. Doppler flow meter.
4. Tourniquet (recommended but optional).
5. A second set of instruments for the harvest team.

Surgical Procedure

1. A normal preoperative arteriogram of bilateral lower extremities demonstrating three-vessel runoff of the right and left popliteal artery with normal patency of all distal vessels.
2. The patient is placed in a supine position. The knee is flexed to 90°, and the hip is internally rotated with the use of a hip bump. The heel is then placed on a gel bumper, which is secured to the table. The patient is prepped and draped in a sterile fashion. A sterile tourniquet is applied.
3. Anatomic landmarks are palpated and marked (Figure 59.1) to include the head of the fibula and the lateral malleolus of the ankle. The dorsalis pedis and posterior tibial pulses are palpated and marked with Doppler accordingly. With a surgical pen, a mark is placed 6–8 cm inferior to the head of the fibula and 6–8 cm superior to the lateral malleolus. This allows the proximal and distal 6–8 cm of the fibula and its ligamentous

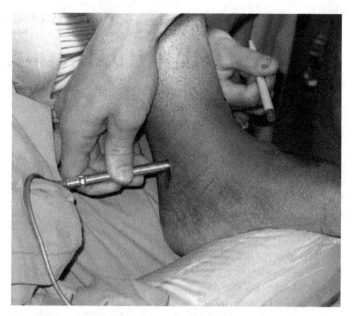

Figure 59.2.   The dorsalis pedis and posterior tibial pulses are palpated and Dopplered accordingly and marked for future reference.

attachments to be preserved. A line is drawn along the posterior crural septum connecting the two marks.
4. If a skin flap is to be harvested in conjunction with the fibula, the flap should be designed along the posterior septal crural. A Doppler will allow for the identification of septocutaneous perforating vessels (Figure 59.2). Typically, the skin flap is designed in the distal one-third of the flap.
5. The extremity is exsanguinated, and the tourniquet inflated to 300 mmHg. Time of inflation must be recorded. Inflation time must be keep under 2 hours to avoid possible ischemic events.
6. A skin incision is made to the depth of the superficial fascia along the length of the incision to include the skin flap (Figure 59.3). A subfascial dissection is

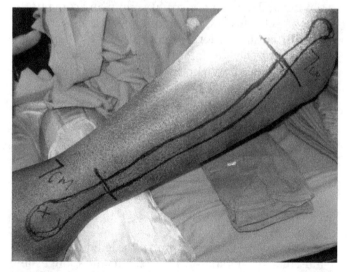

Figure 59.1.   Anatomic landmarks are palpated and marked to include the head of the fibula and the lateral malleolus of the ankle. Marks are placed 6–8 cm inferior to the head of the fibula and 6–8 cm superior to the lateral malleolus. This allows the proximal and distal 6–8 cm of the fibula and its ligamentous attachments to be preserved. A line is then drawn along the posterior crural septum connecting the two marks.

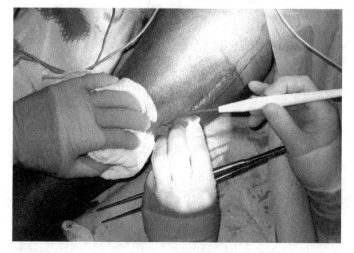

Figure 59.3.   A skin incision is made to the depth of the superficial fascia along the length of the incision to include the skin flap.

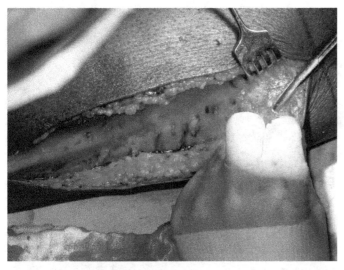

Figure 59.4. A septocutaneous perforator is seen emerging from the posterior crural septum. The superficial fascia is dissected to allow access to the lateral compartment.

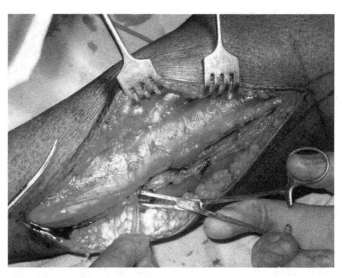

Figure 59.5. The septocutaneous perforator is ligated (a skin paddle was not utilized in this case).

performed to elevate the skin island and expose the posterior crural septum (Figure 59.4). Septocutaneous perforators may be seen emerging from the posterior crural septum (Figure 59.5). If no septocutaneous perforators are seen, a muscle cuff is included to capture any musculocutaneous perforators. Anterior and posterior skin flaps are elevated superficial to the fascia, exposing the peroneus longus muscle anteriorly and the soleus muscle posteriorly. The superficial peroneal nerve should be identified and preserved.

7. The peroneus longus muscle is elevated and retracted anteriorly and medially (Figure 59.6). This provided

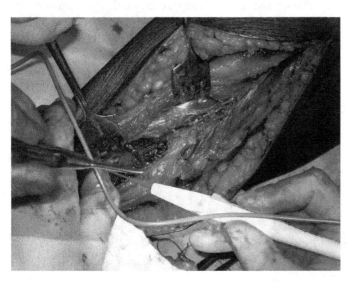

Figure 59.6. The peroneus longus muscle is elevated and retracted anteriorly and medially. This provided the approach through the lateral compartment of the fibula. The peroneus brevis is then identified and divided, maintaining a 5 mm cuff of muscle to protect and preserve the underlying periosteum, while allowing access to the fibular bone.

the approach through the lateral compartment of the fibula. The peroneus brevis is then identified and divided, maintaining a 5 mm cuff of muscle to protect and preserve the underlying periosteum, while allowing access to the fibular bone. Dissection then proceeds anteriorly medially along the fibula to the anterior crural septum marking the anterior compartment of the fibula.

8. The anterior crural septum is divided to expose the extensor digitorium longus and extensor hallucis muscles. Maintaining a 5 mm cuff of muscle around the fibula, the digitorium longus and extensor hallucis muscles are divided to expose the interosseous membrane inferiomedially. The anterior tibialis vessels and the deep peroneal nerve are identified anteriomedial to the fibula in the anterior compartment and retracted medially.

9. The interosseous membrane is incised 5 mm medially from the fibula in the proximal third and extended the length of the fibula. Care must be taken when incising the interosseous membrane due to the close proximity of the peroneal vasculature on the inferior aspect of the membrane.

10. A subperiosteal dissection is performed at the proposed proximal and distal osteotomy sites. Protecting the medial aspect of the fibula and peroneal vessels, the proximal and distal osteotomies are performed with a reciprocating or oscillating saw, ensuring that a minimum of 6–8 cm of fibula remains distal to the fibular head and proximal to the lateral malleolus (Figures 59.7 and 59.8).

11. A bone clamp is used to retract the fibula laterally, allowing visualization of the peroneal vessels distally (Figure 59.9). The posterior tibialis muscle is divided

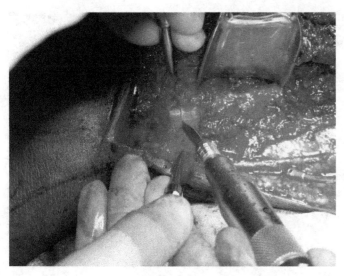

Figure 59.7. A subperiosteal dissection is performed at the proposed proximal and distal osteotomy sites. Protecting the medial aspect of the fibula and peroneal vessels, the proximal and distal osteotomies are performed with a reciprocating or oscillating saw, ensuring a minimum of 6–8 cm of fibula remains distal to the fibular head and proximal to the lateral malleolus.

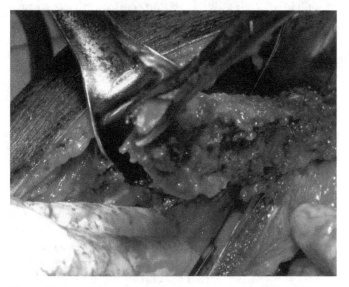

Figure 59.9. A bone clamp is used to retract the fibula laterally, allowing visualization of the peroneal vessels distally. The posterior tibialis muscle is divided distal to proximal to allow the pedicle to be visualized along the entire length of the fibula.

distal to proximal to allow the pedicle to be visualized the entire length of the fibula.

12. The tourniquet is let down and time recorded. The dorsalis pedis and posterior tibialis pulses are verified by palpation or Doppler ultrasound. The flow through the peroneal vessels is also verified. A vessel loop is placed circumferentially around the distal peroneal vessels to occlude flow. The flow through the dorsalis pedis and posterior tibialis vessels was again veri-

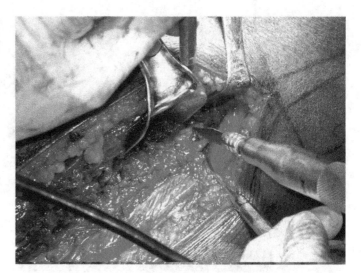

Figure 59.8. Proximal osteotomy performed with a reciprocating saw, ensuring a minimum of 6–8 cm of fibula remains distal to the fibular head.

fied and should demonstrate strong signals. The distal peroneal vascular bundle is then ligated and divided.

13. The dissection proceeds posteriolaterally in the deep and superficial posterior compartments dividing the flexor hallucis longus and soleus muscles while maintaining a 5 mm muscle cuff on the fibula. Doppler is then used to confirm a strong signal of the peroneal vessels. The proximal peroneal vascular bundle is then ligated and divided. The fibula and skin paddle are passed to the reconstruction team (Figure 59.10).

14. After adequate hemostasis is achieved, the deep muscle layers are reapproximated with 2-0 Vicryl interrupted sutures (Figure 59.11). Two suction drains are placed. The dermal layer is reapproximated. The skin is closed with staples or a nonresorbable suture (Figure 59.12). In the event that the skin flap is greater than 4 cm, a split-thickness skin graft may be required.

15. The dorsalis pedis and posterior tibialis pulses are palpated, Dopplered, and marked. The foot is checked for warmth and adequate capillary refill.

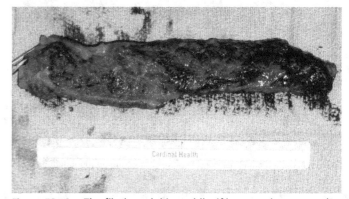

Figure 59.10. The fibula and skin paddle, if harvested, are passed to the reconstruction team for inset.

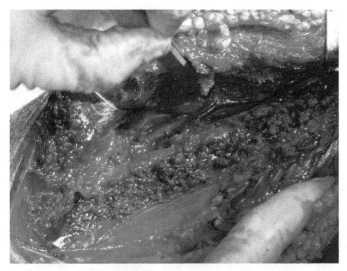

Figure 59.11.   After adequate hemostasis is achieved, the deep muscle layers are reapproximated with 2-0 Vicryl interrupted sutures, and two suction drains are placed.

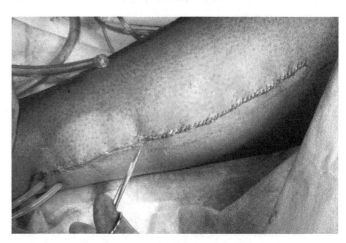

Figure 59.12.   After the dermal layer is approximated, the skin is closed with staples or a nonresorbable suture. In the event that the skin flap is greater than 4 cm, a split-thickness skin graft may be required.

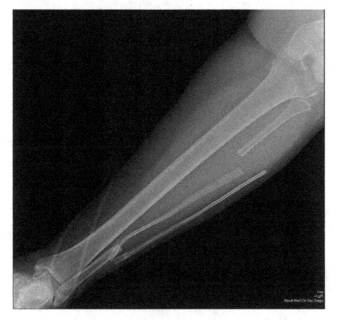

Figure 59.13.   Plain radiographic film taken of the harvest site on postoperative day 2.

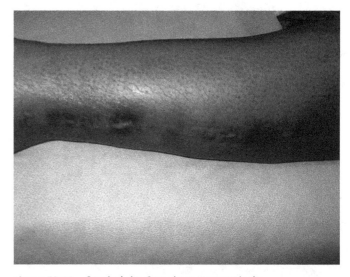

Figure 59.14.   Surgical site 6 weeks postoperatively.

16. Bacitracin is applied to the surgical site, and a Telfa dressing is placed over the incisions. The lower leg is circumferentially wrapped with cotton batting and an Ace bandage. The leg is then elevated. (See Figures 59.13 and 59.14 for postoperative images at 2 days and 6 weeks.)

Complications

Compartment syndrome
Muscle weakness
Ankle instability as the far end of the fibular forms part of the ankle joint and may become less stable

Nerve damage to the peroneal nerves and muscle branches, leading to weakness and limitation of the range of motion of the foot
Neurosensory damage with resultant numbness on the dorsal aspect of the foot
Lower leg blood vessel damage to anterior or posterior tibia vessels
Infection
Chronic pain of lower extremity
Loss of limb

Key Points

1. Flap harvest requires meticulous dissection of the vascular pedicle. Magnification and an experienced, microvascular-trained assistant surgeon are ideal.
2. Preoperative verification of collateral blood flow is required prior to flap harvest. Potential necrosis with loss of lower extremity function may occur with no collateral circulation.
3. Perioperative antibiotic coverage is continued for 72 hours postoperatively. Sterile technique is used to change any dressings associated with the wound. Lower extremity infections can cause significant morbidity and disability.

References

Eisele, D., 2009. *Complications in head and neck surgery*. 2nd ed. St. Louis, MO: Mosby.

Grabb, W.C. and Strauch, B., 2009. *Grabb's encyclopedia of flaps*. 3rd ed. Philadelphia: Lippincott Williams & Wilkins.

Urken, M., 2010. *Multidisciplinary head and neck reconstruction: a defect-oriented approach*. Philadelphia: Lippincott Williams & Wilkins.

Wei, F-C., 2009. *Flaps and reconstructive surgery*. Philadelphia: Saunders Elsevier.

60

Radial Forearm Free Flap

Christopher M. Harris[1] and Remy H. Blanchaert[2]

[1]Department of Oral and Maxillofacial Surgery, Naval Medical Center Portsmouth, Portsmouth, Virginia, USA

[2]Private Practice, Oral and Maxillofacial Surgery Associates, Wichita, Kansas, USA

A means of obtaining free tissue transfer for the replacement of moderate to large soft tissue defects associated with ablative wounds.

Indications

1. Utilized for the reconstruction of moderate to large soft tissue defects related to traumatic, congenital, and benign or malignant defects
2. Most commonly utilized for the replacement of oral and oropharyngeal soft tissues due to ablative treatment of malignancies

Contraindications

1. Vascular anatomy disruption due to prior surgical procedures or trauma in the area of interest
2. Anatomical variants precluding the use of a radial forearm flap: aberrant or no radial artery, absent branching from the superficial arch to the index finger and thumb, and lack of connections between the superficial and palmar arches
3. Hereditary or acquired coagulopathy, which may lead to flap loss
4. Inability of the patient to medically tolerate anesthesia and a prolonged surgical procedure

Anatomy

Vascular supply: The radial artery supplies the arterial flow to the flap. The radial artery runs the length of the arm and terminates in the deep palmar arch. The ulnar artery supplies the superficial palmar arch. Anastomoses occur between the two that supply collateral circulation to the hand. The radial artery gives off multiple perforating branches to the skin, subcutaneous tissue, muscles, and radius bone of the volar forearm. The lateral intermuscular septal perforators are found between the flexor carpi radialis and the brachioradialis muscles. Venous drainage of the flap is from the deep radial veins and the superficial system. The superficial system allows for better anastomosis due to a larger caliber, but it may be unreliable with small flaps. The arterial vessel caliber (2–3 mm) and vein caliber (1–4 mm) allow for

easier anastamosis. A long vascular pedicle is available for most oral cancer defect reconstructions.

Radial Forearm Flap Landmarks

1. Proximal wrist crease
2. Antecubital fossa
3. Superficial veins (cephalic)
4. Flexor carpi radialis tendon
5. Brachioradialis muscle
6. Flexor carpi ulnaris
7. Palmaris longus tendon (when present)

Radial Forearm Flap Layers

1. Skin
2. Subcutaneous tissue
3. Antebracial fascia
4. Superficial veins
5. Radial artery and venae comitantes; lateral intermuscular septum
6. Paratenon
7. Forearm tendons

Radial Forearm Flap Technique

1. Preoperatively, a history of wrist surgery or trauma needs to be ascertained, as certain conditions may restrict safe flap harvest. An Allen's test is performed to verify collateral circulation from the ulnar artery. Questionable findings dictate that other vascular studies (e.g., color Doppler) be performed to verify adequate circulation prior to performing the procedure. Inadequate circulation between the superficial and deep palmar arches increases the risk of vascular insufficiency to the hand and thumb if the flap is harvested. Preoperatively, the patient is instructed to not allow intravenous attempts or venipuncture in the chosen arm. This is also recorded as an order within the patient's medical record.
2. The flap design is drawn on the volar forearm with a surgical skin marker. Superficial veins and the radial artery are also marked for identification. The distal margin is 2–3 cm proximal to the wrist crease. The ulnar margin is typically the flexor carpi ulnaris. The radial margin is

Atlas of Operative Oral and Maxillofacial Surgery, First Edition. Edited by Christopher J. Haggerty and Robert M. Laughlin

typically the brachioradialis muscle, but can extend over to the dorsal surface. The proximal extent is dependent on the size of flap needed for the reconstruction. The entire volar surface skin can be harvested if needed.

3. Surgical prep and draping are performed. A sterile tourniquet is applied to the upper arm.
4. The limb is exsanguinated with an elastic wrap, and the tourniquet is inflated to 250 mmHg. The tourniquet "uptime" is recorded. The dorsal wrist has a rolled lap sponge placed underneath, and an open lap sponge across the palm is secured with clamps to the arm board. This is used to extend the wrist slightly and secure the arm.
5. The dissection is carried out on the distal end of the flap. Skin and subcutaneous tissue are incised. The dissection is carried down to the flexor tendons of the forearm. Subfascial dissection proceeds to identify the radial artery, venae comitantes, and any potentially usable superficial veins.
6. The radial artery is identified between the flexor carpi radialis tendon and the brachioradialis (Figure 60.2). A small section of the radial artery and its two venae comitantes is exposed. These are ligated and divided.
7. The dissection at this point can be advanced from the ulnar or radial side. The paratenon of the underlying tendons must be maintained. The skin paddle and pedicle are attached to the deeper tissues. Dissection should identify the palmaris longus tendon. In some cases (e.g., lip reconstruction), this may be included with the flap to use as a suspensory mechanism. Care is taken to not damage the superficial sensory branch of the radial nerve during the dissection. Damage may leave neurosensory dysfunction of the dorsal thumb and index finger.
8. The intermuscular septum separates the brachioradialis and the flexor carpi radialis. The intermuscular septum contains the vascular pedicle. The deep margin of the pedicle is released by ligating and dividing branches to the deeper musculature and radius bone.
9. The proximal edge of the skin paddle is incised, and a wavy proximal skin incision is made to a point just distal to the antecubital fossa and connects with the proximal end of the skin paddle. The proximal tissue flaps are elevated in the subdermal plane to expose the underlying musculature.
10. The pedicle is dissected along the intermuscular septum to the point where the brachioradialis and flexor carpi radialis intersect. The fascia between the two muscles are separated proximally, taking care not to damage the pedicle underneath. The brachioradialis muscle and flexor carpi radialis are retracted. The dissection of the pedicle continues in a proximal direction. Multiple perforators are ligated and divided to free up the vascular pedicle. The recurrent radial artery is typically the endpoints of proximal dissection. The venae comitantes frequently are larger or co-join in this region.

11. The tourniquet is released, and "downtime" is recorded. The flap is allowed to reperfuse for 15 to 20 minutes (Figure 60.3). Hemostasis of the flap and the forearm wound bed is achieved with microclips or bipolar cautery during this reperfusion. Verification of adequate vascular supply to the flap and hand is verified during this time.
12. The proximal pedicle is divided and moved to the oral cavity for inset and anastomosis (Figure 60.4).
13. The wound bed is closed with dermal sutures and staples. Attempts to cover tendons of the forearm with muscle are made prior to closure. A suction drain is placed in the forearm prior to closure.
14. The defect is reconstructed with a full-thickness or split-thickness skin graft. The authors typically utilize a full-thickness skin graft, which provides thicker coverage of the forearm tendons. A wound vacuum-assisted closure (VAC) and a 45° dorsal wrist splint are applied. The authors typically utilize a dorsally placed arterial line wrist splint, cast padding, Kerlix gauze, tape, and an Ace wrap to secure the wrist and finger position. The fingers are checked for adequate capillary refill, and the wrist should be in a functional position. Poor capillary refill indicates a vascular compromise. If noted, the splint and dressing should be removed and replaced. The VAC and splint are left in place for 7 days prior to evaluating the amount of skin graft success. The suction drain is removed when drain output is less than 25 mL over 24 hours.

Complications

1. **Damage to the vascular pedicle**: May result in flap loss, but may be repaired if a small side wall defect occurs.
2. **Ischemia to hand and digits**: Signs include pallor, diminished capillary refill of the hand and thumb after flap harvest, and pain. Late signs may be frank ischemia and necrosis. Reconstruction of the radial artery with a vein graft may be required. Regular vascular checks of the hand and fingers intraoperatively and postoperatively (once each hour) are needed to verify adequate vascular supply. Forearm dressing should be loosened or removed and changed if poor vascular supply is noted due to possible compression in the postoperative period.
3. **Skin graft loss**: Partial loss or total loss is possible with any shearing movements of the graft postoperatively. Dorsal wrist splints are used to minimize hand movement. VAC therapy is used to improve graft success as well. Partial graft loss is managed with local wound therapy, but it may require further attempts at grafting or rotational flaps to close the defect over the flexor tendons.
4. Hematoma of the forearm
5. Wound infection
6. Neuroma, or neurosensory dysfunction of the hand or digits
7. Wrist stiffness and grip strength decrease, and loss of range of motion

1. Flap harvest requires meticulous dissection of the vascular pedicle. Magnification and an experienced, microvascular-trained assistant surgeon are ideal.
2. Preoperative verification of collateral blood flow is required prior to flap harvest. Potential necrosis with loss of digit hand function may occur with no collateral circulation.
3. Wound complications with tendon exposure are the most commonly seen complication. Careful graft technique, full-thickness graft use, adequate wrist immobilization, and early recognition and management of graft failure are imperative to minimize postoperative issues.
4. Perioperative antibiotic coverage is continued for 72 hours postoperatively. Sterile technique is used to change any dressings associated with the wound. Forearm infections can cause significant morbidity and disability of the arm and hand.

Case Report

Case Report 60.1. A 68-year-old patient presents with a chief complaint of a large palatal opening, food impaction, and halitosis 2 years status post gunshot wound. On clinical examination and on review of the computed tomography scan, a large oronasal communication extending through the palate and left alveolus and chronic maxillary sinusitis was identified. The patient was treated with a "medallion" radial forearm flap to close the defect. The flap pedicle was tunneled through the soft tissue of the cheek, and anastomosis with the facial vessels was utilized. (See Figures 60.1 through 60.6.)

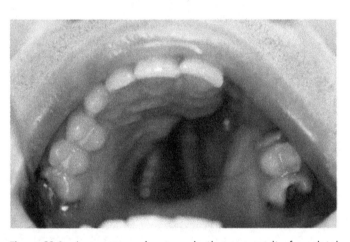

Figure 60.1. Large oronasal communication as a result of a palatal and alveolar gunshot wound.

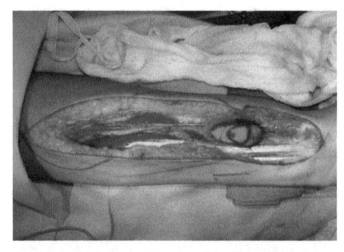

Figure 60.2. Dissection and elevation of the skin paddle and vascular pedicle. The radial artery is identified between the flexor carpi radialis tendon and the brachioradialis.

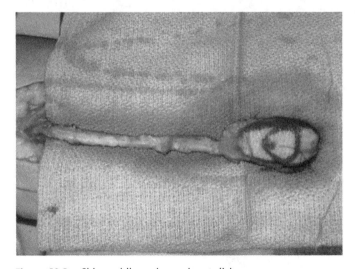

Figure 60.3. Skin paddle and vascular pedicle.

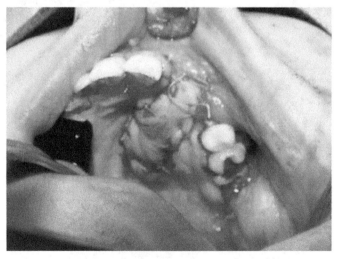

Figure 60.4. The inset of the skin paddle into the oronasal defect providing separation of the oral cavity and nasal cavity.

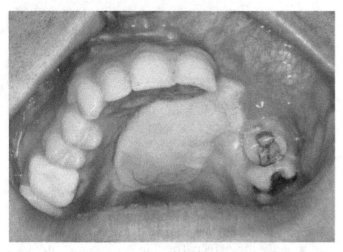

Figure 60.5.   The reconstructed palate and alveolus at 6 months postoperatively.

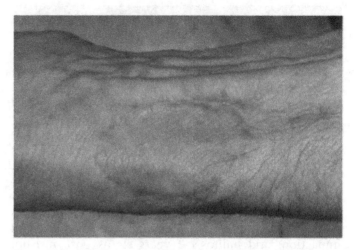

Figure 60.6.   The donor site at 6 months postoperatively.

References

Eisele, D., 2009. *Complications in head and neck surgery*. 2nd ed. St. Louis, MO: Mosby.

Grabb, W.C. and Strauch, B., 2009. *Grabb's encyclopedia of flaps*. 3rd ed. Philadelphia: Lippincott Williams & Wilkins.

Urken, M., 2010. *Multidisciplinary head and neck reconstruction: a defect-oriented approach*. Philadelphia: Lippincott Williams & Wilkins.

Wei, F-C., 2009. *Flaps and reconstructive surgery*. Philadelphia: Saunders Elsevier.

CHAPTER 1

Anterolateral Thigh Perforator Free Flap

Melvyn S. Yeoh and Stavan Patel

Department of Oral and Maxillofacial Surgery, Louisiana State University Health Science Center, Shreveport, Louisiana, USA

A method of reconstructing soft tissue defects to various regions of the body. The anterior lateral thigh (ALT) perforator free flap has the ability to provide either individual components or any combination of skin, fascia, and muscle to reconstruct soft tissue defects of the head and neck region. The ALT flap can be harvested as cutaneous, fasciocutaneous, fascial, adipofascial, or musculocutaneous based on the vastus lateralis muscle (VLM) perforators, and a chimeric flap based on the ascending, transverse, and descending branches of the lateral circumflex femoral artery (LCFA) combined with the VLM, rectus femoris muscle (RFM), tensor fascia lata (TFL), and anteromedial thigh (AMT) skin paddle.

Indications

1. Reconstruction of soft tissue defects created by pathologic resection or traumatic avulsions involving the tongue, oral, maxillofacial, skull base, head, and neck regions
2. Desire for a two-team approach as flap harvest does not require patient repositioning for most oral, maxillofacial, and head and neck defects
3. Need for a large skin paddle for extensive reconstructions
4. Desire for a sensate flap
5. Reconstruction of combined hard and soft tissue defects when used as a flow-through flap in combination with a fibula osteocutaneous free flap for reconstruction of larger defects requiring extensive osseous and soft tissue reconstruction

Contraindications

1. History of previous traumatic injury to the upper thigh
2. Patients who have limited blood supply to the lower extremity (e.g., a history of vascular surgery [femoral-femoral bypass or aorto-femoral bypass])
3. Hypercoagulable conditions
4. Intramuscular dissection of the perforators is technically challenging and has a steep learning curve. Surgeons not well versed in ALT free flaps may elect for other reconstructive procedures

5. Severe obesity: Due to the large amount of subcutaneous fat in severely obese patients, it may be difficult to dissect the flap and close the donor site primarily. Due to its bulkiness, it is challenging to inset the flap without secondary thinning
6. Relative contraindication: Patients with claudication due to peripheral vascular disease and no palpable popliteal pulse
7. Relative contraindication: ALT skin is usually lighter in color and thicker when compared to tissues of the head and neck region. ALT free flaps may provide poor color and skin-thickness matches in certain instances

Anatomy

The musculocutaneous and septocutaneous perforators of the ALT free flap region are supplied by the descending branch of the LCFA, which is the largest branch of the profunda femoris artery. The region is drained by two venae comitantes of the lateral circumflex femoral system, which eventually drain into the femoral vein. Less commonly, other variations exist and the perforators of the ALT free flap may arise from the transverse branch of the LCFA, directly from the profunda femoris artery or the femoral artery.

The vascular pedicle to the ALT free flap lies in the muscular groove between the VLM and RFM. The vascular pedicle consists of the descending branch of the LCFA, two venae comitantes, and the motor nerve to the VLM, which is a branch of the posterior division of the femoral nerve. The neurovascular pedicle length has a range of 8–16 cm, with arterial and venous vessel diameter greater than 2 mm.

The descending branch of the LCFA gives several perforators to the skin of the ALT as it travels within the intermuscular space between the VLM and RFM. These perforators most commonly have a musculocutaneous course or, less commonly, a septocutaneous course.

The dominant perforator is generally located within a 3 cm radius circle at the midpoint between a line drawn from the anterior superior iliac spine (ASIS) to the superiolateral aspect of the patella. Typically, the perforator to the skin is found in the inferiolateral quadrant of this circle.

Atlas of Operative Oral and Maxillofacial Surgery, First Edition. Edited by Christopher J. Haggerty and Robert M. Laughlin.
© 2015 John Wiley & Sons, Inc. Published 2015 by John Wiley & Sons, Inc.

The lateral femoral cutaneous nerve provides sensory innervation to the skin in the ALT region and allows for its use as a sensate flap.

Preoperative Management

1. A thorough history and physical examination, appropriate laboratory studies, and a radiographic workup should be completed prior to surgery. Evaluation should include an estimation of the size of defect and the type of tissue required for its reconstruction (skin, fascia, muscle, bone, and nerves), the length of the vascular pedicle required, and the possible recipient vessel locations for anastomosis of the free tissue flap.
2. Preoperative evaluation for ALT free flap typically does not require angiography of the lower extremities, but it should include a physical examination of the thighs for previous surgery scars.
3. ALT free flap harvest is contraindicated in patients who have had previous vascular bypass procedures in the lower extremities. It is relatively contraindicated in patients who have claudication due to peripheral vascular disease and no palpable popliteal pulse. In this subset of patients, lower extremity angiography must be performed prior to planning an ALT free flap.
4. Due to the variable nature of the ALT skin perforators, patients should be consented for modification of the flap design and for flap harvest from the contralateral thigh.

Surgical Technique

1. The patient is positioned supine on the operating table with both legs in a neutral position.
2. Both legs are prepared circumferentially and in entirety from the hips to the lower legs and draped in a sterile fashion. This will allow for manipulation of the legs if the original flap design requires modification or if harvest from the contralateral thigh is necessary.
3. The anterior superior iliac spine (ASIS) and the superiolateral aspect of the patella are identified, and a straight line is drawn connecting these two points (Figure 61.3). The straight line denotes the intermuscular septum between the VLM and RFM.
4. The midpoint of this line is identified, and a 3 cm radius circle is drawn around this midpoint. The encircled area is where the most dominant skin perforator is usually encountered, commonly in the inferior-lateral quadrant of the circle.
5. Using a handheld Doppler probe, the skin perforators within the circled area are mapped and marked. Typically, 1–3 perforators are identified along the line, and the flap is centered over these vessels.
6. Depending on the size of the defect, flap dimensions are determined and marked on the thigh. Care is taken to center the flap on the identified skin perforators. Depending on the body habitus of the patient,

a flap size of up to 35 cm × 25 cm can be harvested for the ALT region. Large flap harvests will require closure with a split-thickness skin graft (STSG) as primary closure will be unobtainable.
7. Most commonly, the ALT free flap is harvested as a fasciocutaneous flap. Dissection is initiated by making the skin incision on the medial border of the flap design, which is commonly located over the RFM. This allows for identification and preservation of the skin perforators.
8. The incision is carried through the subcutaneous fat and the deep fascia overlying the RFM. The incision is extended laterally within a subfascial plane until the intermuscular septum between the VLM and RFM is reached. During the lateral subfascial dissection, perforators to the skin are identified and preserved (Figure 61.4).
9. Upon lateral retraction of the flap, the perforators can be identified as either septocutaneous or musculocutaneous and are traced back to the descending branch of the LCFA, which lies within the intermuscular septum and can be visualized by gentle medial retraction of the RFM.
10. In cases where a septocutaneous perforator is identified, the perforator is used as a guide to trace and dissect back to the vascular pedicle deeper in the intermuscular septum.
11. In cases where a musculocutaneous perforator through the VLM is identified (Figure 61.5), it is necessary to map out its course through the muscle by gently unroofing the overlying muscle and tracing it back to the main vascular pedicle. The VLM over the perforator is dissected, lifted away, and incised. The posterior and lateral branches from the perforator to the muscle are ligated. Muscle dissection over the musculocutaneous perforator is achieved in a distal-to-proximal direction until the perforator is traced back to the descending branch of the LCFA (Figure 61.6). A small cuff (5–10 mm) of VLM can be left around the vessel to protect the perforating vessel. Muscle dissection should be executed under loupe magnification, using tenotomy scissors for dissection and hemoclips, bipolar electrocautery, or ultrasonic shears for hemostasis.
12. If a thinner, more pliable cutaneous perforator flap is required for the defect, the initial skin incision on the medial border of the flap design is carried through the subcutaneous fat until the deep fascia is reached. Further dissection of the skin paddle is extended laterally within a suprafascial plane until the marked skin perforator is identified. To avoid kinking of the cutaneous perforator, a small 2 cm radius cuff of deep fascia is maintained around the perforator and resected with the flap. To prevent necrosis of the cutaneous flap margins, a minimum tissue thickness of 5 mm should be maintained.

13. If no viable cutaneous perforators are identified by the medial skin incision, the ALT dissection can be converted to a TFL flap, an AMT flap, or a VLM only flap, or the medial thigh incision can be closed primarily and a contralateral thigh ALT free flap can be harvested.

14. Once the appropriate perforators are identified via the medial incision, another skin incision is made on the lateral border of the flap design. Lateral-to-medial dissection can be performed in a subfascial plane for fasciocutaneous flaps or in a suprafascial plane for thinner cutaneous flaps, until the perforators are identified. During this lateral dissection, if needed, the fascia lata can be included in the flap design and harvested with the flap. Fascia lata can be used for reconstruction of the oral commissure and skull base dural defects.

15. After the perforators are identified via both medial and lateral incisions, they are traced back via retrograde dissection through the muscle for musculocutaneous perforators or through the septum for septocutaneous perforators, until they split off from the descending branch of the LCFA. The motor nerve supplying the vastus lateralis muscle is dissected free from the vascular pedicle and preserved if possible. The vascular pedicle is dissected in the intermuscular septum until adequate caliber of vessels and appropriate pedicle length are achieved (Figure 61.7).

16. If a sensate flap is to be lifted, care must be taken to preserve the lateral femoral cutaneous nerve. The lateral femoral cutaneous nerve enters the thigh close to the ASIS and deep to the inguinal ligament. The lateral femoral cutaneous nerve travels inferiorly within the deep subcutaneous fatty tissue just superficial to the deep fascia and close to the line connecting the ASIS and the superiolateral patella.

17. If a bulkier flap is desired for a deeper defect, the VLM (up to 20 cm) can be included in the flap, and a musculocutaneous flap can be harvested. If septocutaneous perforators to the skin are found, then the skin and the muscle can be harvested on different vessels of the same pedicle, but if a musculocutaneous perforator to the skin is found, then the path of the perforator through the muscle to the vascular pedicle must be mapped by unroofing the muscle fibers over the vessel. Due to the variable anatomy of this area, this step is crucial to prevent accidental injury to the perforator during resection of the muscle in a musculocutaneous flap. For even larger defects, a chimeric flap can be designed based on the same vascular pedicle to include the AMT flap or TFL flap.

18. Once the flap and vascular pedicle are dissected completely, multiple skin paddles can be created based on the separate perforators to allow for favorable inset of the flap within 3D defects. To reconstruct through-and-through cheek defects, a bipaddled flap can be used based on individual perforators. However, if only one perforator is available, the flap can be de-epithelialized in the middle and folded to reconstruct the defect.

19. For defects smaller than 8 cm, primary closure of the ALT donor site can be executed in a layered manner, initially by reapproximating muscles that were dissected and suturing the superficial fascia, followed by the subcutaneous tissue and skin. Resorbable sutures are used for closure of the deep edges and staples for the skin. A closed suction drain is placed in the intermuscular septum between the VLM and RFM to prevent formation of a hematoma or seroma. In donor defects wider than 8 cm, a split-thickness skin graft (STSG) or a V-Y perforator-based local rotational flap is required for closure of the donor site. In cases where a skin graft is required, after suturing the STSG to the defect with resorbable sutures, the graft is perforated to prevent fluid accumulation under the graft. A cotton and 3% bismuth tribromophenate petroleum gauze bolster dressing is applied to keep the graft in place. A non-adherent dressing is applied to the incision edges, and the entire wound is dressed in the usual manner.

Postoperative Management

1. Postoperatively, the patient is typically kept intubated and transferred to the intensive care unit (ICU) for monitoring of the flap. Extreme hypotension or hypertension must be avoided to prevent hypoperfusion of the flap and hematoma formation, respectively. It is important to keep pressure off of the vascular pedicle and to avoid kinking of the pedicle postoperatively. This can be achieved by keeping the neck in a neutral position, avoiding any type of neck ties, and keeping the patient on the ventilator and sedated. If stable, patients are weaned from the ventilator and sedation after 24 hours and transferred from the ICU after 48–72 hours.

2. The flap should be evaluated with a clinical examination every 2 hours postoperatively for the first 72 hours. After 72 hours, the flap is evaluated clinically every 6 hours for the next 48 hours, followed by every 8 hours until the patient is discharged. Clinical examination of the flap should include evaluation of color, warmth, skin turgor, and capillary refill time, and a pinprick test if needed. A handheld Doppler probe may be used as an adjunct to the clinical exam to evaluate the viability of the flap tissue.

3. Postoperatively, the patient is given intravenous maintenance fluids, which are tapered once enteral tube feeds are tolerated. Feeds via nasogastric, orogastric, gastrostomy, or jejunostomy tube are initiated 36–48 hours postoperatively. Oral intake is allowed once satisfactory integration of the flap and wound healing have occurred.

4. Intravenous corticosteroids are administered for the first 72 hours. Intravenous antibiotics are administered for 5–7 days, depending on the surgeons' preference.

Patients are typically discharged with a 7-day course of enteral antibiotics.

5. Closed suction drains are stripped and recorded every 4 hours postoperatively. Drains are removed once the output is less than 30 mL in 24 hours.

6. Patients are allowed to bear weight as tolerated on the donor leg once they are transferred from the ICU, typically 72 hours postoperatively.

7. Dressing on the ALT area is maintained for 5–7 days postoperatively. If a bolster dressing is used for a STSG, it is removed after 5–7 days, and the area is dressed with non-adherent 3% bismuth tribromophenate petroleum gauze daily until the skin graft is completely integrated. Skin staples at the donor site are removed 10–14 days postoperatively, usually at the first postoperative outpatient clinic visit.

Early Complications

1. **Infection, bleeding, and paresthesia**: Although infrequent, immediate donor site complications of localized wound infection, hematoma, seroma, and decreased sensation in the ALT area can occur. Localized infections and small bleeds can be minimized with the use of perioperative antibiotic and meticulous technique and treated with local conservative management.

2. **Flap failure**: Recipient site complication of free flap failure and partial necrosis can be minimized by following standard protocols for free tissue transfer, including avoiding kinking of the vessels, preventing excess pressure on the vascular pedicle, and maintaining adequate perfusion of the flap.

3. **Compartment syndrome**: May occur in patients who have undergone ALT free flap harvest and subsequent primary closure of donor defects with a width greater than 8 cm. Patients with compartment syndrome should undergo immediate surgical decompression of the donor site to prevent permanent damage to the lower extremity.

Late Complications

1. **Leg weakness**: Patients typically have minimal long-term complications associated with the donor site. Patients who have had large segments of the VLM resected with the ALT free flap or extensive dissection of the motor nerve innervating the thigh muscles have reported some weakness and fatigue of the operated limb, but are still able to perform daily activities and have sufficient range of motion at both the hip and knee joints. When compared to the sites that are primarily closed, sites with skin grafts have limited range of motion at the hip and knee joints due to the development of adhesions between the underlying muscle and the overlying skin graft. Recovery of the operated limb for normal daily function can be achieved with early postoperative outpatient physical therapy.

2. **Scarring**: Patients are commonly satisfied with the aesthetic results of the donor site, but if wound dehiscence occurred within the postoperative period creating an unsightly scar, a scar revision surgery can be performed to improve aesthetics.

3. **Color mismatch**: A thorough description of the color mismatch between the ALT skin and the skin of the head and neck region should be reviewed with the patient prior to the procedure to minimize postoperative dissatisfaction.

4. **Excess hair**: In males, there can be substantial hair growth on the transferred ALT skin paddle. Standard methods of hair removal can be applied to correct this issue.

5. **Excess bulk**: After integration of the flap into the surrounding tissue, there may be excess tissue bulk that can interfere with function or may not be aesthetically ideal. In such cases, a debulking procedure can be carried out to provide a more functional and pleasing aesthetic result.

Key Points

1. The ALT free flap has become the workhorse perforator free flap for head and neck reconstruction cases that require versatility in skin paddle size and variable soft tissue bulk.

2. The ALT free flap provides a long vascular pedicle with good-caliber vessels for anastomosis away from the defect site.

3. The major perforator to the skin paddle can be identified using portable Doppler within a 3 cm radius circle drawn at the midpoint of the line connecting the ASIS and the superiolateral point of the patella.

4. The majority of the skin perforators are musculocutaneous, whereas a minority are septocutaneous in nature. Most perforators to the skin paddle originate from the descending branch of the LCFA.

5. It is important to unroof the musculocutaneous perforators and trace their trajectory in all cases because a small minority of the perforating vessels may have a tortuous trajectory to the flap paddle and could be injured when incising the VLM fibers.

6. A meticulous dissection of the perforator under loupe magnification (2.5×) and preservation of a 2 cm radius cuff of fascia will minimize shearing or kinking injury to the perforator vessel.

7. In overweight patients with thick subcutaneous tissue, it is more challenging to harvest and inset the flap. In these instances, the flap can be thinned by suprafascial dissection and secondary thinning of the deep fat layer. Caution should be exercised when thinning the flap to a thickness of less than 5 mm, as overthinning the flap may cause marginal flap ischemia and necrosis after the inset.

8. The ALT free flap allows for primary closure of the donor site in cases where the skin paddle width is

8 cm or less. With large flap harvests, closure of the donor site will require a split-thickness skin graft (STSG), as primary closure will be unattainable.

9. A drawback of the ALT perforator free flap is the technically challenging dissection and, in a very small number of cases (1–5%), there are no viable skin perforators originating from the descending branch of the LCFA. In such cases, the surgeon should be familiar with the anatomy of the thigh and be able to raise a TFL or AMT flap if needed, or close the site primarily and lift the ALT free flap from the contralateral thigh.

10. Small defects (<4 cm) in the oral cavity created after resection of T1 or T2 tumors may not be ideal for reconstruction using an ALT free flap due to its subcutaneous tissue bulkiness. For this reason, oral cavity defects are traditionally successfully managed using the more pliable radial forearm free flap.

Case Report

Case Report 61.1. A 38-year-old male presents status post motor vehicle accident resulting in multiple systemic injuries including basilar skull fractures and a complex scalp avulsion injury. Initial attempt of primary closure of the avulsed area using local tissue rearrangement was unsuccessful due to the substantial size of the wound. Due to lack of local tissue available for primary closure, a fasciocutaneous ALT free flap was used to provide coverage and bulk to the area of avulsed scalp. (See Figures 61.1 through 61.10.)

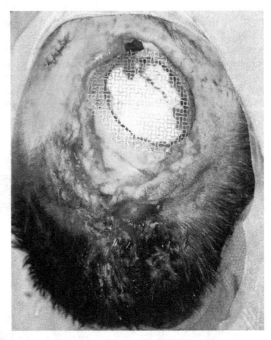

Figure 61.2. Frontal mesh cranioplasty performed, necrotic tissue debrided, avascular bone flap removed, and wound edges refreshed in preparation for free tissue transfer.

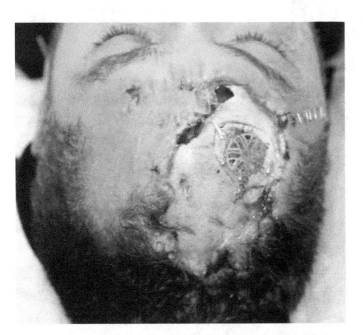

Figure 61.1. Scalp defect after initial debridement and local tissue rearrangement.

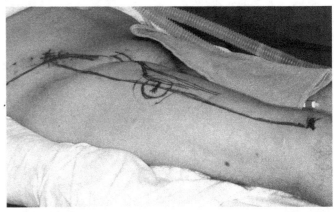

Figure 61.3. The anterior superior iliac spine and the superiolateral patella landmarks are identified and marked by a line connecting the two points. A 3 cm radius circle is drawn from the midpoint of the line and is used as a reference to locate the cutaneous perforator. The descending branch of the lateral circumflex femoral artery and its dominant perforator are identified using Doppler.

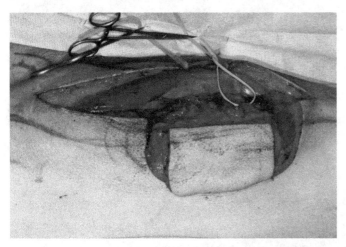

Figure 61.4. A 10 cm × 7 cm elliptical skin paddle is designed centrally based on the cutaneous perforator. The incision is carried down through the subcutaneous fat and the deep fascia overlying the rectus femoris muscle (RFM). The incision is extended laterally within a subfascial plane until the intermuscular septum between the vastus lateralis muscle and RFM is reached. During the lateral subfascial dissection, perforators (marked with vessel loops) to the skin are identified and preserved.

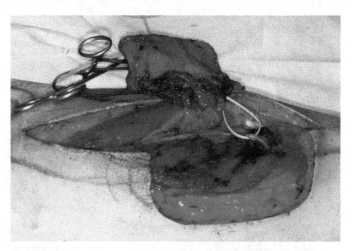

Figure 61.5. The musculocutaneous perforator through the vastus lateralis muscle (VLM) is identified and dissected out of the muscle. A VLM cuff is maintained around the vessel to the skin paddle to prevent injury and kinking of the vessel during inset and also to provide additional bulk to the reconstructed area.

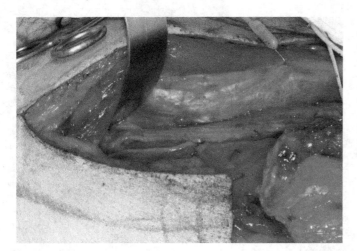

Figure 61.6. After mobilization of the flap paddle based on the musculocutaneous perforator, the perforator is traced back via retrograde dissection to its branching point from the descending branch of the lateral circumflex femoral artery, which lies in the intermuscular septum and was visualized by retracting the rectus femoris muscle medially.

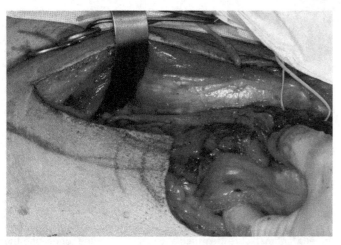

Figure 61.7. The vascular pedicle is dissected in the intermuscular septum, between the vastus lateralis muscle (VLM) and rectus femoris muscle, until appropriate pedicle length and caliber are achieved. The motor nerve to the VLM is dissected free from the pedicle and preserved.

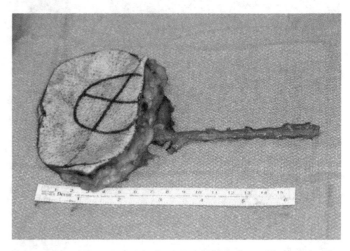

Figure 61.8. Harvested anterior lateral thigh flap with pedicle. The pedicle is divided, and the flap is taken once the recipient site is ready for inset.

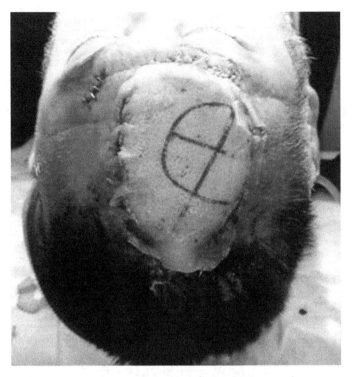

Figure 61.9. Free flap inset into the defect and microvascular anastomosis of the vascular pedicle was performed with the right superficial temporal artery and vein. Flap perfusion was confirmed with SPY and I-C green dye angiography. A closed suction drain was placed within the wound site, and incisions were closed in the usual layered manner.

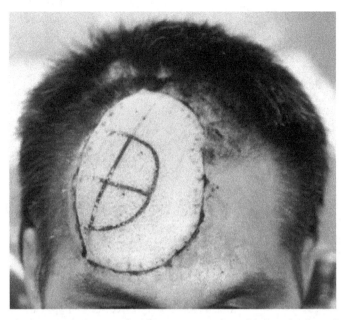

Figure 61.10. Four weeks after reconstruction with anterior lateral thigh free flap. The flap is viable and integrating well in the surrounding tissue. Note color discrepancy and transfer of hair-bearing tissue to the brow.

References

Addison, P.D., Lannon, D. and Neligan, P.C., 2008. Compartment syndrome after closure of the anterolateral thigh flap donor site: a report of two cases. *Annals of Plastic Surgery*, 60, 635–8.

Ayala, C. and Blackwell, K.E., 1999. Protein C deficiency in microvascular head and neck reconstruction. *Laryngoscope*, 109, 259–65.

Ceulemans, P. and Hofer, S.O., 2004. Flow-through anterolateral thigh flap for a free osteocutaneous fibula flap in secondary composite mandible reconstruction. *British Journal of Plastic Surgery*, 57, 358–61.

Hage, J.J. and Woerdeman, L.A., 2004. Lower limb necrosis after use of the anterolateral thigh free flap: is preoperative angiography indicated? *Annals of Plastic Surgery*, 52, 315–8.

Kimata, Y., Uchiyama, K., Ebihara, S., Nakatsuka, T. and Harii, K., 1998. Anatomic variations and technical problems of the anterolateral thigh flap: a report of 74 cases. *Plastic and Reconstructive Surgery*, 102, 1517–23.

Kimata, Y., Uchiyama, K., Ebihara, S., Sakuraba, M., Iida, H., Nakatsuka, T. and Harii, K., 2000. Anterolateral thigh flap donor-site complications and morbidity. *Plastic and Reconstructive Surgery*, 106, 584–9.

Koshima, I., Fukuda, H., Yamamoto, H., Moriguchi, T., Soeda, S. and Ohta, S., 1993. Free anterolateral thigh flaps for reconstruction of head and neck defects. *Plastic and Reconstructive Surgery*, 92, 421–8.

Lin, D.T., Coppit, G.L. and Burkey, B.B., 2004. Use of the anterolateral thigh flap for reconstruction of head and neck. *Current Opinion in Otolaryngology & Head and Neck Surgery*, 2, 300–4.

Mäkitie, A.A., Beasley, N.J., Neligan, P.C., Lipa, J. and Gullane, P.J., 2003. Head and neck reconstruction with anterolateral thigh flap. *Otolaryngology—Head and Neck Surgery*, 129, 547–55.

Shieh, S.J., Chiu, H.Y., Yu, J.C., Pan, S.C., Tsai, S.T. and Shen, C.L., 2000. Free anterolateral thigh flap for reconstruction of head and neck defects following cancer ablation. *Plastic and Reconstructive Surgery*, 105, 2349–57.

Song, Y.G., Chen, G.Z. and Song, Y.L., 1984. The free thigh flap: a new free flap concept based on the septocutaneous artery. *British Journal of Plastic Surgery*, 37, 149–59.

Wei, F.C., Jain, V., Celik, N., Chen HC., Chuang DC., Lin CH., 2002. Have we found an ideal soft-tissue flap? An experience with 672 anterolateral thigh flaps. *Plastic and Reconstructive Surgery*, 109, 2219–26.

Wolff, K.D., Kesting, M., Thurmüller, P., Böckmann, R. and Hölzle, F., 2006. The anterolateral thigh as a universal donor site for soft tissue reconstruction in maxillofacial surgery. *Journal of Craniomaxillofacial Surgery*, 34, 323–31.

Wong, C.H., Wei, F.C., Fu, B.K., Böckmann, R. and Hölzle, F., 2009. Alternative vascular pedicle of the anterolateral thigh flap: the oblique branch of the lateral circumflex femoral artery. *Plastic and Reconstructive Surgery*, 123, 571–7.

62

Nerve Repair

Andrew B.G. Tay[1] and John R. Zuniga[2]
[1]*Department of Oral and Maxillofacial Surgery, National Dental Centre, Singapore*
[2]*Department of Oral and Maxillofacial Surgery, Southwest Medical Center, Dallas, Texas, USA*

Procedure: Trigeminal Nerve Repair

A method of exploring and repairing significant injuries (Sunderland IV to V degree injuries) to injured trigeminal nerve branches: the inferior alveolar nerve (IAN), the lingual nerve (LN), and the infraorbital nerve (ION).

Indications

1. **Witnessed nerve injury**: Partial- or full-diameter nerve damage on direct visual inspection during surgery (including third molar surgery, orthognathic surgery, surgery for maxillofacial trauma, implant surgery, and pathology surgery). Repair at the earliest opportunity under microscopic magnification by a trained microsurgeon offers the best outcomes.

   Primary repair (immediate) is undertaken if conditions are favorable and there is access, microsurgical expertise, facilities, and time available
   Delayed primary repair (3–7 days) may be undertaken if the wound is contaminated or if the patient's condition, lack of microsurgical expertise, or facilities do not permit immediate repair
   Secondary repair (more than 1 week) may be undertaken if there is no improvement in clinical neurosensory testing

2. **Nerve injury with evidence of encroachment or disruption of the nerve canal** (mandibular and infraorbital) on imaging (computed tomography [CT] or cone beam CT).

3. **Nonwitnessed nerve injury**: Loss or alteration of sensation in the nerve distribution after trauma or injury, without visual evidence of damage but confirmed Sunderland IV or V degree injury by clinical neurosensory testing or adjunctive testing (magnetic resonance neurography, trigeminal nerve conduction, etc.).

4. **Nerve injury with neuropathic pain**: Evidenced by a history of spontaneous or stimulus-evoked burning pain or neuralgic pain in the nerve distribution, with or without allodynia, hyperpathia, or hyperalgesia confirmed by neuropathic pain testing.

5. **Chemical nerve injury**: Caustic agents have damaged the nerve (i.e., endodontic irrigation of socket in close proximity to the IAN).

Contraindications

1. Nerve injury with mild or improving sensory loss or with only partial involvement of the nerve distribution
2. Nerve injuries with mild or moderate sensory impairment by clinical neurosensory testing and with no evidence of nerve encroachment or disruption on imaging
3. Nerve injury in the context of life-threatening or more critical injuries, or in unfavorable situations (e.g., a contaminated wound, an unfit patient, or microsurgical expertise or facilities unavailable) for which delayed or secondary nerve repair would be reasonable
4. Nerve injury resulting from local anesthetic injections
5. Neuropathic pain of central trigeminal origin or sympathetically mediated pain source
6. Patient refusal to undergo nerve exploration and repair

Nonsurgical Management

1. Nonsurgical treatment options for nonpainful nerve injuries include observation, medical therapy in the early post-injury phase (e.g., vitamin B complex and steroids), and/or sensory retraining.
2. Nonsurgical treatment options for nerve injuries with neuropathic pain include medication (i.e., Gabapentin, Clonazepam, and Amitriptyline), therapeutic nerve blocks, physical therapy (i.e., TENS), and/or behavioral therapy.

Anatomy

Lingual nerve (LN): The LN is a branch of the mandibular division of the trigeminal nerve and descends between the medial pterygoid muscle and the ramus of the mandible. It is joined by the chorda tympani, a branch from the facial nerve, and 2 cm below the skull base. The chorda tympani carries taste fibers of the anterior two-thirds of the tongue. The LN lies anterior to the IAN and may be located at a variable height from the crest of the mandible (−2 mm to 7 mm). The LN may be located above the lingual plate in 10–17.6% of cases.

Atlas of Operative Oral and Maxillofacial Surgery, First Edition. Edited by Christopher J. Haggerty and Robert M. Laughlin

The LN may be in contact with the surface of the lingual cortex (22.3–62%) a maximum horizontal distance of 7 mm. The LN crosses the lateral surface of the hypoglossus muscle and passes deep to the mylohyoid muscle. It lies superior to the submandibular duct and then crosses downward along the lateral aspect of the duct to turn up along its medial side, on the genioglossus muscle. The LN supplies the tongue as it travels forward along its side. The LN is mono- or oligofascicular proximal to the point where the chorda tympani joins it, and it becomes polyfascicular near the submandibular ganglion. Its fascicular pattern changes every 126 mm on average from this point forward. The LN supplies sensation to the dorsum, lateral and ventral surfaces of the anterior two-thirds of the ipsilateral half of the tongue, mucous membrane of the ipsilateral floor of the mouth, and lingual gingivae of the mandibular teeth.

Inferior alveolar nerve (IAN): The IAN is a branch of the trigeminal mandibular division and descends below the lateral pterygoid muscle curving on the medial pterygoid muscle, to run between the sphenomandibular ligament and mandibular ramus, and to enter the mandibular foramen. The IAN gives off the mylohyoid branch at the mandibular foramen. The IAN travels with the inferior alveolar artery and vein within the mandibular canal, which descends and proceeds anteriorly in a concave curve and ascends to the mental foramen. The mandibular canal wall has a diameter of 2.0 to 2.4 mm and thins near the mental foramen in 60% to 80% of patients. The mandibular canal is located higher in the mandible in patients younger than 20 years of age and older than 60 years; it is, in order of vertical proximity, closest to the roots of the mandibular third molar, then the second molar, then the first molar, and furthest from the second premolar. The horizontal distance of the canal from the buccal cortex, in descending order, is the second mandibular molar, the first molar, and the third molar and second premolar. The mandibular canal curves superiorly and posterior-laterally to reach the mental foramen. The mental foramen is typically located at a third of the height of the mandible from the inferior border, and mesiodistally at the second or first premolar. Just before the mental foramen, the IAN branches into the incisive branch, which continues anteriorly under the apices of the incisors, and the mental nerve, which exits the mental foramen to enter the soft tissue as 1–4 branches (mean 2 branches) at an angle of 36° to the fibers of the orbicularis oris muscle. The IAN tends to be polyfascicular with a decreasing number of fascicles more distally; the fascicular pattern changes every 2 mm. The IAN supplies the ipsilateral lower lip (vermilion, skin, and mucosa), the chin, the labial-buccal alveolar mucosa from the midline to the molar region, and the ipsilateral teeth, with some midline crossover in 31% of cases.

Infraorbital nerve (ION): The ION is a branch of the maxillary division of the trigeminal nerve and enters the orbit through the inferior orbital fissure to progress forward with the infraorbital artery in the infraorbital groove, infraorbital canal, and infraorbital foramen. The infraorbital foramen is located roughly 8 mm (range 6.2–10.7 mm) below the infraorbital rim and is most commonly located in the same vertical plane as the first maxillary premolar. The foramen has a mean diameter of 4.5 mm (range 1–7 mm) and may present as multiple foramina (2–4) in 15% of cases. The ION exits the infraorbital foramen to lie between the levator labii superioris and the levator anguli oris muscles. Outside the foramen, the ION divides into several branches, including the inferior palpebral branches supplying the lower eyelid and cheek, the nasal branches supplying the lateral aspect and alar of the nose, and the superior labial branches supplying the upper lip and labial-buccal gingivae from the midline to the second premolar. While in the infraorbital canal, the ION gives off the anterior and middle superior alveolar branches that supply the maxillary incisors, canines, and premolars.

Surgical Technique for Trigeminal Nerve Repair

1. The patient is positioned supine. The surgical table is positioned to allow two surgeons to site on either side of the patient's head with an operating microscope (two operator eyepieces, microscope focal distance at 250 mm) over the patient's head.
2. General anesthesia via nasal endotracheal intubation with the tube pointing toward the patient's forehead. A throat pack should be placed.
3. For lingual nerve repair, a sandbag is placed under the patient's shoulders to elevate the mandible.
4. The skin and oral cavity are prepped, and local anesthetic containing epinephrine is injected within the operation site for pain control and hemostasis.

Lingual Nerve Repair

Access Phase

1. The operating surgeon sits on the same side as the operation site.
2. A modified Dingman mouth gag is utilized to position the mouth open, using the tongue blade to keep the tongue away from the operative site (Figure 62.1).
3. An intraoral mucosal incision is initiated with a No. 15 Bard–Parker scalpel over the ascending ramus to the distal of the mandibular second molar. A buccal extension from the distal of the molar to the buccal sulcus and a lingual extension to the lingual sulcus curving forward to the mandibular first molar are made. The buccal and lingual supraperiosteal flaps are raised with a periosteal elevator and Metzenbaum curved dissecting scissors.

The flaps are secured to the modified Dingman frame with 3-0 or 4-0 black silk sutures (Figure 62.2).

Preparation Phase

4. The operating microscope is positioned over the operative field.
5. The LN is exposed beginning at the healthy nerve proximal and distal to the injury site. Identification of the LN may be aided by locating its surrounding pouch of fat.
6. The proximal and distal nerve segments are carefully retracted with a vessel loop at each segment.
7. The nerve is released from the injury site (Figures 62.3 and 62.9), which is usually adherent to the lingual surface of the mandible, with careful microdissection using curved microscissors.
8. A modified background (1 × 1 inch neuropatty with the tubing of a small-gauge butterfly venipuncture system inserted and secured with silk sutures; the venipuncture needle is inserted into the lumen of an active suction tubing) is placed beneath the nerve injury site.
9. The nerve injury is examined under microscopic magnification (25×). The nerve injury may be a complete transection with a neuroma at each end of the nerve stump or a partial transection with a neuroma in continuity.
10. Excision of the neuroma is carefully performed with straight microscissors. The nerve ends are trimmed to expose the fascicular surfaces (Figure 62.4). The nerve site is irrigated with heparin–saline periodically.
11. The nerve segments are reapproximated using 6-0 or 7-0 monofilament sutures (Figure 62.5) passed through the epineurium of each segment to the adjacent muscle, so as to facilitate nerve repair without undue tension. A nerve gap of approximately 1 cm or more usually cannot be coapted without tension and will require a nerve graft (Figure 62.10).

Microsuture Phase

12. The trimmed nerve endings are coapted using the vasa nervorum as a guide to align the nerve segments. 8-0 or 9-0 monofilament sutures on a cutting needle are used to place sutures through the epineurium, including a little perineurium. The first suture is placed at the 12 o'clock position, leaving a longer strand. A second suture is placed at the 4 o'clock position. The suture strands are held in position with microforceps and "flip" the nerve over for access to the other side of the nerve. A similar suture is placed at the 8 o'clock position.
13. Sutures are placed within the intervening gaps at regular intervals in the coaptation site circumferentially. Typically, 6–8 sutures are required.
14. The repair site is examined, and excess suture length is trimmed.

15. Once nerve repair has been completed, the approximating suture and background are carefully removed. Gelfoam may be wrapped around the repaired nerve, and the nerve is placed carefully into its bed.

Wound Closure

16. The operating microscope is moved from the operative field.
17. The black silk sutures retracting the buccal and lingual mucosal flaps are released and removed.
18. The operative site is irrigated with saline and carefully suctioned.
19. The mucosal flaps are released, and the site is closed with 4-0 Vicryl interrupted sutures.
20. The modified Dingman mouth gag and the throat pack are removed.

Case Report

Case Report 62.1. A 20-year-old patient presents 4.5 months after loss of sensation after third molar surgery at an outside institution. On review of the cone beam CT, a small perforation of the lingual plate was noted, likely due to bur penetration. Conservative medical management was unsuccessful in relieving the patient's symptoms. Magnetic resonance imaging (MRI) was obtained that revealed a lingual nerve neuroma. The patient underwent successful left lingual nerve neuroma resection and neurorrhaphy with partial resolution of anesthesia. (See Figures 62.1, 62.2, 62.3, 62.4, and 62.5.)

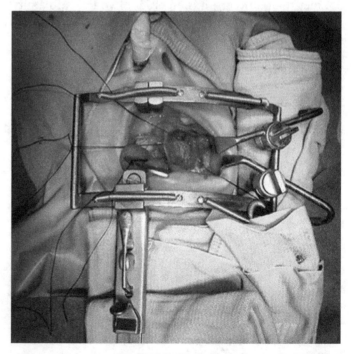

Figure 62.1. Access to the left lingual nerve using a modified Dingman–Zuniga mouth gag.

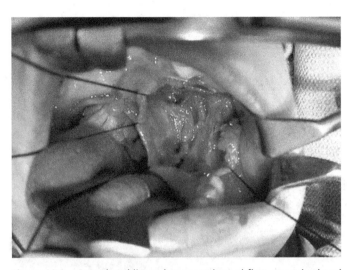

Figure 62.2.   Buccal and lingual supraperiosteal flaps are raised and secured to the modified Dingman–Zuniga frame with 3-0 black silk sutures.

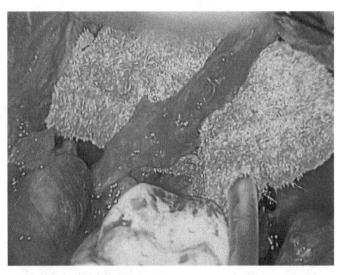

Figure 62.3.   The lingual nerve is released from its position adherent to the lingual surface of the mandible and isolated with a neuropatty as background. A neuroma-in-continuity is visible as a bulge along the lingual nerve.

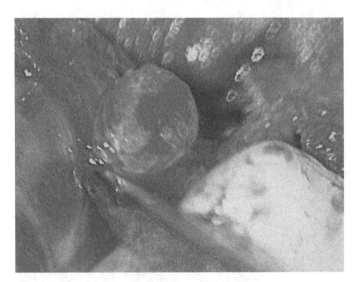

Figure 62.4.   The neuroma is resected, and the cut end of the nerve stump with its fasicles is visible.

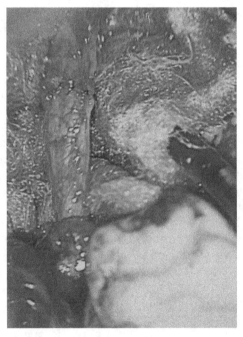

Figure 62.5.   The stumps of the lingual nerve are approximated with 7-0 Ethilon sutures and coapted with eight 8-0 Ethilon microsutures.

Inferior Alveolar Nerve Repair

Access Phase

1. The operating surgeon is positioned on the opposite side of the operation site. The patient's head is turned to the side opposite of the operation site.
2. An incision is initiated with a No. 15 Bard–Parker scalpel just above the mandibular sulcus from the midline of the lower lip posteriorly to the ascending ramus.
3. A subperiosteal flap is raised to expose the mandible from the alveolus to the inferior border, including the mental foramen. The mental nerve is carefully preserved.
4. A window is created circumferentially around the mental foramen by using a small round bur to make grooves that radiate outward from the mental foramen, then are joined to form windows (Figure 62.6). The windows are carefully fractured with either a Coupland or Warwick–James elevator, taking care to avoid the mental nerve. A window is created within the buccal bone over the course of the IAN until the nerve is exposed to 1 cm beyond the injury site (Figure 62.7).
5. A scalpel is used to sharply divide the incisive branch and carefully dissect the IAN free from its bed.

Preparation Phase

6. The operating microscope is positioned over the operative field.
7. The proximal and distal nerve segments are lifted from the mandibular bone with a nerve hook, and a modified neuropatty background is placed beneath the nerve segments.
8. The nerve injury is examined under microscopic magnification. The nerve injury may be a complete transection or a partial transection with a neuroma in continuity.
9. The neuroma is carefully excised with straight microscissors, and the nerve ends are trimmed to expose the fascicular surfaces. The nerve site is irrigated with heparin–saline periodically.
10. The nerve segments are approximated using 6-0 or 7-0 monofilament sutures (Figure 62.8) passed through the epineurium of each segment to the adjacent muscle, so as to facilitate nerve repair without undue tension. The distal nerve segment can usually be transposed toward the proximal segment, so a nerve graft is less likely to be necessary.

   Microsuture phase: Follow steps 12–15 of the "Microsuture Phase" subsection of the "Lingual Nerve (LN) Repair" section.
   Wound closure: Follow steps 16–20 of the "Wound Closure" subsection of the "Lingual Nerve (LN) Repair" section.

Case Report

Case Report 62.2. A 39-year-old patient presents 5 months after the extraction of full bony impacted tooth #17. The patient developed paresthesia, followed by allodynia. Conservative medical management was unsuccessful in relieving the patient's symptoms. An MRI was obtained that revealed an inferior alveolar neuroma. The patient underwent successful left inferior alveolar nerve neuroma resection and neurorrhaphy with resolution of allodynia. (See Figures 62.6, 62.7, and 62.8.)

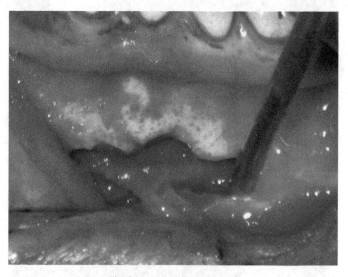

Figure 62.6. Removal of bone around the left mental foramen to expose the distal part of the left inferior alveolar nerve and the incisive branch.

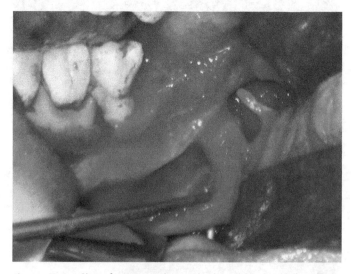

Figure 62.7. Site of neuroma-in-continuity within the left inferior alveolar nerve.

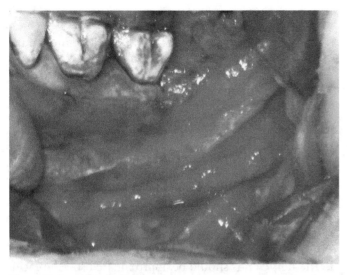

Figure 62.8. Left inferior alveolar nerve neuroma resected and neurorrhaphy completed.

Infraorbital Nerve Repair

Access Phase

The operating surgeon is positioned on the opposite side of the operation site. Depending on the site of the ION injury, two approaches may be used:

1. **Cutaneous approach**: Utilized when the nerve injury site is proximal to the infraorbital foramen
2. **Intraoral approach**: Utilized when the nerve injury site is distal to the infraorbital foramen.

Cutaneous Approach

1. The globe is protected with a temporary tarsorrhaphy using a 4-0 silk suture or a scleral shell.
2. The subciliary incision line is marked with a skin marker approximately 2 mm inferior to the eyelashes along the length of the lower eyelid. The incision may be extended laterally 2 cm beyond the lateral canthus, curving inferior-laterally along a skin crease.
3. The subciliary incision is initiated with a No. 15 Bard–Parker scalpel to the subcutaneous layer, so that the underlying orbicularis oculi muscle is exposed.
4. Dissect subcutaneously with sharp curved scissors inferiorly toward the inferior orbital rim. The dissection proceeds through the orbicularis oculi muscle with scissors to the periosteum overlying the inferior orbital rim. A tissue plane between the muscle and septum orbitale is identified.
5. A skin–muscle flap is elevated from the lower eyelid. The periosteum over the inferior orbital rim is incised with a No. 15 Bard–Parker scalpel a few millimeters below the inferior orbital rim edge. The periosteum is elevated with a periosteal elevator until the infraorbital foramen is reached (7–9 mm inferior to the inferior orbital rim).

6. A groove is created around the infraorbital foramen with a small round bur. Bone is removed from the foramen carefully with Rongeur forceps. The ION is exposed by carefully unroofing the infraorbital canal to 1 cm beyond the nerve injury site.

Intraoral Approach

7. An intraoral vestibular incision is initiated within the unattached mucosa of the maxillary vestibule from the midline to the zygomatic process.
8. A subperiosteal flap is raised from the maxilla to expose the infraorbital foramen.
9. A groove is created around the infraorbital foramen with a small round bur. The bone from the periphery of the foramen is carefully removed with Rongeur forceps.

Preparation Phase

10. The operating microscope is positioned over the operative field.
11. The proximal and distal nerve segments are lifted from the bone with a nerve hook, and a modified neuropatty background is placed beneath the nerve segments.
12. The nerve injury is examined under microscopic magnification. The nerve injury may be a complete transection or a partial transection with a neuroma in continuity.
13. The neuroma is carefully excised with straight microscissors, and the nerve ends are trimmed to expose the fascicular surfaces. The nerve site is irrigated with heparin–saline periodically.
14. The nerve segments are approximated using 6-0 or 7-0 monofilament sutures passed through the epineurium of each segment to the adjacent muscle, so as to facilitate nerve repair without undue tension.

    Microsuture phase: Follow steps 12–15 of the "Microsuture Phase" subsection of the "Lingual Nerve (LN) Repair" section.

Wound Closure

15. The operating microscope is removed from the operative field.
16. The operative site is irrigated with saline and suctioned carefully.
17. The periosteum is closed with 4-0 Vicryl interrupted sutures. The skin is reapproximated with 4-0 silk interrupted sutures or with a running 6-0 monofilament suture.
18. The intraoral mucosal flap is closed with 4-0 Vicryl interrupted sutures.
19. The throat pack is removed.

Postoperative Management

1. Analgesics are prescribed routinely, especially if bone was involved.
2. Antibiotics are not routinely prescribed, unless a concurrent infection, wound contamination, or systemic risk of immunosuppression is present.
3. Chlorhexidine mouth rinse is prescribed.
4. Patients are advised to maintain a soft diet for the first week postoperatively.
5. Patients are typically discharged the same or next day after surgery, and they return to normal activities after 1 week.

Complications

1. **Intraoperative bleeding**: More common if the mandibular cancellous bone is entered. Bleeding can usually be arrested with local measures such as diathermy or packing hemostatic agents within the site of concern.
2. **Infection**: Managed with antibiotics and chlorhexidine rinse. Incision and drainage are indicated if an abscess is identified.
3. **Wound dehiscence**: Often due to excessive flap tension on closure. Managed with regular irrigation or rinsing with chlorhexidine.
4. **Pathologic fracture of the mandible**: The presence of sudden onset of pain, malocclusion, and/or swelling should alert one to the possibility of a fracture. A fracture should be excluded or confirmed via a thorough examination and radiographs. Depending on the clinical requirements, observation with antibiotics and a nonchew diet, closed or open reduction, and fixation may be necessary.
5. **Trismus**: A common sequela of surgery and typically self-limiting, with a return to normal mouth opening after 2–3 weeks. Analgesics, a soft diet, and passive jaw-opening exercises may be helpful.
6. **Inability to locate one nerve segment**: If the proximal nerve segment cannot be found, the distal nerve segment may be connected via nerve share to another nerve (i.e., a cross-mental nerve graft using the sural nerve from the distal IAN segment to the contralateral incisive branch). If the distal nerve segment cannot be found, the proximal nerve segment should be repositioned (i.e., nerve end buried in muscle to avoid neuroma formation).
7. **Failure to gain sensory improvement**: Occurs in 20–40% of nerve repair patients with nonpainful injuries. Persistence of neuropathic pain may be seen in 30–40% of nerve repair patients with painful injuries.
8. **Neuropathic pain**: The development of neuropathic pain after nerve repair is exceedingly rare.

Key Points

1. Appropriate patient positioning at the beginning of the procedure is key to maintaining microsurgeon comfort throughout the surgery.
2. The use of an operating microscope with two operator eyepieces, a video feed (preferable), and the appropriate focal distance of 250 mm is ideal for most microsurgery procedures.
3. Appropriate microsurgical instruments with a bayonet design and 18 cm in length should be utilized. Microsurgical instruments should be demagnetized before surgery. Bipolar diathermy and two suction tubings should be available.
4. Locate the nerve and release the injury site with careful microdissection under microscopic magnification.
5. The nerve ends should be approximated so as to facilitate coaptation without tension.
6. A nerve graft is necessary if the nerve gap is long, usually 1 cm or more.

References

Epker, B.N. and Gregg, J.M., 1992. Surgical management of maxillary nerve injuries. *Oral and Maxillofacial Surgery Clinics of North America*, 4, 439–45.

Gregg, J.M., 1992. Surgical management of lingual nerve injuries. *Oral and Maxillofacial Surgery Clinics of North America*, 4, 417–24.

LaBanc, J.P. and Van Boven, R.W., 1992. Surgical management of inferior alveolar nerve injuries. *Oral and Maxillofacial Surgery Clinics of North America*, 4, 425–37.

Robinson, P.P., et al., 2004. Current management of damage to the inferior alveolar and lingual nerves as a result of removal of third molars. *British Journal of Oral and Maxillofacial Surgery*, 42, 285–92.

Zuniga, J.R. and Essick, G.K., 1992. A contemporary approach to the clinical evaluation of trigeminal nerve injuries. *Oral and Maxillofacial Surgery Clinics of North America*, 4, 353–67.

Procedure: Nerve Graft and Harvest

A method of bridging nerve injuries with long gaps (usually 1 cm or more) that cannot be approximated without excessive tension.

Indications

1. As for nerve repair, but where the nerve gap is too large for coaptation of nerve stumps without tension.
   A. *Intermediate-span nerve injuries* (1 to 3 cm gap) may occur from direct rotary instrument injury (i.e., bur penetration of the lingual mandibular bone to catch the lingual nerve), lacerative or crush injury (i.e., implant surgery or rigid fixation for fracture or orthognathic surgery), chemical injury (i.e., inadvertent injection of endodontic chemicals through a root canal into the mandibular canal), or thermal

injury (i.e., diathermy for hemostasis in close proximity to a nerve)

B. *Long-span nerve injuries* (more than 3 cm gap) may occur from avulsive maxillofacial trauma (i.e., gunshot wound), ablative surgery for intraosseous tumors, or multiple-point injury (i.e., bone plate or screw fixation)

Contraindications

1. Recipient site is infected or contaminated, is significantly scarred, or has poor vascularity (e.g., previously irradiated). Delayed nerve grafting may be considered after recipient site infection or contamination has been resolved
2. Donor site was previously operated on, injured, or diseased
3. Neuropathic pain of central trigeminal origin or sympathetically mediated pain source
4. Patient refusal to undergo nerve grafting

Autogenous nerve grafting remains the gold standard for bridging a significant nerve gap. The most common autogenous donor nerves for trigeminal nerve repair are the sural nerve (SN) and the great auricular nerve (GAN). Other potential donor nerves are the saphenous dorsal cutaneous branch of the ulnar nerve, the medial antebrachial cutaneous nerve, and the lateral antebrachial cutaneous nerve.

Where a nerve graft is necessary but autogenous nerve grafting is not possible, other alternatives include:

A. Autogenous vein grafts
B. Autogenous frozen-thawed muscle grafts
C. Nerve allografts

   Avance (human decellularized nerve allograft; AxoGen Inc., Alachua, FL, US)

D. Resorbable nerve conduits or guides

   Neurotube (polyglycolic acid; Synovis Life Technologies, St. Paul, MN, US)
   Neurolac (polylactide-caprolactone; Polyganics Inc., Groningen, the Netherlands)
   NeuraGen (semipermeable collagen; Integra Life-Sciences, Plainsboro, NJ, US)

Autogenous vein or muscle grafts may be considered for intermediate-length nerve gaps that are between 1 and 3 cm. For nerve gaps longer than 3 cm, a nerve allograft is the preferred method of treatment.

Anatomy

Sural nerve (SN): The SN is located in the posterior aspect of the lower leg, commencing at the popliteal fossa, between the heads of the gastrocnemius muscle. The SN classically forms from the confluence of the medial sural cutaneous nerve and the peroneal communicating branch (60% of the time), which arises from the lateral sural cutaneous nerve (or, less commonly, the common peroneal nerve). The SN may continue directly from the medial sural cutaneous nerve alone (37% of the time), or, rarely, from the lateral sural cutaneous nerve (3% of the time). The SN continues inferiorly from the medial to lateral aspect of the posterior lower leg to lie consistently in the space between the lateral malleolus and the calcanean (Achilles') tendon. The SN distal to the level of the lateral malleolus gives off branches in the foot. The median length of the SN measured from the distal point of the lateral malleolus proximally to the confluence of the medial sural cutaneous nerve and peroneal communicating branch measures 20 cm (Riedl *et al.*, 2008). The SN average diameter is 2.1 mm, about 88% of the IAN and 66% of the LN. It is oligofascicular with small-diameter fascicles. The axon number and axon size are significantly lower (approximately 50% or less) than those of the IAN and LN; its axon density is lower but comparable to that of the IAN and LN. The SN supplies the cutaneous sensation of the posterior and lateral aspect of the distal lower leg, the lateral aspect of the heel and foot, and the little toe.

Great auricular nerve (GAN): The GAN forms from the second and third cervical nerves and emerges at about midheight of the neck from behind the posterior border of the sternocleidomastoid muscle (SCM). The GAN then travels superiorly, just posterior and parallel to the external jugular vein on the lateral surface of the SCM, and enters the lower pole of the parotid gland. The GAN lies deep to the platysma muscle and superficial to the superficial layer of the cervical fascia. The GAN branches in its distal third 37% of the time and measures 6.5 cm on average (range 5.5–9.0 cm). Its average diameter is 1.5 mm, about 63% of the IAN and 47% of the LN. The GAN is oligofascicular with fewer fascicles than the IAN and LN. Its axon number is significantly lower than that of the IAN and LN, but its axon size and axon density are comparable to those of the IAN and LN. The GAN supplies part of the facial skin over the parotid gland, the parotid fascia, and the auricular skin (cranial surface and lower lateral surface [earlobe] below the external acoustic meatus).

Surgical Technique for Trigeminal Nerve Graft Repair

1. The choice of the donor nerve graft site, the anticipated sensory loss, and the side are discussed with the patient prior to surgery. For a sural nerve graft, the nonmaster (usually left) leg is selected as the donor site.
2. Patient positioning, general anesthesia via nasal endotracheal intubation, preparation, and local anesthesia are dependent on the operative site (i.e., LN, IAN, or ION).

3. For a sural nerve graft and if resources allow, a second surgical team may be used to harvest the sural nerve graft once its need is confirmed.

4. The recipient injured nerve should be exposed and prepared, with excision of any neuroma or damaged nerve tissue, so that the recipient nerve stumps are ready for coaptation with the nerve graft. The nerve gap is measured to determine the length of nerve graft required prior to graft harvest.

Sural Nerve Graft

Access

1. The donor leg is flexed and turned, exposing the lateral aspect of the lower leg to the surgeon. The location of the sural nerve is surface marked with a skin marker.

2. A 2 cm horizontal incision is created with a No. 15 Bard–Parker scalpel 1 fingerbreadth distal and superior to the lateral malleolus of the ankle.

3. The skin edges are retracted, and a pair of curved artery forceps is utilized to dissect the subcutaneous tissues to expose the sural nerve and the small saphenous vein and artery superficial to the fascia of the posterior tibialis muscle.

4. The sural nerve is isolated from the vein and artery using vessel loops and dissected with a nerve hook distally and proximally to the desired length (Figure 62.11) (nerve gap distance + 25%). Normally, a 20 to 30 mm length of sural nerve can be harvested through a single incision (Figure 62.12).

5. If a greater length is required, a second incision is made proximal and parallel to the first incision, at about the distance equal to the desired length of nerve.

Harvesting

6. The distal end of the sural nerve is transected sharply, and the nerve is exteriorized to the length required for grafting the measured nerve gap. The distal donor nerve end can be allowed to retract in place.

7. The proximal end of the sural nerve is transected sharply, leaving at least 1 cm of proximal nerve.

8. The harvested sural nerve graft is measured and transferred to the recipient site in saline-soaked gauze. The ends of the nerve graft are inspected under microscopic magnification, and any excess tissue is trimmed so that the ends are prepared for coaptation. The nerve graft is microsutured to the recipient nerve ends using 8-0 or 9-0 monofilament sutures on a cutting needle, in a similar technique as for direct nerve repair, taking into account any difference in size between the graft and recipient nerve ends.

   Donor stump burial: The proximal stump of the donor sural nerve is repositioned into muscle to avoid painful neuroma formation.

9. A U-shaped incision is made with a No. 15 Bard–Parker scalpel within the posterior tibialis muscle fascia, thus creating a "trapdoor" with its "hinge" on its distal edge.

10. The fascial "trapdoor" is elevated to expose the tibialis muscle.

11. The proximal nerve stump end is sutured to the muscle using 5-0 or 6-0 resorbable sutures.

12. The fascial "trapdoor" is closed over the sutured stump.

Wound Closure

13. The subcutaneous layer is closed with 4-0 resorbable sutures, and the skin is closed with subcuticular continuous 6-0 resorbable sutures.

14. The wound edges are reinforced with steri-strips.

15. The wound is covered with a dressing, gauze, and a light bandage.

Case Report

Case Report 62.3. A 33-year-old patient with witnessed complete transection of the left lingual nerve (Sunderland V) during third molar surgery. A primary LN repair was attempted by the operating surgeon, and the patient was followed with weekly neurosensory testing. The patient developed a complete loss of sensation and was referred to a microsurgeon for evaluation and repair. The left LN was explored, and a neuroma-in-continuity (Figure 62.9) was identified and resected, resulting in a 9 mm nerve gap (Figure 62.10). An interpositional graft was performed with harvest of the SN (Figures 62.11 and 62.12) and a tension-free repair (Figure 62.13). Figure 62.14 shows the scar of the nerve donor site 1 year posteratively.

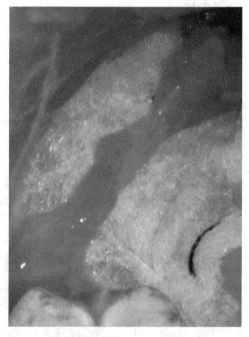

Figure 62.9. Left lingual nerve isolated showing a neuroma-in-continuity.

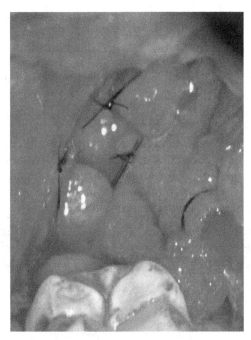

Figure 62.10. Left lingual nerve neuroma resected, leaving a 9 mm gap that could not be approximated without excessive tension.

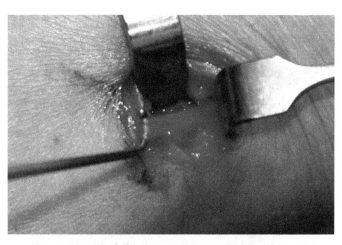

Figure 62.11. Left sural nerve has been exposed and isolated.

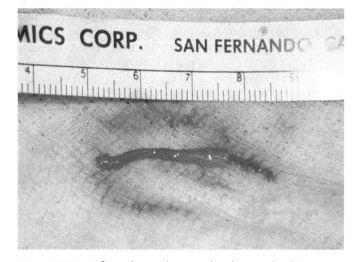

Figure 62.12. Left sural nerve harvested and measuring 25 mm.

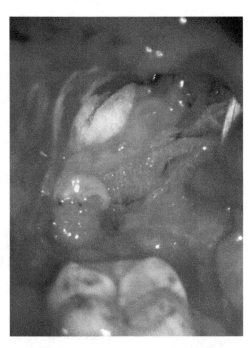

Figure 62.13. Left sural nerve microsutured to bridge the gap in the left lingual nerve.

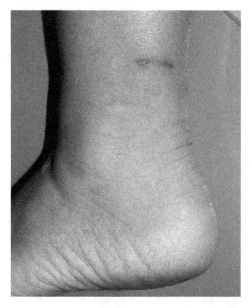

Figure 62.14. Scar of left sural nerve donor site 1 year after surgery.

Great Auricular Nerve Graft

Access

1. The surgeon sits on the same side as the donor neck, and the patient's head is turned to the opposite side. The location of the GAN is surface marked with a skin marker.
2. A 2 cm horizontal incision is created with a No. 15 Bard–Parker scalpel in a skin crease two-thirds of the way up the neck, over the posterior margin of the sternocleidomastoid muscle. Alternatively, if there is already submandibular access to the mandible, the skin incision can be extended posteriorly to the neck.
3. The skin edges are retracted, and curved artery forceps are utilized to dissect the subcutaneous tissues to expose the GAN, taking care to avoid damaging the external jugular vein.
4. The GAN is isolated using vessel loops and dissected superiorly to the desired length (nerve gap distance + 25%). Normally, a 20–40 mm length of GAN can be harvested. Because the GAN diameter tends to be smaller than that of the recipient nerve, it may be necessary to harvest twice the length of the nerve gap for a cable graft.

Harvesting

5. The distal (superior) end of the GAN is transected sharply, then followed by the proximal end, leaving a short stump.

6. The harvested nerve graft is measured and transferred to the recipient site. The ends of the nerve graft are inspected under microscopic magnification, and any excess tissue is trimmed so that the ends are prepared for coaptation. The nerve graft is microsutured to the recipient nerve ends using 8-0 or 9-0 monofilament suture on a cutting needle, in the same method as a direct nerve repair.
7. If a cable graft is necessary, the harvested nerve graft is measured and sharply divided into two equal segments. The nerve graft segment ends are inspected and prepared for coaptation, laid side by side in the recipient site, and microsutured to the recipient nerve ends.

Donor stump burial: The proximal stump of donor nerve is repositioned into muscle to avoid painful neuroma formation. (See Figures 62.15, 62.16, and 62.17.)

8. A U-shaped incision is made with a No. 15 Bard–Parker scalpel in the superficial cervical fascia over the sternocleidomastoid muscle, thus creating a trapdoor.
9. The fascial trapdoor is elevated to expose the sternocleidomastoid muscle.
10. The proximal nerve stump end is sutured to the muscle using 5-0 or 6-0 resorbable sutures.
11. The fascial trapdoor is closed over the sutured stump.

Wound Closure

12. The subcutaneous layer is closed with 4-0 resorbable sutures, and the skin closed with interrupted 6-0 monofilament sutures.

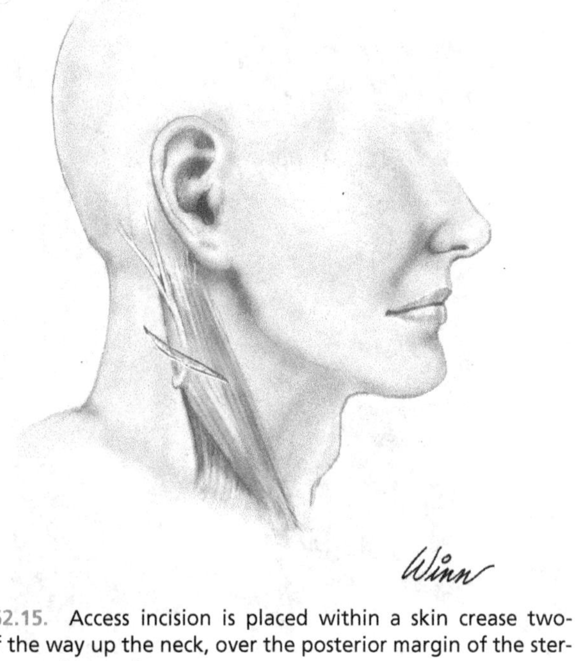

Figure 62.15. Access incision is placed within a skin crease two-thirds of the way up the neck, over the posterior margin of the sternocleidomastoid muscle.

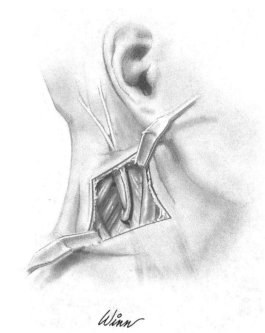

Figure 62.16. Exposure of the great auricular nerve. Care should be taken to avoid damage to the external jugular vein.

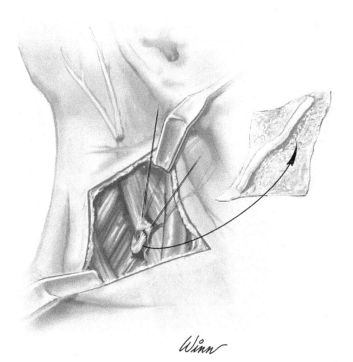

Figure 62.17.   The distal (superior) end of the great auricular nerve is transected sharply, followed by the proximal end, leaving a short stump. The proximal stump of the donor nerve is repositioned into muscle to avoid painful neuroma formation. A U-shaped incision is made in the superficial cervical fascia over the sternocleidomastoid muscle, thus creating a "trapdoor." The proximal nerve stump end is sutured to the muscle, and the fascia is closed.

13. The wound is covered with antibiotic ointment and a dressing.

Postoperative Management

1. Analgesics, antibiotics, and chlorhexidine mouth rinse are prescribed.
2. Patients are advised to maintain a soft diet for the first week.
3. Patients are typically discharged the next day and can return to normal activities after 1–2 weeks.
4. Patients who have undergone sural nerve grafting are given walking aids and instructed to avoid weight bearing on the donor leg for 2 weeks.

Complications

1. **Intraoperative bleeding**: Controlled by diathermy or by tying off any bleeding vessels.
2. **Infection**: Managed with antibiotics and chlorhexidine rinse. Incision and drainage are indicated if an abscess is identified.
3. **Wound dehiscence**: Managed with daily wound care and dressing.

4. **Hypertrophic scar formation**: Treated with steroid injections and/or scar revision after 6 months.
5. **Neuroma formation**: May require revision surgery to remove the neuroma and to bury the nerve stump in muscle to prevent recurrent neuroma formation.
6. **Failure to gain sensory improvement**: Sensory improvement with a nerve graft is generally not as good as with direct nerve repair as there is the greater impediment of a double repair site and additional distance for axonal regeneration.
7. **Loss of sensation in donor nerve distribution**: Expected outcome. For sural nerve grafts, the area of sensory loss involves the lateral surface of the heel and foot and sometimes the little toe. SN sensory loss does not involve the sole of the foot; therefore, there should be no impediment to normal function of the foot after recovery. For GAN grafts, the area of sensory loss usually involves the earlobe and the skin around it.

Key Points

1. The possibility of donor nerve graft and the choice of donor site and side, including the risks of nerve grafting (i.e., loss of sensation in the donor nerve distribution), should be discussed with the patient prior to surgery.
2. Prep and drape the donor site when prepping the main operation site.
3. Use a separate set of instruments for nerve graft harvesting from those used in the oral cavity.
4. If resources permit, have a second surgical team available to harvest the sural nerve graft.
5. It is advised to harvest a nerve graft with an additional 25% of length than the nerve gap distance because the harvested graft will contract. However, excessively long nerve grafts yield a lower predictability due to the longer distance for axonal regeneration.
6. The GAN tends to be smaller than the recipient IAN or LN, and a longer length (double that of the recipient nerve gap) may be required for a cable graft.
7. The recipient bed must be well vascularized for the nerve graft to be successful.
8. The nerve graft should be oriented in the same functional direction from which it was harvested (i.e., the donor proximal end should be connected to the recipient proximal stump).
9. A lower quality of sensory improvement should be expected when a nerve graft is used, compared to direct nerve repair, because there are two repair sites instead of one. The age and health of the patient, the nature of the nerve injury, and the quality of microsurgery will also influence the quality of sensory improvement.

References

Brammer, J.P. and Epker, B.N., 1988. Anatomic-histologic survey of the sural nerve: implications for inferior alveolar nerve grafting. *Journal of Oral and Maxillofacial Surgery*, 46, 111–17.

Eppley, B.L. and Synders, R.V., Jr., 1991. Microanatomic analysis of the trigeminal nerve and potential nerve graft donor sites. *Journal of Oral and Maxillofacial Surgery*, 49, 612–18.

Rayatt, S.S., et al., 1998. Histological analysis of the greater auricular nerve and its use as a graft. *Clinics in Otolaryngology*, 23, 368–71.

Riedl, O., et al., 2008. Sural nerve harvesting beyond the popliteal region allows a significant gain of donor nerve graft length. *Plastic and Reconstructive Surgery*, 122, 798–805.

Schultz, J.D., et al., 1992. Donor site morbidity of greater auricular nerve graft harvesting. *Journal of Oral and Maxillofacial Surgery*, 50, 803–5.

Wolford, L. and Rodrigues, D.B., 2011. Peripheral trigeminal nerve injury, repair, and regeneration. Autogenous grafts/allografts/conduits for bridging peripheral trigeminal nerve gaps. *Atlas of Oral and Maxillofacial Surgery Clinics of North America*, 19, 91–107.

Antibiotic Chart

Matthew W. Hearn, Christopher T. Vogel, Robert M. Laughlin, and Christopher J. Haggerty

Antibiotic	Brand name	Class	Route	Dosage	Interval	Bacteriostatic or bacteriocidal	Cost per dose	Pregnancy category	Pediatric dose (>28 days)
Amoxicillin	Amoxil	Aminopenicillin	PO	500 mg	q8h	Bacteriocidal	$0.08–0.16	B	25–50 mg/kg/day divided TID
Amoxicillin–clavulanate	Augmentin	Aminopenicillin and beta-lactamase inhibitor	PO	875/125 mg	q12h	Bacteriocidal	$0.75	B	45–90 mg/kg/day divided BID
Azithromycin	Zithromax	Macrolide	PO	250 mg (Z-Pack)	As instructed	Bacteriostatic	$26.00/pack	B	10 mg/kg q24h
Cephalexin	Keflex	First-generation cephalosporin	PO	500 mg	q6h	Bacteriocidal	$0.125	B	25–50 mg/kg/day divided q6h
Clindamycin	Cleocin	Lincosamide	PO	300–450 mg	q6–8h	Bacteriostatic	$0.16–0.50	B	20–40 mg/kg/day divided q8h
Doxycyline	Vibramycin	Tetracycline	PO	100 mg	q12h	Bacteriostatic	$2.50	D	2–4 mg/kg/day divided q12h; not recommended for children <8 years of age
Levofloxacin	Levaquin	Fluoroquinolones	PO	750 mg	q24h	Bacteriocidal	$0.25–0.50	C	Not recommended
Metronidazole	Flagyl	Nitroimidazole	PO	500 mg	TID	Bacteriocidal	$0.33	B	30 mg/kg/day divided q8h
Moxifloxacin	Avelox	Fluoroquinolones	PO	400 mg	q24h	Bacteriocidal	$9.10	C	Not recommended
Pencillin VK	Pen V-K	Natural penicillin	PO	500 mg	q6h	Bacteriocidal	$0.125–0.25	B	25–50 mg/kg/day divided q6–8h
Trimethiprim–sulfamethoxazole (TMP-SMX)	Bactrim DS	Sulfonamides and trimethoprim	PO	160/800 mg	q12h	Bacteriostatic	$0.25	C	6–12 mg/kg/day divided q12h (greater than 2 months of age)
Clindamycin	Cleocin	Lincosamide	IV	900 mg	q8h	Bacteriostatic	$2.66–5.33	B	20–40 mg/kg/day divided q8h
Meropenem	Merrem	Carbapenem	IV	1 g	q8h	Bacteriocidal	$11.00	B	60–120 mg/kg/day divided q8h
Penicillin G	Penicillin G	Natural penicillin	IV	2–4 MU	q4h	Bacteriocidal	$8.33–16.66	B	50,000 U/kg/day

(continued)

Atlas of Operative Oral and Maxillofacial Surgery, First Edition. Edited by Christopher J. Haggerty and Robert M. Laughlin
© 2015 John Wiley & Sons, Inc. Published 2015 by John Wiley & Sons, Inc.

Antibiotic	Brand name	Class	Route	Dosage	Interval	Bacteriostatic or bacteriocidal	Cost per dose	Pregnancy category	Pediatric dose (>28 days)
Ceftriaxone	Rocephin	Third-generation cephalosporin	IV	1–2 g	q24h	Bacteriocidal	$1.50–2.50	B	50 mg/kg/day
Ampicilllin-Sulbactam	Unasyn	Aminopenicillin and beta-lactamase inhibitor	IV	3 g	q6h	Bacteriocidal	$3.50	B	100–300 mg/kg/day divided q6h
Vancomycin	Vancomycin	Glycopeptide	IV	15–20 mg/kg	q8–12h	Bacteriocidal	$13.00–20.00	C	40 mg/kg/day divided q6h
Piperacillin–tazobactam	Zosyn	Ureidopenicillin and beta-lactamase inhibitor	IV	3.375 g	q6h	Bacteriocidal	$4.37	B	100 mg/kg/day divided q6h
Penicilin G	Bicillin L-A	Natural penicillin	IM	1.2 MU	Once	Bacteriocidal	$36.07	B	50,000 U/kg one time dose

Note: q6h, every 6 hours; q8h, every 8 hours; q12h, every 12 hours; q24h, daily; BID, twice daily; TID, three times daily. Cost reflects price to pharmacy directly from manufacturer. Cost to patient will vary depending on providing pharmacy.

References

Bertlett, J.G., Auwaeter, P.G. and Pham, P.A., 2012. *Johns Hopkins ABX Guide 2012.* 3rd ed. Burlington, MA: Jones & Bartlett Learning.

Gilbert, D.N., Moellering, R.C., Jr., Eliopoulos, G.M., Chambers, H.F. and Saag, M.S., eds., 2012. *The Sanford Guide to Antimicrobial Therapy 2012.* 41st ed. Sperryville, VA: Antimicrobial Therapy, Inc.

Salkind, A. and Kallenberger, M., eds., 2014. *Truman Medical Center 2014 Antimicrobial Guide.* Truman Medical Center Antimicrobial Stewardship Team.

2 Craniofacial Surgery Timing Chart

Jeremiah Jason Parker and Christopher T. Vogel

Age	Procedure	Timing	Comments
3 months	Repair of cleft lip	3 months	Historically performed after 10 weeks, when weight is greater than 10 lbs. and hemoglobin is greater than 10 dl/mg. This "rule of tens" was originally based on anesthetic risk. Traditionally, however, most cleft lip repairs are undertaken around 3 months of age as no significant benefit has been identified with earlier repair.
7–18 months	Repair of cleft palate	7–18 months	The timing of palatal surgery must balance the need for normal speech development against potential growth disturbances encountered after early surgery. There is an increased risk for developing maxillary hypoplasia when palatal repair is performed prior to 9 months of age. However, by 18 months of age, most children will require an intact palate for normal speech development.
3–5 years	Pharyngoplasty	3–5 years	The diagnosis of velopharyngeal insufficiency (VPI) may not be possible before the age of 3 as a result of testing difficulties in such young children. In most cases, reliable testing can be accomplished between 3 and 5 years of age. Surgical intervention is based on the individual child's speech and phonemic age, however, rather than simply chronologic age.
6–9 years	Orthodontics	6–9 years (initiated)	Interceptive orthodontics may begin during the primary dentition stage, but it is more commonly started in mixed dentition, between 6 and 9 years of age, after the first molars have erupted. Traditional orthodontics typically begins after exfoliation of the primary dentition. Completion depends on the need for orthognathic surgery, dental arch maintenance and grafting, and restorative options.
6–9 years	Dentoalveolar cleft repair	6–9 years (based on dental development)	Although it remains a subject of controversy, secondary bone grafting of maxillary dentoalveolar clefts appears to be best accomplished in the stage of mixed dentition before canine eruption, ideally between ages 6–9 years. In addition, higher success rates have been achieved when grafting is performed prior to the eruption of the tooth located distal to the cleft.
14–16 years (F); 16–18 years (M)	Orthognathic surgery	14–16 years (female); 16–18 years (male)	Best accomplished after cessation of facial-skeletal growth to avoid complications with relapse. Most females undergo surgical correction between 14 and 16 years of age, whereas males typically undergo surgery between ages 16 and 18 years. Exact timing is based on individual growth characteristics.
16–18 years	Dental implant placement	16–18 years	Best accomplished after orthognathic surgery once the dentoalveolar arches have been established and facial-skeletal growth is complete. Additional bone grafting may be indicated prior to implant placement.
18–21 years	Rhinoplasty	18–21 years	Ideally, the dental arch should be established, skeletal maturity achieved, and maxillary hypoplasia corrected before surgical repair of most nasal deformities. As such, correction is typically performed after orthognathic surgery.
	Revision of cleft lip	Varies	Cleft lip and nasal revisions may be accomplished at any time after 5 years of age, as most lip and nasal growth is complete by this age. However, surgical revision may be attempted earlier when severe deformities exist. In addition, surgeries performed before 3 years of age have the advantage of being completed prior to the development of facial image and before the child has memory of the operations.

Note: References for Appendix 2 are located at the end of Chapter 25.

Atlas of Operative Oral and Maxillofacial Surgery, First Edition. Edited by Christopher J. Haggerty and Robert M. Laughlin
© 2015 John Wiley & Sons, Inc. Published 2015 by John Wiley & Sons, Inc.

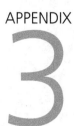

Pathology Chart

Michael J. Isaac, Patrick Lucaci, Robert M. Laughlin, and Christopher J. Haggerty

	Lesion	Location	Radiographic appearance	Treatment	Key points
Odontogenic cysts	Periapical cyst	Attached to the apical aspect of a tooth root showing signs of pulpitis.	Well-demarcated unilocular radiolucency associated with the apex of a tooth root.	Lesions smaller than 1 cm are often treated with involved-tooth root canal therapy or extraction. Lesions larger than 1.0 cm are treated with enucleation and curettage, in addition to endodontic therapy or extraction.	Associated with tooth root with evidence of pulpitis.
	Dentigerous cyst	Most commonly associated with maxillary and mandibular third molars. Second most common location is associated with maxillary canines.	Well-demarcated unilocular radiolucency associated with the clinical crown of an unerupted tooth. Frequently results in involved tooth displacement. Adjacent root resorption not seen.	Smaller lesions are treated with enucleation and currettage of cyst. Larger cysts or cysts adjacent to key anatomical structures may benefit from marsupilization to decrease cyst size prior to a definitive enucleation and currettage procedure.	Aspiration typically yields a clear or straw-colored fluid. Marsupilization should be considered only in large lesions due to the risk of ameloblastoma in situ or neoplastic transformation of the cyst lining.
	Keratinizing odontogenic tumor (*odontogenic keratocyst* [OKC])	Most commonly associated with maxillary and mandibular third molars. Second most common location is associated with maxillary canines.	Variable radiographic appearances. May present as unilocular or multilocular cysts, or as a solid tumor.	Smaller lesions are treated with enucleation and currettage of entire cyst. Larger cysts or cysts adjacent to key anatomical structures may benefit from marsupilization to decrease cyst size prior to enucleation and currettage. Consider resection for recurrent lesions.	If multiple OKCs are present, consider Gorlin's syndrome. Aspiration typically yields a clear or straw-colored fluid. Wide surgical access is key to total removal of cystic lining.
	Calcifying odontogenic cyst (*Gorlin's cyst* [COC])	More common in the maxilla than in the mandible.	Typically appears as a well-demarcated, unilocular, mixed radiolucent-radiopaque lesion.	Enucleation and curettage.	Mixed radiolucent-radiopaque radiographic appearance.

Atlas of Operative Oral and Maxillofacial Surgery, First Edition. Edited by Christopher J. Haggerty and Robert M. Laughlin.
© 2015 John Wiley & Sons, Inc. Published 2015 by John Wiley & Sons, Inc.

	Lesion	Location	Radiographic appearance	Treatment	Key points
	Idiopathic bone cyst (*traumatic bone cyst*)	More common in the mandible, specifically within the mandibular body region.	Appears as a scalloped radiolucency between teeth.	Aspiration, exploration, and curretage. Curretage causes bleeding within the cavity, which stimulates bone formation.	Not a true cyst as there is no discernible epithelial lining. Not caused by trauma as previously believed. Teeth are vital. Commonly presents in childhood or early adolescence as an incidental radiographic finding.
	Nasopalatine duct cyst (*incisive canal cyst*)	Presents as a soft tissue swelling posterior to the maxillary central incisors.	Appears as a heart-shaped unilocular radiolucency (>5 mm).	Enucleation and curettage.	May cause tooth displacement and incisor root resorption.
Odontogenic tumors (benign)	Ameloblastoma	Most commonly located within the posterior mandible, but may occur at any location within the jaws.	Variable radiographic appearance dependent on the type of ameloblastoma. Commonly well-demarcated unilocular or multilocular radiolucencies that may show thinning or perforation of the cortices of the jaws. Commonly associated with tooth displacement, inferior alveolar nerve displacement, and root resorption.	Varies depending on the nature of the ameloblastoma as determined upon biopsy. Luminal and intraluminal unicystic ameloblastomas may be treated with enucleation and curettage. Multicystic and invasive ameloblastomas are treated via resection with 1.0–1.5 cm margins. Lesions that perforate the cortical plates should include an univolved anatomical barrier (i.e., periosteum). Ameloblastic carcinoma is treated with larger resection margins (2.0–3.0 cm), neck dissecton, and frequently postoperative radiation therapy.	Does not cause paresthesia or anesthesia of associated compressed nerves. Treatment guidelines are adjusted based on the histopathological presentation of the lesion from the incisional biopsy.
	Calcifying epithelial odontogenic tumor (*Pindborg tumor*)	Typically located within the posterior jaws (mandible > maxilla).	Radiographic appearance varies depending on the maturity of the tumor. Most early tumors are completely radiolucent. As the lesion matures, it typically demonstrates a mixed radiolucent-radiopaque appearance. Lesions may be either unilocular or multilocular in appearance.	Resection with 1.0 cm bony margins. An uninvolved anatomical barrier (i.e., periosteum) is recommended for lesions that have perforated the cortical plates.	Classically defined by their mixed radiolucent-radiopaque appearance. Often associated with the crown of an impacted tooth.

(continued)

	Lesion	Location	Radiographic appearance	Treatment	Key points
	Odontogenic adenomatoid tumor (*adenomatoid odontogenic cyst*)	Most frequently associated with the maxillary canine.	Well-demarcated unilocular radiolucency, typically associated with an unerupted or impacted maxillary tooth. Often with areas of calcification noted within the lesion.	Removal of involved tooth and enucleation of the associated cyst.	Referred to as the *two-thirds tumors*. Two-thirds occur within the maxilla, two-thirds occur in association with a canine tooth, two-thirds occur in association with an unerupted or impacted tooth, and two-thirds occur in young females within the first three decades of life.
Benign mesenchymal odontogenic tumors	Odontogenic myxoma	Evenly distributed throughout the maxilla and the mandible.	Soap bubble appearance on radiograph with ragged, ill-defined borders. May also present as unilocular lesions.	Marginal or segmental resection with 1.0–1.5 cm margins and an uninvolved anatomic boundary.	
	Cementoblastoma	More common in the mandible than in the maxilla.	Circular radiopaque mass associated with the apical one-half of a tooth root. Radiographic halo may be present around the mass.	Treatment consists of removal of the tooth and associated mass.	Teeth are vital. Typically presents within the first three decades of life.
	Ameloblastic fibroma	Most commomly associated with the mandibular molar region, but may occur at any location.	Presents as a unilocular or multilocular radiolucent lesion with well-demarcated borders. 75% associated with an unerupted crown. May mimic dentigerous cyst.	Treatment involves enucleation and curettage.	Typically occurs within the first two decades of life. Consider ameloblastic fibrosarcoma in workup. Requires long-term follow-up due to potential malignant transformation.
	Odontoma	May occur at any location within the jaws. Compound odontomas are more common within the anterior mandible. Complex odotomas are more common within the posterior mandible.	Compound odontomas resemble a mass containing tooth-like structures or gravel. Complex odontomas resemble a calcified, amorphous mass.	Treatment involves enucleation and curettage.	Incompletely removed odontomas may lead to wound infection as the retained tissue or residual odontoma often contains inadequate blood supply.
	Osteochondroma	Typically associated with the condyle or coronoid process.	Radiopaque enlargement of the condlye or coronoid process with tapered extension to the lateral pterygoid (condlye) or temporalis (coronoid) muscles. Osteochondromas involving the condyle may resemble a "shredded flag" on orthopantomogram, with the flag representing the extension to the lateral pterygoid muscle.	Treatment involves complete excision of the affected condyle or coronoid process.	Typically presents as a nontender hard mass associated with trismus and jaw deviation on opening within the first three decades of life.

Lesion	Location	Radiographic appearance	Treatment	Key points
Central giant cell granuloma (CGCG)	Typically located within the posterior mandible, but may occur at any location. Lesion may cross the midline.	May present as a unilocular or multilocular radiolucent lesion that may displace associated teeth, expand and erode cortices, and cause root resorption.	The injection of intralesional steroids has shown early success in the initial management of CGCGs. Curettage has a highly variable recurrence rate. CGCGs that are aggressive, recurrent or refractory to intralesional steroid injections may be treated with peripheral ostectomy or resection with 0.5–1.0 cm margins.	Aggressive CGCGs are associated with pain and rapid cortical expansion due to continued growth. Nonsurgical treatment modalities frequently do not stimulate complete resolution of CGCGs, but may decrease the size and associated morbidity of future definitive procedures.
Osteosarcoma	More common in the mandible than in the maxilla.	"Sun-ray" appearance due to periosteal reaction, widening of the periodontal ligament of involved teeth (Garrington sign), resorption of involved tooth roots, cortical bone expansion or destruction, and a mixed radiopaque-radiolucent expansile mass.	Definitive treatment involves the initiation of chemotherapy, followed by surgical resection with 3 cm bony and 2 cm soft tissue margins, followed by additional chemotherapy and close follow-up.	Neurosensory changes to involved nerves. 5-year survival rate of 50%. Close follow-up is required due to the frequency of metastasis to distant sites (i.e., lung and brain).
Salivary gland tumors Pleomorphic adenoma	70% of parotid masses (most commonly within the superficial lobe). 60% of submandibular gland masses. 50% of minor salivary gland masses.		Varies depending on the location of the pleomorphic adenoma. Parotid pleomorphic adenomas are treated with 1 cm extracapsular excision versus superficial or deep parotidectomy based on the size and location of the mass. Submandibular pleomorphic adenomas are treated with gland excision to include surrounding tissue if extracapsular extension. Palatal pleomorphic adenomas are treated with 1 cm margins, including periosteum of the hard palate and fascia of the soft palate.	Typically present as a painless, indurated, mobile mass located in regions of salivary glands, such as the parotid gland, the submandibular gland, and areas of minor salivary glands (i.e., palate). Does not metastasize or invade bone. Cut-potato specimen morphology.
Warthin's tumor (*papillary cystadenoma lymphomatosum*)	Most commomly identified within the superficial lobe of the parotid gland.	Increased uptake of Technicium 99.	Superficial parotidectomy.	May occur bilaterally.

(continued)

Lesion	Location	Radiographic appearance	Treatment	Key points
Mucoepidermoid carcinoma	Most common parotid gland malignancy.		A biopsy or fine-needle aspirate (parotid mass) is required to establish the histological grading of the lesion, and a CT scan is required to establish the depth of invasion. Histological grading and adjacent structure invasion will dictate the definitive treatment and recurrence rate.	Infiltration of the facial nerve may cause facial muscle paralysis. Treatment and recurrence rates are based on the histological grading classification (low grade, intermediate grade, and high grade).
Adenoid cystic carcinoma (ACC)	Most common minor salivary gland malignancy. Also occurs in major salivary glands.		Treatment involves resection of the lesion with wide surgical margins, nerve extirpation, and radiation therapy.	Demonstrates perineural invasion and spread, and skip lesions. Palatal ACCs require 3 cm bony margins (typically, hemi- or total maxillectomy) and complete extirpation of the pterygomaxillary space contents. Parotid ACCs require total parotidectomy with or without facial nerve sparing depending on whether perineural invasion has occurred. 5-year survival rate is 75%. 10-year survival rate is 20%.
Polymorphous low-grade adenocarcinoma	May occur at any location where minor salivary glands are identified. Most commonly associated with the palate. Typically do not exceed 4 cm in size.		1.5 cm soft tissue margins. Lesions located within the palate are treated with removal of periosteum as well. Palatal lesions that show bony invasion are managed with involved bone resection.	A malignancy associated with slow growth and rare metastasis involving only the minor salivary glands. 10-year survival rate of 80%.

CT, computed tomography.

References

Božič, M. and Ihan Hren, N., 2006. Ameloblastic fibroma. *Radiology and Oncology*, 40 (1), 35–8.

Leiser, Y., Abu-El-Naaj, I. and Peled, M., 2009. Odontogenic myxoma—a case series and review of the surgical management. *Journal of Craniomaxillofacial Surgery*, 37(4), 206–9.

Marx, R.E. and Stern, D., 2002. *Oral and maxillofacial pathology: a rationale for diagnosis and treatment.* Hanover Park, IL: Quintessence.

Mendenhall, W.M., Amdur, R.J., Hinerman, R.W., Werning, J.W., Villaret, D.B. and Mendenhall, N.P., 2005. Head and neck mucosal melanoma. *American Journal of Clinical Oncology*, 28 (6), 626–30.

Papathanassiou, Z.G, Alberghini, M., Thiesse, P., Gambarotti, M., Bianchi, G., Tranfaglia, C. and Vanel, D., 2011. Parosteal osteosarcoma mimicking osteochondroma: A radiohistologic approach on two cases. *Clinical Sarcoma Research*, 1 (1), 1–8.

Pazdera, J., Kolar, Z., Zboril, V., Tvrdy, P. and Pink, R., 2012. Odontogenic keratocysts/keratocystic odontogenic tumours: biological characteristics, clinical manifestation and treatment. *Biomed Pap Med Fac Univ Palacky Olomouc Czech Repub*, 158 (2), 170–4. doi: 10.5507/bp.2012.048

INDEX

CPSIA information can be obtained
at www.ICGtesting.com
Printed in the USA
JSHW040755190922
30428JS00002B/57

9 781118 442340